CONVERSION TABLE FOR WEIG...

(Gram equivalents for pounds and ounces)

For example, to find weight in pounds and ounces of baby weighing 3315 grams, glance down columns to figure nearest 3315 = 3317. Refer to number at top of column for pounds and number to far left for ounces = 7 pounds, 5 ounces. *Maureen - Scranton 79908*

Pounds→ Ounces↓	3	4	5	6	7	8	9	10
0	1361	1814	2268	2722	3175	3629	4082	4536
1	1389	1843	2296	2750	3203	3657	4111	4564
2	1417	1871	2325	2778	3232	3685	4139	4593
3	1446	1899	2353	2807	3260	3714	4167	4621
4	1474	1928	2381	2835	3289	3742	4196	4649
5	1503	1956	2410	2863	3317	3770	4224	4678
6	1531	1984	2438	2892	3345	3799	4252	4706
7	1559	2013	2466	2920	3374	3827	4281	4734
8	1588	2041	2495	2948	3402	3856	4309	4763
9	1616	2070	2523	2977	3430	3884	4338	4791
10	1644	2098	2551	3005	3459	3912	4366	4819
11	1673	2126	2580	3033	3487	3941	4394	4848
12	1701	2155	2608	3062	3515	3969	4423	4876
13	1729	2183	2637	3090	3544	3997	4451	4904
14	1758	2211	2665	3118	3572	4026	4479	4933
15	1786	2240	2693	3147	3600	4054	4508	4961

OR, to convert grams into pounds and *decimals* of a pound, multiply weight in grams by .0022. Thus, $3317 \times .0022 = 7.2974$, i.e., 7.3 pounds, or 7 pounds, 5 ounces.

To convert pounds and ounces into grams, multiply the pounds by 453.6 and the ounces by 28.4 and add the two products. Thus, to convert 7 pounds, 5 ounces, $7 \times 453.6 = 3175$; $5 \times 28.4 = 142$; $3175 + 142 = 3317$ grams.

Mary Therese Baloga   "55"
Mercy Hospital
School of Nursing
W.-B., Pa.

NURSES HANDBOOK
OF OBSTETRICS

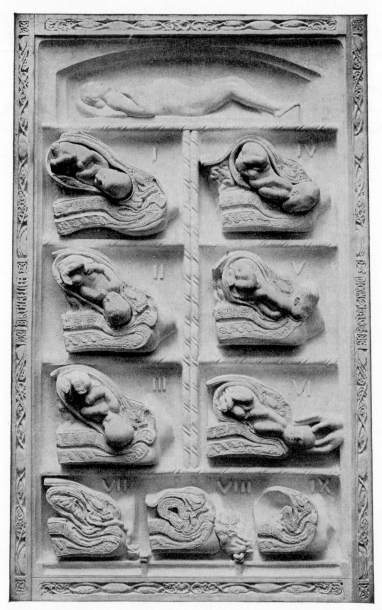

"The Birth Relief"

This distinguished sculptured relief is reproduced through the courtesy of the late Robert Latou Dickinson, M.D., famous gynecologist, obstetrician, and artist; and Abram Belskie, artist and sculptor.

Nurses Handbook of
OBSTETRICS

LOUISE ZABRISKIE, R.N.

Formerly Night Supervisor Lying-In Hospital, New York City, and
Field Director Maternity Center Association, New York City; Director
Maternity Consultation Service, New York City; Lecturer in the
School of Education, Department of Nurse Education, New York
University, New York City

AND

NICHOLSON J. EASTMAN, M.D.

Professor of Obstetrics in the Johns Hopkins University and
Obstetrician-in-Chief to the Johns Hopkins Hospital

377 Illustrations
Including 8 Color Plates

Ninth Edition—Completely Revised

Philadelphia   London   Montreal
J. B. LIPPINCOTT COMPANY

PRINTED IN THE UNITED STATES OF AMERICA

Preface to the Ninth Edition

Every new edition is the result of much investigation in an effort to present new material of value to the student and to delete the outmoded matter. Obstetrics is really concerned with human life from the time of conception to delivery, and from delivery to the termination of the postpartum period. Today, obstetricians with vision are even considering the premarriage and preconception periods as essential foundations for better obstetrics. They do not consider their responsibility ended with the termination of the postpartum period but continue their supervision to the examination a year after delivery.

The subject of obstetrics is very closely interrelated with all others in the course of study and is not only a part of public health education but also, due to present-day emphasis on prenatal care, becomes definitely a part of the preventive medicine program. In this constantly expanding field of science and human relationship the obstetric service continues to offer progressive opportunity and responsibility for the care of the patient by means of the follow-up work of the social worker and the public health nurse as well as having the out-patient departments of many hospitals manned by the public health nurse.

Many hospitals also provide ready access to the clinics (dental, cardiac, skin, chest, diabetic, toxemia, etc.); air conditioned rooms; frozen breast-milk storage; laboratory services (including metabolism and other various tests); roentgenology and blood banks. There is also available the nutritionist, or, better still, the nutrition clinic, to study the relationship between the inadequacies in the maternal diet and the occurrence of congenital malformations, prematurity, stillbirths and toxic conditions. Co-operating, too, are the units for the study of endocrinology, biochemistry and pathology. All these resources are continuing to contribute greatly to the goals for better fundamental health as well as reduced morbidity and lowered mortality. The statistical results are of value only when complete records are kept and made available for analysis and comparison with previous years. In this, the hospital record room, for the collection of facts, plays an important part. All these correlated services constitute an endeavor to give the student a perspective of the far-reaching effects of comprehensive obstetric care.

Since this book is designed primarily for student nurses, simplicity and clarity have been the objectives. The basic principles of obstetrics and obstetric nursing have been stressed rather than any special details of technic which may be used in this or that hospital. However, an effort has been made to include material culled from routines and procedures used throughout the country. To incorporate the new developments the book has been entirely reset in a different format. Chapters have been rearranged to provide more logical sequence. We believe that the present arrangement will aid the student in locating readily any particular subject; at the same time, for the instructor, there is ample opportunity for flexibility in planning the course of study.* Some chapters have been shortened and some lengthened; and one new chapter has been added.

The text is well illustrated throughout to offer clear visualization of the many obstetric processes and procedures. Many of these are new and have been chosen because the authors believe that they convey the concepts involved in structural relationships so much more clearly and succinctly than even the most skillful description. Several illustrations have been designed especially to clarify phases of the subject which, experience has shown, are difficult for beginners to understand. Some have the advantage of color photography, which permits the reproduction of the color and the changes involved.

Since the majority of deliveries in this country now occur in hospitals, special attention has been given to hospital management of obstetric cases. However, the basic principles of good obstetrics are the same whether the delivery is conducted in the home or in the hospital. Nevertheless, in this country, there are more than 600,000 mothers delivered annually in the home, and there are still many mothers who are delivered unattended. For this reason, home and emergency technics are included.

More and more, doctors, nurses and patients have become conscious of the need for more "parent instruction." This has led to an increasing demand for nurses to be prepared to conduct these classes for mothers and also for fathers—classes which include the exercises that some doctors recommend in conjunction with the procedure "childbirth without fear." Public health organizations as well as hospitals provide these opportunities. The chapter "Teaching Aids" has been planned with the idea of furnishing a basis from which students might develop their own teaching outline.

Although the study of embryology is a complete course in itself, it is necessary for the student to recall some of the important phases in the development of the embryo and fetus to correlate embryology with obstetrics; therefore, special thought has been devoted to clarifying and simplifying the material dealing with the very early stages in the formation of the embryo, the mechanism of its implantation in the uterus and the correlated changes in the reproductive organs of the mother.

The chapter on prenatal care has been amplified with greater emphasis on the normal physiologic reactions to pregnancy and the vital importance of adequate care during this period—the period of greatest potential development and growth of the fetus. The preparations for the mother and baby during this period have been systematically arranged. The material in the chapter on prenatal complications has been reorganized, the Rh factor and

---

* The time given by the instructor to different portions of the text will vary with the teaching facilities available, other courses offered and special needs that may be felt.

blood groupings have been clarified and new material has been added on the diseases affecting or affected by pregnancy. The chapter on mental hygiene, submitted by Dr. Leo Kanner, is timely. The use of the newer analgesics and anaesthesias with their procedures and methods has been brought up-to-date. In the chapter on delivery new illustrations have been utilized to elucidate these technics. Subjects that are vital and timely have been added and others expanded to include the important role of nutrition and control of weight during pregnancy, rooming-in and early ambulation. Throughout the complete maternity cycle there are suggestions relating to the integration of posture and body mechanics, with the aim of preventing discomforts and promoting convalescence.

The material on premature care has been entirely rewritten, and current procedures have been incorporated. The immediate care and the after-care of the baby has been enlarged to include rooming-in and the role of the father and how he may share this exciting experience. Emphasis also has been placed on posture in relation to growth and development of the infant as well as the importance of proper clothing, furniture and equipment. Bathing and dressing the baby are illustrated in detail. Current ideas relating to routines and schedules have been enumerated. The chapter on the disorders of the newborn has been completely reorganized and considerably more material added to bring it up-to-date.

Research continues with new methods and new medications, the latter changing so rapidly it is difficult to keep up-to-date with these innovations. However, experience has repeatedly demonstrated that some innovations are transitory and only a step in the progress of our knowledge. To disregard immediately the tried method for the new seems not always to be justified. Time and experience will prove the value; and, with modifications, new ideas relating to maternity care may be incorporated or discarded.

The subject matter in the book is arranged in units with an orientation preceding and revised questions following each unit. Mrs. McManus has entirely revised the "Student Self-Examination Questions" (which have proved so helpful in previous editions) to coincide with present-day plans in nursing education. In addition to covering the factual data concerning obstetric nursing, the questions will test the student's ability to meet real nursing situations.

The authors, artists and publishers have made a co-ordinated effort to present a clear, orderly, well-illustrated textbook. It is the hope of the authors that both students and teachers will find in this edition the fundamental principles necessary in this interesting and vital subject. It is hoped, also, that the new bibliographies may prove an invitation to students to pursue questions and studies that arouse their interest in better care for mothers and babies.

L. Z.

N. J. E.

Preface to the First Edition

The purpose of this textbook on obstetrics is to provide teachers and pupil nurses with a concise, present-day, practical picture of the underlying anatomic and physiologic facts and the approved routine principles and practices of the nursing arts, in relation to this speciality of medicine, both in hospitals and in homes.

The aim has been to avoid the pitfall of overemphasis on complications which concern the doctor rather than the nurse, and to assure stressing the principles and technics of the purely nursing phases upon which the pupil nurse must depend in order to meet the exacting requirements of the present nursing school curriculum.

The approach is from an inclusive angle starting with the beginning of pregnancy, carrying through to the after-care and well into the life of the baby. Motherhood and human welfare are always kept prominently in the forefront.

The important teaching value of pictures has been fully appreciated and the abundant illustrations have been prepared with maximum care to amplify the text. Original photographs, emphasizing specific teaching points, have been taken, under the personal supervision of the author, to visualize numerous technics, to picture in detail setups in hospitals, also in private homes, and to illustrate for the nurse in training many essential points in handling and providing for the comfort of the newborn. Knowledge has advanced rapidly in the field of obstetrics and the preventive side of nursing care is now recognized to be of utmost importance, hence this phase has been stressed throughout.

Many helpful hints on adapting and utilizing available utensils and materials have been incorporated.

It is in the important psychologic phases that the nurse can aid in making a specific contribution to maternal welfare, through her intimate and continued association with the mother. Emphasis is therefore placed on this part of her work, through the understanding contributions of Dr. McIlroy, of the Royal Free Hospital, of London, and Dr. Kenworthy, of the New York School of Social Work.

Since the mother frequently confers with the nurse as to the clothing and general care of the infant for the first few weeks of life, much helpful information along this line has been included, which the nurse can share with the inexperienced mother before transferring the full responsibility to her.

LOUISE ZABRISKIE

New York City

Acknowledgments

When a textbook reaches the ninth edition, the debts of gratitude continue to grow in number and variety. The helpful co-operation of many has made possible the writing of this text. The authors are deeply indebted to Mrs. R. Louise McManus, R.N., A.M., Director of Nursing Education Division, Teachers College, Columbia University, New York, for her "Student Self-Examination Questions." To Miss Ranice Birch, medical artist to the Department of Obstetrics, Johns Hopkins University, Baltimore, the book and its authors owe much. Her illustrations, quite apart from their consummate artistry, are based on precise knowledge of obstetric anatomy and on her many years of study in the delivery room. Likewise, the authors wish to express their appreciation to Miss Elizabeth Cone, Medical Photographer to the Johns Hopkins Hospital, for the many distinguished photographs which she has made.

To Little, Brown and Company, thanks are due for the use of material from *Expectant Motherhood*, by Nicholson J. Eastman. We continue to use several illustrations created by the late Robert L. Dickinson, M.D., and will always be especially indebted to him for his never-failing interest and co-operation, which we have missed so much during this revision. We wish to thank Mr. Abram Belskie for the photographs of his beautifully sculptured models. To Arthur Mitchell Reich, M.D., New York University-Bellevue Medical Center; R. Gordon Douglas, M.D., New York Hospital-Cornell Medical Center; M. Edward Davis, M.D., Chicago Lying-In Hospital; Rudolph Skarda, R.A., University of California Medical Center, San Francisco; Edith B. Jackson, M.D., and Herbert Thoms, M.D., of Yale University; Mrs. Mary Breckinridge, The Frontier Nursing Service, Kentucky; Miss Georgia Hukill, formerly of Chicago Lying-In Hospital; Miss Gertrude Garran, formerly of Boston Lying-In Hospital; Miss Lottie Morrison, Sloane Hospital for Women, New York; Miss Verda Hickox, New York Hospital-Cornell Medical Center; Miss Rose Coyle, Margaret Hague Maternity Hospital, Jersey City; The Misses Hazelmarie Purpi and Marion Scott, Methodist Hospital, Brooklyn; Miss Helen G. McClelland, Pennsylvania Hospital, Philadelphia; Miss Ann Kirchner, Chicago Lying-In Hospital; Miss Cornelia Macpherson, The Directory for Mothers' Milk, Boston; Miss Julia Smith, Childrens' Welfare Federation, New York; and to many others, gratitude is due for their stimulating interest and generous assistance. We wish to thank the New York City Department of Health and the Eastman Kodak Company for photographs used in this edition. The book continues to owe much to Mr. Percy Byron for his expert photography.

We are greatly indebted to Dr. Leo Kanner, Director, Children's Psychiatric Service, Johns Hopkins Hospital, and Associate Professor of Psychiatry, John Hopkins University School of Medicine, for his willingness to take over this responsibility. The chapter on Mental Hygiene has been written by an authority in that field.

To Amey Elizabeth Bardens, who has collaborated on the entire text, we are deeply indebted. Professor Emeritus Jean Broadhurst, Teachers College, Columbia University, has given inspiration and editorial assistance to this edition.

The authors take this opportunity to thank Mr. Ellis W. Bacon, Mr. Walter Kahoe and Mr. Stanley A. Gillet of the J. B. Lippincott Company for their continued co-operation, interest and help.

THE AUTHORS

Contents

UNIT TWO

NURSING IN PREGNANCY

ORIENTATION

UNIT FOUR

NURSING DURING THE PUERPERIUM

ORIENTATION

UNIT FIVE

THE NEONATAL PERIOD

ORIENTATION

UNIT SIX

ADDITIONAL MATERNITY INFORMATION

UNIT ONE

HUMAN REPRODUCTION

ORIENTATION

What is obstetrics? What are its aims? How can nurses further these aims? In order that the student nurse may appreciate early the immeasurable importance of obstetrics to the women and the children of our country, as well as the contributions which she herself can make to this field, these fundamental questions are considered in the first chapter.

The subsequent chapters of this Unit survey the anatomy and the physiology of the female reproductive organs and the development of the unborn baby (the fetus). Since childbirth entails the passage of the infant through an unyielding bony canal, the pelvis, the anatomy of this structure is of the utmost importance in obstetrics. The physiologic mechanism by which conception takes place and a new human being develops is not only a fascinating story in itself but also one which has far-reaching practical implications in respect to the welfare of both mother and child.

The study of obstetrics includes not only the mechanics of anatomy and physiology but also, in its full meaning, the study of human development and relationships. All that a human being comes to be depends upon many factors present at the time of his birth: heritage, care before birth, care at birth, and his care and training in infancy and childhood.

The Unit concludes with a consideration of the various positions which the fetus in utero may occupy. A clear grasp of the material in this Unit, including as it does many basic definitions, is essential to any intelligent understanding of obstetrics. The illustrations should be studied in close correlation with the text, and every effort should be made to visualize the anatomic relationships and the physiologic phenomena described.

1

Aims of Obstetric Nursing

OBSTETRICS DEFINED

Obstetrics is the art and science of caring for the childbearing woman and her newborn baby. It deals essentially with three distinct periods: pregnancy (from the time of conception to the beginning of labor); labor (the process by which the baby and the placenta are expelled from the mother's body into the outside world); and the puerperium (the period during which the organs of reproduction are restored to approximately their former size and condition).

The word "obstetrics" is derived from an old Latin verb *obsto,* which means to "stand by." Thus, in ancient Rome, a person who cared for women at childbirth was known as an "obstetrix," or a person who "stood by"

the laboring mother. While the original employment of the term doubtless referred to the physical act of standing beside the woman, scholars point out that the word also means to "stand by" in the sense of "to protect"—as one ship stands by another in possible danger. Accordingly, it may be said that by the very derivation of the term, obstetrics involves standing by and protecting the childbearing woman throughout pregnancy, labor and the puerperium. The viewpoint that this branch of medicine has to do with protecting the expectant mother throughout her course is a most important one for the nurse to grasp early in the course, for obstetrics is largely concerned with preventing possible dangers and hence is truly a phase of preventive medicine.

3

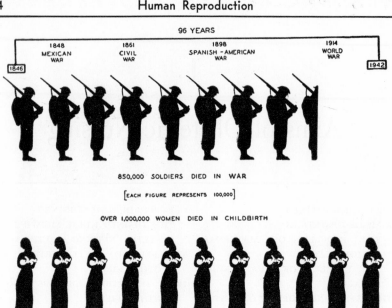

CHART 1. Magnitude of maternal mortality in the United States during a 96-year period as compared with mortality of soldiers. Based on figures contained in an article by Mrs. Mary Breckinridge. The figures are estimates only but are believed to be fairly accurate approximations (Quart. Bull. Frontier Nursing Service, **18**:4, 1942, No. 2). Nurses will find this an inspiring article.

AIMS OF OBSTETRICS

THE PROBLEM OF MATERNAL MORTALITY

It is the aim of obstetrics to reduce to a very minimum the huge toll which women pay in childbearing; to minimize the discomforts of pregnancy, labor and the puerperium; and at the same time, so to safeguard the whole process that mother and child will conclude the experience in a healthy condition.

In a study made by Mrs. Mary Breckinridge, R.N., director of the Frontier Nursing Service, a comparison was made between the number of American women who have died in childbirth during the 96-year period and the number of American men who have died in battle during the same period (Mexican War, Civil War, Spanish-American War and World War I). Her calculations, which are most meticulous and conservative, show that the number of soldiers who died over this period was 858,430, while the number of

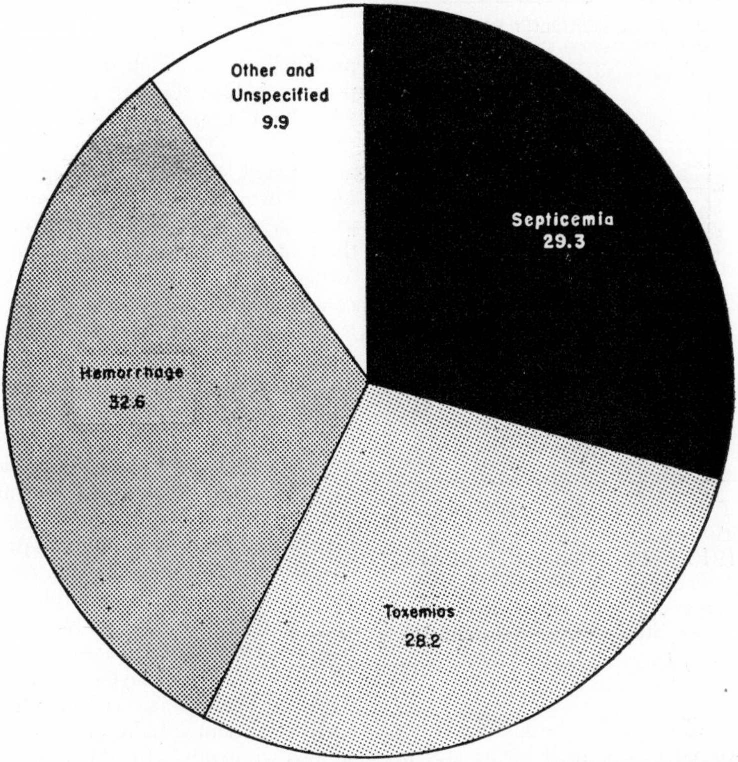

CHART 2. Causes of maternal death; percentage distribution by cause, 1948. (Federal Security Agency, U. S. Public Health Service, National Office of Vital Statistics, Washington, D. C.)

mothers who died in childbirth was over one million. "The young woman has a battlefield of her own," Mrs. Breckinridge concludes, "and that is childbirth. Here the hazards for Americans throughout our years as a nation have been greater than the hazards of war, and with higher casualties. Death and mutilation— mutilation and death, that is the lot of thousands of women every year throughout the generations."

During the year 1948, the number of women who died in the United States from conditions due directly to pregnancy and labor was 4,122 (.12 per cent). Expressed in a different way, for every 10,000 women who become pregnant, 12 die as the result of the process. Dr. Howard C. Taylor, Jr., of the National Research Council, states that in women between the ages of 15 and 45, the process of human birth is the chief

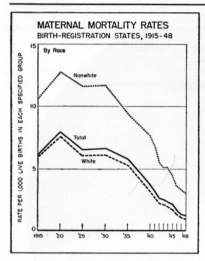

CHART 3. Maternal mortality rates per 1,000 by race, 1915-1948. (Federal Security Agency, U. S. Public Health Service, National Office of Vital Statistics, Washington, D. C.)

cause of deaths in the United States. Maternal deaths, still births and infant deaths amounted to 190,129 in 1948. To this are added 400,000 miscarriages, giving a total of 590,129.

However, if we hope to reduce the number of mothers who die in childbirth, we must first know why these women succumb. They die of three main causes: puerperal infection, toxemia and hemorrhage. Subsequently, these three conditions will be discussed in detail, but it would seem important to stress here the fact that deaths from these causes are for the most part preventable. Puerperal infection is an infection arising in the uterus after childbirth. In most cases it is the result of sheer uncleanliness

on the part of the patient's attendants; in many others it is due to the presence in the delivery room of persons (often doctors and nurses) who have upper respiratory infections. In these instances the bacteria are carried, through coughing, talking, or even exhaling, from the nasopharynx of the affected person to the hands of the attendant, or to the instruments and thence to the birth canal, where inflammation results. It is plain that the nurse can play a most important role in preventing such infections. The toxemias of pregnancy are a group of conditions characterized, in the main, by high blood pressure in pregnancy and in advanced cases by convulsions and coma. If the expectant mother sees her doctor regularly throughout pregnancy (prenatal or antepartal care), the early signs of this complication can be detected, and with suitable treatment the disturbance generally or often can be allayed. Likewise, with the hemorrhagic complications, early treatment usually obviates any serious difficulty. In other words, most deaths in childbirth are preventable and therefore unnecessary.

Statistics

For those students who are statistically minded, figures present a real story. The science of statistics deals with the collection of figures which present a picture of existing facts, by means of the collection, the analysis, the comparison, the interpretation and the presentation of numerical data. Through the keeping of records and the recording of statistics the number and the causes of maternal and infant deaths can be determined and, therefore, pre-

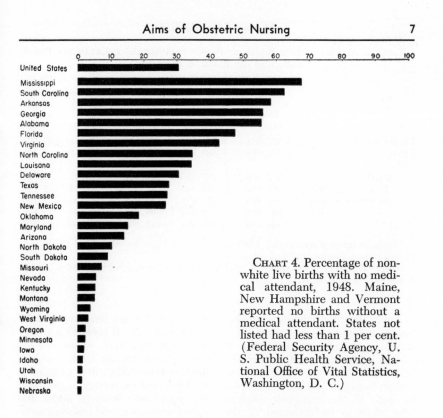

CHART 4. Percentage of non-white live births with no medical attendant, 1948. Maine, New Hampshire and Vermont reported no births without a medical attendant. States not listed had less than 1 per cent. (Federal Security Agency, U. S. Public Health Service, National Office of Vital Statistics, Washington, D. C.)

sent a means of attack to lower the number of deaths by preventive methods. Where funds are necessary this statistical picture offers a convincing argument for financial aid.

During recent years a most gratifying improvement has occurred in maternal mortality rates. Thus, the maternal mortality rate for white women has decreased from 6.0 per 1,000 live births to 0.9, between the years 1931 and 1948, the corresponding figures for nonwhite women being 11.1 and 3.0. This progressive saving of mothers has been no accidental or chance affair but must be attributed to a distinct change in the attitudes of doctors, nurses and

parents. Childbirth is no longer an event to be awaited helplessly by the expectant mother with what fortitude she is able to muster; instead, it is the climax of a period of preparation—a true state of preparedness attained through the co-operation of the physician, the nurse and the expectant mother or parents. As indicated above, this preparation for childbirth, based on careful medical and nursing supervision throughout pregnancy, is called prenatal (sometimes antenatal or antepartal) care.

Prenatal care is the most important advance which has been made in obstetrics during the present century, and it will be of interest to the nurse

TABLE 1. NUMBER OF LIVE BIRTHS BY PERSON IN ATTENDANCE, URBAN AND RURAL: U. S., 1948 (BY PLACE OF RESIDENCE)

		BIRTHS ATTENDED BY			
Area	Total births	Physician (in hospital)	Physician (not in hospital)	Midwife	Other and not specified
United States...........	3,535,068	3,025,206	323,434	156,564	29,864
Urban *................	2,094,018	1,967,915	81,528	38,114	6,461
Places of					
100,000 or more	983,863	946,885	27,377	7,242	2,359
25,000 to 100,000	426,856	404,544	12,552	8,614	1,146
10,000 to 25,000	301,683	279,834	11,969	8,760	1,120
2,500 to 10,000	381,616	336,652	29,630	13,498	1,836
Rural *................	1,441,050	1,057,291	241,906	118,450	24,403

* Includes urban places having 2,500 inhabitants or more according to the 1940 population census. Rural includes all other areas.

Source: Federal Security Agency, U. S. Public Health Service, National Office of Vital Statistics, Washington, D. C.

to know that this salutary contribution to the mother's welfare was initiated by the nursing profession. It had its beginning in 1901, when the Instructive Nursing Association in Boston began to pay antenatal visits to some of the expectant mothers who were to be delivered at the Boston Lying-In Hospital. This work gradually spread until, in 1906, all these women, prior to confinement, were paid at least one visit by a nurse from the association. By 1912 this association was making about three antenatal visits to each patient. In 1907 another pioneer effort in prenatal work was instituted when George H. F. Schrader gave the Association for Improving the Condition of the Poor, in New York City, funds to pay the salary of two nurses to do this work. In 1909 the Committee on Infant Social Service of the Women's Municipal League, of Boston, organized an experiment in prenatal work. The pregnant women were visited every ten days—oftener if necessary. Blood pressure readings and urine tests were made at each visit. This important work was limited because of the effort to make it as nearly self-supporting as possible; therefore, only mothers under the care of physicians and hospitals were accepted. Thus began this movement for prenatal care which has done more than any other single agency to save mothers' lives in our time.

Another important factor in the reduction of maternal mortality has been the development of maternal hygiene programs in State Departments of Public Health, particularly the work of public health nurses in maternal hygiene. These nurses visit a large number of the mothers who otherwise would receive little or no medical care, bringing them much-needed aid in pregnancy, labor and the puerperium. This service fills a great need not only in rural areas but also in metropolitan centers as well. It is hard to realize that a large proportion of our nonwhite mothers have no attendant whatsoever at childbirth (Chart 4). This is an important factor in the much higher maternal death rate in nonwhites. Public health groups, both doctors and nurses, are attacking this problem vigilantly, but much remains to be done.

Still another factor responsible for the decline in maternal mortality is the trend toward hospitalization for childbirth—a trend that is gaining ground every year. In the early years of the century women rarely went to a hospital for such care. In 1935, 37 per cent of the live births occurred in hospitals, and in 1948, 85.6 per cent were hospitalized. This means that the per cent of hospital births has more than doubled during a 10-year period. In our larger cities, 96.2 per cent of the babies are born in hospitals.

THE PROBLEM OF INFANT MORTALITY

Infant mortality comprises two groups of cases: those in which the infant (fetus) dies in the uterus prior to birth (so-called "stillbirth"), and those in which it dies within a short period, usually specified as one month, after birth (neonatal mortality). In the year 1948, 72,838 stillbirths (according to present classification) occurred in the United States, and 72,289 neonatal deaths, or a total loss of 145,127 infant lives in connection with the birth process. This total represents almost 10 per cent of all the deaths which took place in this country in 1948 at all ages and from all causes. The great toll taken in the first day of life

(wholly the result of obstetric causes) is compared in Chart 5 with the number of deaths occurring in the rest of the year.

This staggering number of infant deaths is the result of three main causes: premature birth, brain injury sustained in the birth process, and asphyxiation. Subsequently, these conditions will be discussed in detail. It suffices here to say that the first and most important of them, prematurity, is largely a nursing problem; indeed, in all the wide range of nursing care there is no field which offers such lifesaving possibilities as that of the premature infant.

The welfare of the 3,500,000 babies born annually in the United States is very much the concern of obstetrics and one of its main objectives. To reduce the huge loss of newborn lives, to protect the infant not only at birth but in the prenatal period, and during his early days to lay a solid foundation for his health throughout life—this is the problem and the challenge.

THE EXPANDING SCOPE OF OBSTETRIC NURSING

PUBLIC HEALTH NURSING

In 1912 the Children's Bureau of the United States Department of Labor was created by an act of Congress for the purpose of promoting maternal and child health "among all classes of our people." It was a public health nurse who first conceived the idea of a federal bureau of this kind and originally suggested the plan to President Theodore Roosevelt. The Children's Bureau has stressed continually the importance of public health nursing in maternal welfare. Between the years 1921 and 1929, public health nursing consultants were employed by the Bureau, and their services were offered to the states for maternal and infant hygiene. In rural areas public health nursing services throughout the United States were greatly extended, and 2,978 centers for pre-

natal and child health work were established.

The amount of public health nursing service available in this country has changed only slightly for the past few years. The latest census (1950) showed that 25,081 nurses were employed for public health work (exclusive of industrial nurses) in the United States, in the Terri-

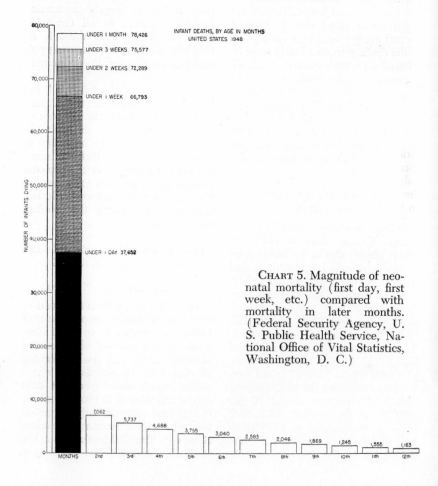

CHART 5. Magnitude of neonatal mortality (first day, first week, etc.) compared with mortality in later months. (Federal Security Agency, U. S. Public Health Service, National Office of Vital Statistics, Washington, D. C.)

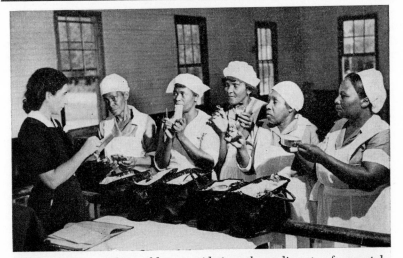

FIG. 1. Nurse teaching old-type midwives the rudiments of prenatal and delivery care. (*Look* magazine)

tories of Hawaii, Alaska, Puerto Rico and the Virgin Islands; and only a small proportion of these rendered maternal and child health care. In fact, many of the 3,070 counties in the United States are still without any public health nursing service.

Public health nursing is concerned not only with the "care of the sick poor in their homes" but also with the education of patients and their families in regard to the basic laws of hygiene and the prevention of disease. As a health teacher, the nurse is in a peculiarly favorable position. Her home visits permit close acquaintance with all members of the family, and in many instances she can gradually and tactfully correct harmful habits of living and instill good ones. In the case of the expectant mother, this instruction is especially important.

THE TRAINED NURSE-MIDWIFE

About 4.5 per cent of all pregnancies and labors in the United States are without benefit of medical attention, and about one half of the nonwhite mothers fall into this neglected group. While it is the ultimate goal to provide all these underprivileged women with complete medical, nursing and hospital care, many years will elapse before that aim can be realized. For this reason it is recognized increasingly that the trained nurse-midwife has a place in maternity programs for certain areas and among certain population groups where medical care is limited.

To the majority of people in this country the term "midwife" means the ignorant, superstitious, and often untrained midwife of the South. In recent years an effort has been made to license these midwives. A teach-

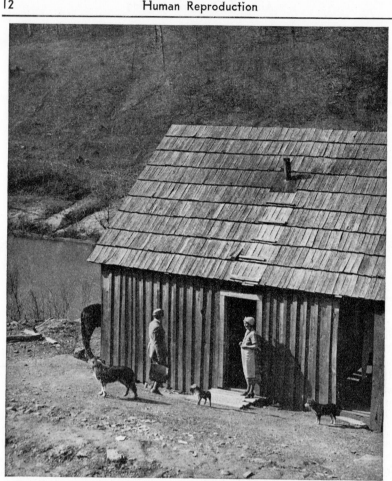

Fig. 2. Prenatal visit. Outside the cabin. (Frontier Nursing Service, Wendover, Ky. Photo by Marvin Breckinridge)

ing and supervisory program for this group is also in effect in several states. By a trained "nurse-midwife" is meant a graduate nurse who has had special postgraduate training at a midwifery school in the actual conduct of home deliveries; she is thoroughly competent to handle normal cases at childbirth. The important contribution which such highly trained nurse-midwives can make to the maternity program of a nation has been demonstrated in certain foreign countries, notably in Norway and Sweden. There some 85 per cent of the deliveries are attended by

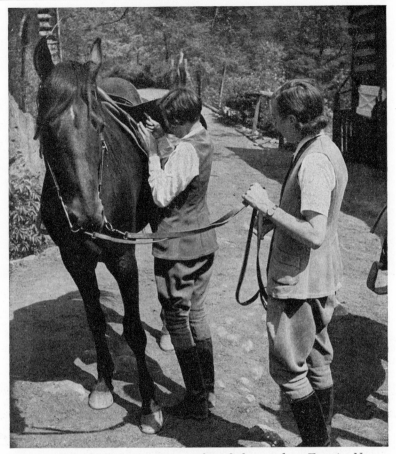

Fɪɢ. 3. Nurse-midwives starting on their daily rounds at Frontier Nursing Service, Wendover, Ky. (Louisville Courier Journal)

such trained personnel with excellent results. Of course, the training, the practice and the supervision of these midwives are regulated most carefully by law, and upon the development of the slightest abnormality in any patient, a physician is summoned at once.

The first use of the trained nurse-midwife in this country was made in 1925 when an organization was established in the mountains of eastern Kentucky to handle the maternity problem in the rural and isolated areas of that territory—the now famous Frontier Nursing Service. The staff is composed not only of nurses but also of trained midwives as well;

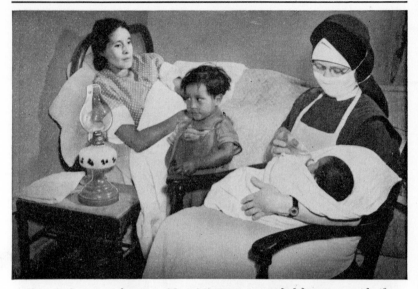

Fig. 4. Care in a home in New Mexico is provided by nurse-midwife service. (Catholic Maternity Institute, Santa Fe, N. Mex.)

a physician is available for consultation in complicated cases. This organization has demonstrated clearly that graduate nurses trained in midwifery can help to lower the maternal mortality rates in rural and isolated areas. Thus, in a series of 5,500 deliveries conducted by the Frontier Nursing Service, there occurred only four maternal deaths, and two of these were not related to the pregnancy. In the fall of 1939 the Frontier Nursing Service inaugurated a course in midwifery for graduate nurses.

In 1931 the Lobenstine Midwifery Clinic was started in New York City to provide a place where graduate nurses could be trained in midwifery. It trains about 12 students a year in a 6-months' course which provides obstetric theory and supervised prac-

tice by an obstetrician and by graduate nurse-midwives.

In October, 1943, the Santa Fe Catholic Maternity Institute School of Midwifery was organized at Santa Fe, New Mexico.

OBSTETRIC NURSING AND THE WAR

The public health nurse and the nurse-midwife always have been needed in our maternity programs. Today this need has definitely multiplied, due to the increase in birth rate, the lack of sufficient maternity hospital beds to meet the need, and fewer doctors preferring rural to urban practice; and, according to the last available statistics (1948), about 509,862 mothers were delivered at home. For vast portions of our population the public health nurse and the trained nurse-midwife represent the only possible solution to the problem. This is a heavy responsibility, but the nursing profession must meet it.

During World War II another obstetric problem was created when millions of women workers took jobs in industrial plants. Since many women are still engaged in industry, the problem persists. In this connection a number of questions arise. Should pregnant women be allowed to work in factories? If so, for how long? What type of work should be forbidden them? How soon may they return to work after childbirth? These and many related questions will be brought to nurses engaged in industrial work, as well as to public health nurses (p. 207).

THE RELATION OF OBSTETRICS TO OTHER FIELDS

Obstetrics is a many-sided subject, and its relationships to the other branches of medicine are numerous and close. Thus, the newborn baby and his problems link obstetrics intimately with pediatrics, and to be a good obstetric nurse one must also be a good pediatric nurse. Moreover, obstetrics may be regarded as a surgical specialty, and a competent obstetric nurse must be thoroughly grounded in the principles of asepsis and in practical operating-room technic. Since a pregnant woman may contract the same diseases as the nonpregnant, the nurse will be confronted with various medical complications of pregnancy, such as tuberculosis, pneumonia, diabetes, etc. In this connection, she must be intimately familiar with the procedures employed for the isolation of communicable diseases, because puerperal infection necessitates meticulous isolation to prevent cross infections. Pregnancy, in many instances, creates an added economic problem, as well as concern about family responsibilities. Since these problems affect the family unit, the obstetric social worker is often the connecting link between the family and the doctor and the nurse (p. 168). Finally, obstetrics is related to psychiatry, since pregnancy sometimes disturbs the mental and emotional balance of the patient; and, in all cases, there is need for emphasis on a cheerful, wholesome mental attitude.

HOW OBSTETRICS DIFFERS FROM OTHER FIELDS

Obstetrics differs from some of the other subjects previously studied by the nurse in that it deals with the normal physiologic processes of the reproductive organs. Under ideal conditions, pregnancy is a constructive period. It has to do with the beginning of a new life. All attitudes and anticipations should point toward a normal outcome. For the patient, any difficulties associated with the experience have the compensation of the new baby to which she looks forward. For the nurse this is a wholly new phase of nursing. Past teachings have been based on the "curative" point of view, and the previous experience of the nurse has been based upon the observation of the symptoms of pain and discomfort, the acquisition of a knowledge of surgical technic, and the art of making patients comfortable. In the earlier courses in her training, the nurse has been given a general idea of the functions of the various systems of the human body, but in this course in obstetrics there is opportunity to pursue the study of the generative organs in detail in order to understand the changes during pregnancy, the climax during labor and delivery, and the adjustments involved during the return to normal in the postpartum period and the months following. She must also have some understanding of the emotional reactions which accompany this whole maternity cycle.

In few fields is so much responsibility placed upon the nurse as in obstetrics. In few, also, are there so many opportunities for originality of thought and initiative. The fact that such monumental advances as our current prenatal care and the related work of the Children's Bureau had their genesis in the nursing profession is proof enough of what can be accomplished in this field by women of vision.

SUGGESTED READING

Adair, Fred L.: Maternity as the frontier of human welfare, The Mother 5:5, 1943.

Breckinridge, Mary: Wide Neighborhoods, New York, Harper, 1952.

Deming, Dorothy: Public health nursing test, Pub. Health Nursing 43:271, 1951.

Fell, Frances: Midwifery delivery services in New Mexico, Am. J. Nursing 45:3, 1945.

Ferguson, E. R.: Nurse midwives serve rural community, Pub. Health Nursing 35:187, 1943.

Gainey, Harold S.: Contribution of the Obstetrician Toward Better Maternal and Newborn Care, Proceedings of the Third American Congress on Obstetrics and Gynecology, pp. 3-7.

Hospital services in the United States, J.A.M.A. 146:109, 1951.

Kamperman, George: An evaluation of the newer obstetrics, Am. J. Obst. & Gynec. 60:239, 1950.

Pastore, J. B., and Thomas, F. K.: How many beds for maternity patients? Hospitals 22:40-43, 1948.

PHS Publication No. 39, International Recommendations on Definitions of Live Births and Fetal Death, Federal Security Agency, Public Health Service, National Office of Vital Statistics, Oct. 1950.

Reid, Duncan E., and Cohen, Mandel E.: Trends in obstetrics, J.A.M.A. 142:615, 1950.

Schwartz, Doris: Nurse-midwives in the mountains, Am. J. Nursing 51:102, 1951.

Special Reports on Maternal and Infant Mortality, U. S. Public Health Service, National Office of Vital Statistics.

Supervision of Maternity Practice in the Home. Proceedings of the First American Congress on Obstetrics and Gynecology, pp. 408-414, 1939.

2

Anatomy as a Basis for Obstetrics

PELVIS

The pelvis, so called from its resemblance to a basin (*pelvis*, a basin), is a bony ring interposed between the trunk and the thighs. The vertebral column, or backbone, passes into it from above, transmitting to it the weight of the upper part of the body, which the pelvis, in turn, transmits to the lower limbs. From an obstetric point of view, however, we have to consider it as the cavity which contains the generative organs, and particularly as the canal through which the baby must pass during birth.

STRUCTURE

The pelvis is made up of four united bones: the two hip bones (or innominate bones) situated laterally and in front, and the sacrum and the coccyx behind. Anatomically, the hip bones are divided into three parts: the ilium, the ischium and the pubis. These bones become firmly joined into one by the time the growth of the body is completed, i.e., at about the age of 20 to 25, so that on examining them in the prepared pelvis no trace of the original edges or divisions of these three bones can be discovered. Each of these bones may be roughly described as follows:

The ilium, which is the largest portion of the bone, forms the upper and back part of the pelvis. Its upper flaring border forms the prominence of the hip or crest of the ilium (hip bone). The ischium is the lower part below the hip joint; from it projects

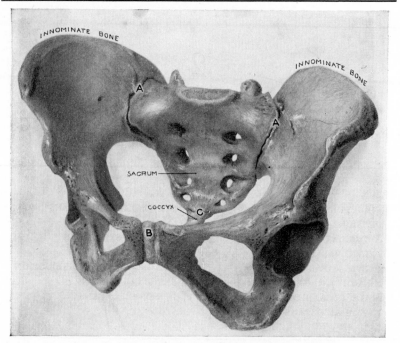

Fig. 5. Pelvis. (A) Sacro-iliac articulations (synchrondroses). (B)
Symphysis pubis. (C) Sacrococcygeal articulation.

the tuberosity of the ischium on which the body rests when in a sitting posture. The pubis is the front part of the hip bone; it extends from the hip joint to the joint in front between the two hip bones, the symphysis pubis, and then turns down toward the ischial tuberosity, thus forming with the bone of the opposite side the arch below the symphysis, the pubic or subpubic arch. This articulation closes anteriorly the cavity of the pelvis.

The sacrum and the coccyx form the lowest portions of the spinal column. The former is a triangular wedge-shaped bone, consisting of five vertebrae fused together; it serves as the back part of the pelvis. The coccyx consists of four very small vertebrae which form a tail end to the spine. The coccyx is usually movable at its attachment to the sacrum (the sacrococcygeal joint) and may become pressed back during labor to give more room for the passage of the fetal head.

Of special importance is the marked projection which is formed by the junction of the last lumbar vertebra with the sacrum; this is known as the sacral promontory and is one of the most important landmarks in obstetric anatomy.

Divisions

Regarded as a whole, the pelvis may be described as a two-storied, bony basin that is divided by a natural line of division (the inlet or brim) into two parts. These parts are called the false pelvis (above) and the true pelvis (below).

The false pelvis, or upper flaring part, is much less concerned with the problems of labor than is the true pelvis, but it is important in obstetrics because it offers certain landmarks for the practice of pelvimetry or pelvic measurements; and because its shape and inclination aid in estimating the nature of the true pelvis and in diagnosing certain forms of pelvic deformity. It also supports the uterus during late pregnancy and directs the fetus into the true pelvis.

The true pelvis, or lower part, forms the bony canal through which the baby must pass during parturition; for convenience in description it is divided into three parts: an inlet or brim, a cavity and an outlet.

Pelvic Inlet

Continuous with the sacral promontory and extending along the ilium on each side in circular fashion is a ridge called the iliopectineal line

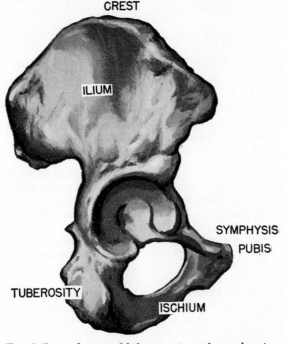

CREST

ILIUM

SYMPHYSIS PUBIS

TUBEROSITY

ISCHIUM

Fig. 6. Lateral view of left innominate bone showing its three constituent parts (standing position).

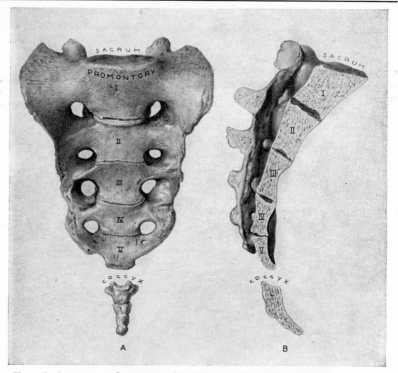

FIG. 7. Sacrum and coccyx. (A) Front view. (B) Median section; note how promontory of sacrum juts forward.

(brim). This bounds an area or plane called the inlet, so named because it is the entry-way or inlet through which the baby's head must pass in order to enter the true pelvis. The pelvic inlet, sometimes also referred to as the pelvic brim or superior strait, divides the false from the true pelvis. It is roughly heart-shaped, the promontory of the sacrum forming a slight projection into it from behind (Fig. 9); it is widest from side to side, and narrowest from back to front, i.e., from the sacral promontory to the symphysis. It

should be noted particularly that the baby's head enters the inlet with its longest diameter (anteroposterior) in the transverse diameter of the pelvis. In other words, as shown in Figure 9, the greatest diameter of the head accommodates itself to the greatest diameter of the inlet. As the inlet is entirely surrounded by bone, the measurements of its diameters can be estimated accurately; and for the same reason, these measurements are very important, since variations from the normal (e.g., smaller in size or flattened) may cause grave difficulty at the time of labor.

Pelvic Outlet

When viewed from below, the pelvic outlet is a space bounded in front by the symphysis pubis and the pubic arch, at the sides by the ischial tuberosities, and behind by the coccyx and the greater sacrosciatic ligaments. It requires only a little imagination to see that the front half of the outlet resembles a triangle, the base of which is the distance between the ischial tuberosities, and the other two sides of which are represented by the pubic arch. From an obstetric point of view, this triangle is of great importance, since the baby's head must make use of this space to gain exit from the pelvis and the mother's body. For this reason Nature has provided a wide pubic arch in females, whereas in males it is narrow (Fig. 16). If the pubic arch in women were as narrow as it is in men, natural childbearing would be extremely difficult, since the baby's head, unable to squeeze itself into the narrow anterior triangle of the

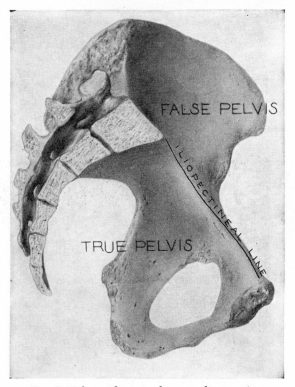

FIG. 8. False and true pelves, median section.

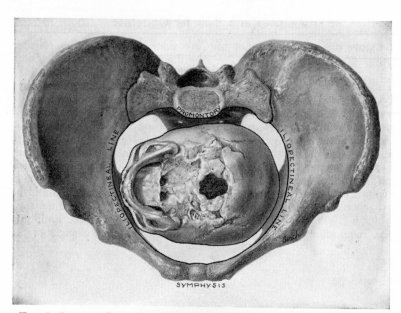

Fig. 9. Largest diameter of baby's head entering largest diameter of inlet. Therefore, it enters transversely.

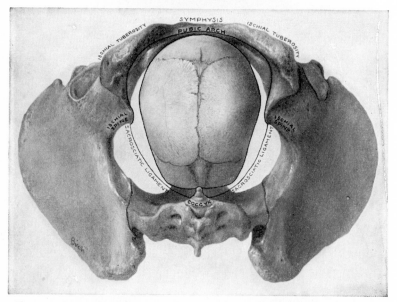

Fig. 10. Largest diameter of baby's head passing through largest diameter of outlet. Therefore, it passes through outlet anteroposteriorly.

outlet, would be forced backward again the coccyx and the sacrum where its progress would be impeded.

As has been stated, the greatest diameter of the inlet is the transverse (from side to side), whereas the greatest diameter of the outlet is the anteroposterior (from front to back). Moreover, the baby's head, as it emerges from the pelvis, passes through the outlet in the antero-posterior position, again accommodating its greatest diameter to the greatest diameter of the passage. Since the baby's head enters the pelvis in the transverse position and emerges in the anteroposterior, it is obvious that the head must rotate some 90° as it passes through the pelvis. This process of rotation of the baby's head is one of the most important phases of the mechanism of labor and will be discussed in more detail later on page 312.

Pelvic Cavity

The pelvic cavity is the space between the inlet above, the outlet below and the anterior, posterior and lateral walls of the pelvis. It is important to note the curved nature of the cavity when viewed from the side. The curved angle of the cavity determines the direction which the

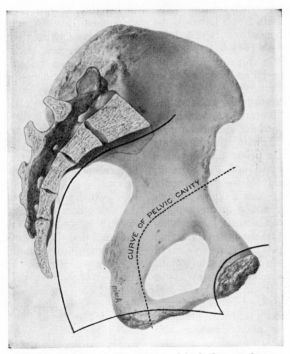

FIG. 11. Pelvic cavity. Heavy black line indicates location of soft parts, vagina, etc.

baby takes through the pelvis in a normal delivery and along which the baby is extracted in a forceps or other abnormal delivery. As might be expected, labor is made more complicated by this curvature in the pelvic canal because the baby has to accommodate itself to the curved path as well as to the variations in the size of the cavity at different levels.

ARTICULATION AND SURFACES

The articulations (joints) of the pelvis, which possess obstetric importance, are four in number. Two are behind, between the sacrum and the ilia on either side, and are termed the sacro-iliac synchondroses (Fig. 5, A); one is in front, between the two pubic bones, and is called the symphysis pubis (Fig. 5, B); and the fourth, of little consequence, is between the sacrum and coccyx, the sacrococcygeal articulation (Fig. 5, C).

All of these articular surfaces are lined with fibrocartilage, which becomes thickened and softened during pregnancy; likewise, the ligaments which bind the pelvic joints together become softened and, as a result, greater mobility of the pelvic bones develops. A certain definite, though very limited, motion in the joints is desirable for a normal labor; however, there is no change in the actual size of the pelvis. From a practical standpoint, one of the most important facts for the nurse to know about these joints is that the increased mobility which they develop in pregnancy produces a slight "wobbliness" in the pelvis and throws greater strain on the surrounding muscles and ligaments. This accounts, in large part, for the frequency of backache

and legache in the latter months of pregnancy.

The pelvis is lined with muscular tissue which provides a smooth, somewhat cushioned surface over which the fetus has to pass during labor; these muscles also help to support the abdominal contents.

PELVIC VARIATIONS

The pelvis presents great individual variations—no two pelves are exactly alike. Even those patients with normal measurements may present differences in contour and muscular development which influence the actual size of the pelvis. These varying differences are due in part to heredity, disease, injury and development. Heredity may be responsible for passing on many racial and sexual differences. Such diseases as tuberculosis and rickets cause malformations. Accidents and injuries during childhood or at maturity result in deformities of the pelvis or other parts of the body which affect the pelvis. Adequate nutrition and well-formed habits related to posture and exercise have a very definite influence upon the development of the pelvis.

It must be remembered also that the pelvis does not mature until between the ages of 20 and 25 years, and until that time complete ossification has not taken place.

There are many so-called borderline cases of abnormal pelvic development. Such pregnant patients should be supervised closely. At periodic intervals the size of the fetus is estimated (by palpation of the abdomen), and definite arrangements are made for the type of delivery indicated.

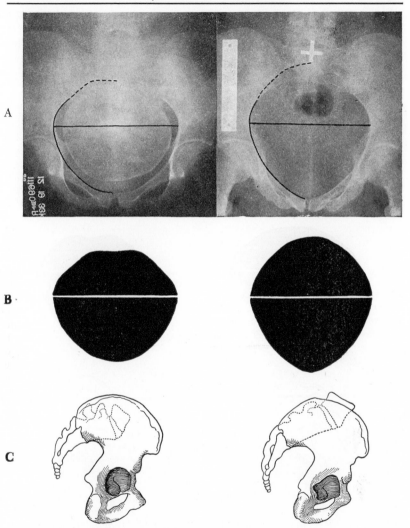

Fig. 12 (*Left*). Gynecoid (normal female) pelvis. Inlet is well rounded in hind- and fore-pelvis (A, B). Sacrosciatic notch is curved, moderate in width and depth (C).

Fig. 13 (*Right*). Anthropoid pelvis. Inlet is deep in hind- and fore-pelvis, increased in anteroposterior diameter (A, B). Sacrosciatic notch is broad, shallow (C).

(Roentgenograms from W. E. Caldwell, M.D., and H. C. Moloy, M.D., Sloane Hospital for Women, New York)

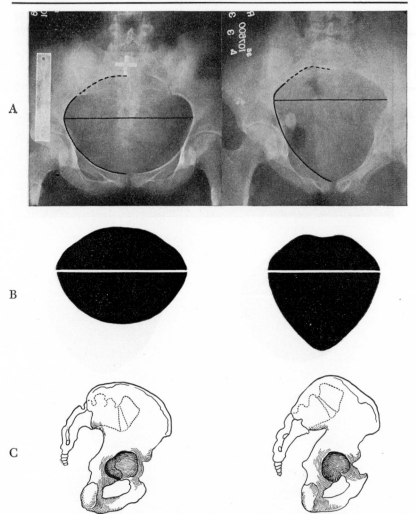

Fig. 14 (*Left*). Platypelloid pelvis. Inlet is a transverse oval, well-curved but decreased in anteroposterior diameter (A, B). Sacrosciatic notch is curved, small (C).

Fig. 15 (*Right*). Android pelvis. Inlet is wedge-shaped with shallow hind-pelvis and pointed fore-pelvis (A, B). Sacrosciatic notch is narrow, deep, pointed (C).

(Roentgenograms from W. E. Caldwell, M.D., and H. C. Moloy, M.D., Sloane Hospital for Women, New York)

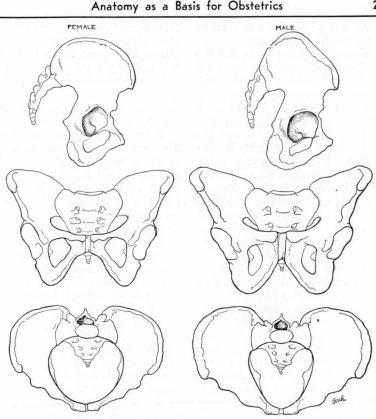

FIG. 16. Female pelvis contrasted with male in lateral, front and inlet views.

There are several types of pelves. Even pelves whose measurements are normal differ greatly in the shape of the inlet, in the proximity of the greatest transverse diameter of the inlet to the sacral promontory, in the size of the sacrosciatic notch, and in their general architecture. Dr. H. C. Moloy and the late Dr. W. E. Caldwell, of the Sloane Hospital for Women, New York City, have utilized these characteristics in establishing a new classification of pelves which has been of great interest and value to obstetricians. The four main types, according to this classification, are shown in Figures 12 to 15. The manner in which the baby passes through the birth canal and consequently the type of labor vary considerably in these several pelvic types.

In addition, of course, there are many pelvic types which result from abnormal narrowing of one or the other diameters. These contracted pelves will be described in a subsequent chapter (see p. 380).

In comparing the male and the female pelves, several differences will be observed. As already emphasized, the most conspicuous difference is in the pubic arch, which has a much wider angle in women. The symphysis is shorter in women, and the border of the arch probably is more everted. Although the female pelvis is more shallow, it is more capacious than the male, much lighter in structure, and smoother. The male pelvis is deep, compact, conical, and rougher in texture, particularly at the site of muscle attachments. The recent findings of Drs. Daniel G. Morton and Charles T. Hayden, of San Francisco, indicate that both males and females start life with pelves which are identical in type, and that the major differences observed in adult male and female pelves do not appear until puberty and are therefore due to the influence of the sex hormones. (For definition and description of the sex hormones, see p. 60.)

PELVIC MEASUREMENTS

Importance of Pelvic Measurements. The entire problem in childbirth centers on the safe passage of the fully developed fetus through the pelvis of the mother. Slight irregularities in the structure of the pelvis may cause a slow or instrumental delivery, while any marked deformity may render the delivery by the natural passages impossible. For these reasons the pelvis of every pregnant woman should be measured carefully early in the prenatal period to enable the physician to determine, before labor begins, whether or not

there is anything in the condition of the mother's pelvis that may complicate the delivery. This examination is a part of the antepartal examination. In addition to a general physical examination, the pelvic measurements are made and compared with the dimensions of the normal pelvis.

Types of Pelvic Measurements. The external pelvic measurements give only an approximate idea of the size of the pelvis. These measurements are taken with an instrument called a pelvimeter. Those most commonly made are: (1) the widest distance between the lateral edges of the iliac crests on either side, the intercristal; (2) the distance between the two anterior superior iliac spines, the interspinous; (3) the external conjugate or distance between the anterior aspect of the symphysis pubis in front and the depression below the spine of the fifth lumbar vertebra behind; (4) the intertuberous diameter or tuber-ischii diameter, sometimes abbreviated as T.I., is the distance between the inner aspects of the ischial tuberosities. In addition, some physicians measure the right and the left oblique external diameters, as well as the intertrochanteric distance (between the trochanters of the femurs). The right oblique diameter is taken from the right posterosuperior spinous process of the ilium to the left anterior superior spine of the ilium. For this measurement the patient lies on her right side, and the position is reversed in taking the left oblique measurement. For all the other pelvic measurements the patient lies on her side or back, according to the diameters to be measured, and with the abdomen exposed.

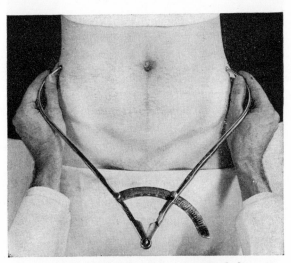

FIG. 17. Method of measuring intercristal diameter.

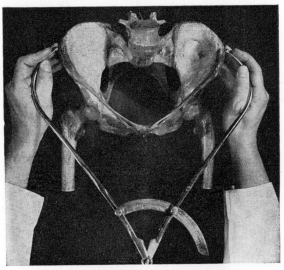

FIG. 18. Intercristal diameter measured on bony
pelvis.

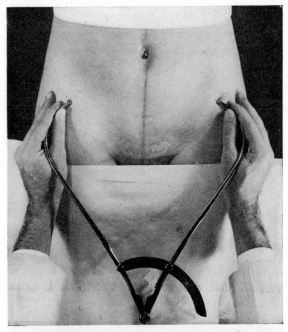

FIG. 19. Method of measuring interspinous diameter.

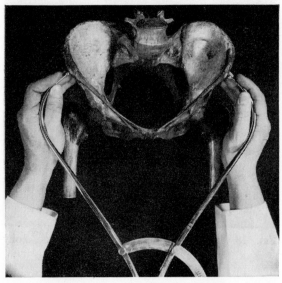

FIG. 20. Interspinous diameter measured on bony pelvis.

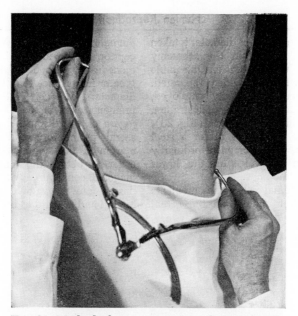

FIG. 21. Method of measuring external conjugate diameter.

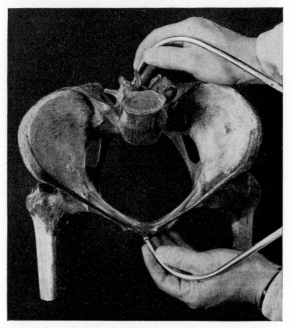

FIG. 22. External conjugate diameter measured on bony pelvis.

The intertuberous diameter is taken with the patient in the lithotomy position, well down on the table and with the legs widely separated. The instrument usually employed, and the one shown in the illustration, is the Williams pelvimeter (Fig. 23), but some physicians prefer a steel tape. This measurement is ordinarily taken on a level with the lower border of the anus.

The internal pelvic measurements are made to determine the actual diameters of the inlet. With the exception of the interischial measurement just described, these are of far greater importance than the external diameters. The chief internal measurement taken is the *diagonal conjugate* or the distance between the sacral promontory and the lower margin of the symphysis pubis. In order to obtain the length of the diagonal conjugate, two fingers are passed into the vagina and pressed inward and upward as far as possible

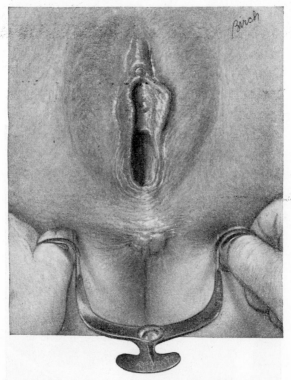

Fig. 23. Method of measuring tuber-ischii or inter-tuberous diameter of outlet, using the Williams pelvimeter. The measurement is made on a line with the lower border of the anus.

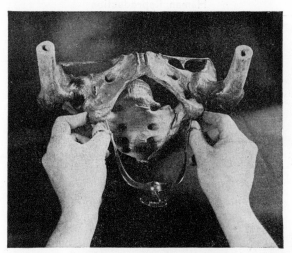

Fig. 24. Tuber-ischii or intertuberous diameter measured on bony pelvis.

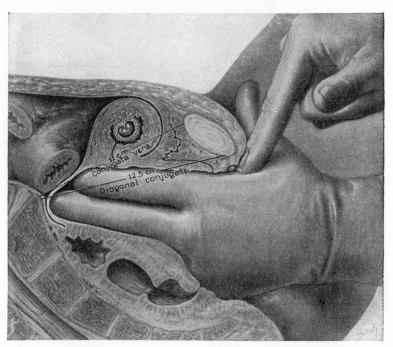

Fig. 25. Method of obtaining diagonal conjugate diameter.

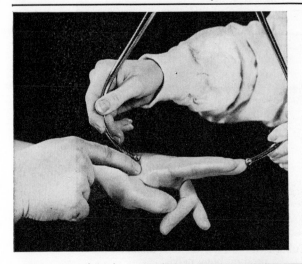

Fig. 26 (*Top*). Method of measuring diagonal conjugate diameter as obtained in Figure 25, using pelvimeter.

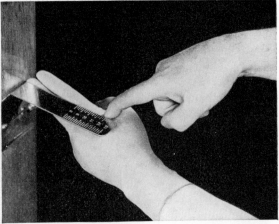

Fig. 27 (*Bottom*). Method of measuring diagonal conjugate diameter as obtained in Figure 25, using wall bracket.

until the middle finger rests on the sacral promontory. The point on the back of the hand just under the symphysis is then marked by putting the finger of the other hand on that exact point, after which the fingers are withdrawn. The distance from the tip of the middle finger to the point marked is the diagonal con-jugate measurement. This distance may be measured with a pelvimeter or by means of a wall bracket (Fig. 27). In common medical parlance this measurement is often referred to as the "C.D." (conjugata diago-nalis).

Another extremely important in-ternal diameter is the true conjugate,

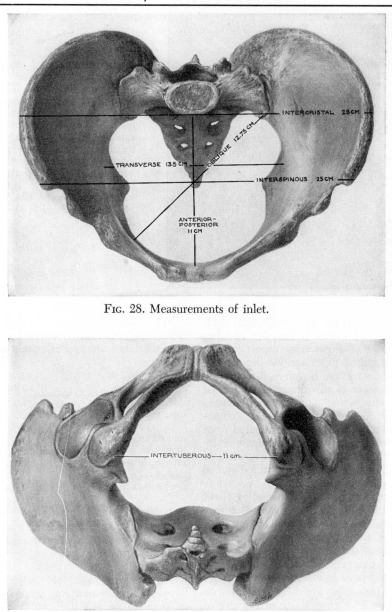

Fig. 28. Measurements of inlet.

Fig. 29. Intertuberous measurement of outlet.

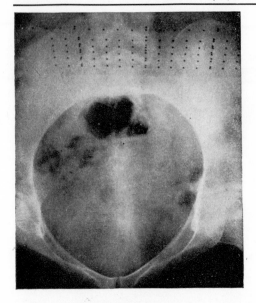

Fig. 30. Pelvis inlet roentgenogram. The scale represents corrected centimeters for various levels of the pelvic canal. The top line is used for measuring the diameters of the inlet. The other levels are established on the lateral roentgenogram. Pelvic morphology is readily established by viewing both lateral and inlet views. (Herbert Thoms, M.D., Yale School of Medicine)

or in Latin, the *conjugata vera* (C.V.), which is the distance between the posterior aspect of the symphysis pubis and the promontory of the sacrum. However, direct measurement of this diameter cannot be made conveniently (except by means of the roentgenogram); consequently, it has to be estimated from the diagonal conjugate diameter by subtracting 1.5 cm., or two thirds of an inch. For instance, if the diagonal conjugate is 12.5 cm., the conjugata vera may be estimated as being about 11.0 cm. The length of the true conjugate, or conjugata vera, is of the utmost importance, since it is about the smallest diameter of the inlet through which the baby's head must pass. Indeed, the main purpose in measuring the diagonal conjugate is to give an estimate of the size of the conjugata vera.

In women with normal pelves, the sizes of the diameters which have been discussed are approximately as follows:

	CENTI-METERS
Intercristal	28.0
Interspinous	25.0
External conjugate	20.0
Intertuberous	11.0
Right and left external obliques	22.0
Intertrochanteric	31.0
Diagonal conjugate	12.5
Conjugata vera	11.0

X-RAY PELVIMETRY

As stated above, there is no manual procedure which permits measurement of the transverse diameter of the inlet. For these reasons both roentgenologists and obstetricians have striven to perfect an x-ray method which will not only yield precise measurements but also will give a clear picture of the entire inlet and of the general pelvic architecture. A number of such methods are now available and are being used more and more frequently, particularly in cases in which pelvic abnormalities are suspected.

Possibly the most widely used method, and one of the simplest, is that of Dr. Herbert Thoms of New Haven, Conn., a pioneer worker in this field. For a complete study two roentgenograms are made as follows: (1) The patient is placed on the x-ray table in a semirecumbent position so that her pelvic inlet is horizontal and as nearly parallel as possible with the plate beneath her. The exact plane in which the pa-

tient's inlet lies, both front and back, is now determined and recorded. After an exposure of the film has been made, the patient is removed from the table, and a lead plate or grid containing perforations, a centimeter apart, is placed in the plane previously occupied by the inlet of the patient. Another exposure is now made on the same film. When the latter is developed, the outline of the inlet is shown, as are also the dots produced by the perforations in the lead plate. Since the projected dots on the film represent centimeters in the plane of the inlet, the diameters of the inlet can be read off directly as centimeters. (2) A somewhat similar procedure is carried out with the

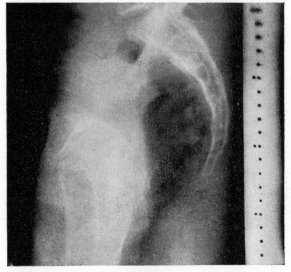

FIG. 31. Lateral roentgenogram. The scale represents corrected centimeters in the midplane of the body. By means of calipers the various diameters may be measured. The lateral morphologic aspects are readily visualized. (Herbert Thoms, M.D., Yale School of Medicine)

patient standing and from the lateral view. Here, however, an upright lead and iron rod, with a centimeter scale notched on its edge, is placed posterior to the patient and close to the gluteal fold. After an exposure has been made, the developed film will show a lateral view of the symphysis pubis, the sacral promontory, other bony landmarks, and in addition, of course, the notched centimeter scale for establishing the dis-

tance between important points—particularly the conjugata vera diameter.

Other technics entail the use of stereoscopic procedures which allow the physician to view the films with three-dimensional vision and thus gain a clear image of all pelvic relationships.

When roentgenograms are made late in pregnancy by any of these methods, it is possible to secure also

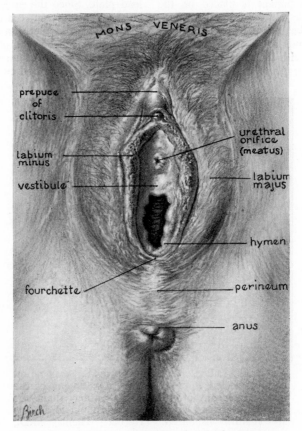

Fig. 32. External organs of reproduction.

an impression of the size of the baby's head. When this is considered in relation to the pelvic picture, helpful information may be obtained in forecasting whether or not this particular pelvis is large enough to allow this particular baby to pass through.

Preventive Care Based on Pelvimetry. The importance of the knowledge gained through skillful performance of external and internal pelvimetry cannot be overestimated. Especially should it never be neglected in the case of a woman pregnant for the first time, nor in any case in which the patient has suffered previously from difficult or tedious labors.

FEMALE ORGANS OF REPRODUCTION

The female organs of reproduction are divided into two groups—the external and internal (Figs. 32 and 34-37).

External Organs

The external organs are the mons veneris, the labia majora, the labia minora, the clitoris, the hymen, and the perineal body in the perineum. The term *vulva* is used sometimes in a broad sense to include all these external parts, but as commonly employed it refers simply to the labia majora and minora. Since the latter structures are folds of skin and mucous membrane which serve to keep the vaginal opening closed, it may be helpful to recall that the word vulva comes from a Latin word, *valva*, meaning "a folding door."

The mons veneris is a firm, cushionlike formation over the symphysis pubis and is covered with hair.

The labia majora are two prominent longitudinal folds of skin which extend downward and backward from the mons veneris and disappear in forming the anterior border of the perineal body. These two thick folds of skin are covered with hair on their outer surfaces but are smooth and moist on their inner surfaces. At the bottom they are not really joined but appear to become lost in this space, ending close to and nearly parallel with each other.

The labia minora are two thin folds of reddish tissue covered entirely with thin membrane and situated between the labia majora, with their outer surfaces in contact with the inner surfaces of the labia majora; the labia minora extend from the clitoris downward and backward on either side of the orifice of the vagina. In the upper extremity each labium minus separates into two branches which when united with those of the opposite side enclose the clitoris. The upper fold forms the prepuce and the lower the frenum of the clitoris. At the bottom the labia minora are smaller and thinner and blend together as a thin fold of skin forming the anterior edge of the perineum or perineal body. This thin edge is known as the fourchette.

The clitoris is a small, highly sensitive projection composed of erectile tissue, nerves and blood vessels; it is covered with a thin epidermis. It is homologous with the penis in the male. The clitoris is so situated that it is partially hidden between the anterior ends of the labia minora.

The hymen marks the division between the internal and the external organs. It is a thin fold of mucous membrane situated at the orifice of

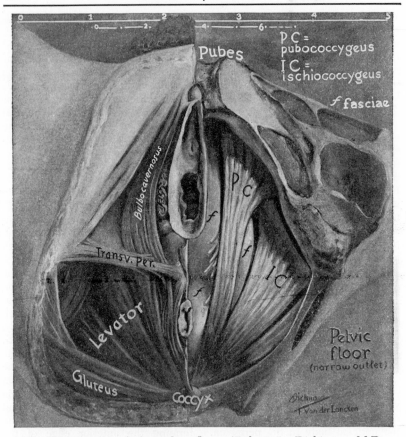

FIG. 33. Muscles of the pelvic floor. (Robert L. Dickinson, M.D., New York)

the vagina. It may be entirely absent or it may form a complete septum across the lower end of the vagina. In women who have had children the irregularity of torn edges remains. The external, triangular area which is enclosed between the clitoris above and the labia minora at the sides is called the vestibule.

The perineal body of the perineum is made up of muscles and fascia which form the support of the pelvic organs from below. The levator ani muscle is the muscle most frequently lacerated during the birth of the baby; therefore, it should be guarded most carefully at this time, for it may be torn to an extent varying all the way from a slight surface "nick" to a deep laceration, extending through the anus and up into the rectum itself, when the baby's head is born.

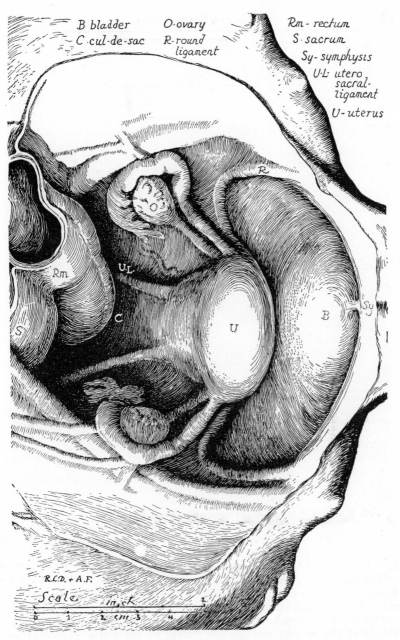

B bladder   O·ovary   Rm - rectum
C·cul-de-sac   R·round   S· sacrum
ligament   Sy- symphysis
U·L· utero
sacral-
ligament
U- uterus

R.L.D. + A.F.

Scale   in.ck

Fig. 34. Pelvic contents from above, showing the position of the pairs of ligaments and the relationship to the uterus, the tubes and the ovaries. (Robert L. Dickinson, M.D., New York)

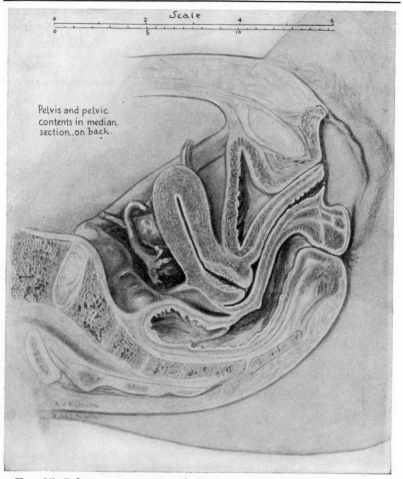

Scale

FIG. 35. Pelvic contents in median section with the subject on her
back. (Robert L. Dickinson, M.D., New York)

INTERNAL ORGANS

The internal organs of reproduction are the ovaries, the fallopian tubes, the uterus and the vagina.

Ovaries. The ovaries are the sex glands of the woman and are homologous with the testes in the male.

They are two small bodies, each about the size of an unshelled almond, situated one on either side of the uterus. They lie embedded in the posterior fold of the broad ligament of the uterus (Fig. 34) and are supported by the suspensory, the

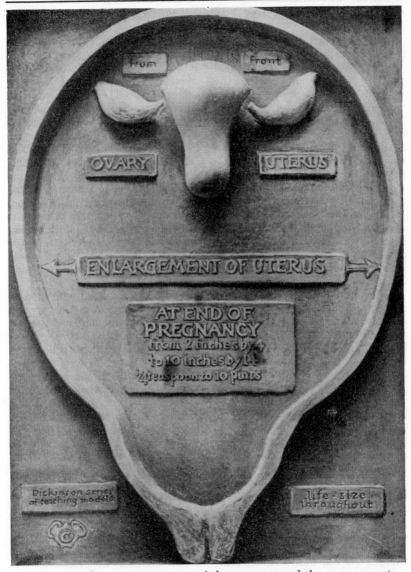

Fig. 36. The comparative size of the pregnant and the nonpregnant uterus. (From the Dickinson-Belskie *Birth Atlas* Series, published by the Maternity Center Association, New York)

ovarian and the mesovarian liga-ments.

Each ovary contains in its sub-stance at birth a large number of germ cells or ovules (primordial ova) (p. 57). Beginning at about the time of puberty one (or possibly two) of the follicles which contain the ovules enlarges each month, grad-ually approaches the surface of the ovary and bursts (Fig. 42). The ovum and the fluid content of the fol-licle are liberated on the exterior of the ovary into the abdominal cavity, then they are swept into the tube and so pass into the uterus. The develop-ment and the maturation of the fol-licles (containing the ova) and the ova continue from puberty to meno-pause; however, their formation commenced from birth.

The arteries which supply the ovary are four or five branches that arise from the anastomosis of the ovarian artery with the ovarian branch of the uterine (Fig. 37). The veins proceeding from the ovary be-come tributary to both the uterine and the ovarian plexus.

The nerves supplying the ovaries are derived from the craniosacral and the thoracolumbar sympathetic sys-tems. The postganglionic and visceral afferent fibers form a plexus sur-rounding the ovarian artery, which in turn is formed by contributions from the renal and the aortic plexuses and corresponds to the spermatic plexus in the male.

Fallopian Tubes. The fallopian tubes (Figs. 37 and 47) are two trumpet-shaped, thin, flexible, mus-cular tubes, about 4½ inches long and somewhat thinner than a lead pencil. They extend from the upper angles of the uterus, just below the fundus, in the upper margin of the broad ligament, toward the sides of the pelvis. They have two openings, one into the uterine cavity and the other into the abdominal cavity. The opening into the uterine cavity is minute and will admit only a fine bristle; the abdominal opening is somewhat larger and is surrounded by a large number of fine fringes; hence the term "fimbriated end." The fallopian tubes convey the dis-charged ova by peristaltic action from the ovaries to the cavity of the uterus; by their tentaclelike proc-esses the fimbriated ends of the tube draw the escaped ova into the tube. Thus, the function of the fallopian tube is to conduct the ovum along the canal by peristaltic action until it reaches the uterus.

The tubes are lined with mucous membrane containing ciliated epi-thelium. The muscular layer is made up of longitudinal and circular fibers which provide peristaltic action. The serous membrane covering the tubes is a continuation of the peritoneum, which lines the whole abdominal cavity.

The fallopian tubes receive their blood supply from the ovarian and the uterine arteries. The veins of the tubes follow the course of these arteries and empty into the uterine and the ovarian trunks. The nerves which supply the uterus supply the tubes (Fig. 37).

Uterus. The uterus is a hollow, thick-walled, muscular organ. It is of about the size and the shape of a flattened pear, weighing from 1 to 2 ounces in its nonpregnant state (Figs. 34 and 36). Due to its mus-cular composition, it is capable of enlarging to the size of a pumpkin;

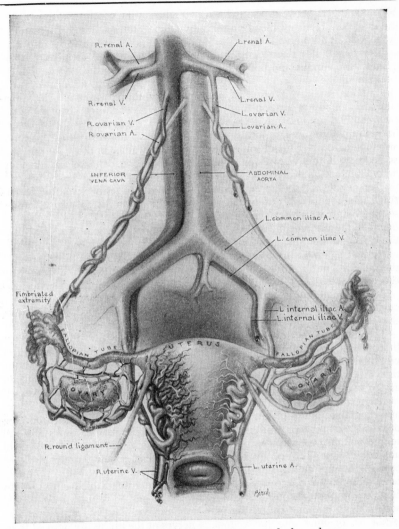

FIG. 37. Blood supply of the uterus and the adnexa.

at the termination of pregnancy it weighs about 2 pounds. It is made up of involuntary muscle fibers arranged in all directions, making expansion possible in every direction to accommodate the products of conception. Due to the nature of this arrangement of the muscle, the uterus is able to expel its contents at the termination of normal labor (Fig.

85). Arranged between these muscular layers are many blood vessels, lymphatics and nerves.

The uterus has three distinct divisions: the fundus, the body of the uterus and the cervix. The fundus is the upper rounded portion of the uterus; the body or cavity is that part between the fundus and the cervix; and the cervix is the lower constricted segment of the uterus which projects into the vagina for about 1 to 1½ inches.

The cavity of the uterus is very small and somewhat triangular in shape, being widest at the fundus, between the very small openings into the canals of the fallopian tubes, and narrowest below at the opening into the cervix. The uterus is lined with mucous membrane (endometrium) and is divided into two parts: the cavity of the body of the uterus and the cavity of the cervix.

The cervix is less freely movable than is the body of the uterus. Its muscular wall is not so thick, and the mucous membrane lining its cavity (cervical endometrium) is different in that it is much folded and contains more glands, which produce mucus and are the chief source of the mucous secretion during pregnancy. The cervix has an upper opening called the internal os, leading from the cavity of the uterine body into the cervical canal, and a lower opening called the external os, opening into the vagina. The cervix is very small in the nonpregnant woman, barely admitting a probe, but at the time of labor it dilates to a size sufficient to permit the passage of the fetus (Fig. 155).

The spaces between the side of that part of the cervix which extends into the vagina and the vaginal walls are termed fornices (plural of fornix), and are divided into four parts. The lateral fornices are the spaces between the cervix and the vaginal walls on either side; the anterior fornix is between the anterior wall of the cervix and the anterior vaginal wall; the posterior fornix is between the posterior vaginal wall and the posterior wall of the cervix. The rectovaginal excavation formed by the peritoneum where it bridges between the rectum and the vagina is called the cul-de-sac of Douglas (Fig. 34).

UTERINE BLOOD SUPPLY. The uterus receives its blood supply from the ovarian and the uterine arteries. The ovarian artery is a branch of the abdominal aorta. The uterine artery branches from the internal iliac vessel. The internal iliac also supplies the external genitals (Fig. 37).

The uterovaginal plexus returns the blood from the uterus and the vagina. These veins form a plexus of exceedingly thin-walled vessels which are embedded in the layers of the uterine muscle. Emerging from this plexus the trunks join the uterine vein, which is a double vein. These veins follow on either side of the uterine artery and eventually form one trunk which empties into the hypogastric vein.

UTERINE NERVE SUPPLY. The nerves of the uterus are derived from the craniosacral and the thoracolumbar sympathetic system. These nerves follow the course of the blood vessels between the folds of the broad ligament and terminate in the involuntary muscle of the uterus.

Since the uterus is a freely movable organ suspended in the pelvic cavity between the bladder and the rectum, the position of the uterus may be influenced by a full bladder or rectum which pushes it backward or forward (Figs. 35 and 40). The uterus also changes its position when the patient stands, lies flat, or turns on her side. There are, also, abnormalities, such as anteflexion where the fundus is tipped too far forward (Fig. 40); retroversion where it is tipped too far backward (Fig. 40); and prolapse, due to the relaxation of the muscles of the pelvic floor and the uterine ligaments.

LYMPHATIC VESSELS. The lymphatic vessels drain into the lumbar lymph nodes.

LIGAMENTS. The uterus is supported in two ways: by ligaments (Fig. 34) and by the muscles of the pelvic floor (Fig. 33). The ligaments which support the uterus in the pelvic cavity are the broad ligaments (2), the round ligaments (2), the uterosacral (2), the uterovesical (1) and the rectovaginal (1). The broad ligaments which extend across the pelvis are really folds of the peritoneum which, between the anterior and the posterior folds, envelop the fallopian tubes, the ovaries, and the round and the ovarian ligaments. This peritoneal tissue contains muscle fibers which enable these ligaments to lend some support to these structures. The round ligaments are two fibrous cords which are attached on either side of the fundus just below the fallopian tubes. They extend forward through the inguinal canal and terminate in the mons veneris and the labia majora. These ligaments aid in holding the fundus forward. The uterosacral ligaments are two cordlike structures which extend from the posterior cervical portion of the uterus to the sacrum. These aid in supporting the cervix. The uterovesical ligament is merely a fold of the peritoneum which passes over the fundus and extends over the bladder. The rectovaginal ligament is a fold of the peritoneum which passes over the posterior surface of the uterus and is reflected on to the rectum.

PELVIC MUSCLES. The pelvic floor is made up of the muscles described below (Fig. 33).

The levator ani and the coccygeus form a partition separating the pelvis from the perineal cavity. The levator ani is the larger and is situated anteriorly, extending from the posterior surface of the body of the os pubis to the spines of the ischium, interlacing in a fascial line which extends between these two points. It descends to be attached to the coccyx posteriorly, continues around the lower portion of the rectum just above the external sphincter, and farther front surrounds the vagina.

The coccygeus muscle, which forms a smaller portion of the pelvic floor, lies just behind the levator ani. It is attached to the spines of the ischium and extends to the coccyx and the sides of the sacrum. It assists the levator ani in its pelvic support and also flexes the coccyx laterally.

The pyriformis muscle helps to complete the pelvic floor in that it lends support to the other muscles. It lies just above the upper border of the coccygeus muscle. It is attached to the anterior surface of the sacrum and passes laterally through the greater sciatic foramen and is inserted into the superior surface of the great trochanter of the femur. This muscle also permits the rotation of the thigh outward. These muscles form a muscular sheet which is perforated by three canals: the urethra in front, the vagina in the middle and the rectum behind. But they are arranged in such a way as to strengthen the pelvic floor as much as possible (Fig. 33). The urethra in front passes through a strong membrane which runs across the upper part of the pubic arch. The vagina runs through it in a very oblique direction, upward and back-

ward, so as to make only a valvular slit. Its walls, too, are in close contact, so that the pressure from above simply presses the anterior wall firmly against the posterior, which in turn is supported by the muscles passing into the perineal body. The anal canal is surrounded at the anus by its sphincter, which binds it to the coccyx behind and to the perineal body in front. Above, the rectum is supported by the muscles passing into it.

There is another group of muscles with which the obstetrician is concerned; for identification they are

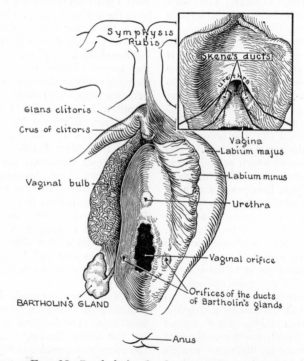

Fig. 38. Bartholin's glands. Insert shows orifices of ducts of Skene's glands which open just within the meatus of the urethra.

named as follows: the transverse perineal, the bulbocavernosus, the pubococcygeus and the gluteus maximus. There are, also, three sphincters which are important: the anal sphincter, the vaginal sphincter and the urethral sphincter.

PERINEUM. The perineum, which lies between the vagina and the rectum, has a central tendon which is the meeting place of the five muscles: the external anal sphincter, the two transverse perineal and the two bulbocavernosi.

Vagina. The vagina is a dilatable passage with muscular walls lined with mucous membrane. It is from 3 to 5 inches in length and leads from the hymen to the uterus; it surrounds the cervix (Fig. 40). Its walls are arranged into thick folds, known as the columns of the vagina. Ordinarily these walls are in contact, so that there is no actual space or canal; but during labor they are smoothed out or stretched so as to permit the baby to be born. The Bartholin, or vulvovaginal, glands (Fig. 38) are situated one on each side of the vaginal orifice; they open by means of a duct into the groove between the hymen and the labia minora.

RELATED PELVIC ORGANS

Bladder. The bladder is a thin, muscular sac which serves as a reservoir for the urine. It is situated in front of the uterus and behind the symphysis pubis. When empty or only moderately distended it remains entirely in the pelvis; but if it becomes greatly distended it rises into the abdomen. Urine is conducted into the bladder by the ureters, two small tubes which extend down from the basin of the kidneys over the brim of the pelvis and open into the bladder at about the level of the cervix. The bladder is emptied through the urethra, a short tube which terminates in the meatus (Fig. 32). Lying on either side of the urethra and almost parallel with it are two small glands, less than 1 inch long, known as Skene's glands. Their ducts empty into the urethra just above the meatus. Often in cases of gonorrhea, Skene's glands and ducts are involved (Fig. 38).

Anus. The anus is the entrance to the rectal canal. The rectal canal is surrounded at the opening or anus by its sphincter muscle, which binds it to the coccyx behind and to the perineum in front. It is supported by the muscles passing into it (Fig 33).

The muscles involved are those that aid in supporting the pelvic floor. The rectum is considered here because of the proximity to the field of delivery.

MAMMARY GLANDS

Breasts. The breasts, or mammary glands, are two highly specialized cutaneous glands located on either side of the anterior wall of the chest between the third and the seventh ribs (Fig. 39). They are abundantly supplied with nerves and are intimately connected, by means of the sympathetic nervous system, with the uterus and other generative organs. The internal mammary and the intercostal arteries supply the breast gland, and the mammary veins follow these arteries. There are, also, many cutaneous veins which become dilated during lactation. The lymphatics are abundant, especially toward the axilla. These breast glands

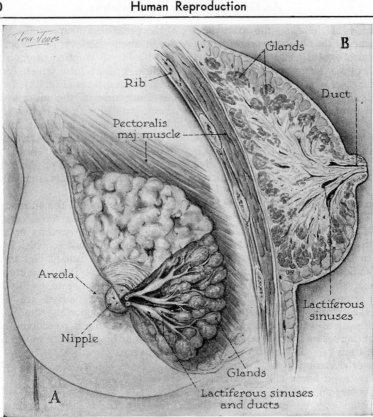

FIG. 39. (A) Mammary gland, showing the lactiferous ducts and sinuses. (B) Cross section of the breast.

are present in the male, but only in the rudimentary state, and are not connected by the sympathetic system to the male generative organs.

INTERNAL STRUCTURE

The breasts of a woman who never has borne a child are, in general, conical or hemispherical in form, but they vary in size and shape at different ages and in different individuals. In women who have nursed one or

more babies they tend to become pendulous. At the termination of lactation certain exercises aid in restoring the tone of the breast tissue.

The breasts are made up of glandular tissue and fat. Each organ is divided into 15 or 20 lobes, which are separated from each other by fibrous and fatty walls. Each lobe is subdivided into many lobules and these contain numerous acini which are lined with a single layer of cells enveloped in a capillary network. By the process of osmosis the products necessary for the milk are filtered from the blood, but the secretion of the milk really begins in the acini cells. As the ducts leading from the lobules to the lobes and from the lobes approach the nipple they are dilated to form little reservoirs in which the milk is stored; they narrow again as they pass into the nipple. The size of the breast is dependent upon the amount of fatty tissue present and in no way denotes the amount of lactation possible.

EXTERNAL STRUCTURE

The external surface of the breasts is divided into three portions. The first is the white, smooth and soft area of skin extending from the circumference of the gland to the areola. The second is the areola, which surrounds the nipple and is of a delicate pinkish hue in blondes and a darker rose-color in brunettes. The surface of the areola is more or less roughened by small fine lumps or papillae, known as the glands of Montgomery (Plate 4, right, bottom). These enlarged sebaceous glands, white in color and scattered over the areola, become more marked during pregnancy. Under the influence of gestation, the areola becomes darker in shade, and this pigmentation, which is more marked in brunettes than in blondes, in many cases constitutes a helpful sign of pregnancy (Plate 5). The nipple or third portion is largely composed of sensitive, erectile tissue and forms a large conical papilla projecting from the center of the areola and having at its summit the openings of the milk ducts. These openings may be from 3 to 20 in number. The care of the breasts (see Chap. 8) constitutes one of the important phases of the nursing care of the maternity patient throughout pregnancy and the puerperium.

MALE ORGANS OF REPRO-DUCTION

The male reproductive system consists of the testes and a system of excretory ducts with their accessory structures (Fig. 41).

EXTERNAL ORGANS

The scrotum and the penis are called the external genitalia. The scrotum contains the testes and may be considered as an evagination of the body wall or a continuation of the abdominal cavity. In the adult male the testes have descended into the scrotal sac, and the canal connecting the sac with the abdominal cavity has closed, although it is open in the fetus.

The penis consists of the urethra, which runs to its tip, and the cavernous bodies (erectile parts) and the skin which covers these structures. The cavernous bodies contain blood spaces which are usually quite empty, and the organ is flaccid. When these spaces fill with blood the organ becomes turgid. The flow of blood is controlled by the automatic nervous system (vasodilator fibers) and varies with sexual activity. The enlarged conical structure at the free end of the penis is called the glans penis which contains the external orifice of the urethra. The glans is almost completely enclosed by a fold of skin called the prepuce.

INTERNAL ORGANS

The internal organs consist of the

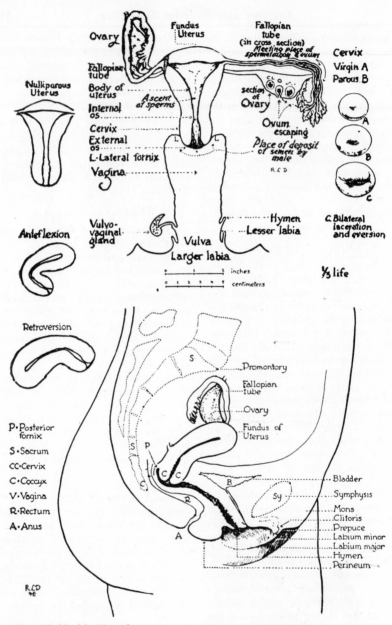

Fig. 40 (*Left*). Female anatomy.   Fig. 41 (*Right*). Male anatomy.
(Dickinson, Robert L.: Human Sex Anatomy, Baltimore, Williams and Wilkins)

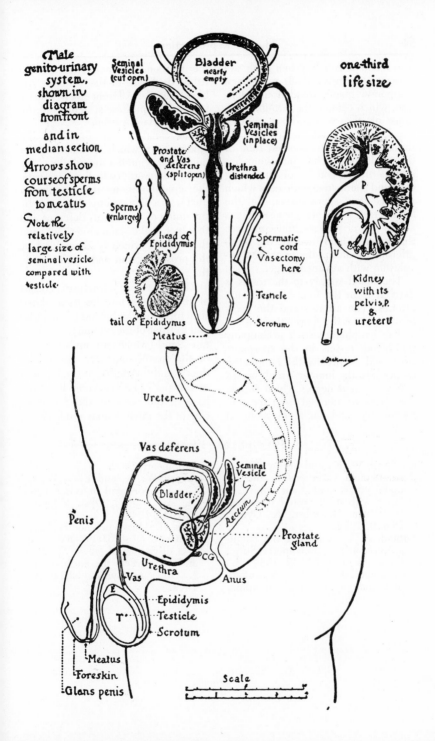

Male genito-urinary system, shown in diagram from front

and in median section

Arrows show course of sperms from testicle to meatus

Note the relatively large size of seminal vesicle compared with testicle.

one-third life size

Seminal Vesicles (cut open)

Bladder nearly empty

Seminal Vesicles (in place)

Prostate and Vas deferens (split open)

Urethra distended

Sperms (enlarged)

head of Epididymis

Spermatic cord

Vasectomy here

tail of Epididymis

Testicle

Scrotum

Meatus

P

Kidney with its pelvis, P. & ureter U

U

U

Ureter

Vas deferens

Seminal Vesicle

Bladder

Rectum

Prostate gland

Penis

Urethra

Vas

CG

Anus

E

Epididymis

T

Testicle

Scrotum

Meatus

Foreskin

Glans penis

Scale

testes and a canal system with accessory structures. Each testis is a compound gland, divided into lobules, which contain the terminal portions of the seminiferous tubules which join repeatedly and eventually form the single much-coiled tube of the epididymis. The epithelium lining the tubules consists of supporting cells and spermatogenetic cells which produce the spermatozoa. In the human testes, spermatogenesis begins at the age of puberty and continues throughout life. However, the seminiferous tubules undergo gradual involution with advancing age.

The blood supply to the testes is derived from the internal spermatic arteries. The arteries and the veins form a part of the spermatic cords.

The lymphatic vessels accompany the blood vessels in the spermatic cord, and eventually the lymphatics empty into the lumbar lymph nodes.

The efferent nerves which supply the testes are derived from the thoracolumbar and sacral divisions of the autonomic system. They are distributed chiefly to the walls of the blood vessels. Afferent fibers convey impulses from these structures to the central nervous system.

The canal system consists of the epididymis (which is made up of numerous seminiferous tubules), the ductus deferens (which passes from the epididymis to the ejaculatory duct), ejaculatory duct (formed by the union of the ductus deferens and the duct of the seminal vesicle), and the urethra, which is surrounded by the prostate gland and terminates in the penis.

The accessory structures consist of the seminal vesicles (sacculated structures located behind the bladder and in front of the rectum), the prostate gland (which surrounds the base of the urethra and the ejaculatory duct), and the bulbo-urethral glands or Cowper's glands (which lie at the base of the prostate and on either side of the membranous urethra).

SUGGESTED READING

Caldwell, W. E., and Moloy, H. C.: Anatomical variations in the female pelvis and their effect in labor with a suggested classification, Am. J. Obst. & Gynec. 26:479, 1933.

Dippel, A. L.: The diagonal conjugate versus x-ray pelvimetry, Surg., Gynec. & Obst. 68:642, 1939.

Greisheimer, Esther M.: Physiology and Anatomy, ed. 6, Philadelphia, Lippincott, 1950.

Mengert, W. F., and Eller, W. C.: Graphic portrayal of relative pelvic size, Am. J. Obst. & Gynec. 52:1032, 1946.

Thoms, H.: Outlet pelvimetry, Surg., Gynec. & Obst. 83:399-402, 1946.

——: A discussion of pelvic variations and a report on the findings, Am. J. Obst. & Gynec. 52:248-254, 1946.

3

Physiology in Relation to Obstetrics

Only a brief statement of the most elementary facts of physiology, the science dealing with the functions of the organs and tissues of the body, can be attempted here, but such a review is essential, in order that the nurse may better understand the special relation of physiology to the problems in obstetrics.

SEXUAL MATURITY

Evidences of sexual maturity in the female begin at the time of puberty with the establishment of the specific reproductive functions of ovulation and menstruation. At puberty certain well-defined changes take place: the establishment of the menses, the monthly bloody discharge from the uterus, is an indication that the internal organs have matured. Changes in the external organs, such as an increase in size, and the appearance of axillary and pubic hair are other evidences of this period of development; the breasts at this time also become larger and more prominent. Along with these physical changes are emotional changes as well.

PUBERTY

Puberty usually occurs between the ages of 12 and 16, although heredity, race, climate and environment may influence its early or late appearance; for example, maturity tends to appear earlier in warm climates and later in cold regions. The reproductive period covers about 30 years, from the beginning of menstruation, at or about the age of twelve, until its cessation during the menopause, at about the age of 45.

55

Ovulation and Menstruation

Ovulation. Each month, with considerable regularity, a blisterlike structure about half an inch in diameter develops on the surface of one or the other ovary. Inside this bubble, almost lost in the fluid about it, lies a tiny speck, scarcely visible to the naked eye; a thimble would hold three million of them. This little speck is the human ovum—a truly amazing structure. It possesses within its diminutive compass not only the potentialities of developing into a human being with all the complicated physical organization entailed, but embodies the mental as well as the physical traits of the woman and her forbears: perhaps her own brown eyes or her father's tall stature, possibly her mother's love of music or her grandfather's genius at mathe-matics. These and a million other potentialities are all wrapped in this little speck, or ovum, so small that it is about one fourth the size of the period at the end of this sentence.

With the exact periodicity which characterizes so many of Nature's works, one blister on one ovary bursts at a definite time each month and discharges an ovum, a process known as *ovulation*. The precise day on which ovulation occurs is a matter of no small importance. For instance, since the ovum can be fertilized (or impregnated by the male germ cell) only within the 36-hour period after its escape from the ovary, this is the only time when a woman is really fertile. During the rest of the monthly cycle, theoretically at least, it is impossible for her to conceive. Evidence of various sorts indicates

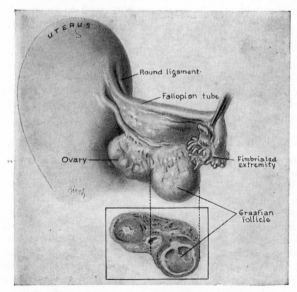

Fig. 42. Ovary with graafian follicle.

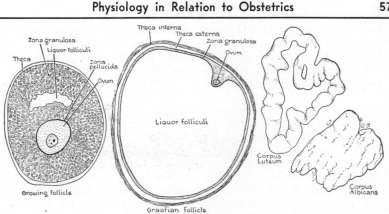

FIG. 43. Development of the graafian follicle.

that ovulation usually occurs between the tenth and the sixteenth days of the menstrual cycle, counting from the day on which bleeding begins. Ordinarily, then, the most fertile time is a week to ten days after the cessation of menstruation. While this is the rule, there are many exceptions, and ovulation may take place at any time between the ninth and the eighteenth days of the cycle. The fact that ovulation rarely occurs during the last ten days of a 28-day cycle has given rise to the birth-control doctrine of the "safe period," or "rhythm," according to which it is impossible to conceive after the eighteenth day. Theoretically, this claim is altogether sound; practically, not a few women appear to have conceived during this period, so that it would seem that occasionally ovulation may take place later than theory would indicate.

Graafian Follicle. In delving further into this process of ovulation, we find that at birth each ovary contains a huge number of undeveloped ova, probably more than 100,000. These

are rather large round cells with clear cytoplasm and a good-sized nucleus occupying the center. Each of these ova is surrounded by a layer of a few small, flattened or spindle-shaped cells. The whole structure —ovum and surrounding cells—is spoken of as a "follicle," while in its underdeveloped state at birth it is referred to as a "primordial follicle." It is the consensus that the manufacture of these primordial follicles ceases at birth or shortly after, and that the large number contained in the ovaries of the newborn represents a lifetime's supply. Nevertheless, the majority of these disappear before puberty so that there are then perhaps 30,000 or so left in each ovary. This disintegration of follicles continues throughout the reproductive period with the result that usually none are found after the menopause.

Meanwhile, from birth to the menopause, a certain few of these primordial follicles show signs of development. The surrounding granular layer of cells begins to multiply rapidly until they are several layers deep, at the same time becoming cuboidal in shape. As this proliferation of cells continues, a very important fluid develops between them, the follicular fluid. After puberty this accumulates in such quantities that the multiplying follicle cells are pushed toward the margin, and the ovum itself is almost surrounded by fluid, being suspended from the periphery of the follicle by only a small neck or isthmus of cells. The structure is now known as the *graafian follicle,* after the famous Dutch physician who in 1672 first described it. While increasing in size so enormously, the graafian follicle naturally pushes aside other follicles, forming each month, as has been said, a very noticeable, blisterlike projection on the surface of the ovary. At one point the follicular capsule becomes thin, and as the ovum reaches full maturity, it breaks free from the few cells attaching it to the periphery

and floats in the follicular fluid. The thinned area of the capsule now ruptures, and the ovum is expelled into the peritoneal cavity.

Changes in the Corpus Luteum. After the discharge of the ovum, the ruptured follicle undergoes a change. It becomes filled with large cells containing a special yellow coloring matter called lutein. The follicle is then known as the corpus luteum or yellow body. If pregnancy does not occur, the corpus luteum reaches full development in about 8 days, then retrogresses and is gradually replaced by fibrous tissue. If pregnancy does occur, the corpus luteum enlarges somewhat and persists throughout the period of gestation, reaching its maximum size about the fourth or fifth month and retrogressing slowly thereafter. The corpus luteum secretes an extremely important substance, *progesterone,* which will be considered in a later section of this chapter.

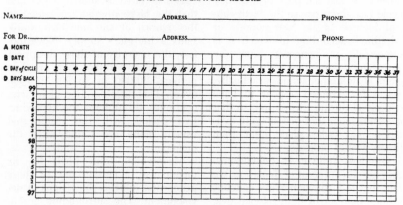

BASAL TEMPERATURE RECORD

NAME_____ADDRESS_____ PHONE_____

FOR DR._____ADDRESS_____ PHONE_____

CHART 6. (*Continued on next page*)

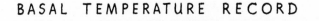

BASAL TEMPERATURE RECORD

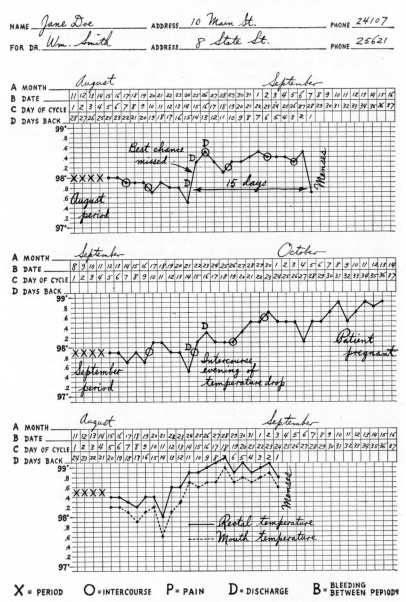

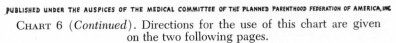

X = PERIOD   O = INTERCOURSE   P = PAIN   D = DISCHARGE   B = BLEEDING BETWEEN PERIODS

PUBLISHED UNDER THE AUSPICES OF THE MEDICAL COMMITTEE OF THE PLANNED PARENTHOOD FEDERATION OF AMERICA, INC

CHART 6 (*Continued*). Directions for the use of this chart are given on the two following pages.

CHART 6

THE USE OF THE BASAL TEMPERATURE GRAPHS

The taking of basal body temperatures is proving a valuable procedure in determining the probable ovulation and in planning a pregnancy. Pregnancy is most likely to occur if intercourse takes place shortly before or after ovulation. In most women ovulation occurs about 14 days before menstruation. It is difficult for patients whose menstrual interval is irregular to calculate the date of ovulation. The use of a temperature graph may help to determine the probable time of ovulation, and hence the time when intercourse is mostly likely to result in pregnancy.

There is a slight rhythm of variation in the normal temperature of a healthy woman. Her temperature is lower during the first part of the menstrual cycle than it is during the latter half. Furthermore, the transition from a lower level to a higher level occurs about the time of ovulation. It is therefore possible to identify the probable date of ovulation by keeping a record of the body temperature. Temperature may vary slightly from day to day from one tenth to one half a degree, so it is essential that the temperature be taken and recorded accurately according to the following directions:

DIRECTIONS

1. Take the temperature rectally with a well-lubricated blunt-tipped rectal thermometer for *Five* (5) *Minutes by the Clock Immediately After* waking in the morning and *Before* getting out of bed, talking, eating, drinking, or smoking. Take the temperature at about *the Same Time Every Morning*.

2. Read the thermometer to within one tenth of a degree and record the reading accurately.

3. Any known cause for temperature variation should be noted on the chart, for example: if sleep has been interrupted or shortened; a cold; grippe; indigestion; a severe emotional disturbance or even indulgence in alcohol.

4. Some women can recognize ovulation by a characteristic pain in the lower abdomen. Others have slight vaginal bleeding or increased clear, slippery vaginal discharge around the time of ovulation. If any

of these manifestations is present, note it on the chart on the day of occurrence. If the pain occurs on more than one day, record the exact hour when it is greatest.

PLOTTING THE TEMPERATURE

1. The menstrual cycle is counted from the first day of one period to the first day of the next period. (1) Start a new graph at the beginning of the period. The first day of menstruation is marked as the first day of the cycle.

2. (A) MONTH—Write the month on this line.

(B) DATE—Put the day of the month on this line.

Write down the day of the month of the first day of menstruation above 1 on the line for "day of cycle" and continue with the days to the end of the line.

(C) DAYS OF CYCLE—This line shows the days of the menstrual cycle.

(D) DAYS BACK—When the next menstrual period starts fill in this line beginning with the day the period starts and from then on number the days backward to the first day of the past period. This serves to show the number of the day at which ovulation occurred in the cycle and the length of the cycle.

3. Chart the temperature daily with a dot, and with a line connect this temperature dot with the dot of the day before. If intercourse occurs in the morning encircle the dot. If it takes place at night mark the circle on the line between that dot and the temperature dot of the next morning.

4. It is necessary to continue the graph for at least two menstrual cycles before the probable time of ovulation can be judged. Sexual abstinence for several days before ovulation allows time for the male to store up sperm and probably increase the chance of fertilization.

5. The temperature will fall and rise within a range of ½ to 1 degree. Watch for a drop in temperature about 15 days before the expected period. The last drop in the cycle (usually the largest) is the important one and intercourse should take place that day or evening.

MOUTH TEMPERATURE

Temperature may be taken by mouth immediately upon awakening *Before Getting Out of Bed and Before Talking, Eating, Drinking or Smoking.* Mouth temperatures show the same variations as rectal. However, mouth temperatures are not usually as marked as the rectal.

MENSTRUAL CYCLE

Menstruation in Relation to Pregnancy

Menstruation is the periodic discharge of blood, mucus and epithelial cells from the uterus. If the individual is normal, it occurs throughout the reproductive period at fairly regular intervals of about 28 days, except during pregnancy and lactation, when it is usually suppressed entirely. Accordingly, the span of years during which childbearing usually is possible—that is, from the age of about 12 to 45—corresponds to the period during which menstruation occurs. In general, moreover, a woman who menstruates is able to conceive, whereas one who does not is probably sterile. There is good reason for believing, therefore, that these two phenomena are closely interlinked, and, since no process of Nature is purposeless, that menstruation must play some vital and indispensable role in childbearing. What is this role?

If, day by day, we were privileged to watch the endometrium or lining membrane of the uterus, we should observe some remarkable alterations. Immediately following the termination of a menstrual period, this membrane is very thin, measuring perhaps a twentieth of an inch in depth. Each day thereafter it becomes a trifle thicker and harbors an increasing content of blood, while its glands become more and more active, secreting a rich nutritive substance which used to be called "uterine milk." About a week before the onset of the next expected period this process reaches its height; the endo-

metrium is now of the thickness of heavy, downy velvet and has become soft and succulent with blood and glandular secretions. At this time the egg, if one has been fertilized, embeds itself into this luxuriant lining.

All these changes have only one purpose: to provide a suitable bed in which the fertilized ovum may rest, secure nourishment and grow. If an egg is not fertilized, these alterations are unnecessary; accordingly, through a mechanism which even today is obscure, the swollen endometrium disintegrates, the encased blood and glandular secretions escape into the uterine cavity; passing through the cervix they flow out through the vagina, carrying the egg with them. In other words, menstruation represents the abrupt termination of a process designed to prepare board and lodging, as it were, for a fertilized ovum; it betokens the breakdown of a bed which was not needed because the "boarder" did not materialize; its purpose then is to clear away the old bed in order that a new and fresh one may be created the next month.

Hormonal Control of Menstruation

If, while watching the changes in the endometrium during the menstrual cycle, as described above, it were possible to inspect the ovaries from day to day, it would be noted that the uterine alterations are directly related to certain phenomena which take place in the ovary.

Immediately following menstruation, it will be recalled, the endometrium is very thin. During the subsequent week or so it proliferates markedly. The cells on the surface

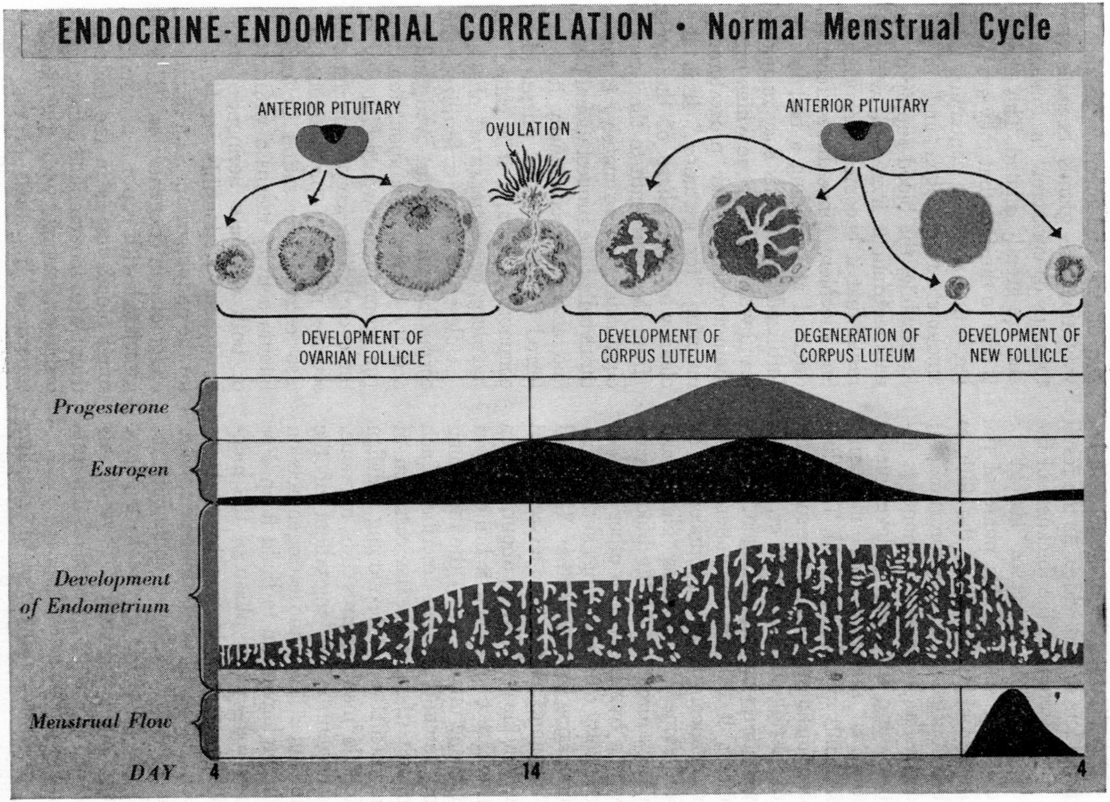

ENDOCRINE-ENDOMETRIAL CORRELATION · Normal Menstrual Cycle

CHART 7. (Therapeutic Notes, Parke, Davis and Co.)

become taller, while the glands which dip into the endometrium become longer and wider. As the result of these changes the thickness of the endometrium increases sixfold or eightfold. During this phase of the menstrual cycle (from the fifth to the fourteenth day, approximately) a graafian follicle each month is approaching its greatest development and is manufacturing increasing amounts of follicular fluid. This fluid contains a most important substance, the estrogenic hormone—or, as it is sometimes called, "estrogen." A hormone, it will be remembered, is a substance which is produced by an endocrine or ductless gland and passes directly into the bloodstream which transports it to other parts of the body where it brings about benefits of one kind or another. The word "hormone" comes from a Greek word which means "I bring about," and in the case of estrogen it brings about (among other things) the thickening of the endometrium described. Each month, then, after the cessation of menstruation, a developing graafian follicle manufactures this hormone, estrogen, as an ingredient of the follicular fluid; and estrogen acts on the endometrium to build it up. For this reason this phase of the menstrual cycle is often referred to as the follicular or estrogenic phase. However, it is more commonly referred to as the *proliferative phase*. The first four or five days of this phase are sometimes called the *resting* or *postmenstrual phase*.

Following rupture of the graafian follicle (ovulation), the cells which form the corpus luteum begin to secrete, in addition to estrogen, another important hormone, progesterone. This supplements the action of estrogen on the endometrium in such a way that the glands become very tortuous or corkscrew in appearance and are greatly dilated. This change is due to the fact that they are swollen with a secretion containing large amounts of glycogen and mucin. Meanwhile, the blood supply of the endometrium is increased, with the result that it becomes very vascular and succulent. Since these effects are directed at providing a bed for the fertilized ovum, it is easy to understand why the hormone which brings them about is called "progesterone," meaning "for gestation." It is also clear why this phase of the cycle (from the fourteenth to the twenty-eighth day, approximately) is sometimes called the progestational phase, and also why occasionally it is referred to as the luteal phase. More commonly, perhaps, it is called the *secretory,* or *premenstrual, phase*.

Unless the ovum is fertilized, the corpus luteum is short-lived, and its activity ceases after about ten days (or around the twenty-fifth day of the cycle). Since corpus luteum cells secrete not only progesterone but also estrogen, cessation of corpus luteum activity means a withdrawal of both of these hormones which have been responsible for building up the endometrium. As a result, the endometrium degenerates. This is associated with rupture of countless small blood vessels in the endometrium with innumerable minute hemorrhages. Along with the blood, superficial fragments of the endometrium, together with mucin from the glands, are cast away, and all this constitutes the menstrual discharge. Naturally, this phase of the cycle (the first to the fifth day, approximately) is called the *menstrual phase.*

What brings about this remarkable rhythmic cycle in the ovary with the resultant monthly changes in the uterus? The "master clock" is in the anterior lobe of the pituitary body. This little structure secretes, among many other hormones, two hormones whose function is to produce, month in and month out, these ovarian alterations. One is called the follicle-stimulating hormone (sometimes abbreviated as FSH), active from the fifth to the fifteenth day of the cycle; and the other the luteinizing hormone (LH), active during the luteal phase. The nurse must be careful not to confuse these anterior lobe hormones of the pituitary with the hormone of the posterior lobe which is also very important in obstetrics but has altogether different functions. A third hormone, gonadotrophin, derived from the chorion, is discussed on page 144.

In addition to their role in controlling menstruation, these two ovarian hormones, estrogen and progesterone, have other far-reaching and important functions. Estrogen is responsible for the development of the secondary sex characteristics, that is, for all those distinctive sex manifestations which are not directly concerned with the process of reproduction. Thus, the growth of the breasts at puberty, the distribution of body fat, the appearance of pubic hair, the size of the larynx and its resulting influence on the quality of the voice, as well as mating instincts are all the result of estrogenic action. We may almost say, therefore, that a woman is a woman be-

cause of estrogen. Often this hormone is used therapeutically. When the nurse is called upon to administer estrogen, intramuscularly, she should understand that it may be labeled on the ampule or other container by various trade names devised by the several pharmaceutical companies. Among these are: Theelin, Theelol, Amniotin, Oestrin, Follicular Hormone and Progynon B. During recent years a synthetic (artificially manufactured) form of estrogen, named stilbestrol, has been used widely. Its effects are essentially the same as estrogen.

Aside from its action on the endometrium, progesterone plays a most important role in preserving the life of the embryo during the first two or three months of pregnancy. It also has a relaxing action on the uterine muscle. For these two reasons, sometimes it is employed therapeutically in cases in which there is a tendency to abort (miscarry—see p. 236). In this connection, the nurse will usually encounter it under the trade name Prolutone.

CLINICAL ASPECTS OF MENSTRUATION

From what has been said concerning the underlying mechanism of menstruation, it is clear that the monthly flow of blood is only one phase of a marvelous cyclic process which not only makes childbearing possible but also profoundly influences both body and mind. For this reason the time of the onset of menstruation, or *puberty,* is a critical period in the life of a young woman. Not only do notable bodily changes occur, but a radical transformation takes place in the mental attitude of the girl. She matures rapidly in mind, and her interests broaden. Nevertheless, her emotions are often unstable, with the result that she may laugh or cry without reason. This transition period from girlhood to womanhood is sometimes a most trying one, but instruction concerning the physical bodily changes and careful observance of the rules of general hygiene, together with tolerance, sympathy and understanding on the part of parents and those closely associated with the adolescent, will do much to secure a normal adjustment.

The average age of the onset of menstruation is 14 years, but not infrequently it begins as early as 11 or as late as 16. Although the duration of the menstrual cycle, counting from the beginning of one period to the onset of the next, averages 28 days, there are wide variations even in the same woman. Indeed, there is scarcely a woman who menstruates exactly every 28 or 30 days. This question has been the subject of several studies on normal young women, chiefly student nurses, who have conscientiously recorded the time and the nature of each period. These investigations show that the majority of women (almost 60 per cent) experience variations of at least 5 days in the length of their menstrual cycles; differences in the same woman of even 10 days are not uncommon and may occur without explanation or apparent detriment to health. The flow normally persists from 3 to 7 days, the average being 5 or 6 days. Although the total amount of menstrual discharge is approximately 2 ounces, the actual blood loss is not much more than an ounce. For reasons which even today are obscure, menstrual blood does not clot.

Normal menstruation should not be accompanied by pain, although quite often there is some general malaise, together with a feeling of weight and discomfort in the pelvis. Frequent, also, are such disturbances as a sense of fatigue, headache, backache, sensitivity in the breasts and unstable emotional reactions. If there is great irregularity or extremely profuse flow or marked pain, a pathologic condition may be present. Painful menstruation is known as *dysmenorrhea*. Absence of the menses is known as *amenorrhea*. The most common cause of amenorrhea is pregnancy, but sometimes it is brought about by emotional disturbances, such as fear, worry, fatigue or disease (anemia, tuberculosis), and occasionally it may be the result of a decided change in climate.

INFERTILITY

Dr. Abraham Stone states that the United States Census Bureau's records show that more than 15 per cent of all married women never bear any children, and most of this childlessness is involuntary. Within the last quarter of a century many very important scientific advances have been made in the field of human infertility. Two newer concepts are of particular significance. One is that impaired fertility is most often due not to a single cause but to a multiplicity of factors. Systemic, local, nutritional, glandular and emotional conditions affect both the husband and the wife; therefore, in each instance it is necessary to make a complete study of the history of the health situation and mode of life of the couple. The second concept is that the husband bears a far greater responsibility as a factor in sterile matings than had been recognized previously. Indeed, modern investigations indicate that about 40 per cent of cases of sterility are attributable to deficiencies on the part of the husband.

A few of the causes in women may be failure of ovulation, obstructions in the genital tract, especially in the cervix or the fallopian tubes, or disturbances in the development of the uterus and its lining which interfere with the implantation and the growth of the fertilized ovum. In the male the causes may be deficiency in the seminal fluid and particularly in the quantity and the quality of the spermatozoa, or obstructions in the seminal ducts which prevent the spermatozoa from passing through. Lack of sperm production may be caused by developmental anomalies, glandular disturbances, local injuries or infections and constitutional diseases.

Due to modern developments in the field of human infertility about 30 per cent of the barren marriages can be rendered fertile. Today there is continued research in the physiologic and psychological aspects of reproduction, and physicians have available better technics and methods for the diagnosis and the treatment of infertility.

MENOPAUSE

Permanent cessation of menstruation usually occurs between the ages of 40 and 50. The period over which this alteration takes place is known as the *menopause,* or *climacteric,* but generally it is referred to by the laity as the "change of life." About 50 per cent of women experience the menopause between the ages of 45 and 50; about 25 per cent between 40 and 45; about 12.5 per cent between 35 and 40; and another 12.5 between 50 and 55. In a general way, the earlier puberty occurs, the later the menopause; conversely, the later puberty is experienced, the earlier the menopause. The menopause is usually a gradual process; the periods first become scanty, then one may be absent, and finally they cease altogether.

The cause of the menopause is cessation of ovarian activity. Having functioned for some 30 years the ovary now shrivels up into a small, flat organ composed mostly of scar tissue. As a consequence, estrogen is no longer produced. This permanent and complete withdrawal of estrogen results in atrophy of the uterus, the fallopian tubes, the vagina and the vulva. The absence of the hormone sometimes produces also certain nervous symptoms, such as flushing of the face and the body, sensations of heat ("hot flashes") and cold, sweating, hyperexcitability and irritability. Estrogen, either as the pure hormone or as stilbestrol, finds its greatest therapeutic usefulness in these menopausal disorders. The better one's general health, the more surely one can look forward to an uneventful menopause.

SUGGESTED READING

Corner, G. W.: The Hormones in Human Reproduction, Princeton, 1942.

Guttmacher, A. F.: Life in the Making, New York, Viking, 1933.

——: Into This Universe, New York, Viking, 1937. (Published also under the title "The Story of Human Birth," Blue Ribbon Books, 1939.)

——: Babies by unknown fathers, Parents Magazine, Feb., 1949.

Kurzrock, Raphael: The menopause, Proceedings of the Third American Congress on Obstetrics and Gynecology, p. 282.

Tyler, Edward T.: Semen studies and fertility, J.A.M.A. 146:307, 1951.

4

Development and Physiology of the Fetus

In all Nature's wide universe of miracles there is no process more wondrous, no mechanism more incredibly fantastic, than the one by which a tiny speck of tissue, the human egg, develops into a 7-pound baby. So miraculous did primitive peoples consider this phenomenon that they frequently ascribed it all to superhuman intervention and even overlooked the fact that sexual intercourse was a necessary precursor. Throughout unremembered ages our own primitive ancestors doubtless held similar beliefs, but now we know that pregnancy comes about in only one way: from the union of a female germ cell, the egg or ovum, with a male germ cell, the spermatozoon. These two gametes, ovum and spermatozoon, become fused into one cell or zygote which contains the characteristics

kinds of sex cells—ovum and spermatozoon. Each motile spermatozoon now has 24 chromosomes in its nucleus; the number at each stage in the formation of the spermatozoon

Enlarged egg showing relative sizes of sperm and egg cells

sperm

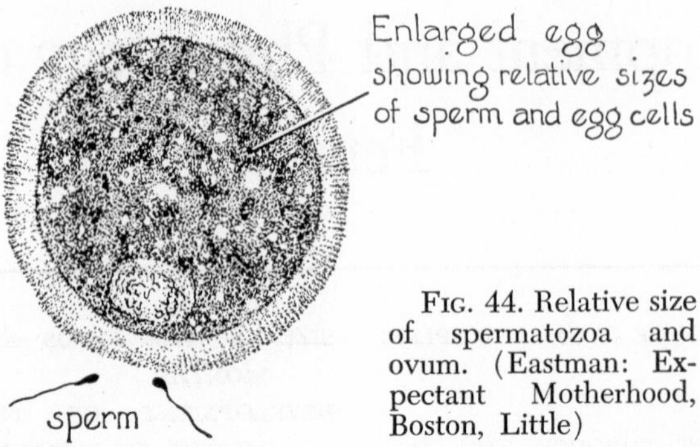

Fig. 44. Relative size of spermatozoa and ovum. (Eastman: Expectant Motherhood, Boston, Little)

of both the female and the male from which these gametes originated.

MATURATION OF OVUM AND SPERM CELLS

By the time the two sex cells or gametes, ovum and spermatozoon, in humans are matured or ready for union a number of peculiar changes have occurred previously as shown in Fig. 45.

Typical cells of the testes and the ovary are shown at the top of the diagram. On the left are shown the steps as a typical testes cell changes into four motile sperm cells or spermatozoa. On the right are seen the stages leading to the development of a single mature ovum. Besides the changes in appearance, very important internal changes have also taken place. The chromosomes, normally 48 in all cell tissues of man, have been reduced in number in both

is indicated by small figures at the lower right at each stage. The ovum, too, contains only 24 chromosomes, its chromosomes having been reduced not by division but by extrusion of chromosome material, called "polar bodies" because they were observed at one pole of the developing ovum. Their remnants are shown in the cells in the top row of Fig. 50. They finally become lost and need not be considered here, as they play no active part in reproduction.

The maturation of the ovum takes place about the time of ovulation and is probably complete before the ovum is discharged from the graafian follicle. The spermatozoon is also fully matured before it is discharged.

The chromosomes differ in form and size, ranging from small spherical masses to long rods which are often bent to resemble the letters V and J.

Every human cell—whatever the tissue—has 48 chromosomes. The re-

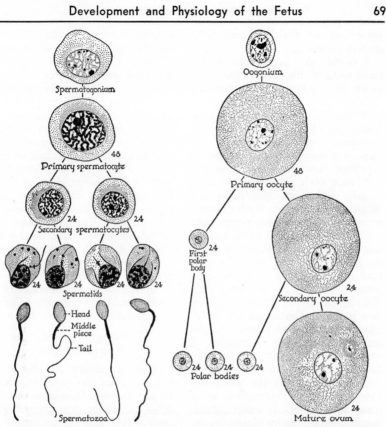

FIG. 45. Diagram of gametogenesis with maturation. The various stages of spermatogenesis are indicated on the left; one spermatogonium gives rise to four spermatozoa. On the right, the oogenesis of the ovum is indicated; from each oogonium, one mature ovum is produced, and three abortive cells. In maturation, the chromosomes are reduced to one half the number characteristic for the general body cells of the species, as indicated; in man, the number in the body cells is 48, and that in the mature spermatozoon and ovum is 24. (Greisheimer, E. M.: Physiology and Anatomy, ed. 6, Philadelphia, Lippincott)

duction to 24 in each gamete means that the fertilized ovum has 48 chromosomes, the number characteristic of all human cells. In every cell division from now on to adulthood and throughout the differentiation of all tissues, each will have 48 chromo-

somes. This is accomplished by an internal change in the cell before division, in which the 48 chromosomes split into halves, and each of the two new cells receives half of the 96 halves or 48 chromosomes. This splitting and halving is continued in all dividing cells until growth ceases.

It is only as a preparation for reproduction by the fertilization of an ovum by a spermatozoon that this number varies, as described above.

Within the chromosomes are contained the ultramicroscopic self-perpetuating bodies called genes, and each gene carries one or more special characteristics. To these genes are attributed such differences as color of hair and eyes, body build and facial characteristics. Each gamete, ovum and spermatozoon comes from a different person with a different ancestral history and different genes in its 24 chromosomes. Since a single gene may carry more than one character, there may be numerous variable results in the offspring of any two parents. The hereditary possibilities discarded or retained in the mature gametes is a matter of chance, but the nature of the combination of the germ plasm which occurs in each generation when two gametes fuse in fertilization is of great significance. If either parent brings defective germ plasm, the result may affect the zygote and the characteristics of the child which results.

Biologists have estimated that at the time of the reduction division some 17 million different combinations are possible due to the interchange of genes. Apparently there is sufficient stability produced during this intricate interchange process to ensure characteristics of the progenitors.

OVA

As described in Chapter 3, ova are normally discharged from the human ovary at the rate of one a month. The ovum at this time is a relatively large cell, measures about 0.2 millimeter ($\frac{1}{125}$ of an inch) and is just visible to the naked eye. The nucleus is small in comparison with the amount of cytoplasm and contains many strands or filaments of deeply staining material. These minute particles are called chromosomes and are the all-important links in the endless chain of heredity; they were discussed in more detail in a previous paragraph of this chapter. The large amount of cytoplasm surrounding the nucleus contains a small quantity of nutritive material in the form of yolk granules. The surface of the ovum is immediately surrounded by a thick membrane, the zona pellucida (translucent belt).

TRANSPORT THROUGH THE FALLOPIAN TUBE

After the ovum has been discharged from the ovary it faces a 10-day journey. Its goal is the cavity of the uterus, more than 3 inches away. The only pathway of approach is the tortuous fallopian tube, whose lining is wrinkled unevenly by the folds of tubal epithelium, and whose passageway at the inner end is no larger than a bristle. Moreover, the ovum has no means of locomotion but must depend upon extraneous forces for propulsion through the fallopian tube. Offhand it would seem to be impossible; actually, the ovum is not only able to make this journey with apparent ease but has been known to reach its destination after the most unbelievable meanderings. For instance, if one fallopian tube has been removed by an operation, the ovum may migrate to the opposite side of the uterus and enter the other tube. This whole "transportation system" is made possible, it seems, through two factors. In the first place, currents in the film of fluid which bathes the lining of the tube waft the ovum downward. If this lining were inspected with a microscope, there would be observed little hairlike projections, called cilia, which wave or beat in such a manner as to direct any overlying fluid (as well as any particle afloat thereon) in the direction of the uterine cavity. Once the ovum has been expelled from the ovary, it is drawn by these currents into the funnel-like opening of the tube and is then propelled down the tube by these same currents. The second factor responsible for the migration of the ovum down the tube is found in the peristaltic action of the tubal musculature. But the ovum is scarcely a third of the way down the tube when the supreme event happens: it meets a spermatozoon, and a new human being is created. As Margaret Shea Gilbert has so happily expressed it in her book, *Biography of the Unborn*, "Life begins for each of us at an unfelt, unknown, and unhonored instant when a minute, wriggling sperm plunges headlong into a mature ovum or egg."

SPERMATOZOA

These minute, wriggling spermatozoa are in some respects even more remarkable than the ova which they fertilize. In appearance they resemble microscopic tadpoles, with oval heads and long, lashing tails

about ten times the length of the head. The human spermatozoon consists of three parts: the head, the middle-piece (or neck) and the tail. The nucleus, and consequently the

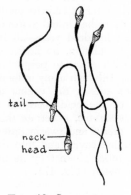

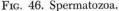

Fig. 46. Spermatozoa.

chromatin material, is in the head; the tail serves for propulsion. They are much smaller than the ovum, their over-all length measuring about one quarter the diameter of the egg, and it has been estimated that the heads of two billion of them—enough to regenerate the entire population of the world—could be placed, with room to spare, in the hull of a grain of rice. As a result of the wriggling motion of the tails, spermatozoa swim with a quick vibratory motion and have been "timed" under the microscope at rates as fast as one seventh of an inch a minute. In ascending the uterus and the fallopian tube they must swim against the same currents that waft the ovum downward; nevertheless, they seem to be able to reach the outer part of the tube within an hour or two. Perhaps the most amazing feature of spermatozoa is their huge number. At each ejaculation, the climax of intercourse in the male, about 300 million are discharged; if each of these could be united with an ovum, the babies which would thus be created would exceed the total number born in the United States during the past hundred years—all from a single ejaculation. So lavish is Nature in her effort to perpetuate the species! Although many million spermatozoa die in the vagina as the result of the acid secretion there, myriads survive, penetrate the neck of the uterus and swarm upward to the uterine cavity and into the fallopian tube. There they lie in wait for the ovum (Fig. 47).

DETERMINATION OF SEX

In the human being, age, state of health and natural physical strength have nothing to do with the determination of sex of the offspring. The sex is determined at the time of fertilization by the spermatozoon—not by the ovum. All spermatozoa and ova have 48 chromosomes originally. Each spermatozoon has 46 regular chromosomes and an "X" and a "Y" chromosome, whereas each ovum contains 46 regular chromosomes and two "X" sex chromosomes. When maturation occurs each spermatozoon and ovum divides into two cells. Each of the two ovum cells contains 23 regular chromosomes and an "X" chromosome, but one half of the spermatozoon cells contain 23 regular chromosomes and an "X" chromosome and the other half of the spermatozoon (or sperm) cells contain 23 regular chromosomes and a

"Y" chromosome. If a sperm cell containing 23 chromosomes and an "X" chromosome fertilizes an ovum, a female will result because in the union of the sperm and the ovum there will be 46 regular chromosomes and an "X" chromosome from the ovum and an "X" chromosome from the spermatozoon. If, on the other hand, a sperm cell containing 23 regular chromosomes and a "Y" chromosome fertilizes an ovum, a male will result because in the union there will be 46 regular chromosomes and an "X" chromosome from the ovum and a "Y" chromosome from the spermatozoon. It is definitely a matter of chance, as far as is known today, whether a sperm with an "X" or a "Y" chromosome will fertilize an ovum. This is evidenced by the fact that almost universally about 94 female babies are born to every 100 male babies in single births. Although many attempts have been made to influence Nature's roulette wheel of sex, to the end that a child of a desired sex may be had, no success has been met. Nor can a physician predict with any degree of assurance, even late in pregnancy, whether the baby will be a girl or a boy.

FERTILIZATION

The process of union of ovum and spermatozoon is known as fertilization. It usually takes place in the outer third of the fallopian tube. As soon as the ovum comes near the army of spermatozoa, the latter, as though they were tiny bits of steel drawn by a powerful magnet, fly at the ovum. One penetrates, but only one. It appears that the entrance of one sperm into an egg causes a

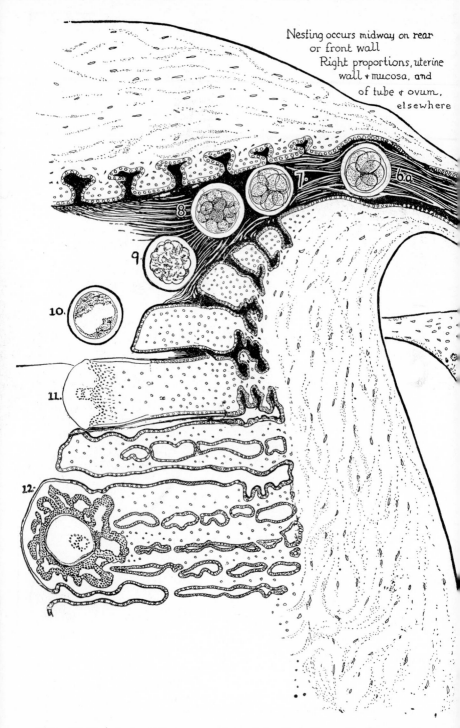

FIG. 47. Travel of egg from ovary through implantation, with alterations en route

licle bursts.
um with adhering
nulosa cells.
st polar body.
l maturation spindle.
rm enters egg.
l maturation division
e and Female pronuclei

5. Pronuclei fusing
Fertilization accomplished
5a. First cleavage division
6-7 Early cleavage
8. Morula.
9-10. Early and later gastrula
11 Ten day monkey egg, showing
yolk sac above and amniotic cavity below
12. Fully implanted growing embryo. (Miller.)

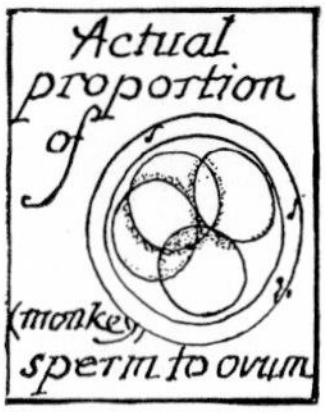

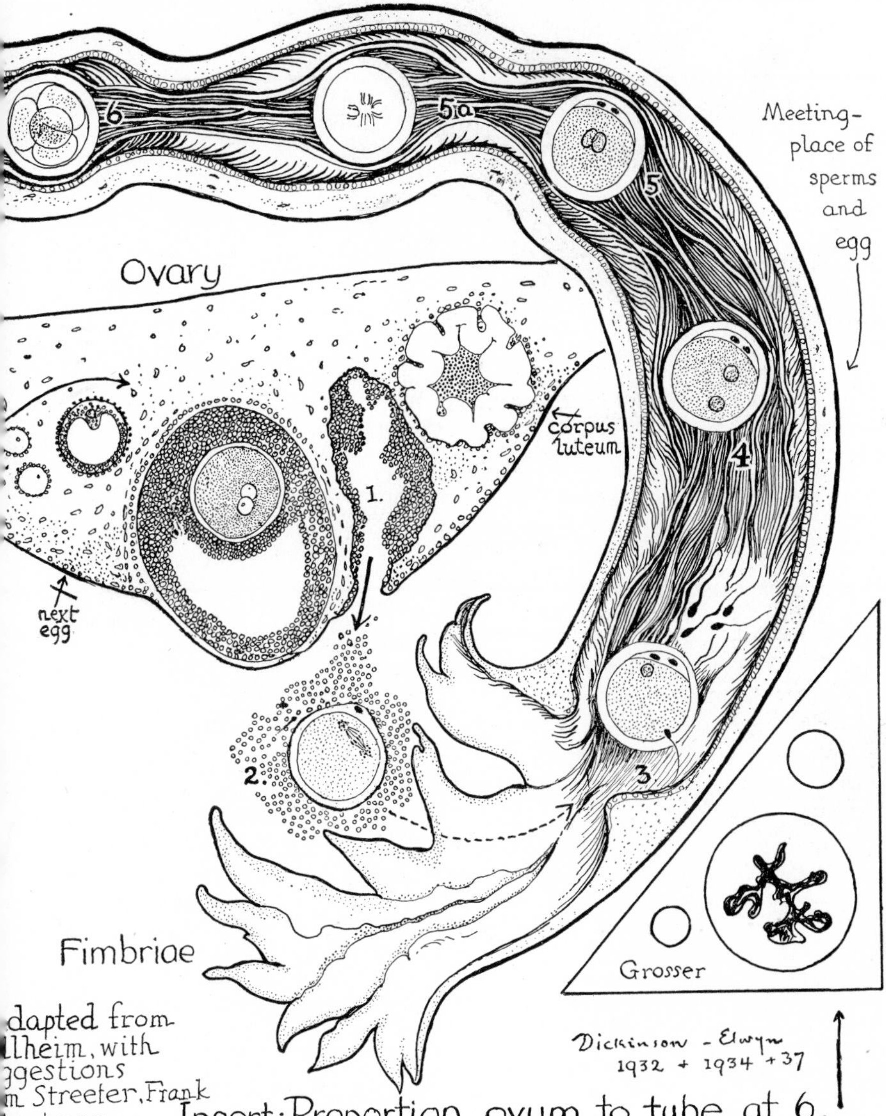

Insert: Proportion ovum to tube at 6.

ys in tube, 7 days in uterus before nesting. (Robert L. Dickinson, M.D., New York)

change in the surface of the egg which prevents entrance of other spermatozoa. The union of ovum and spermatozoon is followed at once by profound changes in the nuclei, which result in cell division and multiplication and the development of a new being. Seemingly electrified, all the particles which make up the ovum (now fused with the sperm) exhibit vigorous agitation, as though they were being rapidly churned about by some unseen force; this becomes more and more violent until it amounts to such an upheaval that the fertilized ovum divides into two cells. Before division the male and the female chromosomes and their genes are mingled and finally split, forming two sets of 48 chromosomes, one set of 48 going to each of the two new cells. This process is repeated again and again, until masses containing 16, 32 and 64 cells are produced successively, and so on endlessly. These early cell divisions produce a solid ball of cells called the "morula," because they resemble a mulberry. It is believed that the 16-cell stage is reached about 96 hours after ovulation. Meanwhile, this growing aggregation of cells is being carried down the fallopian tube in the direction of the uterine cavity.

CHANGES FOLLOWING FERTILIZATION

The journey of the ovum down the fallopian tube is believed to require about 3 days, and then it spends a period of some 6 days in the uterine cavity before actual embedding takes place, a total interval of some 9 days between ovulation and implantation.

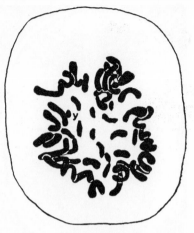

Fig. 48. Human chromosomes, 48 in number, including the small Y chromosome which identifies a male cell. (From Painter)

Meanwhile, important changes are taking place in the internal structure of the fertilized ovum. The cells in the center of the mulberry mass secrete a fluid which pushes the remaining cells to the periphery of the sphere. At the same time it becomes apparent that this external envelope of cells is actually made up of two different layers, an inner and an outer. A specialized portion of the inner layer, after some 260 days, will develop into the long-awaited baby. The outer layer is a sort of foraging unit, called the "trophoblast" (trophectoderm), which means "feeding" layer; it is the principal function of these cells to secure food for the embryo.

While the ovum is undergoing these changes, the lining of the uterus, it will be recalled, is making preparations for its reception. Con-

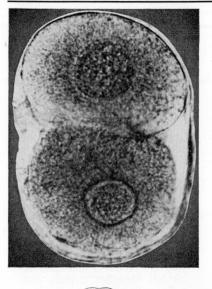

Fig. 49. First baby picture. This human fertilized egg was photographed only 60 hours after fertilization and is the youngest yet seen. It was reported by Drs. Arthur T. Hertig and John Rock, of Harvard, and Carnegie Institution. (Carnegie Institution, through Science Service, Washington, D. C.)

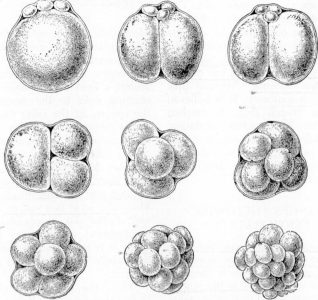

Fig. 50. Segmentation of the fertilized ovum. The ovum divides into two, each of the two into two, making four, and so on indefinitely. (Modified from Sobotta)

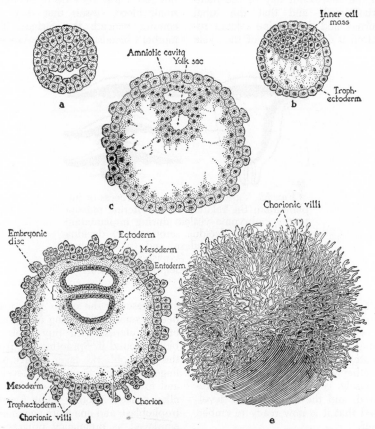

FIG. 51. Early stages of development. (a, b) The cells are separated into a peripheral layer and an inner cell mass; the peripheral layer is called the trophectoderm; the entire structure is called a blastodermic vesicle. (c) The formation of the amniotic cavity and yolk sac is indicated. The former is lined by ectoderm; the latter, by entoderm. (d) The location of the embryonic disk and the three germ layers are shown, together with the beginning of the chorionic villi. (e) The external appearance of the developing mass is shown; the chorionic villi are abundant. (Greisheimer: Physiology and Anatomy, Philadelphia, Lippincott)

Compare with Figure 47: 10 corresponds to b in this illustration; in 11, is shown c, much reduced; in 12, d, with villi well developed.

sidering that ovulation took place on the fourteenth day of the menstrual cycle and that the tubal journey and the uterine sojourn required 9 days, 23 days of the cycle lining and eat out a nest for the ovum but also digest the walls of the many small blood vessels that they encounter beneath the surface. The mother's bloodstream is thus tapped,

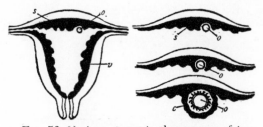

Fig. 52. Various stages in the process of implantation; the relation of the uterine mucosa to the embryonic vesicle during implantation is shown: (s) decidua serotina, (v) decidua vera, (c) decidua reflexa, and (o) the ovum or embryonic vesicle. (Greisheimer: Physiology and Anatomy, Philadelphia, Lippincott)

will have passed before the ovum has developed its trophoblastic layer of cells. This is the period when the lining of the uterus has reached its greatest thickness and succulence. In other words, the timing has been precisely correct; the bed is prepared, and the ovum has so developed that it is now ready to embed itself.

IMPLANTATION OF THE OVUM

The embedding of the ovum is the work of the outer "foraging" layer of cells, the trophoblast, which possesses the peculiar property of being able to digest or liquefy the tissues with which it comes into contact. This process is carried out by means of enymzes. In this manner these cells not only burrow into the uterine and presently the ovum finds itself deeply sunk in the lining epithelium of the uterus, with tiny pools of blood around it. Sprouting out from the trophoblastic layer, quivering, fingerlike projections now develop and extend greedily into the blood-filled spaces. Another name for the trophoblast, and one more commonly employed as pregnancy progresses, is the chorion, and the fingerlike projections mentioned above become known as chorionic villi (Fig. 51). These chorionic villi contain blood vessels connected with the fetus and are extremely important, because they are the sole means by which oxygen and nourishment are received from the mother. The entire ovum becomes covered with villi, which grow out radially and convert the chorion into a shaggy sac.

DECIDUA

The thickening of the uterine endometrium, which occurs during the premenstrual phase of menstruation, has been described already. If pregnancy ensues, this endometrium becomes even more thickened, the cells enlarge, and the structure becomes known as the decidua. It is simply a direct continuation in exaggerated form of the already modified premenstrual mucosa.

For purposes of description, the decidua has been divided into three portions. That part which lies directly under the embedded ovum is known as the decidua basalis, or serotina. That portion which is pushed out by the embedded and growing ovum is called the decidua capsularis or reflexa. The remainder of the decidua, or that portion which is not in immediate contact with the ovum, is known as the decidua parietalis or vera. As pregnancy advances, the decidua capsularis expands rapidly over the growing embryo and at about the fourth month lies in intimate contact with the decidua vera.

THE THREE GERM LAYERS

With nutritional facilities provided, the cells which are destined to form the baby grow rapidly. At first they all look alike, but soon after embedding, groups of cells here and there assume distinctive characteristics and differentiate into three main groups: an outer covering layer, a middle layer and an internal layer. These are called, respectively, the ectoderm, the mesoderm and the entoderm.

From the ectoderm the following structures arise: epithelium of skin, hair, nails, sebaceous glands, sweat glands, epithelium of the nasal and oral passages, salivary and mucous glands of the mouth and nose, enamel of the teeth, and the nervous system. From the mesoderm are derived: muscles, bone, cartilage, dentin of teeth, ligaments, tendons, areolar tissue, kidneys, ureters, ovaries, testes, heart, blood, lymph and blood vessels, and lining of pericardial, pleural and peritoneal cavities. From the entoderm arise: the epithelium of the digestive tract, of glands which pour their secretion into the tract, of the respiratory tract and of the bladder, the urethra, the thyroid and the thymus.

AMNION

Even before these structures become evident, however, a fluid-filled space develops about the embryo, a space which is lined with a smooth, slippery, glistening membrane, the amnion. The space is the amniotic cavity; being filled with fluid, often it is spoken of as the bag of waters; in this the fetus floats and moves (Fig. 54). At full term, this cavity normally contains from 500 to 1,000 cc. of liquor amnii, or the "waters." The amniotic fluid has a number of important functions: it keeps the fetus at an even temperature, cushions it against possible injury and provides a medium in which it can move easily; furthermore, it is known that the fetus drinks this fluid. At the end of the fourth month of pregnancy the bag of waters has enlarged to the size of a large orange and, with the fetus, occupies the entire interior of the uterus.

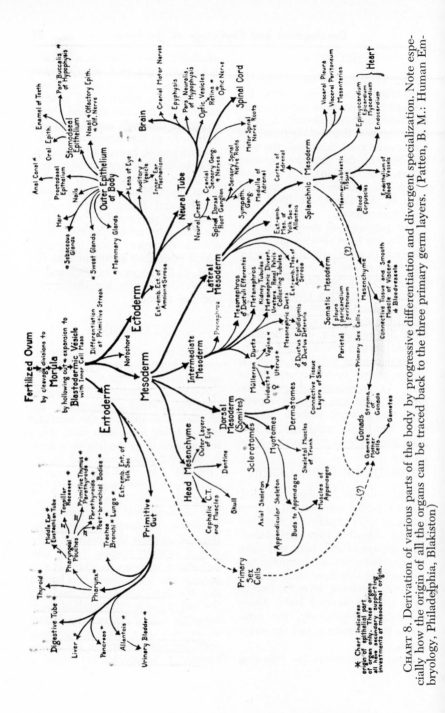

CHART 8. Derivation of various parts of the body by progressive differentiation and divergent specialization. Note especially how the origin of all the organs can be traced back to the three primary germ layers. (Patten, B. M.: Human Embryology, Philadelphia, Blakiston)

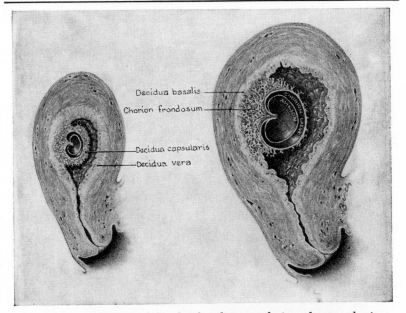

Fig. 53. Development of decidua basalis, capsularis and vera; chorion frondosum.

CHORION

As explained, the early ovum is covered on all sides by shaggy chorionic villi, but very shortly those villi which invade the decidua basalis enlarge and multiply rapidly. This portion of the trophoblast is known as the chorion frondosum (leafy chorion) (Fig. 53). Contrariwise, the chorionic villi covering the remainder of the fetal envelope degenerate and almost disappear, leaving only a slightly roughened membrane. This latter is called the chorion laeve (bald chorion). The chorion laeve lies outside of the amnion, of course, with which it is in contact on its inner surface, while its outer surface lies against the decidua vera. The fetus is thus surrounded by two membranes, the amnion and the chorion, and in ordinary clinical discussions these are usually referred to simply as "the membranes."

PLACENTA

By the third month another important structure has formed, the placenta. This is a fleshy, disklike organ; late in pregnancy it measures about 8 inches in diameter and 1 inch in thickness. It receives its name from a Latin word meaning cake, which this structure resembles somewhat in shape. The placenta is formed by the union of the chorionic villi and the decidua basalis. An analogous situation is seen when a

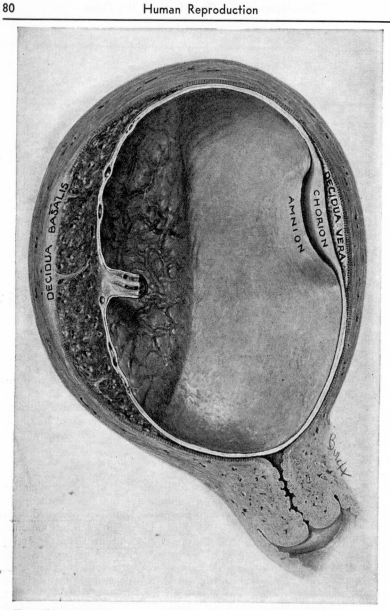

Fig. 54. Amniotic cavity, placenta and membranes (amnion and chorion).

PLATE 1

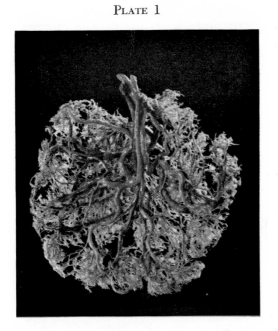

Placenta stripped to the main vessels. Arteries are red; veins, blue. (Life Magazine. Picture taken by Rudolph Skarda Research Anatomist, University of California, San Francisco, Calif.)

PLATE 2

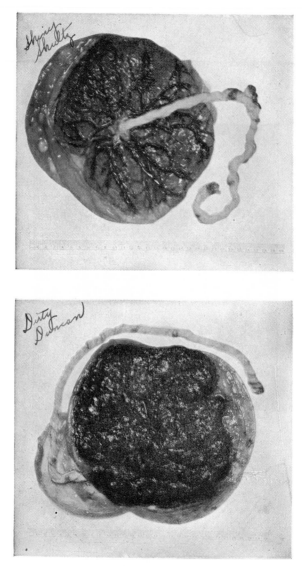

(*Top*) Fetal surface of placenta.
(*Bottom*) Maternal surface of placenta.

tree or a plant sends down its roots into a bed of earth for nourishment; when the plant is removed a certain amount of the earthy bed clings to the interlocking roots. Similarly, a thin layer of the uterine bed clings to the branching projections of chorionic villi, and together they make up this organ, which supplies food to the fetus as the roots and the earth provide nourishment for a plant. At term the placenta weighs about 500 Gm., or one pound. Its fetal surface is smooth and glistening, being covered by amnion, and beneath this membrane may be seen a number of large blood vessels. The maternal surface is red and fleshlike in character, and is divided into a number of segments, about an inch in diameter, called cotyledons.

The placenta and the fetus are connected by means of the *umbilical cord*, or funis, which is usually about 20 inches in length and about three quarters of an inch in diameter. The cord leaves the placenta near the center and enters the abdominal wall of the fetus at the umbilicus, a trifle below the middle of the median line in front. It contains two arteries and one large vein, which are twisted upon each other and are protected from pressure by a transparent, bluish-white, gelatinous substance called Wharton's jelly.

SIZE OF THE FETUS AT VARIOUS MONTHS

The physician, as well as the nurse, is sometimes called upon to estimate the intra-uterine age of a fetus which has been expelled prematurely. For clinical purposes the length of the embryo in centimeters may be approximated during the first 5 months by squaring the number of the month to which the pregnancy has advanced; in the second half of pregnancy, by multiplying the month by 5. Conversely, the approximate age of the fetus may be obtained by taking the square root of its length in centimeters during the first 5 months, and thereafter by dividing its length in centimeters by 5. For instance, a fetus 16 cm. long is about 4 months old; a 35-cm. fetus is about 7 months old.

DEVELOPMENT OF THE FETUS MONTH BY MONTH

Most women consider themselves one month pregnant at the time of the first missed menstrual period, two months pregnant at the second missed period, and so on. Since conception does not ordinarily take place until some 14 days after the onset of menstruation, it is obvious that an embryo does not attain the age of one month until about a fortnight after the first missed period (assuming a 28-day cycle) and its "birthday" by months regularly falls two weeks or so after any numerically specified missed period. This should be remembered in reading the month development of the fetus. Thus, in speaking of the age of a pregnancy in "months," physicians refer to "lunar months," that is, periods of four weeks. Since a lunar month corresponds to the usual length of the menstrual cycle, they find it easier to "figure" in this way.

Month by month the development of the fetus is something as follows:

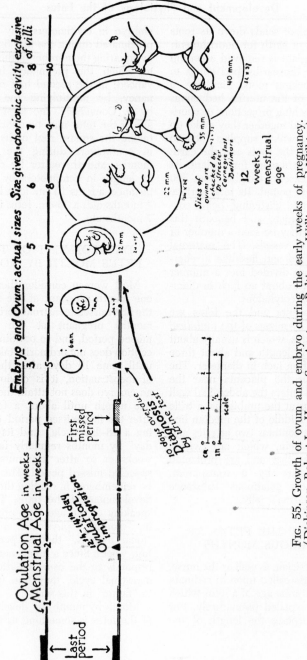

Fig. 55. Growth of ovum and embryo during the early weeks of pregnancy. (Dickinson, Robert L.: Human Sex Anatomy, Baltimore, Williams and Wilkins)

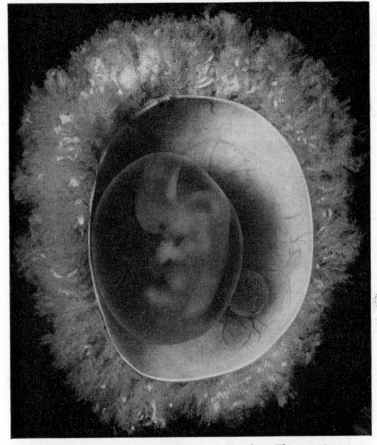

Fig. 56. Human embryo by Chester F. Reather. This specimen represents about 40 days' development and is shown in the opened chorion. H is reproduced at a magnification of 1.7. (Carnegie Institution, Washington, D. C.)

END OF FIRST LUNAR MONTH

The embryo is about one quarter of an inch long if measured in a straight line from head to tail—for it does have a tail at this early stage. The backbone is apparent but is so bent upon itself that the head almost touches the tip of the tail. At one end of the backbone the head is extremely prominent, representing almost one third of the entire embryo. (Throughout intra-uterine life the head is always very large in proportion to the body, a relationship which is still present, although to a lesser degree, at birth.) The tube which will form the future heart has been formed, producing a large, rounded bulge on the body wall; even at this early age this structure is pulsating regularly and propelling blood through microscopic arteries. The rudiments of the future digestive tract are also discernible—a long, slender tube leading from the mouth to an expansion in the same tube which will become the stomach; connected with the latter the beginnings of the intestines may be seen. The incipient arms and legs are represented by small nubbins that resemble buds.

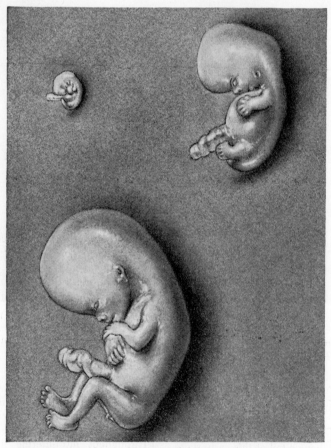

FIG. 57. Actual size drawing of fetus at approximately one month, two months and three months, respectively. (Eastman: Expectant Motherhood, Boston, Little)

END OF SECOND LUNAR MONTH

The embryo now begins to assume human form and hereafter until birth is referred to as a "fetus." It has an unmistakably human face and also arms and legs, with fingers, toes, elbows and knees. During the past 4 weeks it has quadrupled in length and measures about one inch from head to buttocks; its weight is approximately one thirtieth of an ounce. The sex organs become apparent, but it is difficult to distinguish between male and female. During the second month the human tail reaches its greatest development, but by the end of the month it is less prominent and then undergoes retrogression.

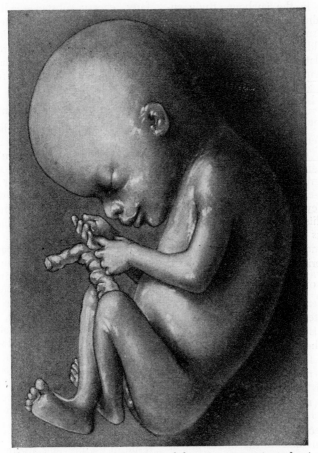

FIG. 58. Actual size drawing of fetus at approximately 4 months.

END OF THIRD LUNAR MONTH

The fetus now measures somewhat over 3 inches in length, and weighs an ounce. The sex can now be distinguished by the presence or absence of the fetal uterus. The fingernails and the toenails appear as fine membranes. Early in this month buds for all the temporary "baby" teeth are present, and sockets for these develop in the jawbone. Rudimentary kidneys have developed and secrete small amounts of urine into the bladder which in all probability escape later into the amniotic fluid. Movements of the fetus are known to occur at this time, but they are too weak to be felt by the mother.

END OF FOURTH LUNAR MONTH

The fetus from head to toe is now six and one-half inches long and about four ounces in weight. A fine, downy growth of hair appears on the skin (so-called lanugo hair) and perhaps a few hairs on the scalp. At the end of this period faint movements of the fetus (quickening) may be felt by the mother, but usually these are not experienced until the next month.

END OF FIFTH LUNAR MONTH

The length of the fetus now approximates 10 inches, while its weight is about 8 ounces. At this period the physician is often able to hear the fetal heart for the first time, and the mother, as we have noted, first feels the baby move. If a fetus is born now it may make a few efforts to breathe, but its lungs are insufficiently developed to cope with conditions outside the uterus and it invariably succumbs within a few hours at most.

END OF SIXTH LUNAR MONTH

The length of the fetus is 12 inches, and its weight 1½ pounds. It now resembles a miniature baby with the exception of the skin, which is wrinkled and red with practically no fat beneath it. At this time, however, the skin begins to develop a protective covering called "vernix caseosa," which means "cheesy varnish." This fatty, cheesy substance adheres to the skin of the fetus and at term may be an eighth of an inch thick. Although a few cases are on record in which fetuses of this size have survived, the outlook must be regarded as practically hopeless.

END OF THE SEVENTH LUNAR MONTH

The fetus measures about 15 inches in length and weighs approximately 2½ pounds. If born at this time it has some chance of survival, perhaps one in ten. There is a widespread notion, quite incorrect, that infants born at the seventh month are more likely to survive than those born at the eighth month. This is another of those old superstitions which have descended through more than two thousand years from the time of the ancient Greek physicians. They believed that the fetus is born by means of its own effort, that is, it pushes with its legs against the upper part of the womb and wriggles out into the world. It was their opinion that the fetus first attempts to escape from the uterus at the seventh month and, if strong, it succeeds. If the attempt fails, it is repeated at the eighth month. However, if it now succeeds it is so exhausted as the result of the previous attempt that it is more likely to die than if it had been successful in the prior attempt

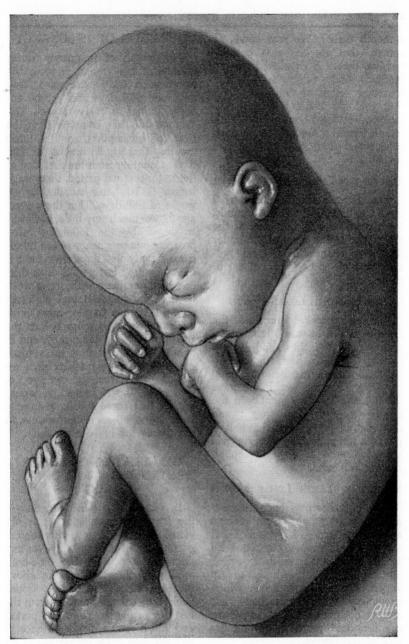

Fig. 59. Actual size drawing of fetus at approximately 5 months.

a month earlier. We now know, of course, that the fetus is entirely passive, that it is expelled from the mother's body solely through the muscular action of the uterus, and that this old belief is wholly fallacious. The fetus born at the eighth month stands a much better chance of survival than one born at the seventh.

END OF THE EIGHTH LUNAR MONTH

The fetus measures about 16.5 inches and weighs some 4 pounds. With good care infants born at the end of the eighth month have better than even chances of survival, possibly as high as two chances out of three.

END OF NINTH LUNAR MONTH

For all practical purposes the fetus is now a mature infant, measures some 19 inches, and weighs around 6 pounds. As though to improve its appearance before making its debut into the world, the fetus devotes the last two months in the uterus to putting on weight and during this period gains a half a pound a week. Its chances of survival are now quite as good as though born at full term.

MIDDLE OF TENTH LUNAR MONTH

Full term has now been reached, and the fetus weighs on an average about 7 pounds if a girl and 7½ if a boy; its length approximates 20 inches. Its skin is now white or pink and thickly coated with the cheesy vernix. The fine, downy hair which previously covered its body has largely disappeared. The fingernails are firm and protrude beyond the end of the fingers.

DURATION OF PREGNANCY

The length of pregnancy varies greatly; it may range, indeed, between such wide extremes as 240 days and 300 days and yet be entirely normal in every respect. The average duration, counting from the time of conception, is 9½ lunar months, that is, 38 weeks, or 266 days. Counting from the first day of the last menstrual period, its average length is 10 lunar months, or 40 weeks or 280 days. That these average figures mean very little, however, is shown by the following facts. Scarcely one pregnancy in ten terminates exactly 280 days after the beginning of the last period. Less than one half terminate within one week of this two hundred and eightieth day. In 10 per cent of cases birth occurs a week or more before the theoretical end of pregnancy, and in another 10 per cent it takes place more than two weeks later than we would expect from the average figures cited above. Indeed, it would appear that some fetuses require a longer time, others a shorter time, in the uterus for full development.

CALCULATION OF THE EXPECTED DATE OF CONFINEMENT

In view of the wide variation in the length of pregnancy, it is obviously impossible to predict the expected day of confinement with any degree of precision. The time-honored method, based on the above "average figures," is simple. Count back three calendar months from the first day of the last menstrual period and add seven days. For instance, if the last menstrual period began on

PLATE 3

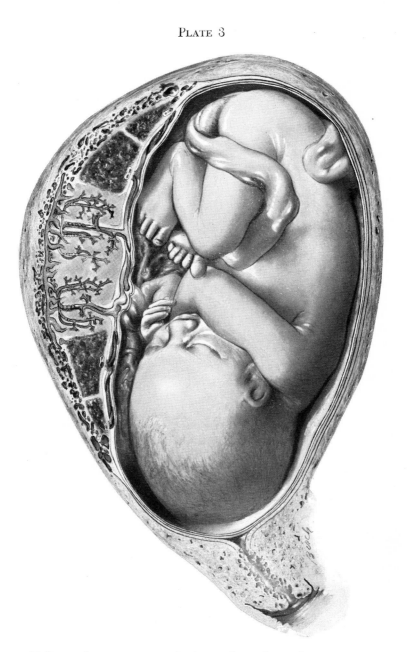

Full-term fetus in utero, with placental circulation shown in color.

June 10, we would count back three months to March and, adding seven days, arrive at the date of March 17. While it may be satisfying to the curiosity to have this date in mind, it must be understood that the likelihood of labor's occurring even within a week of this day is less than 50 per cent. There is one chance in ten that it will come at least two weeks later (Table 6).

Yet, whether pregnancy terminates a week before or two weeks later than the day calculated, the outlook for mother and baby is usually as good as though it had ended at "high noon" on the due date. Actually, women seldom go "over-term"; in most of these cases it is the above system of calculation and not Nature which has erred. For example, ovulation and hence conception may have occurred some days later than calculated; this error would make the beginning and the end of pregnancy that many days later. If, superimposed on this circumstance, we were dealing with a baby which required a slightly longer stay in the uterus for complete development, it would be clear that the apparent delay was quite normal and for the best.

PHYSIOLOGY OF THE FETUS

NUTRITION; PLACENTAL TRANSMISSION

During the period when the ovum lies unattached in the uterine cavity, its nutriment is provided by an endometrial secretion, which is rich in glycogen and has been called "uterine milk." With the burrowing of the ovum into the endometrium, it lies in a lake of fluid representing the broken-down product of endometrial cells and obtains nourishment from this source (Fig. 52).

Very early in pregnancy, certainly by the third or the fourth week, the chorionic villi have blood vessels within them (connected with the fetal bloodstream) and since these villi have already opened up the maternal blood vessels, nourishment is available from the maternal blood by the process of osmosis. In this connection it must be clearly understood that the maternal and the fetal bloods are never in contact and never intermingle. Indeed, even such substances as oxygen and glucose in the maternal blood must diffuse through several layers of tissue of the chorionic villi to reach the fetus. These layers are the cellular epithelium covering the villus, the loose connective tissue within it, and finally the endothelium of the capillary blood vessel in the center of the villus. In this manner oxygen passes into the fetal circulation while the fetal waste product, carbon dioxide, diffuses in the opposite direction. The placenta thus serves as the "lungs" of the baby in utero. Simple food substances, such as glucose, salt, calcium, phosphorus, iron, amino-acids and fatty acids, all diffuse through the chorionic villus to the fetus by this process of osmosis.

It is particularly important to note that most drugs pass readily to the fetus and, if given to the mother very shortly before birth, may affect the behavior of the newborn baby (p. 320). It is interesting to observe in addition that estrogen is transmitted to the fetus and produces certain effects in the newborn which may be very striking. In the first place, as the result of the action of this hormone, the breasts of both boy and girl babies may become markedly enlarged during the first few days of life and even secrete milk—the so-called "witch's milk" (p. 527). Secondly, estrogen causes the endometrium of the female fetus to hypertrophy, as it does that of an adult woman. After birth, when this hormone is suddenly withdrawn, the endometrium breaks down, and sometimes bleeding occurs. For this reason perhaps one girl baby in every 15 manifests a little spotting on the diaper during the first week of life. This is entirely normal and clears up of itself within a few days.

FETAL CIRCULATION

Since the fetus receives its oxygen through the placenta, the lungs do not function in utero. To meet this situation the fetal circulation contains certain special vessels which may be regarded as "by-passes" or "detours" which shunt the blood around the lungs, with only a small amount going through them for nutritional purposes.

The arterial (oxygenated) blood flows up the cord, through the umbilical vein, and passes into the ascending vena cava, partly through the liver, but chiefly through the special fetal structure, the ductus venosus, which connects these two vessels. It is because of the fact that the liver receives a considerable supply of freshly vitalized blood direct from the umbilical vein that it is, proportionately, so large in a newborn baby.

From the ascending vena cava the current flows into the right auricle and directly on to the left auricle through a special fetal structure, the

foramen ovale, thence into the left ventricle and out through the aorta. The blood which goes up the arms and the head returns through the descending vena cava to the right auricle again, but instead of passing through the foramen ovale, as before, the current is deflected downward into the right ventricle and out through the pulmonary arteries, partly to the lungs (for purposes of nutrition only), but mainly into the aorta, through the special fetal structure, the ductus arteriosus.

The blood in the aorta, with the exception of that which goes to the head and the upper extremities, which has been accounted for, passes downward to supply the trunk and the lower extremities. The greater part of this blood finds its way through the internal iliac, or hypogastric arteries, and so back through the cord to the placenta, where it is again oxygenated; but a small amount passes back into the ascending vena cava to mingle with fresh blood from the umbilical vein and again make the circuit of the entire body.

CIRCULATION CHANGE AT BIRTH

The fetal circulation is so arranged that this passage of blood to the placenta through the umbilical arteries and back through the umbilical vein is possible up to the time of birth, but it ceases entirely the moment the baby breathes and so begins to take its oxygen directly from its own lungs. During intra-uterine life, the circulation of blood through the lungs is for the nourishment of the lungs and not for the purpose of securing oxygen.

In order to understand, even in a

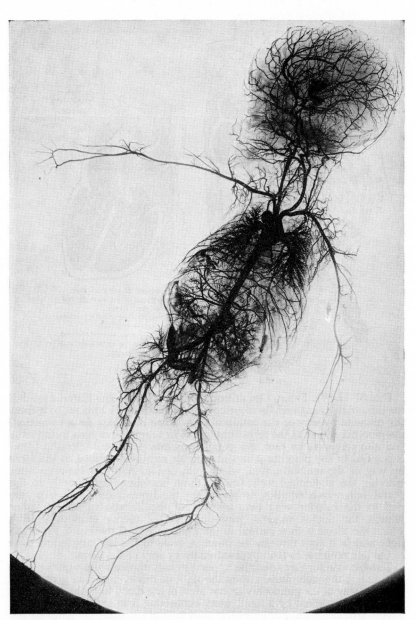

FIG. 60. Anteriogram showing the fetal circulation of a 7-month fetus, male, injected by Rudolf Skarda, Research Anatomist. (Univ. of Calif., Med. Center, San Francisco, Calif.)

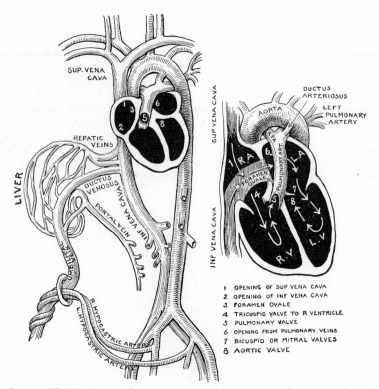

1. OPENING OF SUP VENA CAVA
2. OPENING OF INF VENA CAVA
3. FORAMEN OVALE
4. TRICUSPID VALVE TO R VENTRICLE
5. PULMONARY VALVE
6. OPENING FROM PULMONARY VEINS
7. BICUSPID OR MITRAL VALVES
8. AORTIC VALVE

FIG. 61 (*Left*). FETAL CIRCULATION BEFORE BIRTH. The material needed for the nourishment and the development of the fetus is brought to it from the placenta by way of the umbilical vein. Since the lungs do not function, the placenta serves as the respiratory organ in supplying oxygen to the fetus and also serves as an excretory organ for waste products. After the blood is purified in the placenta it is sent with its nutritive material to the fetus by way of the umbilical vein, which vein divides into two branches after entering the abdominal wall. One of these branches joins directly to the portal vein which empties its blood into the liver, from which it is carried to the inferior vena cava by way of the hepatic veins. The other branch, the ductus venosus, joins directly the inferior vena cava, from which the blood is then carried to the right auricle of the heart. From the right auricle it goes through the foramen ovale to the left auricle and then to the left ventricle to the upper extremity by way of the aorta.

The blood returning from the upper extemity through the superior vena cava enters the right auricle, then the right ventricle, and then goes to the lungs by way of the pulmonary artery. Most of the blood from the pulmonary artery is side-tracked by a small artery connecting it to the aorta called the ductus arteriosus. This, of necessity, must take place, since the lungs do not function before birth.

FIG. 62 (*Right*). FETAL CIRCULATION AFTER BIRTH. Pulmonary circulation becomes established with birth. The umbilical cord circulation ceases.

[*Cont. on next page*

general way, the course of the blood current and how it differs from the circulation after birth, it must be borne in mind that in infants after birth, as in the adult, the venous blood passes from the two venae cavae into the right auricle of the heart, thence to the right ventricle and through the pulmonary arteries to the lungs, whence it gives up its waste products and takes up a fresh supply of oxygen. After oxygenation, the so-called arterial blood flows from the lungs, through the pulmo-nary veins to the left auricle, thence to the left ventricle, and out through the aorta, to be distributed through the capillaries to all parts of the body and eventually collected, as venous blood, in the venae cavae and discharged again into the right auricle.

CIRCULATION PATH AFTER BIRTH

As soon as the baby is born and breathes, the function of the lungs is established, and the placental circulation ceases (the baby no longer is dependent upon his mother's blood

CHANGES IN FETAL CIRCULATION AFTER BIRTH

Structure	Before Birth	After Birth
Umbilical vein	Brings arterial blood to liver and heart	Obliterated. Becomes the round ligament of liver
Umbilical arteries	Bring arteriovenous blood to the placenta.	Obliterated. Become vesical ligaments on anterior abdominal wall
Ductus venosus	Shunts arterial blood into inferior cava	Obliterated. Becomes ligamentum venosum
Ductus arteriosus	Shunts arterial and some venous blood from the pulmonary artery to aorta	Obliterated. Becomes ligamentum arteriosum
Foramen ovale	Connects right and left auricles (atria)	Obliterated usually. At times open
Lungs	Contain no air and very little blood	Filled with air and well supplied with blood
Pulmonary arteries	Bring little blood to lungs	Bring much blood to lungs
Aorta	Receives blood from both ventricles	Receives blood only from left ventricle
Inferior vena cava	Brings venous blood from body and arterial blood from placenta	Brings venous blood only to right auricle

(Williams, J. F.: Anatomy and Physiology, ed. 7, Philadelphia, Saunders.)

Cont. from preceding page]
The arteries and the vein become obliterated immediately at the body junction. Shortly the hypogastric arteries, which are a continuance of the umbilical arteries after entrance into the body, become obliterated at their distal ends, followed by occlusion and obliteration of the umbilical vein and ductus venosus. The ductus arteriosus and the foramen ovale undergo a slower metamorphosis, finally occluding the circulation through the ductus arteriosus and closure of the foramen ovale. (Philips J. Carter, M.D., Louisiana State University, New Orleans)

for oxygen but is a separate being and breathes to oxygenate his own blood). This change not only alters the character of the blood in many vessels but also makes many of these vessels of no use as such; the umbilical arteries within the baby's body become filled with clotted blood and ultimately are converted into fibrous cords, and the umbilical vein within the body becomes the round ligament of the liver, after occlusion of the vessel. After the umbilical cord is tied and separated, the large amount of blood returned to the heart from the lungs, which are now functioning, causes more or less equal pressure in both of the auricles—this pressure causes the foramen ovale to close. The foramen ovale remains closed and eventually disappears, and the ductus arteriosus and the ductus venosus finally shrivel up and are converted into fibrous cords or ligaments, in the course of two or three months. The instantaneous closure of the foramen ovale changes the entire course of the blood current and converts the fetal circulation into the adult type.

The changes in the fetal circulation after birth may be tabulated as given on the preceding page.

PERIODS OF DEVELOPMENT

Human life may be divided into periods. The successive periods, with the duration of each, are indicated below.

The period of the ovum extends from fertilization to implantation, about the close of the second week of prenatal life. (The term ovum is used in a strict sense to denote the female germ cell and also to indicate the developing zygote [fertilized ovum] previous to implantation.)

The period of the embryo extends from the implantation to the third month.

The period of the fetus extends from about the third month, when the developing individual resembles the human form, to the time of birth.

The period of the newborn (neonatal) extends from birth to the close of the first month of postnatal life.

The period of infancy extends from the close of the first month to the close of the first year, or until the assumption of the erect posture, usually in the thirteenth or the fourteenth month.

The period of childhood extends from the close of the first year to about the fourteenth year in females and to about the sixteenth year in males. Puberty ends the period of childhood.

The period of adolescence extends from puberty to the last years of the second decade (late teens) in females, and to the first years of the third decade (early twenties) in males.

The period of maturity extends from the end of the adolescent period to senility (old age).

Development goes on throughout life; during senility, retrogressive or degenerative changes occur.

MATERNAL IMPRESSIONS

One of the commonest superstitions relating to childbearing is the old belief that the mental condition of the mother may modify the development of the unborn infant or, as they used to say, "mark it." For instance, if a pregnant woman were frightened by some ugly beast, let us say, it used to be thought that when the baby was born it might be "marked" or distorted in the likeness of the animal. Very often the "marking" took the form of reddish blotches on the skin of the infant, which, in the mother's imagination, seemed to resemble the beast. Or, sometimes it was thought that the blotch resembled some article of food which the pregnant woman particularly craved.

This belief, like most obstetric superstitions, is of hoary antiquity: the Biblical story of Jacob and the "speckled and spotted" cattle and goats and the "brown" sheep reflects it, while dramatists and novelists from Shakespeare to Dickens have perpetuated the idea in stirring plots. The facts are these. There is no nervous connection between mother and fetus—in other words, no possible pathways along which any such impulses, pleasant or otherwise, could travel. The blood of the mother is likewise separate and distinct from that of the fetus. Furthermore, the fetus is completely formed at the end of the sixth week of pregnancy,

that is, at a period when most women scarcely realize that they are pregnant; and, almost without exception, the causative mental shock or experience which is alleged to have brought about the "marking" occurred much later, long after the organ in question was in its final state of formation. Lastly, all modern experience refutes the belief. Obstetricians of vast experience, as well as maternity hospitals with thousands of deliveries annually, never have reported an authentic case.

How, then, is this age-old superstition to be explained? A number of factors probably contribute to it, chiefly coincidence. Approximately one baby in every 200 is born with some kind of blemish. In the event that such a blemish is present—let us say a reddish blotch on the buttocks of the baby—would it not be easy for an introspective mother, who had been told of this legend, to think finally of some object, some animal, or possibly some article of diet that she craved during pregnancy and, in her imagination, correlate it with the little red blotch?

SUGGESTED READING

Arey, L. B.: Developmental Anatomy, Philadelphia, Saunders, 1946.

Cook, Robert C., and Burks, Barbara S.: How Heredity Builds Our Lives, Washington, American Genetic Association.

Corner, G. W.: Ourselves Unborn; An Embryologist's Essay on Man, New Haven, Yale, 1944.

Davis, M. E., and Potter, Edith: Intrauterine respiration of the human fetus, J.A.M.A. 131:1194-1201, 1946.

Gilbert, M. S.: Biography of the Unborn, Baltimore, Williams & Wilkins, 1938.

Greisheimer, Esther M.: Physiology and Anatomy, Philadelphia, Lippincott, 1950.

Patten, Bradley M.: Human Embryology, Philadelphia, Blakiston, 1946.

Potter, Edith: Fundamentals of Human Reproduction, New York, McGraw-Hill, 1947.

Scheinfeld, Amram: You and Heredity, Philadelphia, Lippincott, 1950.

Snyder, Lawrence A.: The Principles of Heredity, Boston, Heath, 1946.

5

Presentations and Positions

FETAL HABITUS

By habitus, or attitude, of the fetus is meant the relation of the fetal parts to one another. The most striking characteristic of the fetal habitus is flexion. The spinal column is bowed forward, the head flexed with the chin against the sternum, and the arms flexed and folded against the chest. The lower extremities are also flexed, the thighs on the abdomen and the calves of the lower legs against the posterior aspect of the thighs. In this state of flexion the fetus assumes a roughly ovoid shape, occupies the smallest possible space, and conforms to the shape of the uterus. In this attitude it is about half as long as if it were completely stretched out. However, there are times when the fetus assumes many other positions.

FETAL HEAD

From an obstetric viewpoint, the head of the fetus is the most important part. If it can pass through the pelvic canal safely there is usually no difficulty in delivering the rest of the body, although occasionally the shoulders may cause trouble.

The cranium, or skull, is made up of 8 bones. Four of the bones—the sphenoid, the ethmoid and the 2 temporal bones—lie at the base of the cranium, are closely united and are of little obstetric interest. On the other hand, the 4 bones forming the upper part of the cranium are of great importance; these are the frontal, the occipital and the two parietal bones. These bones are not knit closely together at the time of birth but are separated by membranous interspaces called *sutures*. The

96

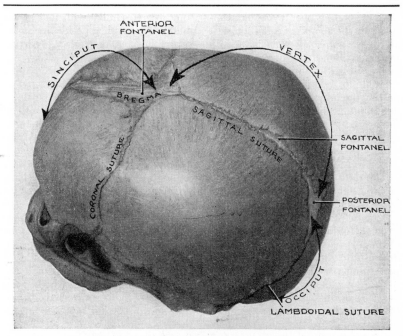

Fig. 63. Fetal skull, showing sutures and fontanels.

intersections of these sutures are known as *fontanels.*

By means of this formation of the fetal skull the bones can overlap each other somewhat during labor and so diminish materially the size of the head during its passage through the pelvis. This process of overlapping is called "molding," and after a long labor with a large baby and a snug pelvis, the head is often so definitely molded that several days may elapse before it returns to its normal shape.

The most important sutures are: the sagittal, between the two parietal bones; the frontal, between the two frontal bones; the coronal, between the frontal and the parietal bones; and the lambdoid, between the pos-

terior margins of the parietal bones and the upper margin of the occipital bone. The temporal sutures, which separate the parietal and the temporal bones on either side, are unimportant in obstetrics, because they are covered by fat parts and cannot be felt on the living baby.

The fontanels of importance are the anterior and the posterior. The anterior fontanel, large and diamond-shaped, is at the intersection of the sagittal and the coronal sutures, while the small triangular posterior fontanel lies at the junction of the sagittal and the lambdoidal suture. The sutures and the posterior fontanel ossify shortly after birth, but the anterior fontanel remains open until the child is over a year old, constituting the familiar "soft spot" just above the forehead of an infant. By feeling or identifying one or another of the sutures or fontanels, and considering its relative position in the pelvis, the physician is enabled to determine accurately the position of the head.

PRESENTATION

The term "presentation" is used to designate that portion of the infant's body which lies nearest the internal os, or, in other words, that portion which is felt by the examining fingers of the physician when they are introduced into the cervix. When the presenting part is known, it is easy to determine the relation between the long axis of the baby's body and that of the mother. Head, or cephalic, presentations are the most common, being present in about 97 per cent of all cases at term. In cephalic presentation the vertex almost always presents, but occasionally the face may be the presenting part, depending upon the degree of flexion of the infant's neck. Next to the head, the breech is the most common presenting part, being present, however, in only about 3 per cent of all cases. In breech presentation, the buttocks or one or both feet may first appear, the latter constituting a single or double "footling." Both head and breech presentations are designated as longitudinal, since the long axis of the baby corresponds to the long axis of the mother's body.

In transverse, or shoulder, presentation the baby lies crosswise in the uterus, and before delivery is possible it must be turned so that its long axis is parallel with that of the mother. Transverse presentations are relatively uncommon, occurring about once in every 200 cases.

POSITIONS

Besides knowing the presenting part of the baby, it is important to know the exact position of this presenting part in relation to the pelvis. This relationship is determined by finding the position of certain points on the presenting surface with regard to the four imaginary divisions or regions of the pelvis. For this purpose the pelvis is considered to be divided into quadrants: left anterior, left posterior, right anterior and right posterior. These divisions aid the physician in indicating whether the presenting part is directed toward the right or the left side and toward the front or the back of the pelvis. Certain points on the presenting surface of the baby have been arbitrarily chosen as points of direction in determining the exact relation of the presenting part to the quadrants of the pelvis. In vertex presentations the occiput is the guiding point; in face presentations, the chin (mentum); in breech presentations, the sacrum; and in transverse, or shoulder, presentations, the scapula (acromion process).

Position, then, has to do with the relation of the presenting part of the fetus to the pelvis. Thus, in a vertex presentation, the back of the head (occiput) may point to the front or to the back of the pelvis. The occiput rarely points exactly forward or backward in the median line but is usually directed to one side or the other.

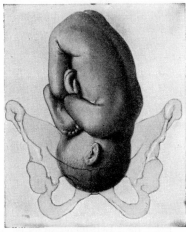

FIG. 64. Left-occipito-anterior position (L.O.A.).

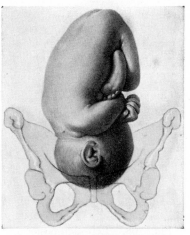

FIG. 65. Right-occipito-anterior position (R.O.A.).

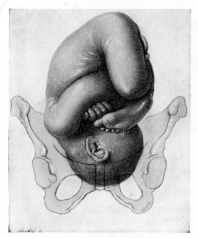

FIG. 66. Right-occipitotransverse position (R.O.T.).

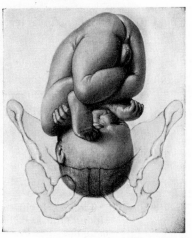

FIG. 67. Right-occipitoposterior position (R.O.P.).

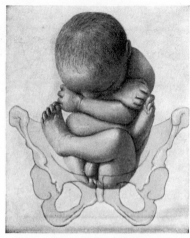

Fig. 68. Left-sacroposterior position (L.S.P.).

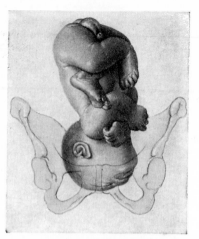

Fig. 69. Left-mento-anterior position (L.M.A.).

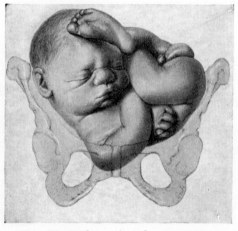

Fig. 70. Right-acromiodorsoposterior position (R.A.D.P.). This means that the *acromium* lies toward the *right* side of the mother and that the back (dorsum) of the infant lies toward the *posterior* part of the pelvis.

The various positions are usually expressed by abbreviations, using the first letter of each word which describes the position: thus, left-occipito-anterior is abbreviated L.O.A. This means that the head is presenting with the occiput directed toward the left side of the mother and toward the front part of the pelvis. If the occiput were directed straight to the left with no deviation toward front or back of the pelvis, it would be termed left-occipitotransverse, or L.O.T. The occiput might also be directed toward the back or posterior quadrant of the pelvis, in which case the position would be left-occipito-posterior, or L.O.P. There are also three corresponding positions on the right side: R.O.A., R.O.T. and R.O.P.

The occipital positions are considered the most favorable for both mother and baby, and of these, the L.O.A. position is preferred. The same system of terminology is used for face, breech and transverse presentations, as indicated in the following list of abbreviations (S, indicating breech; M, chin or face; and A, shoulder).

POSITIONS—VERTEX PRESENTATION

L.O.A.—Left-occipito-anterior
L.O.T.—Left-occipitotransverse
L.O.P.—Left-occipitoposterior
R.O.A.—Right-occipito-anterior
R.O.T.—Right-occipitotransverse
R.O.P.—Right-occipitoposterior

POSITIONS—BREECH PRESENTATION

L.S.A.—Left-sacro-anterior
L.S.T.—Left-sacrotransverse
L.S.P.—Left-sacroposterior
R.S.A.—Right-sacro-anterior
R.S.T.—Right-sacrotransverse
R.S.P.—Right-sacroposterior

POSITIONS—FACE PRESENTATION

L.M.A.—Left-mento-anterior
L.M.T.—Left-mentotransverse
L.M.P.—Left-mentoposterior
R.M.A.—Right-mento-anterior
R.M.T.—Right-mentotransverse
R.M.P.—Right-mentoposterior

POSITIONS—TRANSVERSE PRESENTATION

L.A.D.A.—Left-acromio-dorso-anterior
L.A.D.P.—Left-acromio-dorso-posterior
R.A.D.A.—Right-acromio-dorso-anterior
R.A.D.P.—Right-acromio-dorso-posterior

Figures 71 and 72 show the principal measurements of the fetal skull. The most important transverse diameter is the biparietal; it is the distance between the biparietal protuberances and represents the greatest width of the head. It measures, on an average, 9.25 cm. There are three important anteroposterior diameters: the sub-occipitobregmatic, which extends from the under surface of the occiput to the center of the anterior fontanel and measures about 9.5 cm.; the occipitofrontal, which extends from the root of the nose to the occipital prominence and measures about 12.0 cm.; and the occipitomental, which extends from the chin to the posterior fontanel and averages about 13.5 cm.

In considering these three anteroposterior diameters of the fetal skull it is important to note that with the head in complete flexion and the chin resting on the thorax, the smallest of these, the suboccipitobregmatic, enters the pelvis, whereas if the head is extended or bent back (with no flexion whatsoever), the greatest anteroposterior diameter presents itself to the pelvic inlet. Herein lies the great importance of flexion; the more the head is flexed the smaller is the anteroposterior diameter which enters the pelvis. Figures 73 to 75 show this basic principle in diagrammatic form.

DIAGNOSIS OF FETAL POSITION

Diagnosis of fetal position is made in five ways: (1) inspection; (2) palpation; (3) vaginal and rectal examination; (4) auscultation; and (5) roentgenogram.

INSPECTION

Nurses are expected to be able to determine whether a presentation is normal or otherwise, as work in rural, sparsely settled localities may often require of her knowledge not demanded in her hospital experience. Only under most unusual conditions would she be expected to ascertain this in any other way than by the first two methods, inspection and palpation; and with these two she should thoroughly familiarize herself. Auscultation, while not wholly dependable, may be helpful. Inspection includes a general survey of the shape of the abdomen and must be gained by actual observation. Palpation, on the contrary, demands knowledge of certain specific procedures for the determination of fetal position.

PALPATION

For palpation the patient should lie flat on her back, with her knees flexed, to relax the abdominal muscles; the nurse should lay both hands gently, and at first, flat upon the abdomen. If done in any other manner than this, or if her hands are not warm, the stimulation of her fingers

will cause the abdominal muscles to contract. She should accustom herself to palpate the uterus in a definite, methodical way, and it will be found best to carry out successively the following four maneuvers:

First Maneuver. The nurse should ascertain, facing the patient, what is lying at the fundus of the uterus by feeling the upper abdomen with both hands; generally she will find there a mass, which is either the head or the buttocks (breech) of the fetus. She must decide which pole of the fetus this is by observing three points (Fig. 76):

1. Its relative consistency: the head is harder than the breech.

2. Its shape: if the head, it will be round and hard, and the transverse groove of the neck may be felt. The breech has no groove and usually feels more angular.

3. Mobility: the head will move independently of the trunk, but the breech moves only with the trunk. The ability of the head to be moved back and forth against the examining fingers is spoken of as ballottement.

Second Maneuver. Having determined whether the head or the breech is in the fundus, the next step is to locate the back of the fetus in relation to the right and the left sides of the mother. Still facing the patient, the nurse places the palmar surfaces of both hands on either side of the abdomen and makes gentle but deep pressure. On one side is felt a smooth, hard, resistant plane, the back, while on the other numerous angular nodulations are palpated, the small parts; these latter represent the knees and the elbows of the fetus.

Third Maneuver. This maneuver consists in an effort to find the head

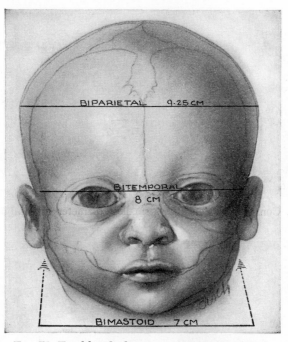

FIG. 71. Fetal head, showing transverse diameters.

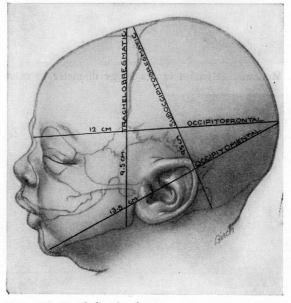

FIG. 72. Fetal head, showing anteroposterior diameters.

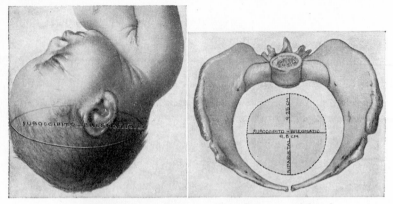

FIG. 73. Complete flexion allows smallest diameter of head to enter pelvis.

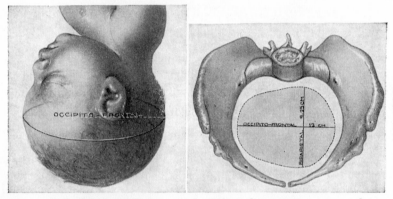

FIG. 74. Moderate extension causes larger diameter to enter pelvis.

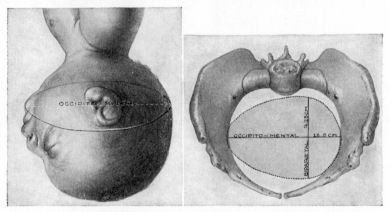

FIG. 75. Marked extension forces largest diameter against pelvic brim, but it is too large to enter.

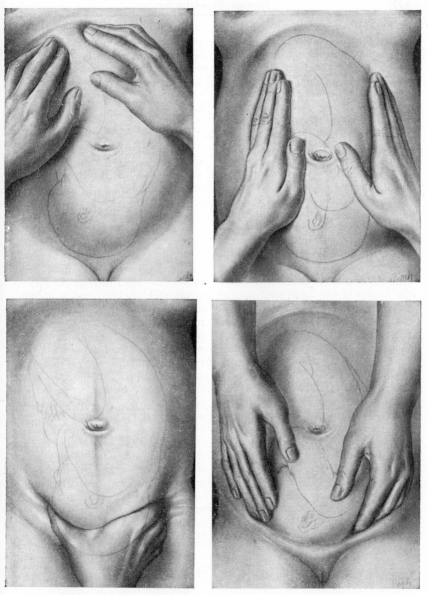

FIG. 76. Palpation: (*top, left*) first maneuver; (*top, right*) second maneuver; (*bottom, left*) third maneuver; (*bottom, right*) fourth maneuver.

at the pelvic inlet and to determine its mobility. It should be conducted by placing the fingers over the middle of Poupart's ligament on one side and the thumb on the corresponding place on the opposite side and by pressing together. If the presenting part is not engaged, a movable body will be felt, which is usually the head.

Fourth Maneuver. In this maneuver the nurse faces the feet of the patient and places the tips of her first three fingers on both sides of the midline, about 2 inches above Poupart's ligament. Pressure is now made downward and in the direction of the birth canal, the movable skin of the abdomen being carried downward along with the fingers. It will be found that the fingers of one hand meet no obstruction and can be carried downward well under Poupart's ligament; these fingers glide over the nape of the baby's neck. The other hand, however, usually meets an obstruction an inch or so above Poupart's ligament; this is the brow of the baby and is usually spoken of as the "cephalic prominence." This maneuver gives information of several kinds:

1. If the findings are as described above, it means that the baby's head is well flexed.

2. Confirmatory information is obtained about the location of the back, as naturally the back is on the opposite side from the brow of the baby, except in the uncommon cases of face presentation, in which the cephalic prominence and the back are on the same side.

3. If the cephalic prominence is very easily palpated, as if it were just under the skin, a posterior position of the occiput is suggested.

4. The location of the cephalic prominence tells how far the head has descended into the pelvis. This maneuver is of most value if the head has engaged and may yield no information with a floating, poorly flexed head.

Vaginal Examination

Vaginal examination is done by the physician and consists in identifying the fontanels and the suture lines of the fetal skull. In experienced hands this gives helpful information about the position of the baby and the degree of flexion.

Auscultation

The location of the fetal heart sounds, as heard through the stethoscope, yields helpful confirmatory information about fetal position but is not wholly dependable. Certainly, it never should be relied upon as the sole means of diagnosing fetal position. In general, however, in L.O.A. and L.O.P. positions the fetal heart sounds are heard loudest in the left lower quadrant. A similar situation applies to the R.O.A. and R.O.P. positions. In posterior positions of the occiput (L.O.P. and R.O.P.) often the sounds are heard loudest well down in the flank toward the anterior superior spine. In breech presentation the fetal heart sounds usually are heard loudest at the level of the umbilicus or above (Figs. 91 and 92).

Roentgenograms

Roentgenograms are employed in the diagnosis of fetal position only in doubtful cases, particularly when twins are suspected. Of course, they give complete and accurate information concerning position, flexion and descent of the fetal head (Fig. 93).

SUGGESTED READING

Adair, F. L.: Obstetrics and Gynecology, Philadelphia, Lea & Febiger, 1941.

Beck, A. C.: Obstetrical Practice, ed. 4, Baltimore, Williams & Wilkins, 1947.

DeLee, J. B., and Greenhill, J. P.: The Principles and Practice of Obstetrics, ed. 9, Philadelphia, Saunders, 1951.

Eastman, N. J.: Williams Obstetrics, ed. 10, New York, Appleton-Century, 1950.

The books listed above are among the standard American works on obstetrics. One of these, at least, will be found in any nurses' library and all in most medical libraries. The nurse will do well to augment her reading by consulting one or another of these volumes from time to time.

CONFERENCE MATERIAL

1. What would be your responsibility to a friend who is pregnant yet has not registered for delivery with either a doctor or a clinic?

2. How would you present the subject of human reproduction to a group of Girl Scouts or high school students?

3. What illustrative material and reference readings would you select for a group conference of young parents or those about to be married?

4. How would you go about looking up the costs of obstetric care in your community?

5. If a patient appealed to you to secure information about the best obstetric care in a certain city in the United States, how would you get this information for her?

6. What authentic sources are available for obtaining maternal and infant mortality statistics?

7. What is the status of the midwife in this country? How does this situation compare with other countries?

8. What forces are in operation to improve the maternity situation?

9. How can you stimulate the interest of a lay group in the community who are willing to give time and some financial support to help with an educational program for the less fortunate?

SITUATION OF NURSING ATTAINMENT

After each unit of this book, some objectively scorable test questions are provided to aid you in making immediate *use* of the information and the knowledge that you have gained through studying each of these units. The questions are planned to enable you to see how some of the important facts function in the nursing care of patients and how knowledge of the facts enables you to (1) recognize, analyze and interpret the nursing needs of obstetric patients, (2) plan to meet these needs, (3) carry out the plan and (4) evaluate both the plan and the results.

These tests represent only a few sample instances where information, facts and principles presented in the units function in nursing care. If you are successful in these samples, you may be in many more instances, but you should not assume that success here guarantees success in all. Likewise, failure on many of these items does not necessarily mean complete lack of understanding, but it is a rather good indication that you need to restudy the unit more carefully.

Use these tests as a study device. After you believe that you have mastered the important points in the unit, fill out the objectively scorable test questions at the end of the unit. Think through each question and response carefully. Complete the entire unit test and then (and not until then) turn to the key on page 643, where you will find the right answers. See how many you had correct. Look up the answers to those that you answered incorrectly.

You will observe that many of the questions demand that you use your previously acquired knowledge of anatomy and physiology, bacteriology, chemistry, pharmacology, psychology, nursing arts and nutrition, together with obstetric nursing knowledge, for all nursing care demands the simultaneous functioning of facts and principles from many of these fields along with those of the special clinical field.

In some judgment and debatable questions the answer given in the key may conflict with the current practice in your institution or locality. Ask your teacher how she thinks you should score yourself on these points.

Since the purpose of these self-scoring tests is to aid you in learning, you will be defeating that purpose and penalizing yourself if you misuse them and look at the key before you have carefully thought through the question. *No one but you is interested in how well or how poorly you do on these tests.* When you have discovered how well or how poorly you have done, you will know better what and how much more to study.

Your teacher's evaluation of your ability to use the material presented in each unit may sample some of these and many other points presented in the unit. Your best preparation for your teacher's appraisal in class and on the ward is your own evaluation of your attainment and study in light of your accomplishment. But, more important, your best preparation for giving skilled professional nursing care to obstetric patients is to have a complete understanding of and ability to use the important facts and principles that relate to that care, an understanding that is largely within your own power to obtain through your own efforts.

Situation Questions

UNIT ONE: HUMAN REPRODUCTION

Read through the entire question and place your answers in the parentheses.

1. To which of the following causes of maternal mortality does careless nursing contribute most frequently?
   a. Cardiac complications
   b. Toxemia
   c. Miscarriage
   d. Hemorrhage during deliveries
   e. Postpartum hemorrhage
   f. Puerperal infection (_____)

2. What improvement is believed to be the greatest single factor for decreasing maternal deaths during the past half century?
   a. Prenatal care
   b. Management of labor
   c. Analgesia during delivery
   d. Nursing care during delivery
   e. Care by the physician during delivery
   f. Care during the puerperium (_____)

3. A patient in the clinic, in the latter part of her pregnancy, reported to the nurse that she was suffering from backache and wanted to know the cause. What would be the most likely reason that the nurse could give her?
   a. The larger size of the fetus tires her more easily.
   b. Increased mobility of joints throws greater weight on surrounding muscles.
   c. She must have some abnormality in pelvic structures.
   d. The enlargement of the abdomen causes a forward tilting of the body.
   (_____)

4. In each of the following write the term or the phrase by which the pelvic measurement described is commonly called.
   a. Between the symphysis pubis and the depression below the fifth lumbar vertebra   a. (_____)
   b. From the lower margin of the symphysis pubis to the sacral promontory   b. (_____)
   c. Between the lateral edges of the iliac crests   c. (_____)
   d. The posterior portion of the symphysis pubis to the promontory of the sacrum   d. (_____)
   e. From the inner aspects of the ischial tuberosities e. (_____)

5. By using the letter or letters of the measurements described in Question 4 indicate:

   a. Those that would be obtained by the physician
      when using a pelvimeter   a. (_____)
   b. Those to obtain by use of gloves   b. (_____)
   c. The one which must be estimated rather than
      measured directly   c. (_____)
   d. The one which represents the smallest diameter   d. (_____)
   e. The one which represents the largest diameter   e. (_____)

6. A patient's chart shows pelvic measurements of 11 cm. for the diagonal conjugate and 9.5 cm. for the true conjugate; therefore, the nurse caring for the patient in the labor room should anticipate that the patient might have:

   a. An easy, rapid delivery
   b. A delivery of reasonable duration
   c. A protracted labor with difficult delivery   (_____)

7. To give adequate care to the patient during and after delivery, the nurse should fully understand the structure of the uterus. Which of the following are true of the uterus?

   a. Its muscular tissue is:

      1. Chiefly striated   3. Entirely striated
      2. Chiefly nonstriated   4. Entirely nonstriated
                                               (_____)

   b. Its muscle fibers are arranged to run:

      1. Circularly
      2. Longitudinally
      3. In all directions
      4. In three layers, the inner and the outer circularly, the other longitudinally   (_____)

   c. Its blood is supplied directly from:

      1. Ovarian and uterine arteries
      2. Abdominal aorta and uterine arteries
      3. Internal iliac and ovarian arteries
      4. Internal iliac and uterine arteries   (_____)

   d. Normally, it is:

      1. Attached anteriorly to the bladder wall
      2. Suspended freely movable in the pelvic cavity
      3. Suspended between the bladder and the rectum
      4. Attached posteriorly to the anterior wall of the sacrum
                                               (_____)

8. Every effort is made to prevent the tearing of the perineum during childbirth. This structure has:

   a. A single, strong elastic muscle
   b. A strong elastic tendon
   c. A tendon to which 5 muscles are attached
   d. Two strong muscles, the anal and the transverse perineal
                                             (_____)

9. The chief hazard to the patient from destruction of the perineum by tearing would likely be:
   a. Infection of the birth canal
   b. Postpartum hemorrhage
   c. Perineal abscess
   d. Prolapsed uterus   (_____)

10. A patient with small breasts in her first pregnancy was worried about her ability to feed her baby.
   a. The nurse could respond correctly to the patient by telling her that:
       1. She probably would be unable to feed her baby.
       2. The size of the breasts does not influence the amount of lactation possible.
       3. Mothers with small breasts usually have less difficulty feeding their babies.
       4. Her baby would be fed better by means of a formula.
                                                          (_____)
   b. Milk is produced by the process of:
       1. Dialysis
       2. Osmosis
       3. Secretion   (_____)
   c. The structures most directly involved in the production of milk are:
       1. Papillae
       2. Glands of Montgomery
       3. Acini cells
       4. Lactiferous sinuses
       5. Areola
       6. Lactiferous ducts   (_____)

11. What are the ovarian hormones produced by the Graafian follicles and the cells of the corpus luteum?
   a. Progesterone and gonadotrophin
   b. Estrogen and progesterone
   c. Gonadotrophin and FSH
   d. FSH and estrogen   (_____)

12. A young mother-to-be told a nurse that she was sure that she would have a boy because her husband was such a strong, physically developed man. The nurse could respond correctly by saying:
   a. "It is the female cell which determines the sex of the child."
   b. "It is unlikely because there are more girls born than boys."
   c. "Physical strength does not influence the sex of the child."
   d. "You are probably right."   (_____)

13. A patient expelled a fetus of 16 cm. prematurely. What would be the approximate age of the fetus?
   a. 2 months
   b. 3 months
   c. 4 months
   d. 5 months   (_____)

14. Although the exact date of delivery cannot be predetermined, if a pregnant woman's last menstrual period began on September 10, the estimated due date would be nearest:

   a. May 6
   b. May 10
   c. June 10
   d. June 17

15. The only direct connection between the fetus and any other structure is through the umbilical cord. The umbilical cord contains which of these important structures?

   a. Umbilical artery
   b. Umbilical arteries
   c. Umbilical vein
   d. Umbilical veins
   e. Umbilical nerves
   f. Umbilical lymphatic duct
   g. Liquor amnii
   h. Wharton's jelly
   i. Amniotic tissue
   j. Chorion   (_____)

16. Arrange each of the following structures in rank order to indicate the sequence of the structures through which the blood must pass from the mother's uterine artery to the fetal liver and heart and return to the uterine veins. Assume the shortest possible return route. On the lines provided add the name or the names of any important structure not mentioned and include in the proper sequences.

a. Uterine artery and branches	1.	_____
b. Ascending vena cava	2.	_____
c. Placental capillaries	3.	_____
d. Right auricle	4.	_____
e. Left ventricle	5.	_____
f. Aorta	6.	_____
g. Foramen ovale	7.	_____
h. Portal artery	8.	_____
i. Liver	9.	_____
j. Uterine veins	10.	_____
k. Umbilical vein	11.	_____
l. Umbilical artery	12.	_____
m. Capillaries in uterine wall	13.	_____
n. Ductus venosus	14.	_____
o. Tissue spaces, uterus	15.	_____
p. Tissue spaces, placenta	16.	_____
q. Right ventricle	17.	_____
r. Left auricle	18.	_____
s. Internal iliac artery	19.	_____
t. Portal vein	20.	_____

u. _____   21. _____
v. _____   22. _____

17. After a protracted labor and a difficult delivery the mother, upon seeing the child, was shocked at the elongated appearance of the child's head. The nurse could correctly reassure the patient by saying:

    a. "The child's head is molded during delivery and will return to normal in a few days."

    b. "All newborn babies' heads are shaped this way."

    c. "The child's head shape was changed during delivery, and it will take six months for it to return to normal."

    d. "After the 'soft spot' closes the head will return to normal."

                                              (_____)

18. Indicate the abbreviations that might be used on a patient's chart to represent each of the positions and the presentations described:

    a. Back of head directed straight to the left   a. (_____)

    b. Back of head directed toward the left side and the front quadrant of the pelvis   b. (_____)

    c. Back of head directed toward the right side and the back quadrant of the pelvis   c. (_____)

    d. Breech presentation, buttocks at the left back quadrant   d. (_____)

    e. Face presentation, chin at the right front quadrant   e. (_____)

    f. Transverse position, shoulder at the right back quadrant   f. (_____)

Note: The key to the correct answers to these questions is given on page 643.

UNIT TWO

NURSING IN PREGNANCY

ORIENTATION

The previous chapters, dealing with the anatomy and the physiology of the generative organs and the developing fetus, have been a foundation for the study of normal pregnancy and its possible discomforts and complications. The importance of prenatal care cannot be overemphasized. The future health of the mother, as well as the foundation for the health, the growth and the development of the baby, are dependent upon adequate care during this period. During this period the patient, the doctor and the nurse must assume the responsibility for securing a well mother and a well baby at the termination of the maternity cycle. The nurse, by means of her contacts with the patient in the clinic and in the home, is able to observe the teaching methods and supervision suited to this difficult and trying situation. During the nurse's surgical experience she may have the opportunity of watching her patient from diagnosis through the operation and complete recovery. Since the maternity cycle extends throughout the 9-month period of pregnancy and the 6 weeks following, the nurse misses this complete picture in her practical experience. Since it may not be possible for the nurse to see the immediate results of this care, she must be able to look ahead and aim for the results which can be obtained only by adequate prenatal care and good medical supervision.

During the prenatal period, too, the mother has many emotional adjustments to make: sometimes fear, worries (financial as well as physical), apprehension and family difficulties or problems are present. These emotional disturbances in some degree or form accompany each prenatal period, whether it be the first or a subsequent pregnancy. Patients of all status have similar adjustments to make. The fact that delivery must be "faced," that there is no turning back or "changing the mind," is in itself sometimes an overwhelming emotional crisis.

Background and Development
of Prenatal Care

As we know it today, prenatal care developed into its present status through devious avenues of investigation and many by-paths of interrelated activity and work. Individuals, both from the profession and the laity, as well as organizations, private and municipal, contributed time, money and interest until, at last, Government action was obtained.

The background of our present maternity situation is of interest both as a history and a story. Prenatal care in the United States had its beginnings in the days of slavery. The intelligent slaveowners paid special attention to the diet and the care of pregnant slaves. Healthy slaves were more valuable, were worth more money and produced stronger offspring. From this beginning, the chronologic efforts which led to our present-day prenatal care follow:

1866. A story was written which concerned cruelty to a child. Some thoughtful person referred the case to *The Society for the Prevention of Cruelty to Animals*. Henry Bergh, a former diplomat to Russia, was the founder and director of this association and was influential in having the judgment pronounced on the ground that a child was a human animal. This incident stimulated interest in the general treatment of children.

1873. *The New York Diet Kitchen Association*, the oldest public health organization in America, was opened at the request of doctors from "de Milt Dispensary" on the lower East Side of New York City. It was first organized as a soup kitchen, and milk, gruel, beef tea and cooked rice were taken to the sick in their homes, with the idea of restoring health. In 1892 they began to make formulas for sick babies and still later dispensed free milk or sold it at 3 cents a quart. Maria L. Daniels was the first nurse director and contributed much for many years to public health progress. In 1926 this group was organized as *The Children's Health Service of New York*. The organization grew with the times, changing its program from curing the sick to preventive work—keeping well babies well. While the organization devoted its major effort to work with babies and preschool children, it also included prenatal care in its program.

1876. The beginning of child-welfare legislation in the United States was the Act passed by the New York State Legislature, granting to *The Society for the Prevention of Cruelty to Children* a charter giving it wide power with regard to the protection of child life. The inception of this legislation was based on the incident of the "child as a human animal" (1866).

1893. The first *Infant Milk Station* in the United States was established in New York City by Nathan Strauss. Through his persistence milk was finally made "safe" through pasteurization; and many such stations were set up.

1900. *The United States Census Bureau* was made a permanent organization. Up to this time, *vital statistics* were considered to be of so little importance in the United States that, as soon as the population was tabulated and classified, the bureau was disbanded, to be re-established and reorganized every 10 years.

1906. *The United States Census Bureau* published mortality statistics which drew attention to the appalling loss of life among babies and children. Up to this time, very little thought had been given to maternity and infant protection.

1907. Due to the growing interest, Mr. George H. F. Schrader was stimulated to give money to *The Association for Improving Conditions of the Poor* (now the *Community Service Society*) for the salaries of two nurses to do prenatal work. This was the first consistent effort to prevent deaths of babies by caring for the mothers *before* the babies were born. Two reasons were given as to why prenatal care would be of value: (1) nurses in convalescent homes for postpartum mothers thought that if patients had better care during pregnancy, the health of mothers would be improved. (2) Social workers going into the homes felt that they were not adequately prepared to advise pregnant mothers.

1907. *The New York Milk Committee* was organized. Its object was the reduction of infant mortality through the improvement of the city's milk supply. It established milk depots which proved beyond question their great value in the reduction of infant mortality by dispensing clean pasteurized milk and by educating mothers.

1908. In this year the *Division of Child Hygiene* was established in New York City, the first in the United States, and it was important enough to be recognized nationally. Josephine Baker, M.D., was appointed chief. This was a pioneer achievement, and the methods that were evolved had no precedent.

1909 to 1914. At approximately this time, Mrs. William Lowell Putnam, of Boston, promoted a demonstration of organized prenatal care. It was called *The Prenatal Care Committee* of the Women's Municipal League. They worked in co-operation with the Boston Lying-In Hospital through Robert L. DeNormandie, M.D., of Harvard Medical School, Dr. Ruggles, of the then Homeopathic Hospital, and the Instructive District Nurses Association. The committee functioned long enough to establish the fact that good obstetric care was not possible without prenatal care.

1909. In this year *The American Association for the Study and Prevention of Infant Mortality* was organized and held its first meeting in New Haven, Connecticut. This committee was composed of both professional and lay members and devoted itself entirely to problems connected with child life, particularly to studying and trying to correct the high mortality rate. At this time there were no records of births or deaths, and the causes of deaths were unknown. The education of doctors and nurses was shamefully unsatisfactory; there was no public health in the schools, and practically no activity on the part of municipal, state or the Federal Government to prevent infant mortality. The first president of this association was J. H. Mason Knox, M.D., and Gertrude B. Kipp was the first secretary. The committee consisted of the Honorable Herbert Hoover, Livingston Ferrand, M.D., L. Emmet Holt, M.D., Richard Bolt, M.D., and Philip Van Ingen, M.D. The work of this organization was of profound significance. In 1918 its expanding activities caused it to change its name to *The American Child Hygiene Association,* and in 1923 the name was changed to the *American Child Health Association.* In 1935, after having contributed to every angle of this pioneer work, the association was disbanded.

1909. *The First White House Conference,* on "The Dependent Child," was called by President Theodore Roosevelt. These investigations resulted in the establishment of the Federal Children's Bureau in 1912. According to some authorities this conference was called through the influence of a public health nurse.

1910. *The Census Bureau* published another report, this time on the mortality of babies under one year of age and at "special ages." As a result of this report maternity hospitals made an effort to improve the care given to babies.

1911. In New York City *the first strictly municipal baby-health stations* were organized under the jurisdiction of the Department of Health, and the full cost of the work was borne by the municipality. Soon the dispensing of milk was of minor importance, and emphasis was placed on prevention–keeping well babies well. They are now called *Child-Health Stations.*

1911. *The New York Milk Committee* (1907) made an investigation at the baby-health stations and found that 40 per cent of all baby deaths (112 per 1,000) occurred within the first month of life before the mothers registered their babies at the health stations. This indicated the necessity for care *before* birth. The committee then decided to carry on an experiment in prenatal work. (See 1917.) They were convinced that much could be hoped for as a result of organized prenatal care.

1912. *The Babies' Welfare Association* (formerly *The Association of Infant Milk Stations* [1893]) represents the first comprehensive and successful attempt to co-ordinate the various child-welfare agencies in any community. All of the organizations of this type agreed to co-ordinate their activities by preventing duplication and overlapping without interfering with the organizations. In 1922 the name was changed to the *Children's Welfare Federation* of New York City. It continues to act as a clearing house and, among its other activities, manages the *Mother's Milk Bureau.*

1912. The Federal *Children's Bureau* was established. It began in the Department of Commerce and Labor; in 1913 it was made a part of the Department of Labor and, in 1946, was transferred to the Federal Security Agency. This was created by Congress through a Federal Act (Government sanction). This bureau was to set up special machinery to study and protect the child and to study all matters pertaining to the welfare of children and child life among all classes of our people, to assemble and accumulate factual information and to disseminate this information throughout the country. Miss Julia Lathrop was chosen as chief. Much of the success of this bureau is credited to Miss Lathrop's vision. Fortunately, her successor, Miss Grace Abbott, continued the work with equal zeal.

1915. *The Birth Registration Area* was established as a Federal Act. The information is compiled in a uniform manner, giving the birth and the death statistics on which are based our information on mortality rates. The New England States, New York, Pennsylvania, Michigan, Minnesota and the District of Columbia, were the first states to comply. Finally, in 1933, Texas joined, making the registration of the 48 states complete. (See Tables 3, 4 and 5.)

1915. Dr. Haven Emerson, Health Commissioner of New York City, appointed a special committee (Ralph W. Lobenstine, M.D., Clifton Edgar, M.D., and Philip Van Ingen, M.D.), in co-operation with the New York Milk Committee, to make an analysis of the facilities for maternity care in the city. The result of the survey showed that there was little prenatal work and no uniformity and that only a very small number of pregnant mothers were receiving care. It showed also that hospitals took care of 30 per cent of the deliveries, midwives delivered 30 per

cent, general practitioners delivered 30 per cent and private doctors, who might be classified as obstetricians, delivered 10 per cent. Previous to this time little or nothing had been done to regulate or control the midwives.

1916. *The National Society for the Prevention of Blindness* was created after much pioneer work and investigation, locally and throughout the states, by Carolyn Van Blarcom, R.N. She was chosen to be the executive secretary. Through these investigations it was learned that by far the greatest cause of blindness was ophthalmia neonatorum. These findings led to the passing of a law compelling all doctors and midwives to use prophylaxis in newborn babies' eyes. Also, as a direct result of Miss Van Blarcom's surveys, a school for lay midwives was started (Belleview School for Midwives, now out of existence). Miss Van Blarcom took out a midwife's license and was the first nurse in the United States so to register. The first obstetrical nursing textbook to be written by a nurse is to Miss Van Blarcom's credit. Her latest contribution to the better care of mothers and babies has been to secure for Johns Hopkins Hospital the E. Bayard Halsted Fund for medical research.

1917. The Women's City Club of New York City and the New York Milk Committee opened three prenatal centers. The one sponsored by the Women's City Club was organized as the *Maternity Service Association* and, with Frances Perkins as the first executive secretary and Miss Mabel Choate as president, provided stimulating leadership. Dr. Ralph W.

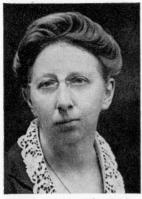

Maria L. Daniels, R.N.

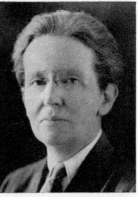

S. Josephine Baker, M.D.

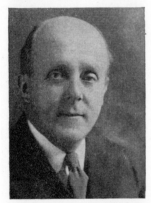

Robert L. DeNormandie, M.D.

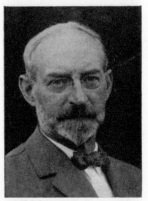

J. H. Mason Knox, Jr., M.D.

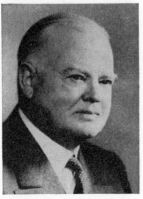

Hon. Herbert Hoover

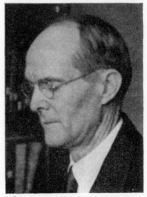

Richard A. Bolt, M.D., Dr.P.H.

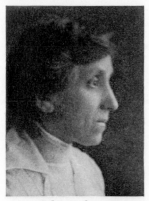

Julia Lathrop

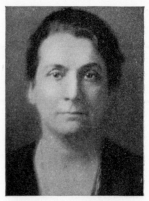

Grace Abbott

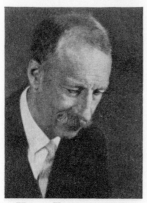

Haven Emerson, M.D.

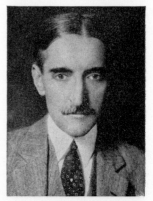

Ralph W. Lobenstine, M.D.

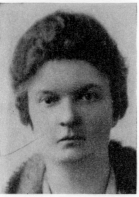

Carolyn Conant Van Blarcom, R.N.

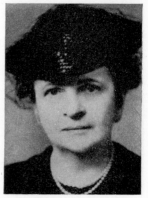

Frances Perkins

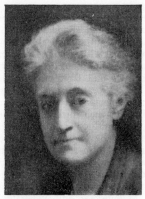

Annie W. Goodrich, R.N.

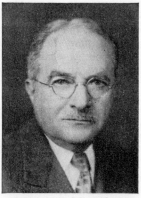

Louis I. Dublin, Ph.D.

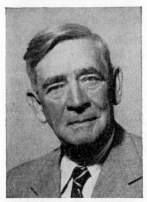

Fred L. Adair, M.D.

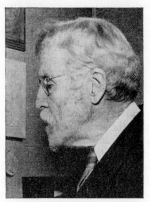

Robert L. Dickinson, M.D.

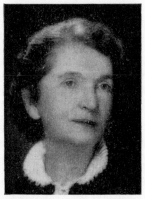

Margaret Sanger, R.N.

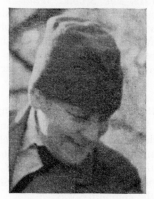

Mary Breckinridge, R.N., Sc.M.

Lobenstine, a famous obstetrician, gave much time, labor, authority and direction as chairman of the medical board. In 1918 this organization was incorporated as the Maternity Center Association and carried out the first extensive piece of organized prenatal work in the United States. Miss Anne Stevens was director. Miss Annie W. Goodrich's wise counsel, as a member of the nursing committee, gave impetus to the organization's accomplishments. Louis I. Dublin, Ph.D., associated with this movement from the beginning, made an analysis of the first 4,000 records collected by the association. This revealed the startling fact that, through prenatal care, 50 per cent of the lives of mothers might be saved, and 60 per cent of the lives of babies. Prenatal training and experience was extended to nurses throughout the world. This piece of intensive prenatal work fired increased interest in the care of mothers and babies. In 1929 the Maternity Center Association opened a school for the training of nurse midwives.

1919. *The Second White House Conference* was called by President Woodrow Wilson, as a result of the activities of the Federal Children's Bureau. It was organized in five sections. Each section was interested in a different phase of maternity and child care.

1920. *The American Committee on Maternal Welfare* was organized with Fred L. Adair, M.D., as chairman, due to his long-time interest in the public health aspects of maternity and child health. The object of the committee was:

To awaken and stimulate the interest of members of the medical profession in cooperating with public and private agencies for the protection of the health of mothers and their offspring before and during pregnancy and labor and after confinement to the end that the conditions which menace and interfere with the health or life of the mother or infant may be improved or prevented, disease and disorder corrected, health promoted and life saved; to teach the principles and practices of general and personal hygiene and health to parents and to improve and generalize the standards and methods of training physicians, nurses and others dealing with the problems of maternity.

This organization publishes the magazine *The Mother;* it also promotes the American Congress of Obstetrics and Gynecology, which has been held irregularly, in 1939, 1942, 1947, 1950 (the first International Congress with 48 countries represented) and 1952.

1921. *The Sheppard-Towner Bill* was passed by Congress, an Act for the Promotion of the Welfare and Hygiene of Maternity and Infancy, to be administered by the Children's Bureau. This bill was introduced in the 65th Congress by Congresswoman Jeanette Rankin of New Jersey. It was reported out of committee favorably but failed to pass. A second bill was introduced in the 66th Congress. It passed in the Senate but, through delays, was not considered by the House. In the first session of the 67th Congress the bill was again introduced by Senator Sheppard and Congressman Towner and, after much agitation, finally passed—an epoch in child-welfare legislation. An appropriation of $1,240,000 per year was granted for five years. The Cooper Bill, passed in 1927, extended it for two more years. This law was accepted by all of the states except three. This legislation gave a tremendous impetus to the education not only of the laity but also of the physicians. Because of this legislation there was created at once, in the states which did not already have them, departments, now quite uniformly labeled Divisions or Bureaus of Maternity and Child Health. In 1935 the Social Security Act was passed, following the plan of the Sheppard-Towner Bill. This Act appropriated $3,800,000. In 1939 the Social Security Act was amended, increasing the appropriation to $5,820,000. The amount has been increased gradually, and by 1952 (82nd Congress), $30,000,000 was appropriated for Maternal and Child Health, Crippled Children and other Child Health Services.

1923. *The National Committee for Maternal Health* was formed with Robert L. Dickinson, M.D., as secretary and later as president. This was a clearing house and a center of information on certain medical aspects of human fertility. The object was to gather and analyze material, to stimulate research, and to issue reports to the medical profession and persuade it to take a leading part in the scientific investigations of these problems in preventive medicine. No other group existed for this purpose. It was dissolved in 1950.

1923. *The Margaret Sanger Research Bureau* came into being, an affiliation of the Planned Parenthood Federation of America, Inc., for research in the field of infertility, contraception and marriage counseling.

1923. Mary Breckinridge began her investigations in Kentucky, which led to the organization of the *Frontier Nursing Service*. With this concentrated effort of all phases of maternity and infant care, the striking results proved the value of prenatal care. Through her vision, determination and unfaltering energy, Mary Breckinridge has made this organization one of world-wide renown. In 1936 the Frontier Nursing Service opened a school for the training of nurse midwives.

1925. *The Joint Committee on Maternal Welfare* was formed. This consisted of the American Gynecological Society, the American Association of Obstetrics and Gynecology and Abdominal Surgeons and the American Child Health Association (1909). Later the section of Obstetrics, Gynecology and Abdominal Surgeons of the American Medical Association was represented. They issued a pamphlet *An Outline of Delivery Care*. This stimulated the Children's Bureau to publish a concise pamphlet *Standards of Prenatal Care* (1925), an outline for the use of physicians, which did much to standardize routine procedures.

1929. *The Third White House Conference* was called by President Herbert Hoover. Mr. Hoover's interest in child welfare was very evident. The conference was very comprehensive and far-reaching and was devoted to all aspects of maternity and child care. The Children's Charter was adopted and became a Federal Act. The 45,000,000 children were analyzed in chart form to show the paramount importance of care during pregnancy and the early years.

1938. *The Conference on Better Care for Mothers and Babies* was called by the Children's Bureau. This was the first time that representatives from the states, private and public organizations, both lay and professional people, met to pool ideas.

1939. The *Maternity Consultation Service* in New York City was organized to further prenatal education and care.

1940. The *Fourth White House Conference* on Children in a Democracy was called by President Franklin D. Roosevelt. It considered the aims of our American civilization for the children in whose hands its future lies; how children can best be helped to grow into the kind of citizens who will know best how to preserve and protect our democracy. By 1940, the 48 states, the District of Columbia, Alaska, Hawaii and Puerto Rico were co-operating with the Children's Bureau in its administration of child welfare services.

1940. *The Cleveland Health Museum* was opened to the public—the first health museum in the Western Hemisphere. It is significant in the maternity field because, in its workshops, it is reproducing the *Dickinson-Belskie models*, acquired in 1945. Dr. Bruno Gebhard, Director, says that, in his belief, the use of this sculptural series in professional and lay education will advance knowledge on this all-important subject more quickly and more accurately than any other visual means thus far available.

1943. *The Emergency Maternity and Infancy Care Program* was launched to care for the wives and the babies of enlisted men in the armed forces. From $17,000,000 to $45,000,000 per year was appropriated. This Act also furthered interest in prenatal and child care.

1946. The *World Health Organization*—an agency of the United Nations—became a reality. At the first meeting in Paris 64 nations signed the constitution. The membership now (1952) totals 79 countries and 3 associated members. The object of the organization is "the attainment of the highest possible level of health of all the peoples." So far, much has been accomplished toward that end. Brock Chisholm is the director general.

1950. *The Fifth White House Conference*, with emphasis on children and youth, was called by President Harry S. Truman.

1950. *The Fred Lyman Adair Foundation* of the American Committee on Maternal Welfare was established. Its purpose is to collect funds from charitable sources to underwrite research and educational projects in this field.

Although there is yet much to be done, encouraging advances have been made over the years. During this seemingly disconnected sequence of activities, from cruelty to a child, care of the sick, keeping the well babies well, mortality studies and then to prenatal care, the aim for well mothers and healthy babies has finally been reached.

Today, in contrast with the past, the general public, including mothers and fathers, through education and publicity, realizes the need for prenatal care. Hospitals have established prenatal clinics with their many clinical facilities. Doctors encourage early supervision in order to keep the mother well and to prevent complications during the maternity cycle.

The credit for the advancement of prenatal care and child care in the United States cannot be assigned to any individual or any one organization. Our present improved conditions are the results of extended public health education, organized efforts through private and public agencies (national, state and local), the intelligent interest and co-operation of public-spirited citizens who gave time and real sums of money, public officials, physicians, nurses, social workers, teachers, dentists and many others who made possible the putting into action of these ideas.

The outgrowth has lead to continuous new researches, technics, and current statistical studies of mortality and morbidity and means of prevention.

6

Normal Pregnancy

PHYSIOLOGIC CHANGES OF PREGNANCY

By the physiologic changes of pregnancy are meant those alterations, both local and general, which affect the maternal organism as the result of pregnancy but subside at or before the end of the puerperium and leave the patient in practically the same condition in which she was before conception occurred. In other words, the physiologic changes of pregnancy are to be regarded as normal, unavoidable and purely temporary; for they are present in varying degrees in every instance, and in the case of a physically healthy woman there should be no traces of them left after convalescence is com-

plete. It must be understood that this statement does not refer to the skin markings which persist (they will be described later); nor does it refer to the slight lacerations of the genital tract, which invariably accompany a first labor. In other words, it refers only to such conditions as would have a tendency to affect temporarily and not permanently the general condition and comfort of the individual.

LOCAL CHANGES

GENITALS

The uterus increases in size to make room for the growing fetus. Naturally, the enlargement of the uterus is the most striking change

128

wrought by pregnancy and, moreover, is directly responsible for other important alterations. The growth of this organ in gestation is phenomenal. Its weight increases from 50 to 1,000 Gm., its length from 7 to some 38 cm., and its capacity from perhaps 2 cc. to about 4,500 cc. (Fig. 36). This tremendous growth is brought about principally by an enlargement of the pre-existing muscle fibers, the length of which increases from 7 to 11 times and the width to 7 times. During the first few months the uterine wall thickens from about 1 cm. to almost 2 cm., but thereafter thins to about 0.5 cm., so that at term the uterus is a rather thin-walled muscular sac.

Between the third and the fourth months of pregnancy the growing uterus rises out of the pelvis and can be palpated above the symphysis pubis, rising progressively to reach the umbilicus about the sixth month and almost impinging upon the xiphoid process at the ninth month. About two weeks before term, in most primigravidae and some multiparae, the head descends into the pelvic cavity. As a result, the uterus sinks to a lower level and at the same time falls forward. Since this relieves the upward pressure on the diaphragm and makes breathing easier, this phenomenon of the descent of the head has been called "lightening" (Fig. 85). By palpating the height of the fundus, experienced examiners can now determine the approximate duration of pregnancy.

Since the full-term pregnant uterus and its contents weigh about 12 pounds, a gravid woman may be likened to a person carrying a heavy basket pressed against the abdomen. Such a person will instinctively lean backward, in order to maintain equilibrium. This backward tilt of the torso is characteristic of pregnancy. From a practical viewpoint, it is important to note that this posture imposes increased strain on the muscles

---

SOME IMPORTANT DEFINITIONS

Gravida: a pregnant woman.

Primigravida: a woman pregnant for the first time.

Primipara: a woman who is pregnant for the first time or has recently given birth to her first child. Some obstetricians employ it only in the later meaning. Usage is not uniform.

Multipara: a woman who has become pregnant two or more times. The term carries the implication that one or more of the previous pregnancies terminated in full-term vaginal deliveries, so that the birth canal, having once been distended, is better prepared for subsequent labors than that of a primigravida.

Para I: a primipara.

Para II: a woman pregnant for the second time (and so on up numerically, Para III, Para IV, etc.)

(The plural of these words is usually formed by adding "e," as "primigravidae.")

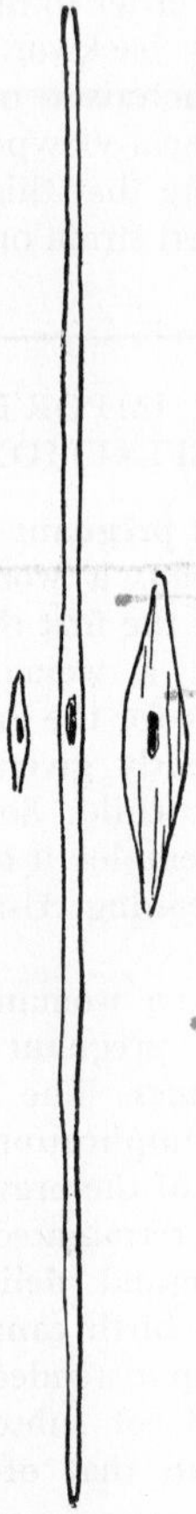

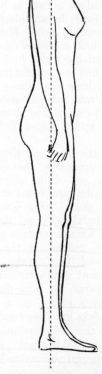

FIG. 77. Size of muscle cells. This illustrates the changes in the size of the muscle cells of the uterus before pregnancy, during pregnancy, and in the puerperium. (After Stieve)

FIG. 78. Pregnancy should and usually does improve posture. The diagram illustrates the correct standing posture showing that a straight line may be drawn from the ear to the ankle. During pregnancy "walk tall, stand tall and sit tall."

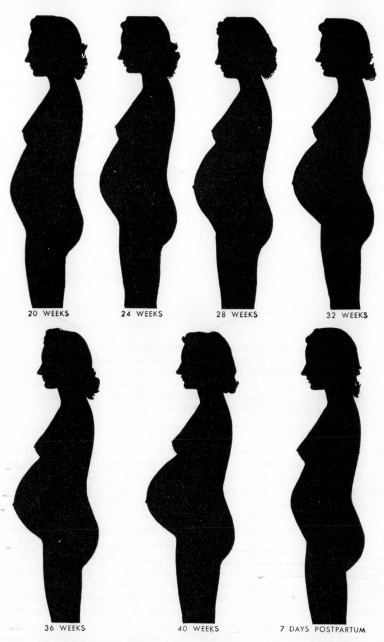

20 WEEKS   24 WEEKS   28 WEEKS   32 WEEKS

36 WEEKS   40 WEEKS   7 DAYS POSTPARTUM

FIG. 79. Changes in abdominal contour in pregnancy. Photographic study of actual patient.

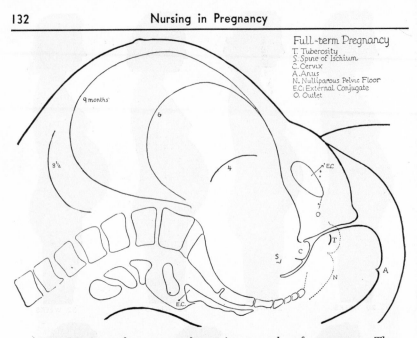

Full-term Pregnancy
T. Tuberosity
S. Spine of Ischium
C. Cervix
A. Anus
N. Nulliparous Pelvic Floor
E.C: External Conjugate
O. Outlet

FIG. 80. Size of uterus at the various months of pregnancy. The fundus (top portion of the uterus) reaches the symphysis at the third month, the umbilicus at the sixth month, and the ensiform cartilage at the middle of the eighth month, after which it "settles" into the pelvis before labor begins. (Dickinson, Robert L.: Human Sex Anatomy, Baltimore, Williams & Wilkins)

and the ligaments of the back and the thighs, and in this way is responsible for many of the muscular aches and cramps so often experienced in late pregnancy.

As shown in Figures 86 and 87, the cervix undergoes certain remarkable changes. The cervical glands become tremendously hypertrophied and distended with mucus. As a result, they form a structure resembling honeycomb and make up about one half of the entire structure of the cervix. This is the so-called "mucous plug" and is of practical importance

for a number of reasons. First, it seals the uterus from contamination by bacteria in the vagina. Second, it is expelled at the onset of labor and along with it a small amount of blood; this gives rise to the discharge of a small amount of blood-stained mucus, which is known as "show." Frequently, the onset of labor is heralded by the appearance of show. Third, since the discharge of the mucous plug removes a substantial portion of the interior of the cervix, it is very helpful in preparing for subsequent dilatation of that organ.

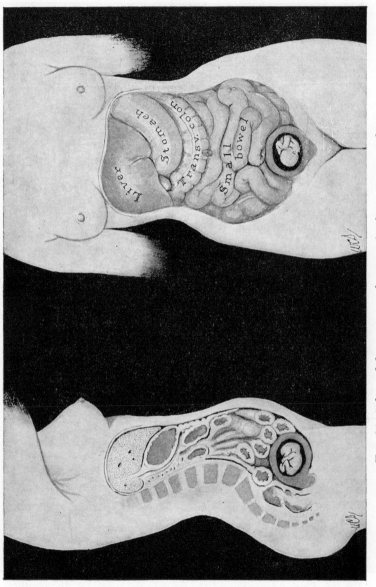

Fig. 81. Side and front views, showing the fetus at 4 months.

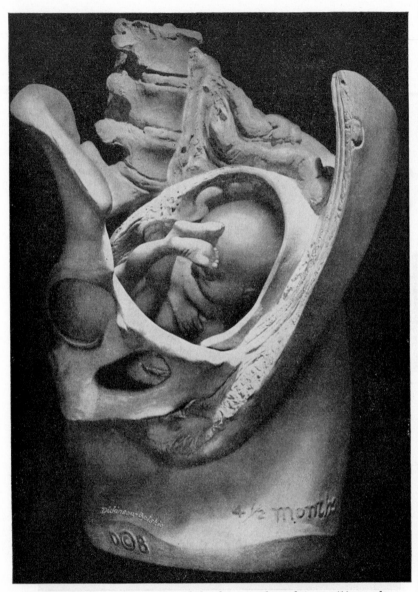

Fig. 82. Size and position of the fetus in the pelvis, at 4½ months. At about this time the mother first feels the fetal movements known as "quickening." (Dickinson-Belskie Birth Atlas Series, Maternity Center Association, New York)

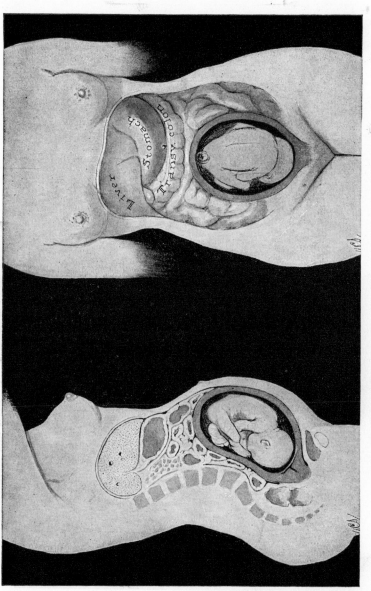

Fig. 83. Side and front views, showing the fetus at 6½ months.

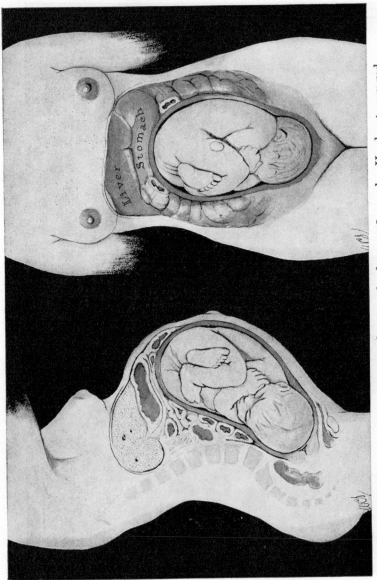

Fig. 84. Side and front views, showing the fetus at 9 months. Head not engaged.

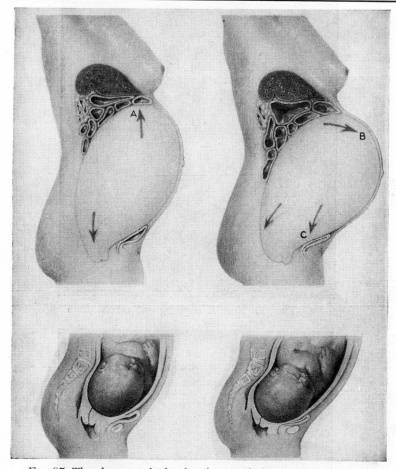

FIG. 85. The changes which take place in "lightening." (A) Pressure exerted on diaphragm before lightening. (B) Pressure relieved by falling forward of uterus. (C) Descent of head causes pressure on pelvic structures, particularly bladder.

While these changes in the uterus and the cervix are taking place, the vagina and the external genital organs are being prepared for the passage of the fetus at the time of labor. These parts become thickened and softened, and their vascularity is greatly increased. This increase in the blood supply of the genital canal gives to the tissues a dark violet hue (Chadwick's sign), in contrast with the ordinary pink color of the parts,

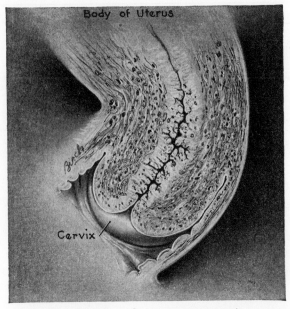

Fig. 86. Normal nonpregnant cervix.

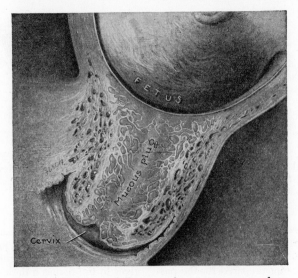

Fig. 87. Cervix at full term, showing mucous plug.

PLATE 4

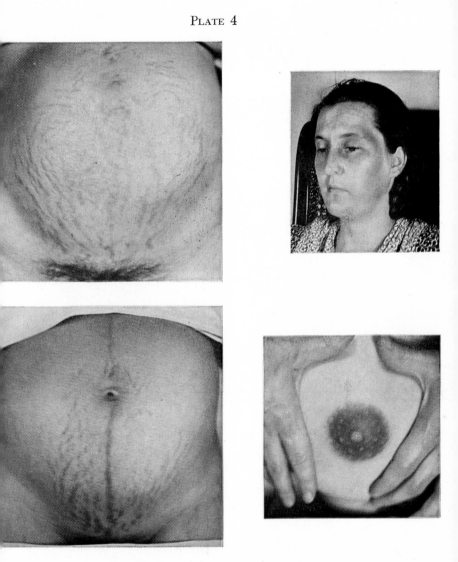

(*Left, top*) Striae gravidarum.
(*Left, bottom*) Linea nigra and also striae gravidarum.
(*Right, top*) Mask of pregnancy (chloasma).
(*Right, bottom*) Montgomery's tubercles.

PLATE 5

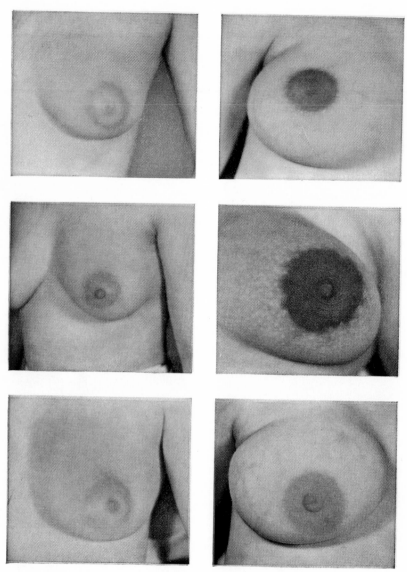

(*Left, top*) Breast in nonpregnant blonde.
(*Right, top*) Breast in pregnant blonde, showing pigmentary changes.
(*Left, center*) Breast in nonpregnant brunette.
(*Right, center*) Breast in pregnant brunette, showing pigmentary changes
and marked secondary areola.
(*Left, bottom*) Breast in nonpregnant red-haired woman.
(*Right, bottom*) Breast in pregnant red-haired woman.

and is often described as a valuable sign of pregnancy. As the result of the succulence of the parts, the vaginal secretions may be considerably increased toward the end of gestation.

Abdominal Wall

The abdomen naturally enlarges to accommodate the increase in size of the uterus. The mechanical effect of this distention of the abdominal wall causes, in the later months of pregnancy, the formation of certain reddish or bluish streaks or striations in the skin covering the sides of the abdomen and the anterior and outer aspects of the thighs. These streaks are known as "striae gravidarum" and are due to the stretching, the rupture and the atrophy of the deep connective tissue of the skin. They grow lighter after labor has taken place and finally take on the silvery whiteness of scar or cicatricial tissue. In subsequent pregnancies new reddish or bluish lines may be found mingled with old silvery-white striae or striations. The number, the size and the distribution of striae gravidarum vary exceedingly in different women, and patients occasionally are seen in whom there are no such markings whatever, even after repeated pregnancies. As the striae are due solely to the stretching of the cutis, they are not peculiar to pregnancy but may be found in other conditions which cause great abdominal distention, such as the accumulation of fat in the abdominal wall or the development of large tumors of rapid growth.

Coincident with the uterine and abdominal enlargement, the umbilicus is pushed outward until, at about the seventh month, its depression is completely obliterated and it forms merely a darkened area in the smooth and tense abdominal wall. Later, it is raised above the surrounding integument and may project, becoming about the size of a hickory nut.

Breasts

Slight temporary enlargement of the breasts, causing sensations of weight and fullness, are noted by most women prior to their menstrual periods. The earliest breast changes of pregnancy are merely exaggerations of these changes. Thus, the breasts become larger, firmer and more tender; a sensation of stretching fullness, accompanied by tingling both in the breasts and in the nipples, often develops, and, in many instances, a feeling of throbbing is also experienced. As time goes on, the nipple and the elevated, pigmented area immediately around it —the areola—become darker in color. The areola tends to become puffy, and its diameter, which in virgins rarely exceeds 1½ inches, gradually widens to reach 2 or 3 inches. Embedded in this areola lie tiny sebaceous glands which take on new growth with the advent of pregnancy and appear as little protuberances, or follicles. These have been called "Montgomery's tubercles" after a famous Irish obstetrician of the nineteenth century who described them very fully and, in summarizing, created a famous medical pun by saying, "They are, in fact, a constellation of miniature nipples scattered over a milky way" (Plate 4, D).

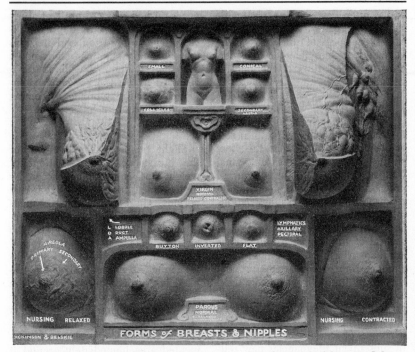

Fig. 88. Forms of breasts and nipples. (Dickinson-Belskie Models, Cleveland Health Museum, Cleveland, Ohio)

These tubercles of Montgomery make their appearance about the eighth week of pregnancy. Needless to say, all these alterations are directed ultimately at furnishing milk for the baby, and as early as the fourth month—the time varies somewhat—a little silvery-white, sticky fluid may be expressed from the nipple; this is a watery precursor of milk, called "colostrum." About the fifth month of pregnancy it is frequently observed that patches of brownish discoloration appear on the normal skin immediately surrounding the areola. This is known as the "secondary areola" and is an almost certain sign of pregnancy, provided that previously the woman never has nursed an infant (Plate 5, D). With the increasing growth and activity of the breasts, it is not surprising that a richer blood supply is needed, and to this end the blood vessels supplying the area enlarge. As a result, the veins beneath the skin of the breast, which previously may have been scarcely visible, now become more prominent and occasionally exhibit intertwining patterns over the whole chest wall.

GENERAL CHANGES

WEIGHT GAIN

During the first 3½ months of pregnancy the weight is usually stationary and may show a slight loss. During the last two thirds of the process, however, there is a steady gain, over some 24 weeks, which averages about a pound a week. The greater part of this 24-pound increment is quite understandable, as shown by the following figures:

Baby	7 pounds
Placenta	1 "
Amniotic fluid	1½ "
Increase in weight of uterus	2 "
Increase in blood volume	1 "
Increase in weight of breasts	1½ "
	—
	14 pounds

The remaining 10 pounds gained by the pregnant woman represent in part general accumulation of fat and in part the increased amount of fluid which tissues tend to retain at this time. Gains between 20 and 25 pounds are natural and in keeping with good health; usually they are lost after the baby is born.

CIRCULATION

The total volume of blood in the body increases during pregnancy about 20 per cent. This means that the pregnant woman at term has between 500 and 1,000 cc. more blood in her circulation than prior to conception. Three aspects of this change in blood volume are of great practical importance. First, it must be realized that the increase in the amount of blood is due largely to an increase in its water content; in other words, the blood is more dilute. For this reason hemoglobin estimations in pregnant women (an important part of the prenatal examination) are likely to be slightly lower than in the nonpregnant. This state is called the pseudo-anemia of pregnancy. It is not a true anemia because there is no diminution in the total amount of hemoglobin in the body but simply a dilution of the quantity previously present. Emphasis must be laid on the fact that such blood dilution never causes any great reduction in the hemoglobin values, never to levels below 70 per cent. When the hemoglobin figure is below 70 per cent, it means that the patient has a true anemia due to inadequate iron in her diet, or to some pathologic state (p. 253). A second extremely important practical point about the change in blood volume is this: although there is an increase in the amount of blood present, it is largely diluted blood; accordingly, the pregnant woman has no excess to lose at delivery. "SAVE BLOOD" is one of the most important axioms of obstetric care and one of which the nurse always should be conscious. The third important aspect of this increase in blood volume relates to its effect on the heart. As a natural result of this change, the heart has more blood to pump through the aorta—about 50 per cent more blood per minute than it did prior to pregnancy. This imposes a 50 per cent increase in the work done by the heart. In women with normal hearts this is of no particular concern, but it causes some slight tendency to shortness of breath. However, in women with heart disease, this increase in the work which the heart has to do may add to the seriousness of the complication. The nurse can be of great help in the care of expectant mothers with heart disease, and it is well that she understand the underlying process by which pregnancy may aggravate the condition.

Palpitation of the heart is not uncommon; in the early months of pregnancy this is due to sympathetic, nervous disturbance, and toward the end of gestation to the intra-abdominal pressure of the enlarged uterus.

RESPIRATION

In the later months of pregnancy the lungs are subjected to pressure from the underlying uterus, and the diaphragm may be displaced upward as much as an inch. As a consequence, shortness of breath at that period is common. It might seem that this upward displacement of the diaphragm would decrease the capacity of the lungs, but a concomitant widening of the thoracic cage occurs which more than compensates for the other change. Actually, indeed, the pregnant woman breathes in much more air than the nonpregnant. This is necessary, since the mother is called upon to oxygenate not only her own blood but, by osmosis, that of her baby as well.

DIGESTION

The digestive and excretory organs are likewise taxed, for the pregnant woman must nourish the baby as well as herself and must also excrete waste for two. During the early months the appetite is likely to be capricious and may be greatly diminished if nausea exists. As pregnancy advances and the digestive apparatus seems to become accustomed to its new conditions, the appetite is increased and may be voracious. Constipation is exceedingly common in pregnancy; at least one half of all gravid women suffer from this disorder. It is due in part to alterations in the nervous control of the bowels and in part to pressure of the growing uterus on the sigmoid and the rectum.

SKIN

Striae gravidarum, which have already been discussed in relation to changes in the abdominal wall, often develop in the breasts, the buttocks and the thighs, presumably as the result of deposition of fat in those areas with consequent stretching of the skin. Certain pigmentary changes are also common, particularly the development of a black line running from the umbilicus to the mons veneris, the so-called *linea nigra* (Plate 4, B). In certain cases, irregular spots or blotches of a muddy brown color appear on the face. This condition is known as *chloasma* or the "mask of pregnancy" (Plate 4, C). These facial deposits of pigment often cause the patient considerable mental distress, but her mind may be relieved by the assurance that they will diminish after delivery. However, the increased pigmentation of the breasts and the abdomen never disappears entirely, although it usually becomes much less pronounced. All these pigmentary deposits vary exceedingly in size, shape and distribution and usually are more marked in brunettes than in blondes.

In addition to the above skin changes, there is a great increase in the activity of the sebaceous and the sweat glands and of the hair follicles. The augmented activity of the sweat glands produces an increase in perspiration, an alteration which is helpful in the elimination of waste material.

URINARY SYSTEM

The urine in pregnancy usually is increased in amount and has a low specific gravity. Sugar is found at times, and while this is usually milk sugar from the breasts and consequently of no significance, the presence of any sugar in the urine always should be reported to the physician, since it may indicate the existence of diabetes, a serious complication. Any trace of albumin in the urine should be regarded as abnormal and likewise reported to the physician at once; although this albuminuria may be transitory, not infrequently it is evidence of another serious complication of pregnancy—toxemia.

The ureters become markedly dilated in pregnancy, particularly the right ureter. This change apparently is due in part to the pressure of the gravid uterus on the ureters as they cross the pelvic brim and in part to a certain softening which the ureteral walls undergo as the result of endocrine influences. These dilated ureters, the walls of which have now lost much of their muscular tone, are unable to propel the urine as satisfactorily as previously; consequently, stasis of urine is common. This stasis, or damming back, of urine is responsible for one of the common complications of gestations—inflammation of the kidney pelvis, or pyelitis.

EFFECTS ON THE NERVOUS SYSTEM

The effect of pregnancy on the nervous system varies greatly; while many women escape nervous manifestations entirely, some patients present more or less altered mental and emotional characteristics, varying all the way from fretfulness and peevishness to rare instances of actual insanity of a melancholy or even maniacal type. In exceptional cases the change is to the opposite extreme, and a woman who is ordinarily of an irritable disposition becomes exceedingly amiable and agreeable. The more unstable emotionally the patient is, the more likely is her nervous system to be affected by the strain of pregnancy; and the nurse who never may have witnessed any such complications during her hospital experience will doubtless encounter women thus affected in the private practice of her profession or in public health work and should be prepared for such emergencies.

ENDOCRINE CHANGES

PLACENTA

In Chapter 4 the placenta is considered simply as an organ designed to transmit nutritive substances from mother to fetus, and waste products in the reverse direction. The placenta has another highly important function: it is one of the most important organs of internal secretion. The early chorionic villi of the implanted ovum secrete a hormone which finds its way into the mother's urine and makes possible the Aschheim-Zondek and the Friedman tests for pregnancy (pp. 151 and 152). This substance is called "chorionic gonadotropin" (meaning gonad-stimulating substance derived from the chorion). It permeates the tissues of the pregnant woman, of course, and is believed by some authorities to be responsible for many changes which take place in the organism during gestation. In addition to manufacturing this new hormone, the placenta takes over from the ovary the production of estrogen and progesterone and augments greatly the amount of those substances present in the body during gestation (p. 60). This increase in estrogen and progesterone is responsible for many important changes associated with pregnancy, such as the development of the breasts and the growth of the uterus. Estrogen, although stimulating breast growth and development, suppresses actual lactation; its removal from the body at delivery, therefore, by releasing this inhibiting force, plays a part in the onset of milk production. This relationship between estrogen and lactation is only one link in the very complicated but beautifully integrated endocrine chain which dominates pregnancy and in which the placenta plays a pre-eminent role.

PITUITARY BODY

The *anterior lobe* of this small gland located at the base of the brain has already been referred to as the "master clock" which controls the menstrual cycle. Its role in pregnancy is likewise very important. It secretes a number of hormones, one of which acts on the breasts, producing lactation (the lactogenic hormone, active only after placenta has been delivered (see previous paragraph)); another acts on the thyroid, another on the ovaries, and still another on the growth process. The last is believed by some observers to be responsible for the rather coarse features which some pregnant women develop.

The *posterior lobe* of the pituitary secretes a substance which has a very strong stimulating effect on the uterine muscle, that is, an oxytocic hormone. This substance is widely employed in obstetrics to cause the uterus to contract after delivery and thereby diminish postpartum hemorrhage. It is usually referred to as "pituitary extract" or by the trade name Pituitrin.

The pituitary body is thus another important link in the endocrine network of pregnancy. As a result of the far-reaching action of its hormones and of those of the placenta, many other endocrine glands show alterations. Thus, the thyroid tends to enlarge, and the parathyroid, the adrenal and the ovary develop characteristic changes.

SUGGESTED READING

Chesley, L. C.: Weight changes and water balance in normal and toxic pregnancy, Am. J. Obst. & Gynec. 48:565, 1944.

Gillespie, Edward Clark: Principles of uterine growth in pregnancy, Am. J. Obst. & Gynec. 59:949, 1950.

Kerr, A., Jr.: Weight gain in pregnancy and its relation to weight of infants and to length of labor, Am. J. Obst. & Gynec. 45:950, 1943.

Potter, Edith: Fundamentals of Human Reproduction, New York, McGraw-Hill, 1947.

7

Signs and Symptoms of Pregnancy

CLASSIFICATION OF SIGNS AND SYMPTOMS

The first visit of the modern expectant mother to her physician is usually prompted by the query, "Am I really pregnant?" Oddly enough, this is the one question which the physician may answer equivocally, because even the most careful examination will rarely reveal clear-cut evidence of pregnancy until two menstrual periods have been missed, and occasionally the diagnosis may remain uncertain for a longer time.

Some of the signs and symptoms of pregnancy can be recognized readily by the nurse, while others can be determined accurately only by one who has had a thorough medical or technical training.

Certain signs are absolutely indicative of pregnancy, but even these may be absent or lacking if the fetus has died in the uterus. Some so-called "positive" signs are not present until about the middle of gestation, and at that time the physician usually can make a diagnosis without them, by the "circumstantial evidence" of a combination of earlier and less significant symptoms.

The signs of pregnancy are usually divided into three groups, as indicated in the following classification:

A. Presumptive Signs
   1. Menstrual suppression
   2. Nausea, vomiting, "morning sickness"
   3. Frequency of micturition
   4. Tenderness and fullness of the breasts, pigmentation, etc.
   5. "Quickening"
B. Probable Signs
   1. Abdominal changes: size, shape, pigmentation, etc.
   2. Fetal outline
   3. Bimanual signs: size of uterus, Hegar's sign, etc.
   4. Changes in cervix
   5. Braxton-Hicks contractions
   6. Violet color of the vaginal mucous membrane (Chadwick's sign)
   7. Pregnancy tests
C. Positive Signs
   1. Fetal heart sounds
   2. Fetal movements felt by examiner
   3. Roentgenogram

PRESUMPTIVE SIGNS

Menstrual Suppression

In a healthy, married woman who has previously menstruated regularly, cessation of menstruation strongly suggests that impregnation has occurred. However, not until the date of the expected period has been passed by ten days or more can any reliance be put on this symptom. When the second period is also missed, the probability naturally becomes stronger.

Although cessation of menstruation is the earliest and one of the most important symptoms of pregnancy, it should be noted that pregnancy may occur without prior menstruation and that occasionally menstruations may continue after conception. An example of the former circumstance is noted in certain Oriental countries, where girls marry at a very early age; here pregnancy frequently occurs before the menstrual periods are established. Again, nursing mothers, who usually do not menstruate during the period of lactation, often conceive at this time; more rarely, women who think they have passed the menopause are startled to find themselves pregnant. Conversely, it is not uncommon for a woman to have one or two periods after conception; but almost without exception these are brief in duration and scant in amount. In such cases the first period ordinarily lasts 2 days instead of the usual 5, and the next only a few hours. Although there are instances in which women are said to have menstruated every month throughout pregnancy, these are of questionable authenticity and are probably ascribable to some abnormality of the reproductive organs. Indeed, vaginal bleeding at any time during pregnancy should be regarded as abnormal and reported to the physician at once.

Absence of menstruation may result from a number of conditions other than pregnancy. Probably one of the most common causes of delay in the onset of the period is psychic influence, particularly fear of pregnancy. Change of climate, exposure to cold, as well as certain chronic diseases such as anemia, likewise may suppress the menstrual flow.

NAUSEA AND VOMITING

About one third of pregnant women suffer no nausea whatsoever. Another third, during the early part of pregnancy, experience waves of nausea for a few hours in the morning, but this does not proceed to the point of vomiting. In the remaining third, the nausea may cause actual vomiting. When this "morning sickness" occurs it usually makes its appearance about 2 weeks after the first missed menstrual period and subsides ordinarily after a month or 6 weeks. Since this symptom is present in many other conditions, such as ordinary indigestion, it is of no diagnostic value unless associated with other evidence of pregnancy. When the vomiting is excessive, when it lasts beyond the fourth month, when it begins in the later months, or when it affects the general health, it must be regarded as pathologic and should be reported at once to the physician. Such conditions are termed "hyperemesis gravidarum" or "pernicious vomiting" and will be discussed with complications of pregnancy in Chapter 10.

FREQUENT MICTURITION

Irritability of the bladder with resultant frequency of urination may be one of the earliest symptoms of pregnancy. It is attributed to the fact that the growing uterus stretches the base of the bladder so that a sensation results identical with that felt when the bladder wall is stretched with urine. As pregnancy progresses, the uterus rises out of the pelvis, and the frequent desire to urinate subsides. Later on, however, the symptom is likely to return, for during the last weeks the head of the fetus may press against the bladder and give rise to a similar condition. Although frequency of urination may be somewhat bothersome, both at the beginning and at the end of pregnancy, it never should constitute a reason for reducing the quantity of fluid consumed, which should be not less than 6 or 8 glasses a day. If, late in pregnancy, frequency of urination disturbs sleep, the full amount of fluid should be taken before 6 in the evening and liquid avoided until morning.

BREAST CHANGES

The breast changes of pregnancy have already been described (p. 139). In primigravidae (women pregnant for the first time) these alterations are helpful adjuncts in the diagnosis of pregnancy, but in women who have already borne children, particularly if they have nursed an infant within the past year, they naturally are of much less significance.

"QUICKENING"

This is an old term derived from an idea prevalent many years ago that at some particular moment of pregnancy life is suddenly infused into the infant. At the time this notion was in vogue, the first tangible evidence of intra-uterine life lay in the mother's feeling the baby move, and the conclusion was only natural that the infant "became alive" at the moment these movements were first felt. As is reflected in the Biblical reference to "the quick and the dead," the word "quick" used to mean "alive" and the word "quickening" meant "becoming alive." Hence, our forbears were accustomed to say that when fetal movements were first felt, "quickening" or "coming to life" of the baby had occurred. We now know that the infant is a living organism from the moment of conception, but the old term "quickening" is still used in obstetric terminology, while among the laity "feeling life" is the common synonym. As used today, quickening refers only, of course, to the active movements of the fetus as first perceived by the mother.

Quickening is usually felt toward the end of the fifth month as a tremulous fluttering low in the abdomen. The first impulses caused by the stirring of the fetus may be so faint as to raise some doubt as to their cause; later on, however, they grow stronger and often become disturbingly active.

Many fetuses, although alive and healthy, seem to move about very little in the uterus, and, not infrequently, a day or so may pass without a movement being felt. Inability to feel the baby move does not mean that it is dead or in any way a weakling but, in all probability, that it has assumed a position in which its movements are not so readily felt by the mother. Moreover, it is a well-established fact that the fetus sleeps in the uterus, and it seems likely that the periods of active movement and quiescence which the mother notices correspond with the phases of somnolence and wakefulness. Should 3 or 4 days pass without movements, the physician should be asked to listen for the fetal heart sounds. If these are heard, it means beyond doubt that the fetus is alive and presumably in good condition. It might seem that the sensations produced by the baby's movements

would be so characteristic as to make this a positive sign of pregnancy, but, oddly enough, women occasionally misinterpret movements of gas in the intestines as motions of a baby and on this basis imagine themselves pregnant. Therefore, the patient's statement that she feels the baby move, cannot be regarded as absolute proof of pregnancy.

PROBABLE SIGNS

ABDOMINAL CHANGES

The size of the abdomen in pregnancy corresponds to the increase in the size of the uterus, which, at the end of the third month, is at the level of the symphysis pubis. At the end of the fifth month it is at the level of the umbilicus, and toward the end of the ninth month at the ensiform cartilage (Figs. 80 to 84). Mere abdominal enlargement may be due to a number of causes, such as accumulation of fat in the abdominal wall, edema, or uterine or ovarian tumors. However, if the uterus can be distinctly felt to have enlarged progressively in the proportions stated above, pregnancy may properly be suspected.

The pigmentation of the abdomen, extending up the median line and surrounding the umbilicus, is, in a woman who never has borne children, almost definitely diagnostic of pregnancy; but, like the pigmentation of the breast, it varies exceedingly in different persons, often being entirely absent in decided blondes and exceptionally well marked in pronounced brunettes. As already mentioned, this pigmentation may remain from former pregnancies and

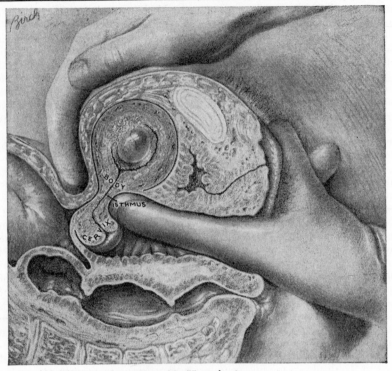

FIG. 89. Hegar's sign.

cannot be depended upon as a diagnostic sign in women who have borne children previously.

FETAL OUTLINE

After the sixth month, the outline of the fetus (head, back, knees, elbows, etc.) usually may be identified sufficiently well to justify a diagnosis of pregnancy. As pregnancy progresses, the outline of the fetus becomes more and more clearly defined. The ability to outline the fetus makes pregnancy extremely probable and, indeed, some physicians consider this a positive sign. In rare instances, however, tumors of the uterus may so mimic the fetal outline as to make this sign fallible.

BIMANUAL SIGNS

Changes in shape, size and consistency of the uterus which take place during the first three months of pregnancy are very important indications. These are noted upon the vaginal examination which shows the uterus to be more anteflexed than normal, enlarged and of a soft spongy consistency. About the sixth week the so-called Hegar's sign, so named for the man who first described it, is perceptible (Fig. 89). At this time the lower uterine segment, or lower part of the body of the uterus, becomes much softer than the cervix. So soft does it become that in its empty state (for it has not yet become encroached upon by the growing embryo) it can be compressed almost to the thinness of paper. This is one of the most valuable signs in early pregnancy. Another valuable sign found on vaginal examination is "ballottement" (from the French "balloter," to toss up like a ball). During the fourth and the fifth months of pregnancy, the fetus is small in relation to the amount of amniotic fluid present; and a sudden tap on the presenting part makes it rise in the amniotic fluid and then rebound to its original position and in turn tap the examining finger. When elicited by an experienced examiner, this response is the most certain of the probable signs.

CERVICAL CHANGES

Softening of the cervix usually occurs about the time of the second missed period. Although the nonpregnant cervix has a consistency approximate to the hardness of the tip of the nose, the pregnant cervix becomes softened like the lips.

BRAXTON-HICKS CONTRACTIONS

Uterine contractions begin during the early weeks of pregnancy and recur at intervals of from 5 to 10 minutes throughout the entire period of gestation. These contractions are painless, and the patient may or may not be conscious of them. They may be observed during the later months

by placing the hand on the abdomen and during the bimanual examination. By means of these contractions the uterine muscles contract and relax thereby enlarging in size to accommodate the growing fetus. These contractions are referred to as the Braxton-Hicks sign, after a famous London obstetrician of the last century who first described them.

VAGINAL CHANGES

The nurse will hardly be called upon to inspect the vaginal mucous membrane for evidences of pregnancy. Owing to pressure and consequent congestion within the pelvis, this mucosa becomes thickened and of a dark violet or purple color instead of its customary pinkish tint in the nonpregnant state. This sign, known as Chadwick's sign, is of no special value in women who have borne children; and as it may be due to any form of congestion or to the presence of new growth of varicosities within the pelvis, it is an unsatisfactory sign for diagnosis.

ASCHHEIM-ZONDEK TEST

Since the very dawn of civilization efforts have been made to devise a satisfactory test for pregnancy. The priest-physicians of ancient Egypt, in the earliest writings handed down to us, tell of a test then in vogue based on the seeming ability of pregnancy urine to stimulate the growth of wheat and barley seeds. The itinerant physicians of classical Greece employed similar tests, while, during the Middle Ages, the omniscient physician merely gazed at the urine and claimed in this way to be able to diagnose not only pregnancy but many other conditions.

Today, thanks to the investigations of two doctors, Aschheim and Zondek, we have at last a sound and trustworthy test for pregnancy, and, interestingly enough, like the tests of old, urine is used for the purpose.

The test is based on the fact that the early chorionic villi of the implanted ovum secrete a hormone which is excreted in the maternal urine, where it can be detected by certain laboratory procedures. The method of its detection is dependent on the fact that this hormone, when injected into immature mice and rats, produces very dramatic and readily visible changes in the ovaries of these animals. Ordinarily, of course, the ovaries of these very immature, 3-week-old animals would be completely quiescent, but when this hormone has been injected the follicles manifest very rapid development, so much so that several of them rupture or ovulate within a few days after the injection. Accordingly, if the urine of a pregnant woman has been injected into one of these animals, mere inspection of their ovaries after a suitable interval (96 hours) will reveal tiny points of follicle rupture; this is a positive test and means that the woman is pregnant. If the woman is not pregnant, the immature ovaries will remain in their quiescent condition and no points of follicle rupture will be seen—a negative test.

If urine for this test is to be obtained, the patient is supplied with a sterile 6- or 8-ounce bottle containing a few drops of some preservative such as toluene to prevent bacterial decomposition of the urine. She is instructed to drink no water after the evening meal and then, upon arising the next morning, to void into a dry, clean basin. The urine then is poured into the bottle, which should be sent to the laboratory without delay. The purpose of withholding fluids the night before is to secure a concentrated urine specimen. If it is impossible to send the bottle to the laboratory immediately, it should be kept cold.

The great value of this test lies in the fact that it becomes positive very early in pregnancy, usually about 10 days after the first missed menstrual period, sometimes even a few days earlier than this. If the test has been carried out properly, it is accurate in more than 95 per cent of cases. It is not, therefore, an absolutely positive sign of pregnancy, but very nearly so.

FRIEDMAN TEST

From a practical viewpoint the Aschheim-Zondek test has certain drawbacks: first, the difficulty of securing immature mice of the correct age for the procedure; and, second, the long 96-hour wait before the result can be obtained. In order to circumvent these difficulties, Dr. M. H. Friedman, of the University of Pennsylvania, introduced an important modification of the test, using adult female rabbits instead of mice. Ten cc. (some authorities recommend 5) is injected into the marginal vein of the rabbit's ear, and 48 hours later the animal is anesthetized, the abdomen is opened, and the ovaries are inspected. The presence of ruptured follicles means that the test is positive.

For the reasons stated, the Friedman test is used in the United States much more widely than the original Aschheim-Zondek test and may be regarded as the standard laboratory test for pregnancy in this country. Its accuracy is about the same as the Aschheim-Zondek test; it likewise becomes positive about 10 days after the first missed period, and the manner of collecting the urine is the same.

HOGBEN, OR TOAD (OR FROG), TEST

Another laboratory procedure which has gained wide popularity in the diagnosis of pregnancy is the South African toad or frog test, more properly called the Hogben test after the British physician who first described it in 1930. The test is based on the fact that female South African toads, when injected with the urine of a pregnant woman, extrude a large number of eggs within 8 to 12 hours. The particular toad employed in any given test is kept in a small glass aquarium with a black paper or cardboard beneath it, and, against this background, the myriad of eggs extruded (in the event the test is positive) are very plainly seen. The accuracy of this test is about the same as that of the Aschheim-Zondek and the Friedman tests, and it possesses the additional advantage that the result of a test can be ascertained much sooner than with the other procedures. It owes its popularity in part also to the fact that the toads are easier and more economical to keep than are rats or rabbits.

OTHER TESTS

Research continues with the hope that a quick, simple, accurate pregnancy test may be developed which will give immediate results and one that may be used in the physician's office. Reports have been made on several of these tests, such as:

1. The prostigmine test (by Drs. Soskin, Wachtel and Hechter, 1940) whereby three doses of prostigmine are given hypodermically either daily or on alternate days. Sometimes only two injections are necessary. Within 3 to 5 days after the last injection, it is usually possible to determine whether or not pregnancy exists. If prostigmine fails to induce menstruation when it is overdue, the patient is undoubtedly pregnant.

2. Colostrum cutaneous test (by Drs. Falls, Freda and Cohen, 1941). A preparation of colostrum is injected into the skin. If pregnancy exists there will be a faint reaction or none at all, while the nonpregnant patient reacts with a prominent wheal typical of an allergic response. Reactions appear within half an hour.

3. The Richardson test (1949). A specimen of urine is examined, and if substantial amounts in sufficient concentration of estrone are found the test indicates pregnancy. Results are available within half an hour after the specimen is analyzed.

4. The 5-minute test for pregnancy (Roland, 1951). Dr. Roland examines mucus from the cervix microscopically. If a fern leaf pattern appears (formed by the crystallization of a substance not yet identified) the patient is *not* pregnant; if the pattern does not appear, ovulation is indicated; the lateness and the absence of the menses are caused by pregnancy.

POSITIVE SIGNS

Although certain of the signs mentioned above—notably, the hormone tests, ballottement, and palpating the fetal outline—are nearly positive evidences of pregnancy, they are not 100 per cent certain; errors in technic occasionally invalidate the hormone tests, while, on rare occasions, the

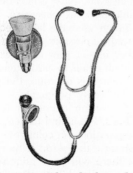

FIG. 90. The dual stethoscope, which consists of the bell and diaphragm, is used for the high-pitched murmurs such as the fetal heart sounds and determinations of blood pressure. (Becton-Dickinson Company)

other signs may be simulated by non-pregnant pathologic states. Using the term "positive" in the strict sense, there are only three positive signs of pregnancy, namely, the fetal heart sounds, fetal movements felt by the examiner, and the x-ray outline of the fetal skeleton.

FETAL HEART SOUNDS

When heard distinctly by an experienced examiner, the fetal heart sounds can leave no doubt about the existence of pregnancy. Ordinarily, they become audible at about the middle of pregnancy, or around the twentieth week. If the abdominal wall is thin and conditions are favorable, they may become audible as

early as the eighteenth week, but obesity or an excessive quantity of amniotic fluid may render them inaudible until a much later date. While the usual rate of the fetal heart is about 140 per minute, it may vary under quite normal conditions between 120 and 150. The use of the ordinary bell stethoscope, steadied by rubber bands, is entirely satisfactory, but in doubtful cases the head stethoscope is superior, since the listener receives bone conduction of sound through the headpiece in addition to that transmitted to the eardrum.

The nurse will do well, while learning the characteristics of the fetal heart sounds, to accustom herself to place one hand on the maternal pulse and feel its rate at the same time that she hears the fetal heart tones through the stethoscope. Occasionally, the inexperienced beginner, particularly when listening high in the abdomen, may mistake the mother's heart sounds for those of the baby. Since the two are not synchronous (fetal 140, maternal 80), the method suggested above will obviate this mistake; in other words, if the rate that comes to your ear through the stethoscope is the same as the maternal pulse, it is probably the mother's heart beat; on the other hand, if the rates are different, it is undoubtedly the sound of the fetal heart.

Two additional sounds may be heard in listening over the pregnant uterus: the funic souffle and the uterine souffle. Since the word "souffle" means a blowing murmur, or whizzing sound, the nature of these two sounds is similar, but their timing and causation are quite dif-

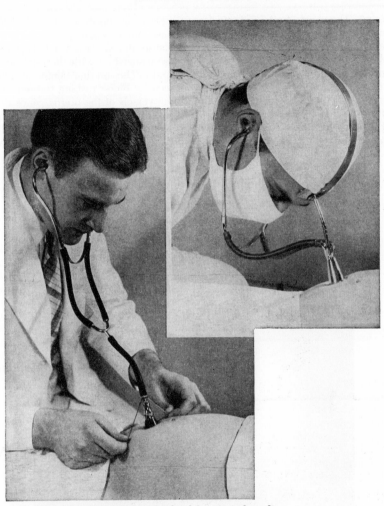

Fig. 91 (*Left*). Listening to fetal heart with ordinary stethoscope.

Fig. 92 (*Right*). Listening to fetal heart with head stethoscope. The head stethoscope gives bone conduction of sound in addition to otic (by ear) and in addition possesses the advantage that it can be used when hands are sterile.

ferent. The word "funis" is Latin for umbilical cord, and, accordingly, the term funic souffle refers to a soft blowing murmur caused by blood rushing through the umbilical cord. Since this blood is propelled by the fetal heart, the rate of funic souffle is synchronous with the fetal heart. It is heard only occasionally, perhaps in one case out of every six. The funic souffle is a positive sign of pregnancy, but it is not usually so listed because almost always it is heard in close association with the fetal heart sounds. The uterine souffle is produced by blood rushing through the large vessels of the uterus. Since this is maternal blood, propelled by the maternal heart, it is synchronous with her heart rate. In other words, the

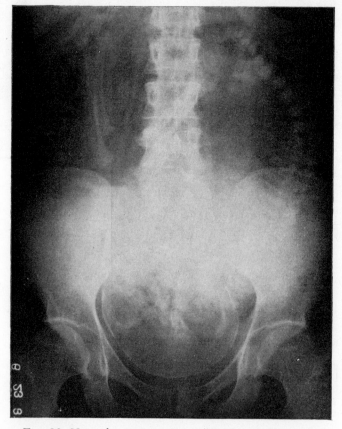

Fig. 93. Normal vertex position. (Bonner, K. P.: Radiography and Clinical Photography, Eastman Kodak Company, Rochester, N. Y.)

rate of the funic souffle is ordinarily around 140 per minute (or the same as the fetal heart rate); that of the uterine souffle, near 80 (maternal heart rate).

FETAL MOVEMENTS FELT BY EXAMINER

As already noted, fetal movements supposedly felt by the patient may be very misleading in the diagnosis

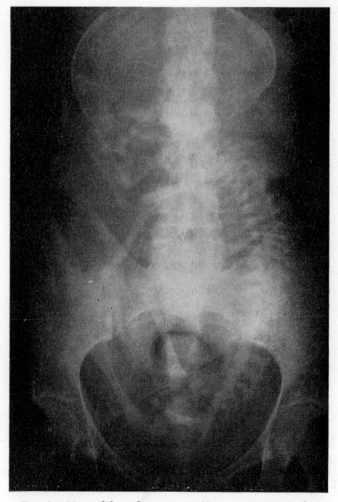

Fig. 94. Normal breech position. (Bonner, K. P.: Radiography and Clinical Photography, Eastman Kodak Company, Rochester, N. Y.)

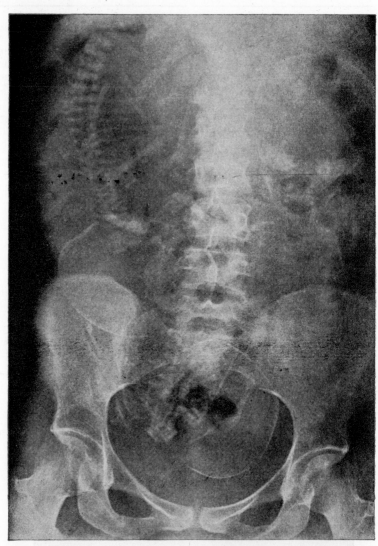

FIG. 95. Roentgenogram of triplets *in utero*. (Bonner, K. P.: Radiography and Clinical Photography, Eastman Kodak Company, Rochester, N. Y.)

of pregnancy. However, when an experienced examiner feels the characteristic thrust or kick of the baby against his hand, this is positive evidence of pregnancy. Often this can be felt after the end of the fifth month.

ROENTGENOGRAM

A roentgenogram showing the outline of the fetal skeleton is, of course, undeniable proof of pregnancy. How early the fetal skeleton will show in the roentgenogram depends upon the thickness of the abdominal wall, the x-ray equipment, and other factors. It has been demonstrated as early as the fourteenth week and is quite easily demonstrated, as a rule, after the twentieth week.

SUGGESTED READING

Foote, E. C., and Jones, G. E. S.: An evaluation of the Hogben pregnancy test, Am. J. Obst. & Gynec. 51:672, 1946.

Galloway, Charles E.: The cervix in pregnancy, Am. J. Obst. & Gynec. 59:999, 1950.

Merkel, Richard L.: A comparative study of chemical tests for the early diagnosis of pregnancy, Am. J. Obst. & Gynec. 60:827, 1950.

Salmon, U. J., Geist, S. H., Salmon, A. A., and Frank, I. L.: A new six-hour test for pregnancy, J. Clin. Endocrinol. 2:137, 1942.

Saunders, C. B.: Frog test for pregnancy, Texas State J. Med. 42:375, 1946.

Schwartz, Harold A.: A simple, accurate pregnancy test, Am. J. Obst. & Gynec. 59:213, 1950.

Weisman, A. I., Snyder, A. F., and Coates, C. W.: Use of the African clawed frog (*Xenopus laevis Daudin*) as a rapid diagnostic test for pregnancy, West. J. Surg. 50:557, 1942.

8

Prenatal Care

DEFINITION

Antepartal or prenatal care is the care and the supervision given to a pregnant woman so that she may pass through pregnancy with the minimum of mental and physical discomfort, and a maximum of mental and physical fitness at its termination, with the reward of a well baby, and the knowledge whereby mother and baby may be kept well. This is accomplished through the combined efforts of the obstetrician, the nurse and the expectant parents.

Prenatal care may be considered the foundation for the normal development, the adequate growth and the good health of the baby. During this formative period the teeth, the bones and the various systems of the body have their beginnings, as well as the foundations for his future health. For the mother adequate prenatal care aids in stabilizing the daily health. As pregnancy advances the demands of the fetus increase. Since individuals react differently to pregnancy, this supervision is of the utmost importance in detecting these reactions. This supervision not only helps to relieve discomforts and to prevent accidents and complications but also aids in ensuring a more rapid convalescence and continued good health.

THE IMPORTANCE OF PREVENTIVE CARE

Prior to the rise of the present-day scientific obstetrics, the physician usually had only one interview with his patient before he saw her in labor, and often at this interview he merely sought to compute the expected date of confinement. When he next saw her she might be in the throes of an eclamptic convulsion or striving vainly to overcome the resistance offered by a contracted pelvis. It is in the prevention of such calamities as these that care and supervision of the pregnant mother has been found to be of such value. Indeed, prenatal care is an absolute necessity if a substantial number of women are to avoid disaster; and it is helpful to all. If it were possible, care should begin as early as the patient conceives or perhaps even earlier than that; not only at the very beginning of her pregnant period, but ideally with her own mother's prenatal state, which likewise had everything to do with the patient's health. In recent years much has been accomplished through premarital and prepregnancy examinations to determine the patient's fitness for pregnancy. More and more doctors are offering this care and encouraging this plan toward positive health.

MEDICAL CARE

Today the emphasis is on positive health, to determine the health status of those anticipating parenthood. Every patient should be under the care of her obstetrician during the entire period of her pregnancy. She should report to him at intervals of at least every 3 or 4 weeks during the earlier months of pregnancy and oftener during the last two months. Each doctor has his own system.

At the first examination the history of the patient is taken, then a general medical examination is carried out, and finally the obstetric examination, which includes an examination *per vaginam,* is given. The examination may be carried out according to the following outline.

PRENATAL RECORD

The name and the address of the patient, her age and parity, and the date of the latest menstrual period are recorded, and the date of delivery is estimated. Inquiries are made regarding the family history, with special reference to any condition likely to affect childbearing, such as tuberculosis or multiple pregnancy. The personal history of the patient is then reviewed not only in regard to previous diseases and operations but particularly in relation to any difficulties experienced in previous pregnancies and labors, such as miscarriages, prolonged labor, death of infant, hemorrhage and other complications. Inquiry is then made into the history of the present pregnancy, especially in relation to nausea, edema of the feet or the face, headache, visual disturbance, vaginal bleeding, constipation, breathlessness, sleeplessness, cramps, heartburn, lower abdominal pain, vaginal discharge, varicose veins, etc. Usually a suitable form for recording these particulars is employed. As a rule obstetricians, hospital clinics and organiaztions have their own forms for recording these details.

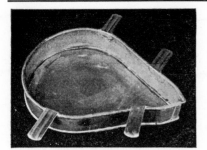

Fig. 96. Metal basin for collecting urine in office. The brackets are allowed to rest on the sides of the toilet bowl, and the seat is placed over them.

General Medical Examination

The general medical examination includes weighing the patient, taking the blood pressure, inspecting the teeth and the throat and making an examination by auscultation and percussion of the heart and the lungs. Opportunity is taken at this time to inspect the breast and the nipples, particularly in relation to their suitability for subsequent nursing. From an obstetric viewpoint one of the important details of the general medical examination is the measurement of the blood pressure, both systolic and diastolic. This is usually carried out first and always should be done when the patient is seen on subsequent visits. As will be explained subsequently, any substantial increase in blood pressure indicates one of the most serious complications in pregnancy—toxemia. A fact for the nurse to keep in mind is that any sudden or gradual rise in the blood pressure is significant and may be alarming.

Obstetric Examination

The obstetric examination is comprised of three parts: (1) palpation and auscultation of the abdomen; (2) estimation of pelvic measurements; and (3) vaginal examination. Palpation and auscultation of the abdomen yield valuable information concerning the size and the position of the fetus. The great importance of careful pelvic measurements has already been emphasized, while the purpose of the vaginal examination (aside from its use in the diagnosis of pregnancy) is to rule out abnormalities of the birth canal (particularly those which might impede labor) and to take the diagonal conjugate measurement.

Laboratory Tests

The laboratory tests carried out in prenatal care are the urine examination, the blood test for syphilis, the estimation of the hemoglobin, tests for the Rh factor and blood type. At the first examination, the urine is tested for albumin and sugar and, at all subsequent examinations, for albumin. A convenient method for collecting urine speciments in the office or clinic is show in the accompanying illustration. If the patient brings the specimen from home she should be instructed to collect a part of the first urine voided in the morning. The blood for the Wassermann or other syphilis test is usually obtained by venipuncture, and a portion of this same blood may be employed for the Rh factor and hemoglobin estimation. Since many pregnant women develop anemia, the latter examination is highly important. If the test for the Rh factor shows the patient to be Rh negative, it may be necessary to check the husband. It is also a wise precaution for the doctor to have the husband's blood type. A metabolism test is routine in the practice of some obstetricians.

The routine estimation of weight at regular intervals during pregnancy is an important detail of prenatal care. Any marked gain or loss in weight will be discussed by the obstetrician. At first the average gain in weight of the fetus is 1 Gm. daily; nine tenths of the weight is gained after the fifth month, and one half of the weight of the fetus is acquired during the last 8 weeks. It is to be expected that most pregnant women have an average gain in weight of between 20 and 25 pounds during pregnancy. In any excessive weight gain, or for a patient who is markedly overweight, one of the low caloric diets may be prescribed in an effort to control the weight. Weight gain should be considered in relation to the patient's general physical condition.

RETURN VISITS

At return visits, careful inquiry is made into the general well-being of the patient, and questions are asked concerning any untoward signs and symptoms, such as edema of the fingers or the face, bleeding, constipation and headache. The patient is then weighed, her blood pressure is taken, and the urine is analyzed for albumin. While an abdominal examination is usually carried out at this time, some physicians limit their abdominal examinations, in so far as

return visits are concerned, to the later months. During these visits the patient should avail herself of the opportunity of asking the doctor any questions which may be of concern to her.

INSTRUCTIONS TO PATIENTS

After the routine examination, the patient is instructed regarding diet, rest and sleep, daily intestinal elimination, proper exercise, fresh air and sunshine, bathing, clothing, recreation and dental care. It is usually possible and always desirable to assure the patient that the findings on examination were normal, and that she may anticipate an uneventful pregnancy followed by an uncomplicated delivery. At the same time, however, she is tactfully instructed regarding certain danger signals which demand immediate report to the doctor. These symptoms are as follows:

1. *Vaginal bleeding, no matter how slight*
2. *Swelling of the face or the fingers*
3. *Severe continuous headache*
4. *Dimness or blurring of vision*
5. *Pain in the abdomen*
6. *Persistent vomiting*
7. *Chills and fever*
8. *Sudden escape of fluid from the vagina*

Pregnancy may swing the balance of a well person to an ill person or a very ill person. In addition to this detailed supervision, the patient needs an explanation of the changes that are taking place within her body. This intelligent instruction will

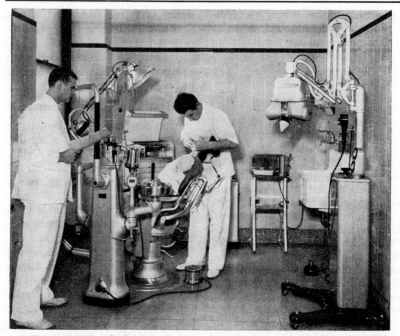

Fig. 97. Dental clinic as a part of an obstetric service. Because of the emphasis today on the preventive care of the teeth during pregnancy, some hospitals have a dental clinic in connection with their prenatal supervision. (Margaret Hague Maternity Hospital, Jersey City, N. J.)

give her greater reassurance and self-confidence. An understanding and sympathetic attitude will do much to buoy the patient's morale.

As the patient approaches full term, she should also be instructed about the signs and symptoms of oncoming labor, so that she may know when the process is beginning and when to notify the doctor. At this time, also, the doctor should know the frequency of contractions and any other pertinent symptoms. If a hospital delivery is planned, the admission routine should have been explained.

DENTAL CARE

Care of the Teeth. At the very beginning of pregnancy, an expectant mother should place herself under the care of a dentist and have her teeth cleaned and have any existing cavities filled, at least temporarily. This is necessary because teeth are important in relation to adequate mastication of food. Some physicians think it advisable to have an x-ray examination of the teeth made as a routine procedure in order to discover any existing foci of infection.

Dental sepsis in the mother is held responsible for many ills. A septic focus "somewhere in the body" is a recognized cause of illness that may arise later. However, before having any extensive dental work the patient should consult her obstetrician. It should be carefully explained to the mother that, if her diet is not supplying the baby with lime salts and other necessities in sufficient amounts to build his bones and teeth, they may be absorbed from her own tissues. She will then understand why such emphasis is placed on this care during pregnancy. The teeth of a pregnant woman are apt to undergo certain destructive changes, which has given rise to the old saying, "For every child, a tooth." But this need not be true, if the proper attention is given to the care of the teeth and nutrition during pregnancy. If, at this time, there may be an increased acidity of the saliva, this condition can be helped by using an alkaline mouthwash of milk of magnesia or sodium bicarbonate. The teeth should be brushed carefully upon arising, before retiring and after each meal, and rinsed with the suggested mouthwash. It is well to explain that a toothbrush with medium or hard bristles should be used and replaced if the bristles become soft.

NURSING CARE

THE PRENATAL CLINIC NURSE

In the prenatal clinic the student nurse has the opportunity to observe and assist in the prenatal examinations. Under supervision the nurse may be permitted to offer nursing advice to the patient. This experience in the outpatient department will also include such details as greeting the patient and making her comfortable while she waits for her appointment with the doctor. In the interim, through these courtesies, there may be an opportunity to find out about any new symptoms or problems that the patient may have and to report them to the proper person. In hospitals where the appointment system is used the waiting time for the patient is minimized. In others, the patient may have to wait longer periods. This waiting time may be utilized by providing the patient with reading material. Visual aids such as posters and charts may be both instructive and diverting. Through these contacts with patients, the nurse can also emphasize the importance of the patient's keeping her return appointment with the doctor or clinic.

THE PUBLIC HEALTH NURSE

The extensive adoption of early antepartum care by various institutions, both lay and medical, is doing much to improve obstetric standards; and, in connection with this movement, the public health nurse has proved to be an invaluable asset. During the period before prenatal care was fully accepted, a case-finding program was a part of some organizations, i.e., the nurse would canvass the district for pregnant mothers. In recent years the demand for hospital deliveries has increased rapidly, so that the trend toward hospital care has exceeded the number of hospital beds to accommodate patients. Therefore, hospitals are not accepting patients unless they register early in pregnancy. This has been a favorable contribution to early registration and, in larger cities espe-

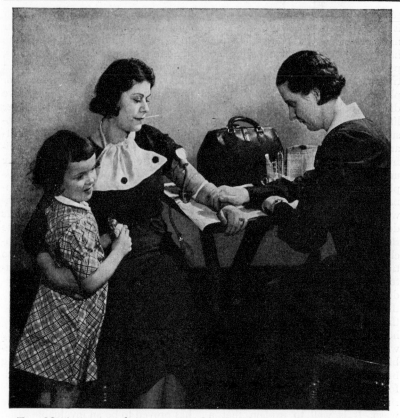

FIG. 98. A nurse making a prenatal visit. The procedure may be the same whether it is done in the medical center or in the home.

cially, has eliminated the necessity for a case-finding program. In some rural areas it is still necessary to work with all available resources, such as the postman, political organizations, newspapers, the church, etc., to reach the delinquent maternity cases.

In a well-organized prenatal program the public health nurse is the intermediary between the physician and his patient. By frequent visits and well-kept records the nurse keeps the obstetrician informed of his patient's condition, thereby relieving him of unnecessary expenditure of time. By these visits the nurse may be the first to note the onset of premonitory symptoms which, if neglected, might lead to serious complications. She is able to stress the importance of regular visits to the physician and to see to it that these visits are made. It now often falls to the nurse to give much of the de-

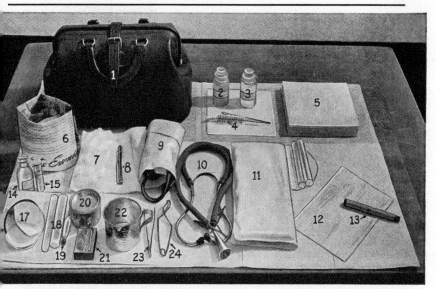

Fig. 99. The articles used in a prenatal visit: 1, prenatal bag, contents removed and bag closed; 2, bottle of green soap; 3, bottle of alcohol; 4, test tube brush on napkin; 5, napkins, enough for one visit; 6, cornucopia for waste; 7, pieces of cotton broken up ready for cleaning thermometers, etc.; 8, thermometer; 9, blood pressure machine; 10, stethoscope; 11, apron (in case), paper, waterproof or muslin; 12, patient's record; 13, fountain pen; 14, dropper bottle of acetic acid; 15, litmus paper; 16, funnel; 17, filter paper arranged in funnel; 18, test tube and urinometer glass; 19, urinometer; 20, sterno; 21, matches; 22, tin cup for urine specimen (a paper cup may be used instead); 23, thumb forceps; 24, test tube holder.

tailed instruction in hygiene and the mode of living, besides teaching the patient how to make some of the necessary preparations for delivery. The patient should learn before the birth of the baby what things will be needed for herself and for the baby and how to prepare them; at this time, too, the expectant mother should take her first lessons in the care of the newborn. In the analysis of this program the nurse's records, through their content, accuracy and value, show the needs to be met. Prenatal care, then, consists of care and advice given by the physician, the complete co-operation on the part of the parents in carrying out this advice, and conscientious follow-up visits on the part of the nurse. The combined efforts of many may be involved in the care of the pregnant mother: doctor, dentist, nurse and social worker, each, in his own field, making a related contribution toward better health.

THE OBSTETRIC SOCIAL WORKER

In recent years the fact that the Social Service Department in the hospital constitutes an important part of the team of a hospital staff has been generally recognized. Previously, there were a few hospitals that appreciated this valuable asset, but today it is accepted as essential. The physical needs of the patient comprise only one of the many responsibilities carried by this department. The Social Service workers are thought of as the individuals able to evaluate and alleviate the so-called social conditions, to make studies, to visit homes, to ascertain the physical and emotional needs of the family. In addition, such a worker is the understanding counselor between the family and the patient during her hospital stay. In many hospitals the social worker takes the patient's history after the initial examination, and, from the physical and social findings, plans are made to meet the patient's needs. Among the many problems encountered are: placing of older children during the mother's hospital stay; arranging for a working housekeeper, if the mother is delivered at home or if the children of school age must be kept at home; planning for convalescent care for the mother and giving financial and material assistance. In her observation of other children in the home, the social worker may be the first person to notice a neglected orthopedic condition, to suspect a need for a chest roentgenogram or to observe a possible sight difficulty.

In the care of the unmarried mother and the problem of illegitimacy there are many aspects to be considered, from planning for a place for the expectant mother to live before delivery to making arrangements for the care of the mother and the baby after delivery. Since these situations often involve the placing of the baby and plans for the re-employment of the mother, the social worker must know about the available approved nursing homes and the suitable employment agencies. Because some unmarried mothers are interested in having their babies adopted, she must be familiar with the legal aspects of adoption, as well as the reputable adoption agencies.

By her observation and experience, the social worker may make it possible for the doctor to see the patient not only as an individual maternity patient but also as an important member of the family, and the family as an integral part of the community. In many hospitals the public health nurse, or the combination social worker and public health nurse, makes a valuable contribution to the patient and to public health.

NUTRITION IN PREGNANCY

Much attention has been given to the diets of the different groups of patients, such as the diabetics, the nephritics, etc.; but until recently little has been said of the diet for the pregnant mother. The reasons for adequate diet during pregnancy are: to maintain the daily strength; to prepare for labor by building up the muscle tone of the body to meet the crisis of labor and delivery; to hasten the patient's convalescence after delivery; to prepare the patient to be better able to nurse the baby; to pro-

284 CASES (216 FIRST SERIES + 68 SIBLINGS)

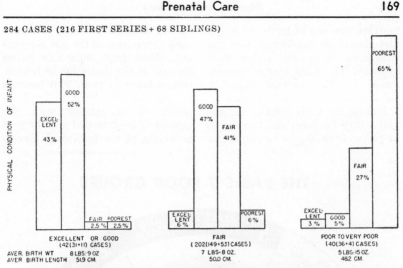

PRENATAL DIETARY RATING (MEAN GENERAL)

CHART 9. Relationship of prenatal dietary rating to the physical condition of the infant at birth. In the study of 284 cases of the physical condition of the baby at birth when the maternal diet was "excellent or good" 95 per cent of the infants were in good or excellent condition, and only 5 per cent were in either fair or poorest physical condition. In contrast, when the maternal diet was "poor to very poor" 65 per cent of the infants were in the poorest physical condition at birth, and 27 per cent were in fair condition, while 8 per cent were in good or excellent physical condition. The consistent shift in physical condition of the infant with each change in dietary rating in either direction is impressive.

The statement still remains true that all of the stillborn infants, all of the neonatal deaths but one, all of the premature infants but one (a neonatal death), all of the functionally immature infants, and most of the congenital defects were found in the group of infants born to mothers with "poor or very poor" prenatal diets. Since no major effort was made to change the dietary habits of these women, it is probable that in the majority of the cases the prenatal dietary rating was representative also of long-established food habits. (Burke, B. S.; Stevenson, S. S.; Worcester, J., and Stuart, H. C.: Nutrition Studies During Pregnancy. Relation of Maternal Nutrition to Condition of Infant at Birth: Study of Siblings, J. Nut. 38:453)

vide the essential building materials for the developing fetus.

During the prenatal state the mother is providing nourishment for two. The second individual is, of course, very tiny by comparison, but because of the rapid formation of new tissue the variety of materials needed for the building of the baby's body (its bones, nervous system, muscles, two sets of teeth, etc.), the diet should be considered from the standpoint of quality rather than quantity. The daily energy requirements for the average pregnant woman are about 2,500 calories.

During the early months the appetite may be poor, and there may be phases of dislike for certain foods. Should there be nausea at this time, close supervision of the diet is necessary. Then, later, there may be an increase in the desire for all food or certain types of food. This increase in appetite may have to be disciplined in accordance with the amount of food needed and the gain in weight of the individual. Sweets

THE BASIC 7 FOOD GROUPS

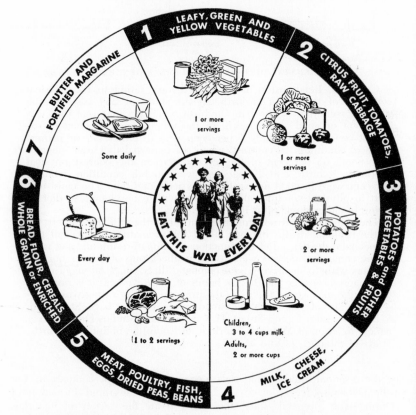

Fig. 100. Poster issued by Bureau of Human Nutrition and Home Economics, U. S. Department of Agriculture, Washington, D. C.

and desserts, as well as the habit of frequent nibbling, should be avoided because of the interference with appetite for the more essential foods and the additional weight added by such foods. The so-called occasional craving for unusual articles of food should be kept in mind; it may mean the lack of a certain element in the dietary that the body seems to demand. Any desires of this nature may be granted with safety if they agree with the patient and are not exceptional in amount or content. If the

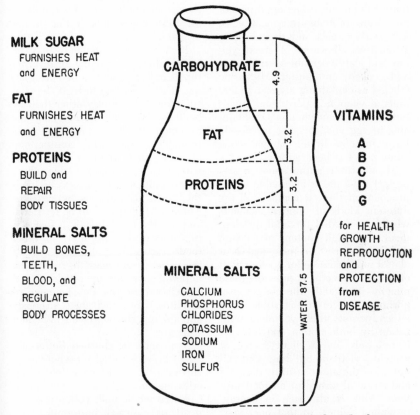

MILK SUGAR
FURNISHES HEAT
and ENERGY

FAT
FURNISHES HEAT
and ENERGY

PROTEINS
BUILD and
REPAIR
BODY TISSUES

MINERAL SALTS
BUILD BONES,
TEETH,
BLOOD, and
REGULATE
BODY PROCESSES

CARBOHYDRATE   4.9

FAT   3.2

PROTEINS   3.2

MINERAL SALTS
CALCIUM
PHOSPHORUS
CHLORIDES
POTASSIUM
SODIUM
IRON
SULFUR

WATER 87.5

VITAMINS

A
B
C
D
G

for HEALTH
GROWTH
REPRODUCTION
and
PROTECTION
from
DISEASE

Fig. 101. Although milk varies somewhat with the breed of cow and the cow's food, the above chart gives a good idea of the reason why milk should be an important part of the diet in pregnancy. Milk is considered nonfattening because it supplies the largest portions of all needed proteins, minerals and vitamins with the fewest number of calories. (Maternity Consultation Service)

diet supplies all the needs of the patient and the growing fetus, such cravings probably will not occur.

The Normal Diet. The physician will regulate the patient's diet according to her condition; but, as a rule, if her previous diet has been nourishing and well balanced, few changes will be necessary. There should be a relatively large proportion of fluids, including one quart of milk daily; proteins from meat, eggs, fish; dark cereals and dark breads; a generous allowance of green, yellow and leafy vegetables; fruits—raw and cooked; and butter. Margarine labeled as containing at least 15,000 units of vitamin A per pound equals butter, except for vitamin D, obtainable in egg yolk, liver or in capsule form; in some brands of margarine vitamin D has been added.

MILK. Milk is nature's most nearly perfect food and is invaluable to the pregnant mother. It contains all the different kinds of mineral elements which are needed for fetal development. The high content of calcium and phosphorus in milk makes it almost indispensable for good growth of bone and teeth; it provides these minerals in exactly the correct proportions and in a digestible form which permits their complete utilization by both mother and fetus. It is not only an excellent source of protein or tissue-building material but also the most readily digested and easily absorbed of all food proteins. Milk is also rich in energy-providing values, so that one quart a day alone furnishes almost one fourth of the total energy requirements. Finally, milk contains some of the most important vitamins, particularly vitamin A, which increases

resistance to infection and safeguards the development of the fetus.

Due to the superb qualities of milk as such, an effort should be made to have the patient drink two glasses of milk a day. The remainder of the quart may be taken in some other form such as soup, cocoa, desserts, etc. Evaporated and dried milk, which have the same food value as the original milk, may be substituted for fresh cow's milk if that is not available.

For some patients, milk may be constipating or fattening, or distasteful. If milk is found to be constipating, it is preferable to treat the constipation in some way other than by omitting the milk. Concerning the fattening effect of milk, the gain probably is due to the consumption of more food than is needed. If weight gain is excessive, the milk is not at fault, but the excess of foods such as bread, potatoes and desserts. These are the articles to be restricted and not the milk. If milk is distasteful, it may be disguised in other foods (soups, cereals, desserts). If the patient were made to realize the importance of this one article of food in relation to the development of this little baby which she is anxiously anticipating, this sacrifice will be met willingly.

Skim milk or churned buttermilk might be substituted for whole milk. However, it would have fewer calories and less vitamin A per quart. Cultured whole milk (often used instead of churned buttermilk) has practically the same caloric value and vitamin content. American cheese may also be used as an occasional substitute. One ounce of cheese contains approximately the same minerals and vitamins as a large glass of whole milk.

PROTEINS. Meat, eggs and seafoods are high in protein, and, during pregnancy, the need for these foods is increased—not only to meet the mother's own demand but also to supply the elements needed by the fetus from conception to birth for the development of all the delicate and intricate systems of his body. These foods contain vitamins and valuable minerals, but their main value is in their amino acids or building stones, as they are sometimes called. Meat, eggs and fish contain complete proteins, proteins which have all of the ten amino acids which are necessary to maintain life and support growth.

Dark cereals and dark breads should replace the white varieties, because they contain more vitamin B. Wheat contains one complete protein, but most cereals do not. When cereals are supplemented by milk they become adequate for growth as well as for maintaining life. Bread should be buttered as a means of increasing the vitamin A intake. The coarse cereals and the dark breads add roughage to the diet. Vitamin B and roughage both help to counteract constipation.

VEGETABLES. (Especially leaf, stem, green and yellow varieties.) These are also daily food necessities for the pregnant mother because they are rich sources of iron, calcium and several vitamins. It is desirable to include at least two of these each day—one raw and the other cooked. At mealtimes there is no reasonable limit to the amount of lettuce, tomatoes, celery, string beans, carrots, beets and asparagus which may be eaten, and by increasing the quantity of such foods to several times the amount ordinarily taken it is usually possible to satisfy the appetite without gaining abnormally in weight. Fresh frozen vegetables are a good alternate. Canned vegetables may be used if fresh are not available. If a good brand is obtained the vitamin content is often higher than that of vegetables cooked at home. The careful preparation and cooking of vegetables will help to retain the maximum of vitamin and mineral content. Some vegetables contain several incomplete proteins which add to the total protein intake.

In addition to their value as nutrient agents, these vegetables deserve an important place in the diet as laxative agents, since their fibrous framework increases the bulk of the intestinal content and thereby stimulates the muscular, eliminative action of the intestines.

FRUITS. Citrus fruits—oranges, lemons and grapefruit—are the best sources of vitamin C. Most of these fruits also supply vitamins A and B. Tomatoes are also an excellent source of vitamin C; the amount, however, must be twice that of the citrus fruits to supply the same amount of vitamin. The other fruits, both raw and cooked (prunes, apricots, etc.), contain important minerals (iron and copper) as well as vitamins. Fruits are not only important for their vitamins, but they may be the means of stimulating a lagging appetite and counteracting constipation (see pp. 182 and 212). Fruit may be used in many ways—as juices, combination salads, additions to cereals or in-between-meal refreshments and desserts, such as gelatins and puddings.

Fruits contain some incomplete proteins but only supplement the other proteins.

FLUIDS. Fluids should be taken freely, averaging 6 to 8 glasses daily. Water aids in the circulation of the blood, body fluids, and the distribution of mineral salts, as well as stimulating the digestion and the assimilation of foods. Fluids help to increase perspiration and to regulate elimination from intestines and kidneys. Tea and coffee may be included in the daily fluid quota if not found to be constipating or sleep-disturbing.

VITAMINS. Vitamins are the *live* elements in food and are essential to life. The best sources are the natural foods. In order to retain the vitamin value in foods they must be fresh, carefully prepared and not overcooked. During pregnancy and lactation the vitamin needs are increased. Some physicians add vitamin preparations to the diet in order to assure an adequate requirement. During the winter months, especially in the northern parts of the United States, the diet is usually supplemented by vitamin D, the antirachitic vitamin. This is usually given in the form of cod-liver oil or concentrates. Some authorities prescribe vitamin K during the last two weeks of pregnancy to prevent hemorrhage in the newborn.

IODINE. Only very small amounts of iodine are needed for the health of the mother and the fetus. These are very readily obtained from seafoods and daily cod-liver oil. However, in certain localities around the Great Lakes and in the Northwest the water supply and the vegetables grown are poor in iodine. This deficiency may be counteracted by the use of iodized salt, or the physician may prescribe small amounts of iodine.

LIME AND OTHER ESSENTIAL SALTS. A leaflet issued by the Health Service Bureau of the Wesleyan and General Assurance Society, Birmingham, on "What Our Foodstuffs Consist Of," puts the mineral salts first on the list of essential constituents and gives a useful little outline of the principal salts, their functions and sources. The following is a summary of the information given on this subject.

Calcium is required by every tissue in the body, especially the bones and the teeth. Without calcium the blood will not clot, the heart will not beat, the muscles will not work, and the clotting of milk in the stomach, which is necessary to enable it to be digested, cannot take place.

Phosphorus is an essential constituent of all the cells and tissues of the body, particularly nervous tissue.

Iron is needed to enable the blood to carry oxygen from the lungs to the tissues.

Chlorine is present in all tissues of the body; consequently, it is an essential constituent of the diet.

Iodine is required, particularly by the thyroid gland situated in the neck, the function of which is to control the combustion of food in the body and to influence growth and body changes, especially before adult life.

The principal foods from which these desirable salts are obtained are: calcium from cheese, eggs, milk, oatmeal, vegetables; phosphorus from cheese, eggs, meats, milk, oatmeal, green vegetables; iron from egg yolk, meat, whole grains, green vegetables; chlorine from table salt; and iodine from fish, and iodized salt.

The value of vegetables is emphasized, especially when they are steamed, or boiled in very little water, to preserve the soluble salts. One of the important but little-understood functions of vegetables is the yielding of basic residues of combustion. The leaflet points out that if the food taken yields excessive acid waste products, a great burden of work is thrown on the kidneys.

Weight Control. Weight gain during pregnancy between 20 and 25 pounds is natural and in keeping with good health. Usually this weight is lost after the birth of the baby. However, increases in weight over 25 pounds are undesirable, for a number of reasons. First, they represent unnecessary poundage for the muscles of the legs and the back to carry about, and this suddenly imposed strain is a common cause of backache, pain in the legs and also easy fatigability. Second, certain serious complications of pregnancy, preeclampsia and eclampsia (see p. 225) are less common in patients whose weight increment is moderate. Third, if weight gain in pregnancy is excessive, it is likely to be a permanent acquisition, so that, if the expectant mother is interested in retaining her figure, she should also be interested in limiting weight gain at this time.

Obstetricians are emphasizing more and more the importance of weight control in pregnancy; some insist on as little as 15 pounds gain. If the patient's weight gain after the third month is of the order of 3 pounds a month it may be regarded as satisfactory, but if it exceeds 4 pounds a month, steps should be taken to control it. Here a nurse can be of the utmost help in advising expectant mothers about certain simple steps which may be taken,

particularly in regard to the curtailment of certain nonessential foods.

Some of the specific suggestions which may be made are as follows.

1. The patient should be acquainted with the amazing fattening potentialities of certain common nonessential foods—foods which, in many people's minds, scarcely deserve that term at all, because most of them are likely to be regarded as mere snacks without appreciable effects on total caloric intake. Actually, these little extras taken between meals or at bedtime constitute one of the most common causes for excessive weight gain in pregnancy and at other times. Even a glass of ginger ale or Coca-Cola averages 100 calories. A chocolate bar approximates more than 300 calories. A single cocktail or highball runs 200 calories. A doughnut (without icing) plus a cup of cocoa yields 400 calories, while the average malted milk served at soda fountains contains some 500 calories. Pie à la mode approximates 600 calories. When it is recalled, as stated on page 170, that 2,500 calories per day is generally recognized as a satisfactory allowance for pregnancy —really, the uppermost limit—it is plain that these "little snacks" mentioned above loom tremendously large in relation to the total caloric allotment. They simply must be eliminated, if the patient is gaining excessively. When hungry between meals, she may take the glass of milk scheduled for dinner, omitting it from her evening meal.

2. The patient should be reminded that the way in which a food is prepared may affect its caloric or fattening value almost as much as the nature of the food itself. Fail-

ure to heed this fact has resulted in many women gaining weight on diets which should cause them, theoretically at least, to lose. Perhaps the simplest way to show how the preparation of a food affects its caloric value is to be found in fried foods. Although the caloric content of a poached or boiled egg is about 80 calories and is so calculated in dietary lists, once that egg is fried, its caloric value jumps to around 120 calories because of the fat absorbed by the egg in cooking. A level tablespoon of fat, let it be emphasized, yields approximately 120 calories. In regard to soups and desserts, it is common knowledge that those made with milk are of much less caloric content than those made with cream, and that those made with skimmed milk are still lower. When flour or cheese in addition to cream is used, as in escalloped or au gratin dishes, the calories soar to unbelievable heights; in general, for this group of foods, the smoother and the more delicious the taste, the higher the caloric value.

The intrinsic caloric value of foods of the same type varies widely. Fruits show considerable variation according to their degree of sweetness. Canned fruit may be very high in calories because of the sugar in the syrup. Likewise, meats vary greatly in their caloric contents, lean meats being low and those with much fat in their substance being high. As an example of the latter, an average serving of linked country sausage may exceed 600 calories. To summarize this aspect of weight control in pregnancy, the patient should be reminded that fried foods invariably possess a high caloric con-

tent and must be curtailed or eliminated altogether; that milk, preferably skimmed milk, should be substituted for cream in preparing soups and desserts; and that lean meat rather than fatty meat must be chosen, and fresh fruit rather than canned.

3. The next suggestion to make to the patients is to substitute skimmed milk for the whole milk included in the recommendation about diet in pregnancy. This reduces forthwith the caloric content of the diet by about 300 calories—no small sum. But be sure that the patient is taking this quart of milk every day. It provides more proteins, minerals and vitamins for less calories (and money) than any other food; and skimmed milk contains, of course, as much protein and minerals (including calcium) as does whole milk.

4. The next suggestion is an easy one to carry out, namely, to substitute saccharin for sugar, not only in coffee or tea, but for cereals and fruits. For cereals, it may be dissolved in the milk used over them, and to sweeten fruits it may be dissolved in a little water. Saccharin should not be cooked, as this makes it bitter.

5. The salt ordinarily added to foods in the kitchen should be reduced drastically or eliminated altogether. If there is any one substance which should be curtailed in any pregnancy, it is salt. First, the amount of salt consumed by the average person is far in excess of human requirements. Second, even if no salt were added to foods either in the kitchen or at the table, this mineral is so widely distributed in food materials that the likelihood of short-

age would be exceedingly remote. Finally, there is a definite relationship between the amount of salt eaten and the amount of water retained by the body; that is, the greater the salt intake the greater the tendency of tissues to absorb water. The tissues of the pregnant woman manifest a particular avidity for water, as is evidenced by the tendency of the face and the fingers to become puffy, and if, superimposed on this tendency, there is an excess of salt in the diet, the tissues may become actually water-logged, with dire consequences. It is a good rule to add no salt to the food at the table and, in the kitchen, to add a little less than one would like, this being the rule for any prenatal patient. In the case of excessive weight gain in pregnancy, it is quite possible that a still further reduction in salt, as recommended above, will reduce superfluous body water and cause a substantial weight loss. At first, this salt-poor diet may seem so bland and tasteless as to constitute something of a hardship; but it is surprising how quickly patients get used to it and after a few days, as a rule, do not object to it appreciably.

6. If the above recommendations do not serve to curtail weight gain, the patient should eliminate all desserts. For these fresh fruits can be substituted, sweetened, if necessary, with saccharin water.

7. It may be necessary to remind the patient to take servings of average size and only one serving.

Because of the importance of the subject the nurse must understand that it will not suffice simply to tell the patients to reduce their food consumption or to eat less fattening foods. Directions, to be effective, must be specific as well as rather comprehensive and should be reviewed with the patients in a sympathetic and understanding way. Above all, it must be emphasized that no curtailment is to be made in food essentials—doubly essential in pregnancy—such as milk, green and yellow leafy vegetables, proteins, minerals and vitamins.

If the simple suggestions listed above are not effective, the case is a special one, and the patient should be under the personal dietary supervision of her physician or a trained nutritionist.

GENERAL HYGIENE

Rest, Relaxation and Sleep. Because rest and sleep are so essential for health, the nurse must emphasize this detail in her teaching during the prenatal period. Pregnant women become tired more readily; therefore, the prevention of fatigue must be stressed very emphatically. The body is made up of various types of cells, each type with a specific function. Depletion of nerve-cell energy results in fatigue, and fatigue causes certain reactions in the body which are injurious. For all body processes, such as digestion, metabolism, working, playing and studying, our nerve-cell energy is utilized. Nature has made provision for some reduction in our normal energy without injury to health. Beyond this limit, the symptoms of fatigue are evidenced in irritability, apprehension, tendency to worry and restlessness. These symptoms are sometimes very subtle and misleading, but, in contrast, human beings are very conscious of tired muscles. It is more important to

avoid fatigue than to have to recover from overfatigue. The pregnant woman should rest to prevent
this fatigue. Rest and sleep replenish
the cell energy. As Dr. Jastrow says
of this code of rest and sleep, they
"must be shaped according to the individual's nervous disposition, habits
of life, age, and circumstances." If
patients cannot sleep, they should
attempt to rest. Rest is the ability to
relax. Patients should learn to relax,
seek diversion and acquire new interests. Even the balanced diet contributes an influence to this habit of
rest and sleep. There is no code so
variable, so necessarily adapted to
the individual, as that of rest and
sleep. The final test is whether the
day's work is done with zest and
energy to spare. Advise the patient
to take a nap or at least to rest for
one half hour every morning and
every afternoon. If this is not possible, advise her to lie down, if for
only a few minutes, several times a
day, using a light, warm covering in
a well-ventilated room. It should be
explained that rest means not only to
lie down or perhaps to sleep, but to
lie down comfortably—to relax—to
rest the body, the mind, the abdominal muscles, the legs and the back
and to stretch out, and so make it
easier for the heart to pump the
blood to the extremities. During the
last months of pregnancy, a small
pillow used for support of the abdomen, while the patient lies on her
side, does much to relieve the discomfort common during this period
and adds materially to the degree of
rest that the patient gets in a given
time.

Suggest to the patient that, instead
of standing, she sit whenever pos-

sible, even while doing her housework.

Often the so-called minor discomforts of pregnancy can be overcome
by rest. Rest and the right-angle position (Fig. 126) are advised for
swelling, edema and varicosities of
the lower extremities. Rest and the
Sims' position (Fig. 128) are advised
for varicosities of the vulva and the
rectum. Even for the more serious
abnormalities, which the nurse may
discover in her routine visit, the
simple aids included in "diet and
rest" may help much until more specific orders from the obstetrician can
be obtained.

The expectant mother should get
as much sleep as she feels she needs.
Some people need more than others.
It is advisable to sleep with open
windows, but out of a draft. Fresh
air, a comfortable bed with light
warm coverings, and a warm bath
with a hot drink before retiring will
aid in producing sleep. With many
women it is the nervous system that
suffers most during pregnancy, and
nervousness is always exaggerated by
loss of sleep. Loss of sleep also lowers individual resistance.

Exercise in the open air during
pregnancy is usually very beneficial,
but for each individual patient the
obstetrician must decide whether the
customary exercise should be increased or diminished. There should
be a difference in the amount of exercise for the early and the late periods
of pregnancy. When pregnancy is
advanced, exercise may be limited in
comparison with the amount advised
previously. Exercise usually means
diversion, and, of course, this phase
is most important. Exercise also
steadies the nerves, quiets the mind,

promotes sleep and stimulates the appetite, all of which are valuable aids to the pregnant mother.

Walking in the fresh air is quite generally preferred to every other form of exercise during pregnancy, because it stimulates the muscular activity of the entire body, strengthens some of the muscles used during labor and is available to all women. Exercise of any kind should not be fatiguing; to secure the most beneficial results it should be combined with fresh air and sunlight, as well as periods of rest.

The woman who does her own housework needs less planned exercise. However, she does need fresh air, sunshine and diversion. It is far better for the patient to be occupied than to sit idly, but standing for long periods of time should be avoided. Lifting heavy objects, moving furniture, reaching to hang curtains, running a sewing machine by foot—all have been blamed for causing miscarriages and should be avoided during pregnancy. Dancing, swimming, horseback riding, tennis, golf and long climbs are all subjects that should be discussed with the obstetrician for his final decision.

One medical authority says: "Laughter is the most wholesome and rejuvenating of all exercises, improving the appetite and digestion, enhancing the freedom of circulation and respiration, giving sparkle to the eye and the glow of youth to the cheek. The man or woman with a mirthful temperament eats well, sleeps well, works well and enjoys life.

"Laughter accomplishes the seeming miracle of both relaxing and resting the tissues while it vigorously exercises certain muscles and organs. When you are laughing heartily you are drawing in large quantities of oxygen to vitalize the blood, and your abdominal muscles are shaking and massaging the digestive organs and stimulating them to greater activity. This vibratory action is also beneficial to the heart. Laughter is an exercise that can be safely indulged in by young and old, regardless of state of health. Mirth is to the human body what sunshine is to vegetation." *

Fresh Air and Sunshine. The expectant mother should have all the fresh air and sunshine that is possible, and both exercise and rest out of doors are most beneficial. It must not be forgotten, however, that many patients have to spend much of their time indoors. The house should be kept well ventilated but free from noticeable drafts.

Much emphasis is now placed upon the beneficial effects of sunlight, and rightly so, because sunlight is helpfully stimulating to the body tissues, as has been demonstrated frequently by its healing effect in treating wounds and tuberculous lesions. These stimulating effects are mainly due to the blue-violet rays present in light, some of which are visible when light is broken up by a prism or in a rainbow. There are, however, very active or stimulating violet rays not visible to the eyes, even when it is so split or broken, and we speak of them as ultraviolet rays (ultra, beyond; therefore, beyond visibility). Clothing, smoke, glass, even air itself, interfere with the passage of light; and in the

* Georgia's Health.

wintertime when the sunlight is not very strong, very little ultraviolet light is available, and the little that might be received is decreased greatly by the extra clothing worn and the greater amount of time spent indoors. It is important, therefore, to emphasize the value of open air, rest and exercise, especially since pregnant women tend to spend too much time indoors. Even two minutes with the windows open is beneficial. Many obstetricians advise cod-liver oil or concentrates as an additional safeguard.

Care of the Skin. The skin may be more active during pregnancy, and there may be increased or decreased perspiration, resulting in irritation or dryness. Since the skin is one of the organs of elimination, bathing is obviously important, and baths should be taken daily because they are stimulating, refreshing and relaxing. They not only act as a tonic and general invigorator, but they favor elimination through the skin as well. Elimination through the skin is thought to lessen the strain of elimination by the kidneys.

During pregnancy, baths may be taken with warm water and soap just before retiring at night, followed with a brisk rub; but, if preferred, a morning bath may be taken, with tepid or cool water (85° to 90° F.). Chilling the body should be avoided, as this interferes with the action of the skin. Cold baths, cold sponges and cold shower baths never should be taken unless approval has been given by the obstetrician. During the last two months of pregnancy, many physicians advise the use of a shower, spray or sponge bath; these are chosen in preference to tub baths

with the idea of avoiding the possible entrance of the bath water into the vaginal canal. This choice is logical and recommends itself. An additional argument against tub baths is that the patient is more awkward at this period, due to the increased weight of the abdomen, and she should take no chance of slipping or falling.

Care of the Breasts and the Nipples. A detail of prenatal care is the care of the breasts and the nipples. It is one of the important preparations for breast feeding. During the prenatal period the breasts often have a feeling of fullness and weight. A well-fitted supporting brassière may relieve these discomforts. There may be sufficient secretion from the nipples to necessitate wearing a pad to protect the clothing. The daily care of the nipples should begin between the sixth and the seventh months; and the reason for it, as well as the actual procedure, should be explained to the patient. Early in pregnancy the breasts begin to secrete, and this secretion often oozes out on the surface of the nipple, and in drying it forms fine imperceptible crusts. If these crusts are allowed to remain, the skin underneath becomes tender; and if left until the baby arrives and nurses, this tender skin area is likely to crack. With this condition there is always a possibility of infection.

Instruct the patient to wash her hands, and then, with a piece of clean cotton, bathe each nipple thoroughly with white soap and clean water, for one or two minutes, making sure that all dried material has been removed. She should then dry them with a clean towel and apply

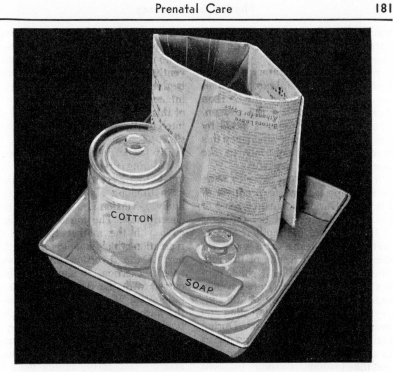

FIG. 102. Breast tray containing soap in a covered dish, cotton, and a paper cornucopia. If the mother will assemble these articles on a tray, it will simplify the care that she should give her nipples after the sixth month of pregnancy. Some obstetricians believe that the nipples should be anointed daily with mineral oil, cocoa butter, lanolin, etc., and others believe that equally good results are obtained by doing nothing other than maintaining simple daily cleanliness. (Maternity Consultation Service, New York)

albolene, lanolin, cocoa-butter, Ortho Massé or petroleum jelly (the lanolin and petroleum jelly may stain the clothes) with the ends of the two fingers and the thumb, so that it is worked into the tiny creases found on the surface of the nipple. This care toughens the nipples and prepares them for the baby's nursing. Some physicians recommend daily bathing with warm water followed by careful drying. If the patient's nipples are flat or inverted, this care should begin earlier, and when applying the albolene, the nipple should be grasped by the thumb and the two fingers and drawn out and held for a moment. This treatment should be given two or three times daily, so that the nipples may be made more prominent for the baby to grasp. In extreme cases where the nipples are badly inverted, the obstetrician will instruct the nurse concerning the care needed.

Elimination: Respiratory, Urinary, Intestinal. *The respiratory system* functions to eliminate the carbon dioxide and to utilize the oxygen. The utilization of foods is aided by this exchange. During pregnancy this is of importance not only to the mother but also to the fetus.

The urinary system excretes some of the important waste products of the body. During pregnancy some of the waste products of the fetus, as well as those of the mother, are excreted. This means extra work for the kidneys. The results of the routine urine examination (which cannot be overemphasized) are not only indices of the efficiency of the kidneys but also means of detecting any overtaxing of these organs. During early pregnancy, the enlarging uterus in the pelvic cavity makes pressure on the bladder, causing frequent urination. This condition is relieved when the uterus rises into the abdominal cavity. Pressure on the bladder may also be experienced in the later months of pregnancy, due to the weight of the uterus.

Intestinal elimination is also important because of the waste products to be eliminated by both mother and fetus. For the patient who has adhered to regular habits of elimination, there usually is little or no change in the daily routine. However, there are individuals whose elimination is affected by the weight and the pressue of the enlarged uterus, and constipation results (p. 212).

Personal habits of intelligent daily hygiene are the best resource that the expectant mother has, and, fortunately, the present-day tendency is to emphasize strongly the preventive value of regular elimination, beginning with the habit-training in infancy and throughout life. The lack of this training must be combated as intelligently and as tactfully as possible.

Diversion. Recreation is a necessity during pregnancy and will do much to divert the mother's mind from thinking about labor and delivery. Diversion also may add to her cheerfulness. The nurse should discuss with the mother the type of recreation which is most relaxing for her. If the diversion involves any special exertion, it should be discussed with the doctor before it is attempted. If a "blue day" comes, the husband should make it his particular responsibility to provide a means of counteracting it. The nurse should also discuss with the father and the rest of the family ways in which they might help to make this period less of a strain. The husband cannot take over the innumerable discomforts that always are associated with pregnancy, but he can do a great deal to help his wife get the much-needed diversion. He can help her to secure the kind of social relaxation that she enjoys most. Good books, radios, music, movies, interest in sports, television, cards, sewing clubs, church functions, visiting, driving, walking and having friends come in are some of the means of providing relaxation and diversion. However, the patient should avoid crowds, chances of infection and all conditions likely to cause a sense of discomfort. Amusements, exercise, rest and recreation at proper intervals help to keep the pregnant mother well and happy. Encourage the mother to provide an environment of happy anticipation for the baby.

Traveling. This is perhaps a detail of prenatal care which most patients think very little about, unless there is a tendency to nausea or the patient has had a previous miscarriage. The general advice is to avoid traveling during the first and the last months of pregnancy and at the times when menstruation would normally occur. The obstetrician should be consulted concerning the advisability of traveling at any time during the entire period of pregnancy.

Mental Attitudes. Pregnancy should be a happy experience. When husbands understand more about the discomforts involved in pregnancy, their helpfulness will be greater. Labor must be faced, and this crisis of the maternity period must create some concern for the mother. Consideration and understanding on the part of the husband, the family, the doctor and the nurse do much to relieve fears, anxieties and uncertainties.

Marital Relations.

The expectant mother should be under the guidance of a good physician from the time pregnancy is suspected. Great care especially should be taken to avoid excess in the sex relationship or to avoid it entirely at the period when menstruation would normally have taken place because of the greater liability of the wife to miscarriage at such times.

The husband is to realize that his wife is under nervous and emotional tensions which call for constant patience and sympathy on his part. If at this time a wife should feel a sudden and unexplained aversion to her mate, let both of them realize that it is an accompaniment of her condition rather than a real change in her attitude. Failing to realize this some young people have drifted into unpleasant and bitter experiences of misunderstanding and conflict entirely out of harmony with their love for each other. Sometimes this happens partly because the nature of the wife calls out all the more at this time, in a way which she may not fully understand, for the full sympathy and support of her husband. If he will help her through the early part of this period by unusual considerateness in every way he will be likely to find that health and happiness are improved, as her whole being meets the call of motherhood.*

Smoking. While most obstetricians disapprove of excessive smoking in pregnancy, there is no reason for believing that a woman who smokes moderately, ten cigarettes or less a day, need change her custom at this time, except as preparation for hospitalization in a ward where smoking is prohibited. This subject should be discussed with the doctor.

* Wood, L. F., and Dickinson, R. L.: Harmony in Marriage, New York, Round Table Press, p. 90.

SUGGESTED READING

American Committee on Maternal Welfare, Inc. (F. L. Adair, Editor): Maternal Care, Chicago, Univ. Chicago Press, 1937.

Becker, J. E., Bickerstaff, H. J., and Eastman, N. J.: Nutrition in relation to pregnancy and lactation, Am. J. Pub. Health 31:1263, 1941.

Bigley, Loretta I.: Community Clinics, Philadelphia, Lippincott, 1947.

Block, Babette: The unmarried mother, Pub. Health Nursing 43: 375, 1951.

Brooks, Ethel G.: Union health departments, Pub. Health Nursing 42:335, 1950.

Burke, Bertha S.: Nutrition during pregnancy, a review, J. Am. Dietet. A. 20:735, 1944.

Burke, B. S., Beal, V. A., Kirkwood, S. B., and Stuart, H. C.: The influence of nutrition during pregnancy upon the condition of the infant at birth, J. Nutrition, June, 1943. (Reprints—Children's Bureau.)

Burke, Bertha S., Stevenson, Stuart S., Worcester, Jane, and Stuart, Harold C.: Nutrition studies during pregnancy, J. Nutrition 38:453, 1949.

Burke, Bertha S., and Kirkwood, Samuel B.: Problems and methods in nutrition services for pregnant women, Am. J. Pub. Health 40: 960, 1950.

Cavanagh, William V.: The effectiveness of a hospital birth control clinic, Am. J. Obst. & Gynec. 59: 883, 1950.

Eastman, N. J.: Expectant Motherhood, ed. 2, Boston, Little, 1947.

Fitzhugh, Mabel L.: Is this part of your antepartal program?, Am. J. Nursing 50:742, 1950.

Jeffers, Frances C.: Preparation for marriage, Am. J. Nursing 51:514, 1951.

Kilander, H. F.: Nutrition for Health, New York, McGraw-Hill, 1951.

Klein, Joseph: The relation of maternal weight gain to the weight of the newborn infant, Am. J. Obst. & Gynec. 52:574-580, 1946.

Loughran, C. H.: Weight control, diet and fluid balance in pregnancy, Am. J. Obst. & Gynec. 52: 42, 1946.

Siegel, Irving: The present status of the prenatal record, Am. J. Obst. & Gynec. 61:683, 1951.

Stare, Frederick J.: Why the science of nutrition?, Nutrition Rev. 8:1, 1950.

Stone, Abraham: Marriage counseling today and tomorrow, Marriage & Family Living 12:39, 1950.

Vilter, C. F., Morgan, D., and Spies, T. D.: Effects of dietary deficiency in pregnancy, Surg., Gynec. & Obst. 83:567-571, 1946.

Williams, P. F., and Fralin, F. G.: Nutrition study in pregnancy, Am. J. Obst. & Gynec. 43:1, 1942.

Worrell, Kathryn E.: The maternal and child health consultant in the hospital program, Pub. Health Nursing 42:329, 1950.

Zabriskie, Louise: Mother and Baby Care in Pictures, ed. 3, Philadelphia, Lippincott, 1946.

——: Prenatal Vision, The Mother, July, 1947.

Zimmerman, Kent A.: The public health nurse and the emotions of pregnancy, Pub. Health Nursing 39:63, 1947.

9

Prenatal Planning

ADVICE TO PARENTS

The nurse has many opportunities to aid in prenatal planning through her contacts with patients in the prenatal clinic, in her visits in the home and in classes where she may meet the fathers and thereby stimulate their interest.

All parents desire healthy radiant children, yet many of them do not realize how much depends on themselves. Babies have no greater heritage than to be wanted, planned for and loved. More and more parents, too, are becoming interested in heredity and environment. This is encouraging. Bearing children is no longer the mother's responsibility alone; it is a joint undertaking of both parents. The baby begins his existence at the moment that conception takes place, and the father should begin to assume his share of the responsibility from this time. Mothers, of necessity, have to accept the discomforts, the burdens and the risks associated with pregnancy, labor and the after-birth period; but a helpful, responsible, understanding and sympathetic father can do much to make this period less of a burden and safer than it otherwise would be. The father should make it his business to know what adequate maternity care is and to see to it that his wife receives the best care available. While the busy housewife continues with her duties in addition to bearing the discomforts that pregnancy involves, the busy husband should assume the responsibility of the heavy work during this time, such as lifting and scrubbing, and he should try to spare her all unnecessary exertion. This will mean much to both the mother and the baby, for the prevention of fatigue is one of the important details of prenatal care.

Fathers can assist in many ways, such as helping in the selection and the preparation of the things needed for the baby's care. An ingenious husband may make many of these articles in addition to various labor-saving devices for his wife. If the delivery is to take place at home the father should know the preparations needed and how they are to be used. This information makes it possible for the husband to be helpful to the doctor and the nurse as well as to his wife. With such consideration during pregnancy fathers continue this helpfulness with the baby and the childhood period. If classes on parenthood are offered, attending classes together will aid the parents in their mutual appreciation of the value of prenatal planning.

CLASSES

Today there are definite courses offered to mothers and fathers, and these clubs and classes are included as part of the programs of Visiting Nurse Associations, Red Cross chapters, and many State Departments of Health and hospitals (see p. 609). The Maternity Consultation Service, New York City, has instituted parents' classes where the expectant mother and father attend together. These classes tend to promote the idea of sharing parenthood. Knowledge of the physiologic changes of pregnancy creates in husbands a desire to be helpful and to assume more responsibility not only for the

care of the mother and baby after delivery but for the prenatal period as well. The teaching material used in any series of classes should be approved by obstetricians, but the details are worked out by nurses to suit the conditions under which the work is conducted. The more each individual patient comes in touch, during her pregnancy, with a competent nurse, trained in this special branch, the more likely will she be to demand the best care at delivery that the family budget will allow.

PREPARATION FOR NATURAL CHILDBIRTH

In order for the principles of natural childbirth to be successfully carried out it is essential that the expectant mother be taught the facts concerning the changes taking place in her body during pregnancy and what is to be expected from the procedure of exercises. She should understand, also, that she will have to be conscientious concerning this effort and that there will be entailed a certain amount of work and discomfort.

CHILDBIRTH WITHOUT FEAR

Childbirth without fear is not entirely a new idea. Many obstetricians have practiced similar methods for many years; of course, not to the extent that Dr. Grantly Dick Read has suggested, but its corollary with relaxation and naturalness. This subject, "childbirth without fear," has been so publicized recently by lay magazines and newspapers that certain misconceptions have crept in, and very often expectant parents inquire about the new method of

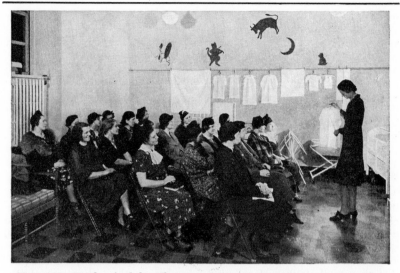

Fig. 103. Mothers' club. The group is receiving instruction on the baby's layette.

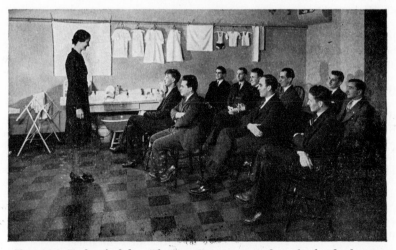

Fig. 104. Fathers' club. The group is interested in the kind of care that their wives and babies should have.

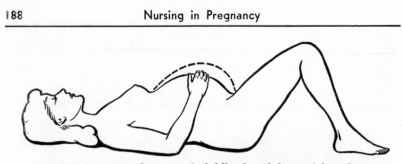

Fig. 105. Exercises for natural childbirth: Abdominal breathing.

"childbirth without pain." The obstetricians who practice these technics do not suggest that labor is without pain or that labor should be conducted without anesthetic aids when needed. However, it is believed that the manifestations of suffering are more often influenced by mental and emotional reactions than by the physical condition.

There is no one method of caring for a patient at the time of delivery, because individuals vary in mental attitudes, physical structure, capacity of the pelvis, muscular condition of the uterine wall, size of the baby as well as whether it is the first or the third pregnancy. Many people tend to be influenced enthusiastically for some new technic that has proved to be successful in a few cases. Each obstetric experience requires individualization. If doctors are chosen because of confidence in their judgment, skill and understanding, certainly the management of labor and delivery should be left to their discretion.

The results of the program, "Training for Childbirth," directed by Dr. Herbert Thoms, of Yale, at the Grace New Haven Community Hospital (University Service), are interesting, informative and convincing. This program started in 1947 and has become known rather widely in lay and professional circles as a "Natural Childbirth Program." In addition to the usual prenatal program, they emphasize the education of the mother, the use of certain exercises primarily aimed at relaxation, the importance of sympathetic continuous attention and care (support) during labor. Dr. Thoms has graciously given his permission to print the exercises taught in his clinical program.

THE EXERCISES °

In the following pages the exercises are explained. A mimeographed copy of this explanation, including the illustrations, is given to each woman at the first exercise class. This material would be better presented in booklet form, adding instructions in prenatal hygiene and so forth—a project that we are now developing.

Exercise No. 1—Breathing

Lie on your back (on a blanket or a pad on the floor, or on a bed that does

° Make certain that the bladder is empty before practicing any of the exercises.

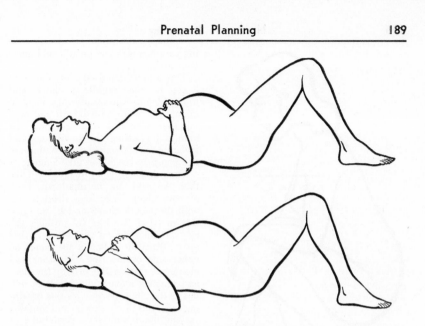

FIG. 105 (*Continued*). Exercises for natural childbirth: (*Top*) Panting. (*Bottom*) Relaxation.

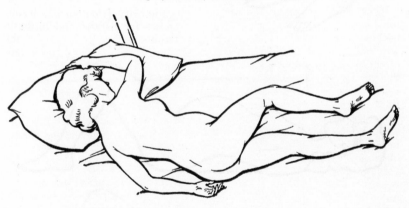

not sag), with the legs bent at the knees and the feet flat on the floor or the bed.

Type 1 (Abdominal Breathing). With the mouth closed, breathe gently in and out, keeping as relaxed as possible. Let the abdominal wall rise with each breath taken in and drop down with each outgoing breath.

If you find this difficult at first, place your hands gently on each side of the abdomen, with the arms and the elbows at rest on the floor or the bed, and imagine that you are raising and lower-

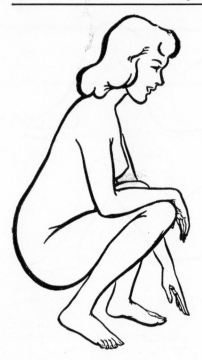

ing your hands as you breathe and move your abdomen.

This is to be practiced every day until it can be done rapidly or slowly and to any depth. Aim at allowing one half minute for taking in a breath and raising the abdominal wall and one half minute for letting the breath go and lowering the abdominal wall. With practice you may be able to take longer.

Type 2. There is an inverted V (like this: Λ) made by the ribs in the front of your chest. Take in a deep breath with the mouth closed and try to open this inverted V wider by pushing the ribs on either side of your chest farther apart. Place the palms of the hands on either side of the ribs with arms and elbows at rest on the bed or the floor and practice moving the hands in and out as the chest moves with this breathing. Do this both slowly and rapidly, varying the rhythm, for a period of 2 or 3 minutes at least 4 times daily.

FIG. 105 (*Continued*). Exercises for natural childbirth: Posture.

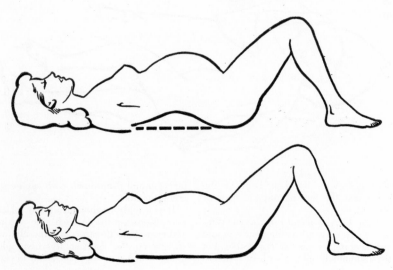

Type 3 (Panting). With the mouth open, breathe in and out, lifting up the sternum, or breast bone, and letting it fall again. This breathing is compared with the panting of a dog—rapid short breaths with the mouth open, using the top of the chest only. Similarly, the hands can be placed lightly on the chest and moved up and down as you pant.

These breathing exercises can be done on the bed before you go to sleep at night or before you get up in the morning. They are important because the mother's most essential work during labor and delivery is accomplished by her controlled breathing.

Exercise No. 2—Relaxation

Lie on either side on the floor or the bed, with your head on one pillow, the neck bent slightly forward, and the pillow at an angle for best support.

Place the under arm behind the back, with the elbow and the wrist slightly bent, and the top arm bent forward to lie at rest on the pillow or on the bed. The back is slightly bowed forward, and the baby rests gently on the bed. The top leg is bent at the hip, the knee and the ankle and is brought forward. The bottom leg is bent also, but behind the top leg. All parts of the body are at rest on a firm support, yet all joints are loosely bent so that no muscle is tense.

Close the eyes and the mouth and start relaxing as follows:

Leg:	Squeeze the toes—relax.
	Bend the foot forward—relax.
	Straighten the leg—relax.
	Tighten the hip—relax.
Other leg:	Same.
Arm:	Make a fist—relax.
	Straighten the elbow—relax.
	Tighten the shoulder—relax.
Other arm:	Same.

Face:	Screw it up—relax.
	Let the facial muscles relax as thoroughly as possible.
Breathing:	Breathe regularly and as slowly as possible, moving the abdomen forward and backward, as you have been practicing in Exercise No. 1 on abdominal breathing.
	Think *only* of breathing in and out; your mind will be at peace, and usually sleep will follow.

After you have learned the relaxation in steps, try relaxing suddenly and instantly so that you will be able to use controlled relaxation during the first stage of labor.

Important: After such complete relaxation, a sudden upright position occasionally may bring slight dizziness. Bring the slowed circulation to normal for activity by moving the feet and the hands, stretching, turning over, and sitting up gradually.

Exercise No. 3—Contraction and Relaxation of the Pelvic Floor Muscles

Lie on the back with the legs crossed at the ankles, and the knees straight.

a. Squeeze together the muscles of the two buttocks, or where you sit, as you count to 5 slowly—1, 2, 3, 4, 5.

b. As you count, press your thighs together at the back and count on to 7—6, 7.

Try not to hold your breath during the two exercises above.

c. While doing a and b try to contract your anus (back passage) by tucking it further in toward your pelvis as if you were trying to keep from having a bowel movement. As you do this, count on to 10— 8, 9, 10.

When these contractive exercises are completed, relax these muscles slowly, then repeat the exercise in the 3 steps *a*, *b*, and *c* 4 or 5 times.

When the exercise is properly done you will feel the "drawing in" sensation as you practice, first only in your anus, then gradually also in your vagina, or birth canal, and finally to the front, up into the region of the uterus. *Relax very slowly!*

A pregnant woman should have good posture and carry her baby well supported and gracefully.

Exercise No. 4—Posture

Squatting. Stand with the feet flat, about 24 inches apart, and squat. Rest the arms on the knees. If you find this difficult, practice squatting by holding lightly to some heavy article of furniture until you can balance yourself.

Pelvic Rocking, Lying Down. Lie on the back with the knees bent and the feet flat on the bed or floor.

a. Push both hands under the lower back to make sure of a hollow, then arch the back. At the same time relax the muscles in the lower abdominal wall and push the abdomen up.

b. Pull the hands out and flatten the back so that there is no space between the back and the floor or the bed. At the same time, tighten the lower abdominal muscles and the muscles of the buttocks.

Pelvic Rocking, Standing. Stand with the feet about 6 inches apart but parallel, and the toes pressed into the floor.

a. As before, make a hollow in the back. Relax the lower abdominal muscles and bring the abdomen forward.

b. Then straighten up the back. Tense or tighten the muscles in the lower abdomen and in the buttocks.

After practicing *a* and *b* until *b* is easier, open out the chest for full chest breathing, lift the head in "proud" position, and walk carrying your baby with good support.

SCHEDULE

The average normal prenatal patient makes her first visit to the clinic in the sixth week of pregnancy. At that time her history is taken, physical and laboratory examinations are made, and instructions are given in the hygiene of pregnancy. The remaining prenatal checkups take place according to the following schedule:

Tenth week	First talk by physician
Fourteenth week	First exercise class
Eighteenth week	Second exercise class
Twenty-second week	
Twenty-sixth week	
Thirtieth week	
Thirty-second week	
Thirty-fourth week	
Thirty-sixth week	Second talk by physician
Thirty-seventh week . .	Third exercise class
Thirty-eighth week . . .	Fourth exercise class

Any time after the thirty-second week, the four classes for fathers- and parents-to-be are given at weekly intervals, usually in the evening. This course is given every two months. A member of the pediatric staff attached to the nursery sees each prenatal patient at some regular visit to acquaint her with the plans for care in the hospital for the coming infant.

As Dr. Thoms says, "We recognize that fear and anxiety play a large part in the creation of tension, which has undesirable effects, but we do not place undue emphasis on this aspect. We prefer to think of our pro-

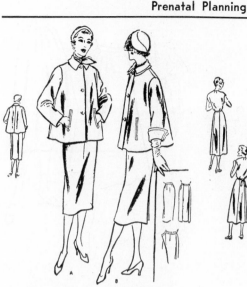

Fig. 106. Maternity dresses. Vogue Patterns: (*Left*) No. 7282; (*right*) No. 6339. (Copyright, 1951, Condé Nast Publications, Inc., New York)

gram in a broad sense as being directed toward childbirth with understanding and support rather than childbirth without fear."

Satisfactory results in connection with natural childbirth is aided by such factors as: attaining good physical health and emotional stability; learning about the baby's development during the prenatal period; understanding the muscular processes that take place during labor and delivery; preparing for labor by attending classes where supervised exercises are practiced and perfected; having sympathetic understanding and "support" during labor; planning for the postpartum period, the physical and emotional adjustment of the mother and the care of the new baby.

CLOTHING FOR THE MOTHER

During pregnancy clothes should be given the same or perhaps even more attention than at other times, as they not only aid in controlling the body temperature (keeping it uniform, etc.) but they afford the patient an added opportunity for diversion.

Top Togs. Increasingly the stores are devoting a department to maternity fashions which is very helpful in settling the problem of suitable clothing during pregnancy. Price ranges are wide to accommodate all economic levels, and the possibility

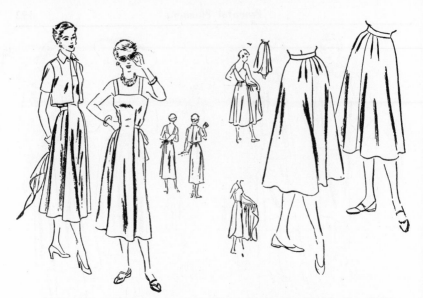

Fig. 107. Maternity dresses. Vogue Patterns: (*Left*) No. 6957; (*right*) No. 7261. (Copyright, 1951, Condé Nast Publications, Inc., New York)

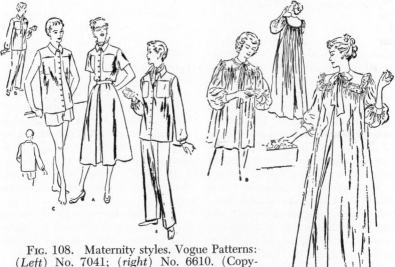

Fig. 108. Maternity styles. Vogue Patterns: (*Left*) No. 7041; (*right*) No. 6610. (Copyright, 1951, Condé Nast Publications, Inc., New York)

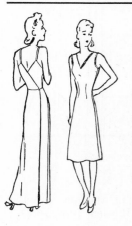

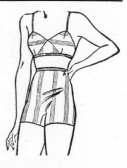

Fig. 109. Slip. An adjustable slip is a convenient and comfortable one to wear during pregnancy. Vogue Pattern No. 8999. (Copyright, *Vogue*)

Fig. 110. Underthings should have no tight bands and should be lightweight, comfortable and easy to launder.

of converting the clothing to later use has been anticipated. Today designers and stylists are giving consideration to the pregnant mother so that she may dress attractively and not be self-conscious about her appearance. Clothing should be made of lightweight materials, it should hang from the shoulders and should be comfortable.

Underthings. The underclothes (slips and briefs) that one has been used to wearing should be worn during pregnancy, provided that they are comfortable and adjustable. The patient should dress according to the climate and the temperature, care being taken not to get chilled or to become overheated.

Abdominal Support. Women who have been unaccustomed to wearing a support will scarcely feel the need of one, especially during the early months of pregnancy. Later, however, a properly fitted maternity girdle often gives the needed support to keep the patient from becoming fatigued.

If the patient's abdomen is large, or if the patient has had babies before, causing the abdomen to be relaxed or pendulous, a properly made and well-fitting maternity corset will give support and comfort.

Breast Support. A brassière that is comfortably snug, holding the breasts in a normal position and avoiding downward pressure or pressure on the nipples, will do much to prevent fatigue. Proper support of the breasts aids in correct posture and helps to prevent backache. There are several excellent models of brassières. The choice should be determined by the individual's size and need for support. During pregnancy it may be more comfortable to use a small pad directly over the nipple to prevent friction and to absorb any secretion. The same brassière may be used during the early postpartum period for the support of the breasts of nursing mothers.

Garters. "Round garters" or any tight bands (rolled stockings, elastic tops on stockings) that encircle the

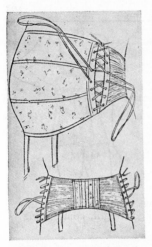

FIG. 111. Circlet maternity girdle for support of abdomen and back during pregnancy. (Kleinert's, New York)

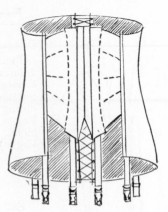

FIG. 113. Maternity corset. (Mary Hayden, New York)

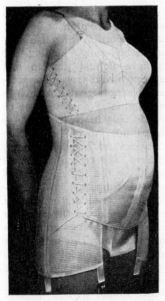

FIG. 112. Maternity corset and brassière. (Spencer, Inc., New Haven, Conn.)

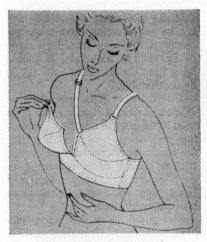

FIG. 114. Maternity brassière for use during and after the nursing period. Special construction allows for sanitary gauze over the nipples and convenient opening for nursing. (Maiden Form Co., New York)

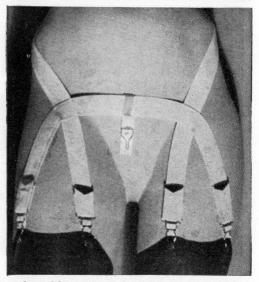

Adjustable garter belt. (Fancee Free Mfg. Co., St. Louis, Mo.)

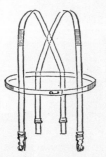

FIG. 115. Shoulder garters made of skirt belting, tape or ribbon, 1½ inches wide. The strap over the front should be attached to the belt far enough to the side to prevent pressure on the breasts.

leg tend to aggravate varicose veins and edema of the lower extremities and should be discarded in favor of suspender garters or some form of stocking supporters attached to an abdominal support. It will be remembered that arteries have muscular tissue in their walls, while veins have little or none, so that arteries are able to resist pressure. The external veins lie close to the surface, while the arteries are embedded deeper in the tissues. Hence, any constriction of any extremity affects the veins far more than the arteries, and blood, which apparently meets with no obstruction whatever in its flow down the extremity through an artery, may on its return through the vein find at the point of constriction sufficient

closure of the vessel to "dam it back" and so stretch the vein wall that a varicosity is formed. There is already a marked tendency toward this condition because the enlarged and constantly enlarging uterus tends to impede the return circulation from the lower extremities by compression of the great abdominal vessels, and round garters definitely tend to aggravate the condition. Garters that encircle the leg never should be worn, even by growing children, for the tendency to varicosities is always present; and, when once formed, they never entirely disappear but later may lead to great discomfort.

Shoes. Comfortable, well-fitted shoes should be worn. As pregnancy advances, the posture changes. The

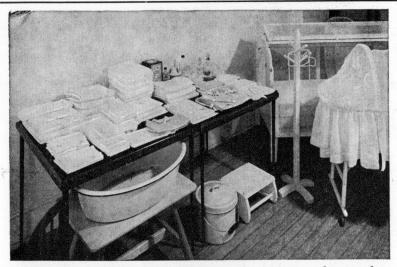

Fig. 116. Suggestions for the layette and equipment, showing the essentials for the care of the baby. (Maternity Consultation Service, New York)

shoulders are thrown back as the enlarging abdomen protrudes, and in order to maintain the body balance, more weight is imposed on the heels. High heels may cause backache and fatigue. They also interfere with a proper poise of the body and throw weight upon the lower abdomen, in addition to the strain which is caused by the enlarging uterus. If the patient is accustomed to very high heels, suggest to her that she change to the solid heels which afford a more substantial support; in so doing she will take less chance of tripping and falling. If a patient changes from high heels to low ones suddenly, she may suffer from pains in the calves of the legs which may add temporarily to her discomfort.

PREPARATIONS FOR THE BABY

The baby's layette and equipment are of real interest to all parents—in fact, interesting to the majority of people. The cost of the layette should be in keeping with the individual economic circumstances. Much or little may be spent in its preparation, but nurses who are teaching parents should know the reasons why certain types of clothes and equipment are preferable. In the selection of clothing the following points should be considered: comfort (few seams); ease in making and laundering; ease in putting on and taking off; very light in weight; and they should be made so that they will hang from the shoulders (because of postural development). The complete outfit of clothes that the baby wears should not weigh more than 12 to 16 ounces.

The new baby is the most helpless of all young. He is very delicately constructed, his bones are still in the process of calcifying, and his development is progressing so rapidly that he doubles his birth weight in the first 5 or 6 months. His clothes should not inhibit his normal activities, because these activities are the means of developing the muscles ~~which he~~ will use later when creeping, sitting and walking.

Layette. During pregnancy it may be interesting as well as diverting for the patient to make many of the articles listed in the layette.

Layette necessities are:

3 or 4 diaper bands (sometimes called sleeveless shirts)

3 or 4 shirts

3 to 4 dozen diapers (if diaper service is not used)

4 squares or receiving blankets

3 nightgowns or kimonos

6 diaper pads (11" x 16")

2 waterproof protectors for under diaper pads

2 or 3 dresses
2 or 3 pettiskirts } (not essential)

2 afghans or blankets

1 bunting

2 bath towels (40" x 40")

2 face towels

2 washcloths

1 bath apron

Nursery equipment:

basket, bassinet, crib, or Kiddie-Koop

mattress

mattress protector (waterproof)

sheets or pillow cases for basket mattress

bathtub

low table for tub (Fig. 317)

low chair for mother

diaper pail

toilet tray—equipped

absorbent cotton—or cotton balls

applicators or Q-tips

baby soap

oil or baby lotion

safety pins

netting (crib and carriage)

rectal thermometer

Additional suggestions for layette and equipment:

sacques

sweaters

kimonos

crib blankets

crib spreads

crib pads

bibs

masks

shirt and sweater driers

clothes drier

complete toidey

chest of drawers

nursery stand

footstool

diaper bag (for traveling)

disposable diapers

nursery light

carriage

If the baby is to be born at home, there will be needed, in addition to the supplies listed above, the following:

4 straight bands 4" x 27" (used as a bandage for the cord dressing)

cord set (tapes, ties, dressings, scissors)

silver preparation (prophylactic for the eyes) (Fig. 154)

Layette Described. BANDS. The 4" x 27" bands are really no more than bandages to keep the cord dressing in place. They are made of fine flannel or flannelette. They should be pinked, not hemmed. These bands may be made from one half yard of 27-inch flannelette, cut in four pieces crosswise; there are, also, several kinds that may be bought ready for use. These first bands are replaced, when the umbilicus has healed, by the diaper band (sleeveless shirt). These are made of cotton or cotton and wool. Even a small amount of wool absorbs moisture and stays warm, while all cotton is cold and clammy when wet or damp. Bands serve as a waist to which to pin the diaper and aid in keeping the abdomen warm. The neckline should be so constructed that it does not slip off the shoulders and that the pull from the pinned diaper comes on the shoulders close to the neck, an important factor in the baby's postural development. The bands may be worn summer and winter.

SHIRTS should be of the same materials as the bands, coat style, with well-shaped neck and sleeves with roomy armholes. This style is easier to put on and take off during this period when the baby's head needs to be supported. If "pull-over" shirts are used, the neck opening should be so constructed that it is large enough to be put on over the feet.

DIAPERS. There are several varieties of diapers. The cotton birds-eye diapers (27″ x 27″), Pant-ease (knitted tubular), Curity (layette cloth) and Chix (gauze) are all satisfactory. Since diapers are worn the entire 24 hours, they should be considered from the point of view of comfort, absorbency, washing, drying qualities and folding.

PADS (11″ x 16″) are used under the baby next to the diaper. They should be backed by a piece of waterproof material to protect the rest of his clothing and bed. They should be made of absorbent material that is easy to wash and dry (huck toweling or layette cloth).

SQUARES OR RECEIVING BLANKETS. These should be made of flannelette one yard square. This square is used to fold loosely about the baby and may be so pinned that he always is covered and protected from drafts. If properly pinned, the baby may lie and kick and at the same time keep his little feet covered and warm. In the early weeks these squares take the brunt of the service and in this way save the fine wool covers from becoming soiled so quickly.

NIGHTGOWNS may be made of soft knitted material or flannelette. They should be lightweight, loose, warm, comfortable and absorbent, easy to wash; they need not be ironed. Some types have a drawstring at the wrist and at the bottom to keep the baby's hands and feet covered.

DRESSES AND PETTISKIRTS. These should be simple, dainty and attractive. The kimono-style dress is easy to make (Fig. 121), put on and take off. To make possible adjustment of the sleeves, there should be a drawstring at the wrist. The armholes and the neck of the pettiskirt should be bound with soft seam binding, and the drawstring at the neck should be tacked in the center of the front to prevent its pulling out. Both dresses and pettiskirts should be fastened in the back with tiny buttons or ties. Dresses and pettiskirts need not be worn except on occasions. This not only conserves the mother's energy but will mean less handling for the baby.

KIMONOS may be made of fine knitted material, flannelette, or flannel, and may be used instead of dresses or nightgowns.

AFGHANS OR BLANKETS. These should be of very lightweight all-wool material. Two lightweight blankets are much warmer than one heavy one. The temperature and the weather will determine the amount of covering needed.

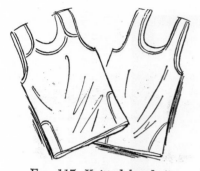

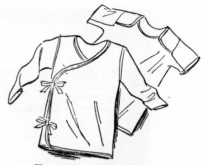

FIG. 117. Knitted band, infant size 2. The band should be without seams except on the shoulder and should be reinforced where diaper is pinned.

FIG. 118. Shirt, infant size 2, coat or wrap-around style and pullover type.

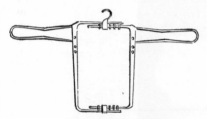

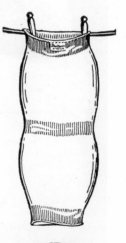

FIG. 119. Plastic frame for drying baby's shirts and sweaters. It is adjustable for larger sizes. Shrinking is avoided, shape is preserved, and unnecessary wear is avoided if these articles are dried on a frame.

FIG. 120. The Pant-ease diaper, soft, comfortable and easily laundered. (Pant-ease Infant Wear Company, Arcade, N. Y.)

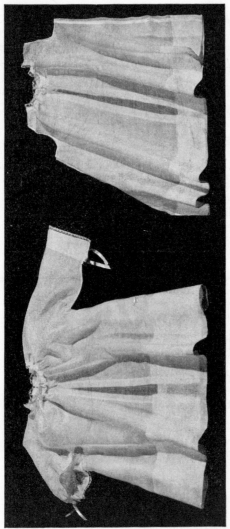

Fig. 121. (*Left*) There are many styles of fine dresses, but the kimono type is more comfortable for the baby and the simplest to iron. All seams should be fine and flat, and the neck should be so finished that it is smooth on the inside. The dress should be opened down the back from neck to hem and fastened with ties or tiny flat buttons. (*Right*) Pettiskirts are needed with sheer dresses. They should be opened all the way down the back, and the armholes should be ample.

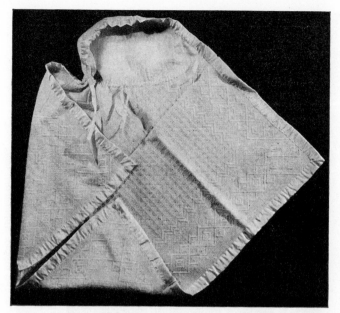

Fig. 122. An afghan converted into a practical bunting by sewing a piece of silk into one corner with shirr strings so that it can be drawn into a hood and allow ventilation around the ears. Tight bonnets never should be worn. (Zabriskie: Mother and Baby Care in Pictures, Philadelphia, Lippincott)

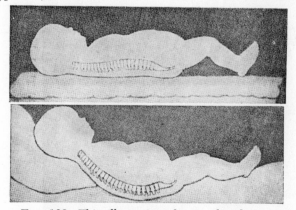

Fig. 123. This illustration shows what happens to a baby's sensitive spine when the mattress of his bed is too soft to support his back, or when a pillow is used. Babies should have a firm mattress to lie on and they should not be propped up with a pillow. (*Trained Nurse* and *Hospital Review*)

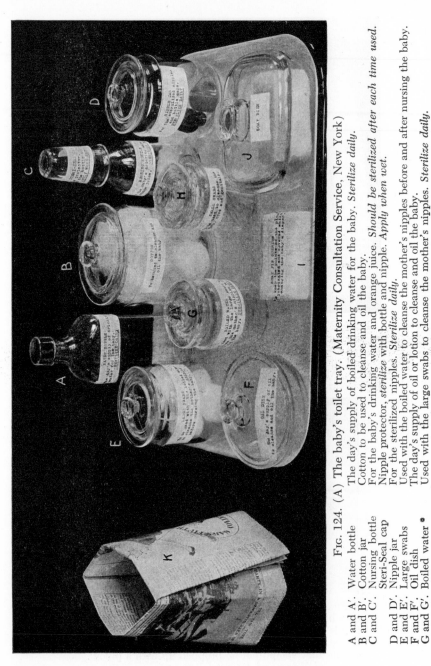

Fig. 124. (A) The baby's toilet tray. (Maternity Consultation Service, New York)

A and A'. Water bottle   The day's supply of boiled drinking water for the baby. *Sterilize daily.*
B and B'. Cotton jar   Cotton to be used to cleanse and oil the baby.
C and C'. Nursing bottle   For the baby's drinking water and orange juice. *Should be sterilized after each time used.*
D and D'. Steri-Seal cap   Nipple protector, *sterilize* with bottle and nipple. *Apply when wet.*
E and E'. Nipple jar   For the sterilized nipples. *Sterilize daily.*
F and F'. Large swabs   Used with the boiled water to cleanse the mother's nipples before and after nursing the baby.
G and G'. Oil dish   The day's supply of oil or lotion to cleanse and oil the baby.
      Boiled water *   Used with the large swabs to cleanse the mother's nipples. *Sterilize daily.*

[242]

I and I'. Soap pin-cushion   A place to stick the safety pins to keep the points lubricated and covered while changing diaper.

J and J'. Soap dish   Mild soap.
K and K'. Cornucopia   For waste.

Additional cotton, toothpicks, oil or lotion and soap are needed to keep the tray replenished.

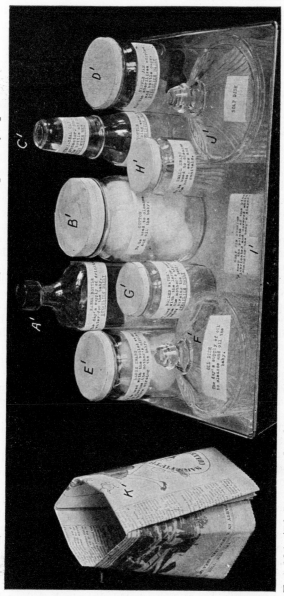

Fig. 124. (B) Improvised toilet tray for baby. A household tray or baking pan may be substituted for the enamel tray. Miscellaneous jars may be utilized. (Maternity Consultation Service, New York)

* There is a difference of opinon as to whether boric acid solution or sterile water should be used. Since the question as to the need for boric acid has been raised, and we find no supporting data to prove its value, we use the simpler method.
† There is also a difference of opinion as to whether toothpick swabs or twisted cotton should be used. Swabs are cleaner and easier to handle and perfectly safe if properly made and used only after the method of holding the baby's head steadily has been learned. Because mothers find it difficult to cleanse baby's nose with twisted cotton, they may neglect this detail of care unless taught to make and use swabs properly. (The end of the toothpick must be blunt and thoroughly covered with cotton.)

SHEETS. Crib sheets are usually 45″ x 72″ and are available in muslin, percale and knitted materials. The knit sheets are practical for bottom sheets and do not need to be ironed. Pillow cases are very usable for the carriage or the basket mattress. Receiving blankets may be used for top sheets.

WATERPROOF SHEETING. *Various* waterproof materials are suitable to protect the mattress and to be used under the pads. Even though the mattress may have a protective covering, it is necessary to have a waterproof cover large enough to cover the mattress completely—something that can be removed and washed. (Waterproof material should not be dried in the sun.)

BUNTING may be a square blanket with a hood in one corner. This type provides protection without too much handling and prevents the habit of wearing bonnets.

WASHCLOTHS should be small and soft, made from terry cloth or some soft used material. If the round-shaped variety is used, there are no dangling wet corners to drag over the baby's face.

FACE TOWELS should be of some soft, absorbent material.

BATH TOWELS should be soft and absorbent. The 40-inch square bath towel is the most practical because it is large enough to cover the baby completely, and he is not so apt to get uncovered.

WATERPROOF OR KNITTED PANTS offer protection for special occasions. The knitted variety should be made of lightweight wool. They are easy to make, more absorbent, warmer in winter and cooler in summer. If the plastic variety is used they should not be tight at the leg or the waist.

BATH APRON. This is a protection for both mother and baby and may be made of plastic material.

Nursery Equipment. In choosing the equipment, again the individual circumstances should be taken into consideration. Expense, space and future plans all influence the selections. Most nurseries are planned for the satisfaction of the parents. Eventually the baby's room becomes the child's room; and if economy must be considered, furniture should be selected that will appeal to the child as he grows and develops.

THE BABY'S ROOM. Preferably, the baby should have his own room. If this is not feasible, a quiet airy place, out of drafts, may be selected. Ventilators (even the homemade kind) may be used in the windows to protect the baby from drafts.

BED. The baby should have his own bed. This may be a basket, a bassinet, a crib, a Kiddie-Koop or a bed designed by the parents. The trimming on the basket or bassinet should be such that it can be removed easily and laundered. A bed may be made out of a box, a bureau drawer, a couch or a large armchair. Many parents may have a carriage that may be used as a bed. The baby needs fresh air; therefore, he should not lie so low in the bed or carriage that the air is limited. This may be remedied by an extra flat pillow under the mattress. At the foot of the crib or basket there should be a roll to protect the baby's feet from the tight top covers (Fig. 315). The baby's bed should be kept clean and should be aired daily when the weather permits.

MATTRESS. The mattress should be firm (not hard) and flat. All mattresses, including the waterproof-covered, should be protected by a waterproof sheeting to prevent the mattress from becoming stained and from absorbing odors. The waterproof sheet is easily washed and dries quickly.

NETTING will be needed for the carriage, the basket or the crib during the insect season. If the Kiddie-Koop is used, it is screened to protect the baby from insects and animals.

BATHTUB. The enamel tub is safe and easy to keep clean.

BATHTUB TABLE. The table on which the tub is placed for the lap bath should be of convenient height (Fig. 317). A coffee table, stool, chair, box or child's table may be used for this purpose.

MOTHER'S CHAIR. The chair should also be a convenient height and comfortable for the individual mother.

DIAPER PAIL. It should be large enough for the day's supply of soiled diapers. It may also be used for boiling the diapers.

TOILET TRAY. This tray should be prepared and ready for use immediately after the delivery of the baby.

PLANS FOR AFTER-CARE OF MOTHER AND BABY

It is always a relief to the patient and her husband when the plans for delivery and the arrangements for care at the time of delivery and the period following have been completed. The parents should make some provision for the mother to be free from other responsibilities until she has regained, in part at least, her physical strength and until lactation has been established. If the patient is to be delivered at home, certain preparations are not only an aid to the doctor and the nurse but also a great comfort to the mother at the time of her labor. These may be prepared ahead of time with a small expenditure of time, strength and money.

The nurse should make an effort to include the father when discussing the details of prenatal care. Often it is only with his help that his wife gets the full care she needs and that the doctor and the nurse wish her to have. (See Chap. 11.)

EMPLOYMENT

The expectant mother who is employed will naturally desire to know how late in pregnancy she may continue her work and how early she may return after the baby is born. Clerical work may be kept up as long as desired. Work which involves much in the way of physical activity, especially heavy lifting or continuous standing, should be avoided altogether. Although employers nowadays are very liberal-minded about such matters, there are naturally certain positions which cannot be held after the pregnancy becomes apparent. If this is a factor, plans should be made to discontinue work when pregnancy becomes evident. Following delivery, 6 weeks are needed for the obstetrician to determine whether or not the reproductive organs are returning to their approximate normal size and position. Accordingly, no commitments should be made until the baby is from 6 to 8 weeks old. At the time of the postpartum examination, the obstetrician will discuss with the patient her future plans. It always must be kept in mind that the first 6 years of a child's life are the most impressionable, and when making these future plans with the mother, this fact must not be ignored because of interest in re-employment.

During the war emergency, millions of women were engaged in war industries. Many women are still employed, and the problem of pregnancy for the working mother is a most important one. In order to safeguard the interests of expectant mothers so engaged, the following "Standards for Maternity Care and Employment of Mothers in Industry" have been recommended by the Children's Bureau and the Women's Bureau of the U. S. Department of Labor.

1. Facilities for adequate prenatal medical care should be readily available for all employed pregnant women; and arrangements should be made by those responsible for providing prenatal care, so that every woman would have access to such care. Local health departments should make available to industrial plants the services of prenatal clinics; and the personnel management or physicians and nurses within the plant should make available to employees information about the importance of such services and where they can be obtained.

2. Pregnant women should not be employed on a shift including the hours between 12 midnight and 6 A.M. Pregnant women should not be employed more than 8 hours a day nor more than 48 hours per week, and it is desirable that their hours of work be limited to not more than 40 hours per week.

3. Every woman, especially a pregnant woman, should have at least two 10-minute rest periods during her work shift, for which adequate facilities for resting and an opportunity for securing nourishing food should be provided.

4. It is not considered desirable for pregnant women to be employed in the following types of occupation, and they should, if possible, be transferred to lighter and more sedentary work:

a. Occupations that involve heavy lifting or other heavy work.

b. Occupations involving continuous standing and moving about.

5. Pregnant women should not be employed in the following types of work during any period of pregnancy, but should be transferred to less hazardous types of work.

a. Occupations that require a good sense of bodily balance, such as work performed on scaffolds or stepladders and occupations in which the accident risk is characterized by accidents causing severe injury, such as operation of punch presses, power-driven woodworking machines, or other machines having a point-of-operation hazard.

b. Occupations involving exposure to toxic substances considered to be extra hazardous during pregnancy, such as:

Aniline
Benzol and toluol
Carbon disulfide
Carbon monoxide
Chlorinated hydrocarbons
Lead and its compounds
Mercury and its compounds
Nitrobenzol and other nitro compounds
    of benzol and its homologs
Phosphorus
Radioactive substances and x-rays
Turpentine

Other toxic substances that exert an injurious effect upon the blood-forming organs, the liver, or the kidneys.

Because these substances may exert a harmful influence upon the course of pregnancy, may lead to its premature termination, or may injure the fetus, the maintenance of air concentrations within the so-called "maximum permissible limits" of State codes, is not, in itself, sufficient assurance of a safe working condition for the pregnant woman. Pregnant women should be transferred from workrooms in which any of these substances are used or produced in any significant quantity.

6. A minimum of 6 weeks' leave *before* delivery should be granted, on presentation of a medical certificate of the expected date of confinement.

7. At any time during pregnancy a woman should be granted a reasonable amount of additional leave on presentation of a certificate from the attending physician to the effect that complications of pregnancy have made continuing employment prejudicial to her health or to the health of the child.

To safeguard the mother's health she should be granted sufficient time off after delivery to return to normal and to regain her strength. The infant needs her care, especially during the first year of life. If it is essential that she return to work, the following recommendations are made:

a. All women should be granted an extension of at least 2 months' leave of absence after delivery.

b. Should complications of delivery or of the postpartum period develop, a woman should be granted a reasonable amount of additional leave beyond 2 months following delivery, on presentation of a certificate to this effect from the attending physician.

SUGGESTED READING

Bigley, Loretta I.: Community Clinics, Philadelphia, Lippincott, 1947.

Children's Bureau: Prenatal Care, Washington, D. C.

——: Infant Care, Washington, D. C.

Cole, Miriam L.: Classes that mothers like, Pub. Health Nursing 43:442, 1951.

Eastman, N. J.: Expectant Motherhood, ed. 2, Boston, Little, 1947.

Goodrich, Frederick, W., Jr.: Natural Childbirth, New York, Prentice-Hall, 1950

Heardman, Helen: A Way to Natural Childbirth, Baltimore, Williams & Wilkins, 1948.

Literature on Class Outlines from State Departments of Health.

Maternity Center Assoc., N. Y.: Public Health Nursing in Obsterics, Part IV.

Peck, Elizabeth, and Carney, Ruth: Guidance programs for new mothers, Am. J. Nursing 51:184, 1951.

Read, Grantly Dick: Childbirth Without Fear, New York, Harper, 1944.

Thoms, Herbert: Training for Childbirth, New York, McGraw-Hill, 1950.

Thoms, Herbert, and Roth, L. G.: Understanding Natural Childbirth, New York, McGraw-Hill, 1950.

Visiting Nurse Assoc. of Brooklyn: Suggested Material for Teaching Mothers' Classes.

Zabriskie, Louise: Mother and Baby Care in Pictures, ed. 3, Philadelphia, Lippincott, 1946.

——: Prenatal Vision, The Mother, July, 1947.

——: How to Bathe and Dress Babies, pamphlet.

10

Complications of Pregnancy

MINOR DISCOMFORTS

The so-called minor discomforts of pregnancy can often be entirely overcome, and many of the serious complications can be prevented if the patient places herself, early in pregnancy, in the hands of a competent obstetrician. Prevention is the most important phase of prenatal care. Fortunately, it demands little more than common sense in daily living.

Nausea and Its Control. Nausea and morning sickness in the early months are so frequent as to be considered an expected discomfort. These symptoms occur in about 60 per cent of the pregnancies and usually appear from about the end of the fourth to the sixth week. The condition varies all the way from the slightest feeling of nausea, when a patient first gets up, to persistent and intense vomiting, a serious condition called penicious vomiting. Usually it occurs in the morning only, but a small percentage of patients may have nausea and vomiting throughout the entire day.

Often this condition can be controlled and frequently it may be greatly relieved. Various "before breakfast" remedies are often used. If, one half hour before rising, the patient takes a dry piece of toast or a cracker or sips of hot water (plain or with lemon juice), hot tea, clear coffee or hot milk, relief may be obtained. In some instances eating an olive has been tried with excellent results. After taking any one of the "before breakfast" remedies, the patient should remain in bed, on her right side, for about one half hour; she should then get up slowly and dress slowly (sitting meanwhile as much of the time as possible). After this she is usually ready for her breakfast.

Other suggested remedies include eating an increased amount of carbohydrate foods during this period of disturbance or eating simple and light food five or six times a day instead of the three regular full meals; unsweetened popcorn during the morning is sometimes advised. The patient may be helped by drinking sweet lemonade, about half of a lemon to a pint of water sweetened with milk sugar. Usually after vomiting, the patient is quite thirsty, and it is not difficult for her to drink lemonade. Ginger ale in small amounts also is often most helpful. This nausea and vomiting, if once established, is difficult to overcome, and so it is especially desirable to prevent the first attack, or at least to control this condition as soon as possible after it develops. It must be remembered that if the patient is unable to retain most of her food her system is being depleted when the daily health should be maintained. Pregnancies may differ, and what may help one person may not benefit another. The "trial and error" method is often necessary to obtain results.

Emotional Disturbances. More and more attention is being directed toward the part that emotions may have in the reactions to pregnancy. Some of this may be due to the internal glandular adjustments that are taking place during the early weeks and months. The emotional stability of the patient before pregnancy may determine how she will adjust to this new experience. Fears, worries and family misunderstandings have their effects, sometimes depleting the body physically as well as affecting the mental attitude. The undesirable state of pregnancy may create a disinterest which may interfere with the daily maintenance of good hygienic care of the patient and the developing baby. However, the happy anticipation of the new baby is so stimulating sometimes that it may interfere with her rest, sleep and even appetite. Fatigue, overwork and increased responsibility also have their physical and emotional results and directly affect the nervous and emotional disposition. If these seemingly unimportant reactions are not recognized they may lead to unfavorable complications.

As far as the nurse is concerned it is a great art to know how little to say or how much not to say. One does not have to be a psychiatrist to achieve this, but thoughtful, sympathetic, understanding care will do much to accomplish a normal balanced reaction on the part of the patient.

Heartburn, a condition peculiar to pregnancy, is a neuromuscular phenomenon which may occur any time throughout gestation. It may be described as a burning discomfort diffusedly localized behind the lower part of the sternum, often radiating upward along the course of the esophagus. Although referred to as heartburn, it really has nothing to do with the heart. Often it is associated with other gastro-intestinal symptoms of which acid regurgitation, belching, nausea and epigastric pressure are most troublesome. Nervous tension and emotional disturbances may be a precipitating cause. The definite cause of heartburn is not known, but worry, fatigue and improper diet may contribute to its intensity.

While fatty foods are especially

aggravating in this disturbance, strangely enough, the taking of some form of fat, such as a pat of butter or a tablespoon of cream, a short time before meals, acts as a preventive. Little or no fat should be included in the diet.

To relieve this condition, some physicians advise a half cup of black coffee containing a teaspoonful of unsalted butter. Others recommend a tablespoon of lime water or milk of magnesia. A small glass of milk before meals is sometimes helpful.

Flatulence is a somewhat common and very disagreeable discomfort. Usually it is due to undesirable bacterial action in the intestines which results in the formation of gas. Eating only small amounts of food which are well masticated may prevent this feeling of distress after eating. Regular daily elimination is of prime importance, as is the avoidance of foods which form gas. Such foods as beans, parsnips, corn, sweet desserts, fried foods, cake and candy should be avoided. If these measures fail to relieve the condition, the physician should be consulted.

Constipation is not unusual during pregnancy. It is due largely to impaired peristaltic motion of the intestine caused by pressure from the gravid uterus. The patient should make sure that at least one satisfactory elimination occurs daily; and, as a routine measure, it is well to drink a glass of hot water each morning before breakfast. The water should be as hot as can be taken, and a pinch of salt may be added to give it taste. In some cases, cold water may be more efficacious. In the discussion of elimination, a number of routine suggestions are made, which, if followed, will materially aid in preventing constipation from becoming uncontrollable. Proper elimination cannot be emphasized too much, and daily regularity of habit aids in preventing constipation. In mild cases of constipation a diet of fruits, vegetables, dark breads and coarse foods, with several glasses of water daily, may relieve the condition.

If a mild cathartic seems to be advisable, the nurse may safely suggest prunes and senna prepared in the following way.

Put 2 tablespoonfuls of senna leaves in a cup and pour boiling water over them. Let stand all night. Wash one pound of prunes and soak them all night. Cook until tender. Just before taking them from the stove, add the senna tea (no leaves) to the prunes, and let the mixture come to a boil. Remove from stove and cool. Adding a slice of lemon often improves the taste. The patient should eat from 4 to 6 of the prepared prunes and some of the juice daily.

Another excellent laxative recipe is a half pound each of prunes, figs and seedless raisins and 2 ounces of senna leaves. Wash and dry the fruits very thoroughly and mix with dry senna before putting through a chopper. If this preparation is made into small balls and rolled in sugar, it will keep almost indefinitely. It is more pleasing than the prunes to the majority of patients. Some obstetricians advise milk of magnesia or cascara for their patients. Cascara is easier to take in the pill form, but it seems to be less effective; when the fluid extract is given, the size of the dose and the frequency of its administration must be determined according to the individual patient's reactions. When the proper dosage

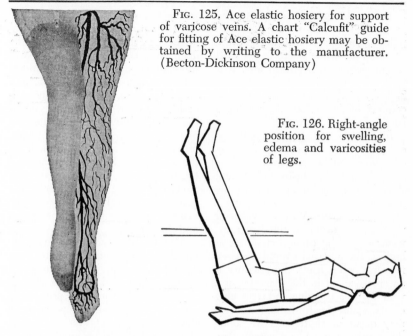

FIG. 125. Ace elastic hosiery for support of varicose veins. A chart "Calcufit" guide for fitting of Ace elastic hosiery may be obtained by writing to the manufacturer. (Becton-Dickinson Company)

FIG. 126. Right-angle position for swelling, edema and varicosities of legs.

has been determined, this drug is generally very satisfactory. The salines are usually reserved for the cases in which they are distinctly indicated, such as certain types of toxemia, and should be given only on the obstetrician's order.

Simple treatments, combined with a largely farinaceous diet, are ordinarily all that is necessary, and the obstetrician should be consulted before even these are used.

Diarrhea occasionally occurs during pregnancy, and its onset should be reported at once to the doctor. Milk boiled for two minutes may be recommended by the nurse, and the patient may be advised to rest. If diarrhea is allowed to persist, it may result in an abortion. either because of severe straining efforts or because of an extension of the existing intestinal contractions. In the latter months of pregnancy diarrhea may cause premature labor.

Dyspnea. Difficult breathing or shortness of breath occasionally results from pressure on the diaphragm by the enlarged uterus and may be sufficient, in the last weeks of pregnancy, to interfere considerably with the patient's sleep and general comfort. Usually it is not a serious condition; but unfortunately it cannot be wholly relieved until after "lightening" (p. 305), the settling of the fetus into the pelvic cavity with relief of the upper abdominal pressure, or after the birth of the baby, when it will disappear spontaneously. It is most troublesome when the patient attempts to lie down, and her comfort may be greatly enhanced by propping her well up in bed with pillows. In this semisitting posture she will at least sleep better and longer than with her head low. It is well for the nurse to demonstrate how these pillows may be arranged comfortably, so that the patient's back is well supported.

In patients with known heart disease, shortness of breath, especially of rather sudden onset, may be a sign of oncoming heart failure and should be reported at once to the physician.

Varicose Veins. Varicose veins or varices may occur in the lower extremities and, at times, extend up as high as the external genitals or even into the pelvis itself. A varicosity is an enlargement in the diameter of a vein due to a thinning and stretching of its walls. Such distended areas may occur at short intervals along the course of the blood vessel; they give it a knotted appearance. They are commonly caused by pressure in the pelvis due to the enlarged uterus, which presses on the great abdominal veins and so interferes with the return of the blood from the lower limbs. Added to this primary cause, any debilitated condition of the patient favors the formation of varicosities in the veins, because of the general flabbiness and lack of tone in the tissues.

Naturally, the greater the pressure in the abdomen, the greater will be the tendency to varicose veins of the legs and the vulva. Therefore, any occupation which keeps a patient constantly on her feet in the latter part of pregnancy causes an increase in abdominal pressure and so acts as an exciting factor.

The first symptom of the development of varices is a dull, aching pain in the legs due to distention of the deep vessels, and inspection will show a fine purple network of superficial veins covering the skin in a lacelike pattern. Later, the true varicosities appear, usually first under the bend of the knee, in a tangled mass of bluish or purplish veins, often as large as a lead pencil. As the condition advances, the varicosities extend up and down the leg along the course of the vessels, and in severe cases they may affect the veins of the labia majora, the vagina and the uterus.

The treatment consists first and chiefly in the prompt abandonment, at the beginning of pregnancy, of round garters and all other articles of clothing that can cause pressure at any part of the body. If varicosities develop in spite of this precaution, the patient should be taught to take the right-angle position, that is, to lie on the bed with her legs extended straight into the air at right angles to her body, her buttocks and heels resting against the wall. At first this position should be taken for from 2 to 5 minutes several times a day, and that will soon demonstrate what can be accomplished. For some patients this position is very uncomfortable at first; but if it is explained and the discomfort is therefore anticipated, the patient is less likely to discontinue the exercise. Late in pregnancy this position may be too difficult to assume because of pressure against the diaphragm.

In order to give support to the weak-walled veins, either an elastic stocking or elastic bandage is often recommended. The initial cost of

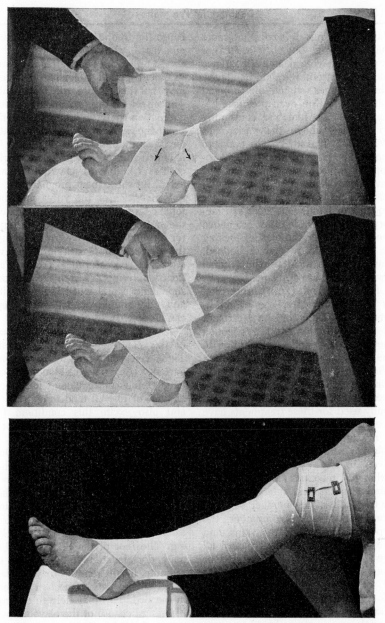

FIG. 127. The method of applying the Ace bandage for varicosities or edema of the legs, which are sometimes treated by the application of Ace, Elastic, Ace adhesive (Becton-Dickinson Company) and Elastoplast bandages (Duke Laboratories).

elastic stockings is somewhat more than bandages, but they are easier to put on, have a neater appearance and longer useful life than bandages. The bandages should be applied spirally with firm even pressure, beginning at the foot and continuing up the leg above the varicosities (Fig. 127). The stocking or bandage should be removed at night and re-applied in the morning, after the legs have been elevated so that the vessels will be less dilated. The longer stocking or bandage is more satisfactory when the varicosities are above the knee. Either the elastic stocking or bandage is washable; indeed, washing helps maintain the original elasticity of these appliances.

INJECTION TREATMENT. According to some authorities, the establishment of a clinic for the treatment of varicose veins by the injection method is a definite contribution in the care of the expectant mother. The pain and the discomfort due to varicose veins may be relieved by these injections. The solutions generally used for these treatments have been sodium monolate, quinine or a mixture of glucose and sodium chloride solution. The treatment is given usually at weekly intervals, although injections may be given more frequently at intervals of two or three days. The number of injections varies with the number, the type and the size of the veins, and the treatment is continued until all the dilated veins are obliterated or until a few weeks before the date of expected delivery. The series of treatments vary with individual doctors. Some obstetricians think that these injections should be postponed until after pregnancy: (1) be-

cause the treatment is one more discomfort for the patient, and (2) the condition of the veins after the convalescent period following delivery may not necessitate the treatment. The effect of this treatment on the circulation routes and on subsequent pregnancies, however, is still a matter of study and observation, and it is hoped that the recurrence of varicosities will be prevented, to some extent, in subsequent pregnancies.

Varicosities of the vulva may be relieved by placing a pillow under the buttocks and elevating the hips for frequent rest periods or by taking the elevated Sims' position for a few moments several times a day. Patients suffering from this condition should not stand when they can sit, and they should not sit when they can lie down.

More important than the treatment of this condition is its prevention. Tight constricting garments, round garters, constipation, standing for long periods of time, and improper amount of rest all tend to aggravate and also excite this condition. In some instances varicose veins seem to be inherited.

RUPTURE OF VARICOSE VEINS. Occasionally, a varicose vein in the vagina may rupture during the prenatal or intrapartum period. The hemorrhage is venous and can be controlled readily by pressure; for example, with the finger or by packing. The foot of the bed should be markedly elevated. If the patient is at home, her extremities may be elevated on the back of a chair placed in the bed. This may help to control bleeding because of the elevated position of the bleeding points. Sometimes the doctor has to put a "tie" around the vein in order to control the bleeding. Incidentally, the same plan of treatment with slight modifications may be employed for a ruptured vein in the lower extremities. If a tourniquet is to be used here, remember to apply it below the bleeding point, because the bleeding is venous, in contrast with arterial bleeding coming from above.

Hemorrhoids. Hemorrhoids are varicosities of the veins about the lower end of the rectum and the anus, and the little lumps and nodules seen in a mass of hemorrhoids are merely the distended portions of the affected vessels. Like varicosities in other areas, they are due to pressure interfering with return venous circulation and are aggravated by constipation. They often cause great distress to the pregnant patient and, due to pressure at the time of delivery, may cause great distress during the postpartum period.

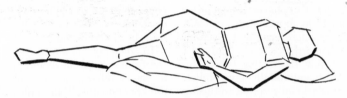

Fig. 128. Sims' position for varicosities of vulva and rectum.

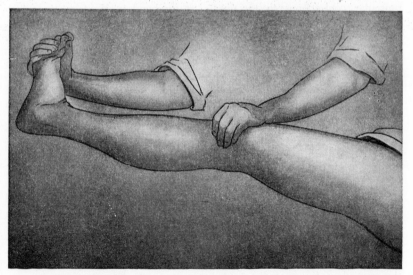

Fig. 129. Showing the nurse helping the patient during a cramp, making pressure on the knee to straighten the leg and forcing the toes upward.

The first step is treatment relieving the constipation. When internal hemorrhoids protrude through the rectum, they should be replaced carefully by pushing them gently back into the rectum. Usually the patient can do this for herself, after lubricating her finger with petrolatum or mineral oil, taking either the knee-chest position (Fig. 252) or elevating her buttocks (Fig. 128) on a pillow. The application of an ice bag, or cold compresses wet with witch hazel or Epsom salts solution, gives great relief. The physician may order tannic acid in suppositories, or compresses of witch hazel and glycerin. If the hemorrhoids are aggravated the first few days after labor, the same treatment usually gives relief. Surgery is seldom resorted to during pregnancy.

Cramps are painful spasmodic muscular contractions in the legs. These cramps may occur at any time during the prenatal period but more generally during the later months due to pressure of the enlarged uterus on the nerves supplying the lower extremities. Other causes have been attributed to insufficient calcium in the diet, fatigue, chilling and tense body posture. Immediate relief may be obtained by forcing the toes upward and by making pressure on the knee to straighten the leg (Fig. 129). Rubbing the affected part also helps. Elevating the feet and keeping the extremities warm are preventives. Cramps, while not a serious condition, are excruciatingly painful for the duration of the seizure. If the husband has been taught the procedure for immediate relief much pain will be prevented.

Edema or swelling of the lower extremities is very common during pregnancy and is sometimes very uncomfortable. It is especially prone to occur in hot weather. Often it may be relieved by a proper abdominal support or by resting frequently during the day. Elevating the feet or taking the right-angle position often gives much relief. If the swelling is persistent, the patient may have to stay in bed, but ordinarily this condition proves to be no more than a discomfort. However, as edema is one of the symptoms of toxemia, it never must be considered as a mere discomfort until all other suspicions have been eliminated.

In edema of the lower extremities, careful investigation should be made to see if other parts are affected—the abdominal wall, the vulva or the back. When positive symptoms are found, or when the edema extends to the hands or the face, the condition should be reported to the physician at once with the findings of the urine examination and a report on the blood-pressure reading. A diet of milk and green vegetables and rest in bed may profitably be advised by the nurse while waiting for orders from the obstetrician.

Vaginal Discharges. In pregnancy vaginal discharges occur frequently, so that a moderately profuse yellowish or white discharge at this time has no particular significance. However, such a condition always should be brought to the obstetrician's attention, for a profuse yellow discharge may be regarded as a possible evidence of gonorrhea, especially when it is accompanied by such urinary manifestations as burning and frequency of urination. A smear may be taken, and the microscopic result will indicate whether or not definite treatment is necessary. If any discharge becomes irritating, the patient may be advised to bathe the vulva with a solution of sodium bicarbonate or boric acid. The application of K.Y. jelly after bathing often relieves the condition entirely. Instructing a patient to wear a perineal pad is sometimes all the advice that is needed. A douche never should be taken unless the obstetrician orders it.

A particularly stubborn form of leukorrhea in pregnancy is caused by the parasitic protozoan known as the trichomonas vaginalis. It is characterized not only by a profuse frothy discharge, white or yellowish in color, but also by irritation and itching of the vulva and the vagina. The diagnosis is easily made by the physician by taking a small quantity of the fresh secretion and putting it under the microscope in a hanging-drop. Here the spindle-shaped organisms, somewhat larger than leukocytes, with whiplike processes attached, can be seen in active motion. Many drugs have been used in the treatment of this condition, the most common being picric acid, either in the form of a 1 per cent aqueous solution or as a suppository.

Pruritus, or itching of the skin, is not uncommon during pregnancy. Some feel that it is due to a mild toxemia, while others think that it may be the result of irritating material being excreted by the skin glands and deposited upon the surface of the body. Proper hygienic measures should be advised. More fluids may be taken so as to promote the activity of the skin, the kidneys and the intestines and thus dilute the

material which may be responsible for the itching. Bathing with a solution of sodium bicarbonate, raw starch or oatmeal water often brings real comfort and may be recommended by the nurse until the condition is reported to the obstetrician.

MAJOR COMPLICATIONS

While the above disorders may be discomforting, they rarely threaten the life of the patient or her infant. However, minor discomforts, if neglected, may lead to a major complication. On the other hand, there are certain complications of pregnancy which do very seriously jeopardize the lives of both mother and child. The more common of these major disturbances fall into four groups:

1. Toxemias.
2. Hemorrhagic complications.
3. Blood groups and the Rh factor.
4. Diseases and pregnancy.

Toxemias

The toxemias of pregnancy are a group of disturbances peculiar to gravid women, characterized (in early pregnancy) by *persistent vomiting;* and (in the middle and the last trimesters) by a variety of signs and symptoms, notably, *elevated blood pressure, albuminuria, edema* and, in certain severe cases, *convulsions* and *coma.* As the name indicates, it has long been supposed that these conditions are due to poisons in the blood, derived presumably from the products of conception, that is, from the fetus, the placenta, the membranes or the amniotic fluid. Since the toxemias of pregnancy occur only in association with pregnancy, this explanation appears reasonable, but as yet no toxin has been demonstrated in the blood or the tissues of such patients, and the actual cause of these disturbances is obscure.

The toxemias of pregnancy are a very common complication of gestation, being seen in 6 or 7 per cent of all gravidae. They rank third to puerperal infection as a cause of maternal death, accounting for almost 2,000 maternal deaths in the United States each year. As a cause of fetal death, they are even more important. Thus, a study carried out by the Children's Bureau in 15 states revealed that 37 per cent of patients with toxemia of later pregnancy had stillborn children. A similar survey carried out in New York City showed that 45 per cent of the babies born from mothers with toxemia were stillborn. Indeed, it can be estimated conservatively that at least 30,000 stillbirths and neonatal deaths each year in this country are the result of toxemia of pregnancy. The great majority of these deaths are due to prematurity of the infant.

This huge toll of maternal and infant lives is in large measure preventable. Proper prenatal supervision, particularly the early detection of signs and symptoms of oncoming toxemia and appropriate treatment, will prevent many cases and so ameliorate others that the outcome for mother and child is usually satisfactory. The nurse is often the first to encounter these signs and symptoms, not only in the clinic but also on home visits, and it is urgently necessary that she be constantly on the lookout for them so that treatment may be instituted at the earliest possible moment.

Classification. The toxemias of pregnancy are usually classified into four main groups: hyperemesis, preeclampsia, eclampsia and chronic hypertensive vascular disease.

DEFINITIONS. *Hyperemesis* is characterized by persistent vomiting of such a degree that little or nothing is retained by the stomach, weight loss ensues, and acetone and diacetic acid appear in the urine. It occurs in the first trimester.

Preeclampsia is characterized by a sudden elevation in blood pressure, albuminuria and edema in a gravida who previously has been normal in these respects. This is a forerunner or the prodromal stage of eclampsia. It is a disease of the last trimester.

Eclampsia is characterized by convulsions and coma, in association with elevated blood pressure, albuminuria and edema. It is a disease of the last trimester.

Chronic hypertensive vascular disease is characterized by chronic, long-standing elevation of blood pressure in gravidae who, as a rule, manifest hypertension whether pregnant or not. Pregnancy aggravates the already existing tendency to hypertension. As indicated by these statements, this disease is seen in all stages of pregnancy, but exacerbations are most common in the second trimester.

HYPEREMESIS GRAVIDARUM. Hyperemesis gravidarum, sometimes called "pernicious vomiting," is simply an exaggeration of the nausea and the vomiting which many pregnant women experience. There is no precise borderline between what is sometimes (and unfortunately) called "normal" nausea and vomiting, and the condition designated as "hyperemesis" or "excessive vomiting." All gradations exist from the gravida who has only slight morning nausea to the unfortunate patient whose persistent, intractable vomiting leads to her death. Indeed, the gravest case of hyperemesis starts originally as "simple" nausea. Accordingly, the woman with "simple nausea" is never to be dismissed as normal but must be regarded as a potential case of hyperemesis, and early treatment should be instituted.

Clinical Picture. Vomiting of sufficient degree to cause weight loss, produce acetone and diacetic acid in the urine, and necessitate hospital treatment occurs about once in every 200 pregnancies. Since these patients usually have been vomiting both food and fluids for weeks, their bodily economy shows marked deviations from the normal. *Dehydration* is pronounced, as evidenced by a dry skin and a dry, cracked tongue; the blood also is low in water, as it were, becomes concentrated and shows a high hemoglobin reading; the urine is scanty. As another result of dehydration, a low-grade fever may be present, and the pulse is usually accelerated. *Starvation,* which is regularly present, manifests itself in a number of ways. Weight loss may vary from 5 pounds to as much as 30 or 40 pounds. This is tantamount to saying that the digestion and the absorption of carbohydrates and other foodstuffs has been so inadequate that the body has been forced to burn its reserve stores of fat in order to maintain bodily heat and energy. When fat is burned without carbohydrates present, the process of combustion does not go on to completion; consequently, certain incompletely burned products of fat metabolism make their appearance in the blood and the urine. These are chiefly acetone and diacetic acid, and their presence in the urine in hyperemesis is common and always indicates a substantial degree of starvation. Then, too, vitamin starvation is regularly present, and in extreme cases, when marked thiamine chloride deficiency exists, disturbances of the peripheral nerves result with loss of function of the legs and arms (peripheral neuritis).

Neurotic Element. It has long been thought that hyperemesis gravidarum is in large measure a *neurosis.* The term "neurosis," it will be recalled, is employed very loosely to designate a large array of conditions in which symptoms occur without demonstrable pathologic explanation, the symptoms being due, it is thought, to a functional disturbance of the patient's psyche. Some psychiatrists estimate that 40 per cent of patients who visit physicians belong in this neurotic class. As many examples show (quite apart from pregnancy), nausea is often psychic in origin. For instance, a repellent sight, or an obnoxious odor, or the mere recollection of such a sight or odor, may give rise to nausea and even vomiting. Our general use of the adjective "nauseating" to depict a repulsive object is further acknowledgment that an upset mind may produce an upset stomach.

In all life's encounters there are probably few experiences which are at first more upsetting, mentally and emotionally, than the realization by a young woman that she is pregnant. At the onset, there are several weeks of anxious uncertainty before she can be sure of the diagnosis. Then, numerous adjustments must be made and plans changed. Emotionally, the implications of pregnancy extend far back into the past when she first met her husband, while its future ramifications are endless. The responsibilities entailed are plain enough, also, and seem on first thought perhaps more than can be assumed. These and a thousand other thoughts crowd themselves into the mind; and in women who cannot adjust themselves to all these new circumstances, it is understandable that the groundwork for a neurosis is laid. Beyond question, there is a large neurotic element in most cases of hyperemesis, a factor which looms large in the treatment of the condition.

The neurotic factor, on the other hand, is not the whole cause of hyperemesis, nor in all probability even the basic cause. In every case an important, underlying organic process is also at work—either the dissemination of toxins into the maternal bloodstream or some maladjustment of the metabolism to the changes wrought by the growing fetus. It is this toxic or organic element which is doubtless the fundamental cause of the disease. To what extent the patient reacts to this underlying process by vomiting seems to be determined in large measure by neurotic factors, that is, by her psychic and emotional stability and by the mental stress and strain which pregnancy has imposed.

Treatment. The principles underlying the treatment of hyperemesis gravidarum are as follows: (1) combat the dehydration by liberal administration of parenteral fluids; (2) combat the starvation by administration of glucose intravenously and thiamine chloride subcutaneously and, if necessary, by feeding a high caloric, high vitamin fluid diet through a nasal tube (Fig. 130); and (3) combat the neurosis by psychotherapy, sedatives and isolation.

Although it may be necessary on occasion to treat cases of hyperemesis in the home, hospitalization is urgently desirable, because isolation from relatives, change of atmosphere, and better facilities for intravenous medication confer unusual benefits in this condition. During the first 24 hours in the hospital, it is customary to withhold all food and fluids by mouth in order to give the gastro-intestinal tract as complete a rest as possible. Glucose solution, usually in 10 per cent concentration, is administered intravenously and, in addition, normal saline solutions subcutaneously or intravenously. The total fluid intake should approximate or exceed 3,000 cc. in the 24 hours. The nurse must keep a careful record of the exact quantity of fluids given, the amount of urine excreted, and the quantity of the vomitus. Sedation is accomplished either by Luminal Sodium hypodermically in dosage of 1 or 2 grains every 4 hours, or by the rectal instillation of some barbiturate drug such as sodium amytal, 3 grains every 6 hours. Thiamine hydrochloride, 50 mg. daily hypodermically, supplies the most urgent vitamin needs during the first 24 hours. All visitors are excluded during this period, including husband and relatives.

After such a regimen for 24 hours, dry toast, crackers or cereal are given by mouth in small quantities every

2 or 3 hours. Fluids are given on alternate hours in small amounts (not over 100 cc. at a time); hot tea and ginger ale usually are tolerated better than plain water. If no vomiting occurs, the amounts and the variety of the food are increased gradually until the patient is on a regular soft, high-vitamin diet. The intravenous administration of fluids may have to be continued for several days, depending on the oral intake.

The success of the treatment will depend in large measure on the tact,

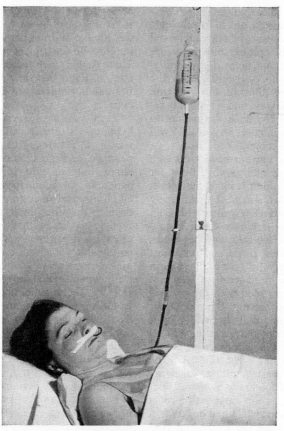

FIG. 130. Levin's tube. The tube is passed through a nostril and the esophagus and into the stomach by the doctor. A variety of nutritious vitamin-rich fluids fill the container above. The glass Murphy drip permits observation of the number of drops per minute introduced into the stomach.

the understanding and the attitude of the nurse. While optimism must be the keynote of the nurse's approach to the patient, this must be coupled with a plainly avowed determination to conquer the complication. The patient must be led gradually to understand that, in the treatment of vomiting, the nurse knows no such word as "failure." Not a few of these patients are in psychologic conflict because of family, financial or social difficulties, and many are averse to the whole idea of pregnancy. If one can only get to the root of these difficulties in a tactful, sympathetic way, and by suitable readjustments reconcile the patient to becoming a mother, a great deal will have been accomplished.

The nurse must exercise great care in preparing and serving trays for patients suffering from hyperemesis. The portions should be extremely small and attractively arranged. Cold liquids such as ginger ale or lemonade must be ice-cold; and hot foods, such as soups, cocoa and tea, must be steaming hot, since lukewarm liquids may be nauseating. It is best not to discuss food with the patient, even when serving the tray, but simply assume that she will enjoy it and talk about other matters. At all times keep the emesis basin out of view, since the sight of it may be enough to start vomiting. Likewise, the smell of food may be nauseating; accordingly, the patient's room should be kept well-aired and should be as far from the kitchen as possible.

If vomiting continues despite these measures, the physician may institute nasal feeding. A small rubber tube (Levin tube) is inserted by the physician through a nostril and on down into the stomach. The tube is strapped to the patient's cheek, connected with an overhanging bottle, and left in place. By this means, large amounts of vitamin-rich liquid foods may be administered. The secret of success with nasal feeding lies in very slow but constant introduction of food into the stomach. The apparatus should be so arranged that the number of drops per minute passing through the tube can be counted. This should not exceed 50 per minute. Even this slow rate, it may be noted, yields about 200 cc. per hour.

Even the most severe cases of hyperemesis usually will respond favorably to the treatment described if patience and persistence are exercised; but, in rare instances, the patient may continue to vomit despite all efforts, and such grave signs may develop that the physician is forced to the conclusion that further continuation of pregnancy will be at the cost of the woman's life. The following signs are grave omens and, especially when several are present, may call for therapeutic abortion: (1) jaundice; (2) delirium; (3) steadily rising pulse rate to levels of 130 or above; (4) fever of 101° or above which persists despite liberal fluid intake; and (5) hemorrhages in the retina, as shown by the physician's ophthalmoscopic examination.

PREECLAMPSIA. As has been stated in the previous classification of the toxemias of pregnancy, preeclampsia is characterized by a sudden elevation in blood pressure, albuminuria and edema in a gravida who previously has been normal in these respects. It is the forerunner or prodromal stage of eclampsia; in other words, unless the preeclamptic process is checked by treatment or by delivery, it is more or less likely that eclampsia (convulsions and coma) will ensue. Characteristically, preeclampsia is a disease of the last 2 or 3 months of pregnancy and is particularly prone to occur in young primigravidae. The underlying disease processes of preeclampsia and eclampsia are probably identical, the chief difference being that the latter goes on to convulsions and coma, while the former does not.

The earliest warning signal of preeclampsia is suddenly developing hypertension. Accordingly, the importance of frequent and regular blood-pressure estimations during pregnancy cannot be emphasized too strongly. The absolute blood-pressure reading is probably of less significance than the relationship it bears to previous determinations and to the age of the patient. For example, a rise from 110/70 to 135/85 * in a young woman is a more urgent danger signal than a rise from 135/85 to 150/90 in a patient of 35.

The next most constant sign of preeclampsia is sudden, excessive weight gain. If cases of preeclampsia are studied from the viewpoint of fluid intake and output, it is at once apparent that these sudden gains in weight are due entirely to an accumulation of water in the tissues. Such weight gains, in other words, represent latent edema and almost always precede the visible face and finger edema which is so character-

* These paired numbers represent the systolic and diastolic blood pressures as measured in millimeters of a column of mercury (Hg).

istic of the advanced stages of the disease. From what has been said, it is apparent that a pair of scales is essential equipment for good prenatal care. Sudden gains of more than 2 pounds a week should be viewed with suspicion; gains of more than 3 pounds, with alarm. Weight increases of the latter magnitude call for more frequent blood-pressure determinations, and if these latter are also abnormal, hospitalization with intensive treatment is indicated. In investigating suspected edema, it is well to ask the patient if her wedding ring is becoming tight, since finger and facial edema is a more valuable sign of preeclampsia than is swelling of the ankles. In the facies of a patient with outspoken preeclampsia, the eyelids are almost swollen shut; and, associated with the edema, marked coarseness of the features develops.

The sudden appearance of *albumin in the urine*, with or without other findings, always should be regarded as a sign of preeclampsia. Usually it develops later than the hypertension and the gain in weight and for this very reason must be regarded as of serious omen when superimposed on these other two findings.

But the very essence of preeclampsia is the lightninglike fulminance with which it strikes. Although the above physical signs of preeclampsia usually give the physician ample time to institute preventive treatment, it sometimes happens that these derangements develop between visits to the office or the clinic, even though they be only a week apart. For this reason it is imperative that all expectant mothers be informed, both verbally and by some form of printed slip or booklet, in regard to certain danger signals which they themselves may recognize. Insofar as the toxemias of pregnancy are concerned, the following symptoms demand immediate report to the doctor: (1) severe, continuous headache; (2) swelling of the face or the finger; (3) dimness or blurring of vision; (4) persistent vomiting; (5) decrease in the amount of urine excreted; and (6) epigastric pain (a late symptom).

For purposes of classification it is customary for physicians to divide cases of preeclampsia into two groups: *Preeclampsia mild* and *preeclampsia severe.* In "preeclampsia mild," the systolic blood pressure ranges between 140 and 160 mm. Hg, not exceeding the latter figure, while the diastolic pressure runs between 90 and 100 mm. Hg. The albumin in the urine is small in amount, often only a trace. Edema is usually slight. "Preeclampsia severe" is characterized by a sustained systolic blood pressure of more than 160 mm. Hg, and usually a diastolic pressure of more than 100 mm. Hg. Albuminuria and edema are marked. In this group many patients present one or more of the signs of impending eclampsia, such as headaches, blurred vision, epigastric pain, vomiting, torpor or irritability. In other words, patients with "preeclampsia severe" are on the verge of convulsions. In "preeclampsia mild," convulsions are much less likely to occur, but the possibility never can be eliminated.

Treatment. In the face of the warnings of developing toxemia, as mentioned above, the physician's first duty is to make arrangements for frequent blood-pressure readings. In milder cases often this is carried out through the help of the public health or visiting nurse who makes daily visits to the home of the patient, takes the blood pressure, notes the presence of other signs and symptoms and then reports her findings to the physician. In many cases, however, certainly in all cases of "preeclampsia severe," hospitalization is necessary.

During this period of preliminary observation the following routine usually is followed. Of first importance is a salt-poor diet, that is, one in which no salt is added, either in the kitchen or at the table. Second, activities should be restricted, complete rest in bed being desirable in most cases. Third, saline catharsis should be administered at the onset of the treatment and repeated twice weekly. Fourth, fluid intake is maintained at about 3,000 cc. daily— that is, 8 to 10 glasses of water. Fifth, sedatives are given, such as Luminal Sodium, the dosage being dependent on the severity of the condition. If convulsions are actually imminent, heavy sedation with paraldehyde may be desirable. Lastly, in regard to the protein content of the diet (this is a debated subject), the balance of opinion seems to be in favor of permitting a full diet of meat, provided that the meat is not salty.

The restriction of salt in the diet of the preeclamptic patient is directed at reducing the edema. Even in normal, nonpregnant persons an increased intake of sodium chloride causes water retention. Pregnant

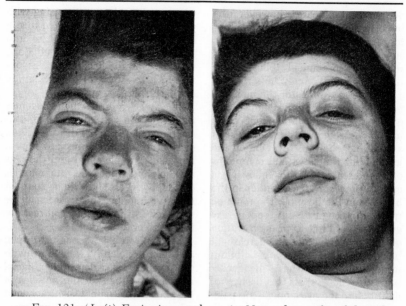

Fig. 131. (*Left*) Facies in preeclampsia. Note edema of eyelids and facial skin and general coarsening of features. (*Right*) Same patient 10 days after delivery.

women, particularly gravidae suffering from preeclampsia, show a marked tendency to retain salt; and there is reason to believe that this tendency of the tissues to retain salt is closely correlated with their tendency to hold water. To superimpose on this already existing salt and water retention, still more salt in the diet is obviously unwise.

By means of the above measures, it is often possible to relieve the signs and symptoms of preeclampsia so that the patient proceeds to term satisfactorily. Not infrequently, however, despite all efforts, the condition persists, and in that event the artificial induction of labor may be-

come necessary. In occasional instances, when the preeclampsia is very severe and fulminating and conditions for artificial induction of labor are not favorable, cesarean section may be the procedure of choice.

The signs and symptoms of preeclampsia usually abate rapidly after delivery, but the danger of convulsions does not pass until 48 hours have elapsed postpartum. Therefore, continuation of sedation throughout this interval is indicated. In the majority of cases the elevated blood pressure as well as the other derangements have returned to normal within 10 days or 2 weeks. In about

30 per cent of cases, however, the hypertension shows a tendency either to persist indefinitely or to recur in subsequent pregnancies. For this reason the prolonged follow-up of these patients is highly important.

The nurse's duties in the management of a case of preeclampsia are manifold. (1) In order that cases may be detected and treated as soon as possible, she must ever be on the lookout for the signs and symptoms of the disease. (2) In following a case of preeclampsia, whether in the home or in the hospital, she must be quick to recognize and report any evidence pointing to an aggravation of the process (sudden increase of blood pressure, edema or albuminuria; also persistent headache, blurred vision, spots or flashes of light before the eyes, epigastric pain, vomiting, torpor, muscular twitchings). (3) Since water retention plays such a large role in the disease, it is essential that she keep a meticulous fluid intake and output chart. (4) She must pay careful attention to excluding salt from the diet, both in the kitchen and on the trays. (5) In severe cases she must protect the patient from external stimuli; the room should be darkened, lights never directed at the patient's face, and noises kept at a minimum. (6) In severe cases she must have ready a mouth-gag to prevent the patient from biting her tongue in the event that a convulsion develops. In some hospitals, nurses are taught to use rolled towels instead of mouth-gags.

ECLAMPSIA. *Clinical Picture.* As indicated, the development of eclampsia is almost always preceded by the signs and symptoms of preeclampsia. A preeclamptic patient, who may have been conversing with you a moment before, is seen to roll her eyes to one side and stare into space with fixed eyes. Immediately, twitching of the facial muscles ensues. This is the *stage of invasion* and lasts only a few seconds.

The whole body then becomes rigid in a generalized muscular contraction; the face is distorted, the eyes protrude, the arms are flexed, the hands are clenched and the legs are inverted. Since all the muscles of the body are now in a state of tonic contraction, this phase may be regarded as the *stage of contraction;* it lasts 15 or 20 seconds.

Suddenly the jaws begin to open and close violently, and forthwith the eyelids also. The other facial muscles and then all the muscles of the body alternately contract and relax in rapid succession. So forceful are the muscular movements that the patient may throw herself out of bed, and almost invariably, unless protected, the tongue is bitten by the violent jaw action. Foam, often blood-tinged, exudes from the mouth; the face is congested and purple, and the eyes are bloodshot. Few pictures which the nurse is called upon to witness are so horrible. This phase in which the muscles alternately contract and relax is called the *stage of convulsion;* it may last a minute or so. Gradually the muscular movements become milder and farther apart, and finally the patient lies motionless.

Throughout the seizure the diaphragm has been fixed with respiration halted. Still no breathing occurs. For a few seconds the woman appears to be dying from respiratory arrest, but just when this outcome seems almost inevitable, she takes a long, deep, stertorous inhalation, and breathing is resumed. Then coma ensues. The patient will remember nothing whatsoever of the convulsion or, in all probability, events immediately before and afterward.

The coma may last from a few minutes to several hours, and the patient may then become conscious; or the coma may be succeeded by another convulsion. The convulsions may recur during coma, or they may recur only after an interval of consciousness, or they may never recur at all. In the average case from 5 to 10 convulsions occur at longer or shorter intervals, but as many as 20 are not uncommon. Convulsions may start before the onset of labor (ante partum), during labor (intrapartum), or any time within the first 48 hours after delivery (postpartum). About a fifth of the cases develop postpartum.

Upon physical examination, the findings of eclampsia are similar to those in preeclampsia, but exaggerated. Thus, the systolic blood pressure usually ranges around 180 mm. Hg, and sometimes exceeds 200 mm. Hg. Albuminuria is frequently extreme, from 10 to 20 Gm. per liter. Edema may be marked but sometimes is absent. Oliguria, or suppression of urinary excretion, is common and may amount to complete anuria. Fever is present in about half the cases.

In favorable cases, the convulsions cease, the coma lessens, and urinary output increases. However, it sometimes requires a day or two for clear consciousness to be regained. During this period eclamptic patients are often in an obsterperous, resistant mood and may be exceedingly difficult to manage. A few develop actual psychoses. In unfavorable cases the coma deepens, urinary excretion diminishes, the pulse becomes more rapid, the temperature rises, and edema of the lungs develops. The last is a serious symptom and usually is interpreted as a sign of cardiovascular failure. Edema of the lungs is readily recognizable by the noisy, gurgling respiration and by the large quantity of frothy mucus which exudes from the mouth and the nose. Toward the end, convulsions cease altogether, and the final picture is one of vascular collapse with falling blood pressure and overwhelming edema of the lungs.

Like preeclampsia, eclampsia is a disease of young primigravidae, more than 80 per cent of the cases occurring in first pregnancies. It is more likely to occur as full term approaches and is rarely seen prior to the last 3 months. Eclampsia is particularly prone to develop in twin gestations, the likelihood being about four times that in single pregnancies.

Prognosis. Eclampsia is one of the gravest complications of pregnancy; the maternal mortality ranges, in different localities and in different hospitals, from 10 to 20 per cent of such cases. The outlook for the baby is particularly grave, the fetal mortality being about 50 per cent. Although it is difficult in a given case to forecast the outcome, the following are unfavorable signs: prolonged coma; a sustained pulse rate over 120; temperature over 103° F.; more than 10 convulsions (but patients with 200 have been known to recover); 10 or more Gm. of albumin per liter in the urine; systolic blood pressure of more than 200; edema of lungs. If none of these signs is present, the outlook for recovery is good; if two or more are present, the prognosis is serious.

Even though the patient survives, she may not escape unscathed from the attack but sometimes continues to have high blood pressure indefinitely. This statement applies both to preeclampsia and eclampsia. Indeed, about 10 per cent of all preeclamptic and 5 per cent of all eclamptic patients are left with chronic, permanent hypertension. It is of even more importance to note that a still larger percentage of these women (about 50 per cent of preeclamptics and 30 per cent of eclamptics) again develop hypertensive toxemia in any subsequent pregnancies. This is known as "recurrent" or "repeat" toxemia. These facts make it plain that careful, prolonged follow-up of these mothers who have suffered from preeclampsia or eclampsia is imperative. Moreover, the prognosis for future pregnancies must be guarded, although, as the figures indicate, such patients stand at least an even chance of going through subsequent pregnancies satisfactorily.

Principles of Treatment. Since the cause of eclampsia is not known, there can be no "specific" therapy, and treatment must necessarily be empirical. By "empirical" treatment is meant the utilization of those therapeutic measures which have yielded the best results in other cases. It is thus based on experience. Since the experience of different doctors and different hospitals varies considerably, the type of therapy employed from clinic to clinic differs somewhat in respect to the drugs

used and in other details. However, the general principles followed are almost identical everywhere. For the nurse to memorize some particular regimen of therapy, as given in this textbook or as used in this or that hospital, will serve little purpose in her later career and conduces to an undesirable rigidity of attitude. However, she should grasp thoroughly the general principles involved. These are enumerated as follows.

1. PREVENTION. Let it be emphasized again that eclampsia is largely (but not entirely) a preventable disease. Vigilant prenatal care and the early detection and treatment of preeclampsia will do more to reduce deaths from eclampsia than the most intensive treatment after convulsions have once started.

2. CONSERVATIVE TREATMENT. Since eclampsia never occurs in nonpregnant women nor in men, it is reasonable to believe that it must be due in some way to the pregnant condition. By the same token it might be concluded that the best way to treat eclampsia would be to terminate the pregnancy at once, that is, empty the uterus. This was the therapy employed in the early years of the century, and is known as the "radical treatment" of eclampsia; either the cervix was forcibly dilated and the baby extracted, or cesarean section was employed. The results were disastrous. A quarter to a third of the mothers died, often on the operating table from shock.

Dissatisfied with the poor results yielded by the radical treatment of eclampsia, about 1910 physicians began treating the convulsions with sedative drugs, ignored the pregnancy and allowed labor to start

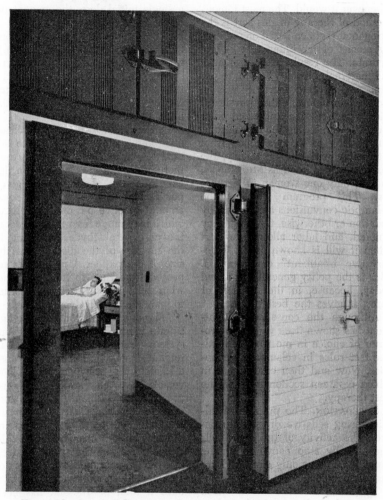

Fig. 132. An outside view of special climate-controlled room for eclampsia patients. Mechanical equipment controlling weather is built into the wall partitions. Two doors prevent any change in the weather when staff enters and leaves room. A control board inside the room makes it possible for the staff to control the humidity from 40 per cent to saturation and the temperature from 50° to 100° F. (Lying-in Hospital and University of Chicago Office of Press Relations. Photo by Hedrich Blessing Studios)

whenever it would. The most famous method of therapy of this sort is the Stroganoff regimen based on sedation by means of morphine and chloral hydrate. The results were dramatic: the maternal mortality fell to 10 per cent, and the fetal mortality was no worse than before. Other physicians tried other sedative drugs and other means of combating the convulsions, but as long as they refrained from interfering with the pregnancy, the results were as good as Stroganoff's, that is, only one woman in ten was lost. This program whereby the eclamptic convulsions are treated by sedation or otherwise, the pregnancy ignored, and labor allowed to start when it will is known as the "conservative treatment" of eclampsia. This is the policy generally followed today, because, in the majority of cases, it gives the best results.

Although the conservative treatment has shown itself to be the program of choice in most cases, hard-and-fast rules in eclampsia are unwise. Now and then cases occur in which cesarean section may be the best therapy.

3. SEDATION. The purpose of administering sedative drugs is to depress the activity of the brain cells and thereby stop convulsions. The drugs most commonly employed are described below.

Morphine. Because of its quick action and readiness of administration, morphine is usually the first drug which the eclamptic patient receives. Thus, it is often given at the patient's home to allay convulsions during transport to the hospital, or in the admission room of a hospital pending the institution of other types of medication. When given as a single initial dose, the amount ordered by the physician is likely to be large, from one quarter to one half a grain (0.016 to 0.032 Gm.). Morphine may also be administered during the subsequent course of the treatment, but the modern tendency is to rely on other drugs for the main sedative program.

Paraldehyde. Although pungent in odor and somewhat difficult to administer, paraldehyde is being used more and more in eclampsia. In this condition it is almost always given per rectum, diluted with an equal amount of olive oil, and in dosages which may range from 20 to 35 cc. of the pure paraldehyde, according to the severity of the disease and the size of the patient. Usually it is repeated from time to time, in somewhat smaller doses perhaps, in order to maintain a fairly deep narcosis.

Magnesium Sulfate. Magnesium sulfate is not only a central nervous system sedative (employed in tetanus) but it is believed to cause a dilatation of the peripheral blood vessels and thus lower the blood pressure. Dr. William J. Dieckmann, director of the Chicago Lying-In Hospital and one of the leading authorities on the toxemias, injects 10 cc. of a 50 per cent solution deep into the gluteal muscles, and 2 cc., or 1 Gm., is given after each convulsion until a total of 10 Gm. has been given. Dr. E. Lazard, of Los Angeles, who was one of the first to use magnesium sulfate in eclampsia, gives 20 cc. of a 10 per cent solution intravenously and repeats it every hour until convulsions are under control.

Barbiturates. The more commonly employed of these are: Luminal

Sodium (0.3 to 1.3 Gm. subcutaneously or per rectum); Pentobarbital Sodium (0.6 to 0.8 Gm. per rectum); and Amytal Sodium (0.6 to 0.9 Gm. per rectum). The drugs produce

rectum. In either case, it usually is repeated every 6 hours, but the dose is decreased to 1.5 Gm.

Ether. In occasional instances, ether may be given by inhalation or

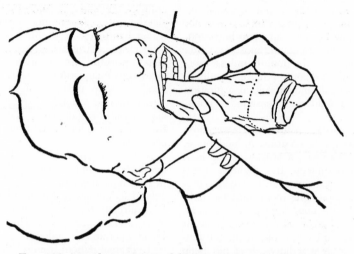

Fig. 133. Mouth gag inserted between jaws of eclamptic patient to prevent tongue injury. The nurse's fingers should be kept away from the teeth, lest they be bitten. (Putnam, Tracy J.: Convulsive Seizures, Philadelphia, Lippincott)

sleep, muscular relaxation, and lowering of the blood pressure.

Chloral Hydrate. As already mentioned, chloral hydrate in conjunction with morphine forms the basis of the Stroganoff treatment. Dr. Henricus J. Stander, the late director of the New York Lying-In Hospital and another outstanding authority on the toxemias, used this drug for 20 years in the treatment of eclampsia and recommended it strongly. If the patient is thoroughly conscious, 2.0 Gm. are given in milk by mouth, but if not, the same amount is administered in 100 cc. of starch water per

by rectum to control convulsions. When given by the latter route, 60 cc. of ether and 120 cc. of olive oil are mixed and injected slowly. Since ether has a tendency to increase pulmonary secretions, it must be employed with caution.

4. PROTECTION OF PATIENT FROM SELF-INJURY. The eclamptic patient must never be left alone for a second. When in the throes of a convulsion, she may crash her head against a bedpost or throw herself onto the floor; or she may bite her tongue violently. To prevent the latter injury, some device should be kept

within easy reach which can be inserted between the jaws at the very outset of a convulsion. A piece of very heavy rubber tubing, a rolled towel, or a padded clothespin is often employed. But the nurse must take care in inserting it not to injure the patient (lips, gums, teeth) and not to allow her own finger to be bitten.

Eclamptic patients must never be given fluids by mouth unless thoroughly conscious. Failure to adhere to this rule may result in aspiration of the fluid and consequent pneumonia.

5. PROTECTION OF PATIENT FROM EXTRANEOUS STIMULI. A loud noise, a bright light, a jarring of the bed, a draft—indeed, the slightest irritation—may be enough to precipitate a convulsion. The room must be darkened, and noise kept at a minimum. If catheterization has to be done, it is well to carry it out about 30 minutes after a sedative drug has been given, so that the patient may be protected against stimulation as much as possible.

6. PROMOTION OF DIURESIS. When an eclamptic patient begins to excrete substantial quantities of urine, the outlook is encouraging. Accordingly, efforts are generally made to stimulate renal activity. This is most often done by the intravenous administration of hypertonic glucose solutions, usually about a 20 per cent solution in amounts ranging from 200 to 500 cc.

7. OTHER THERAPEUTIC PROCEDURES. Although the above principles of treatment may be regarded as more or less standard, the nurse will encounter many experienced obstetricians who secure good results with other procedures.

Venesection, the withdrawal of from 300 to 1,000 cc. of blood, is believed by some authorities to be of great value. Dehydration of the patient through purging with magnesium sulfate (stomach tube), drainage of spinal fluid, hypertonic glucose, etc., is another program which has received attention. Veratrum viride, a drug which lowers the blood pressure, is regarded with favor by many obstetricians. Still another group recommends a regimen centering around gastric lavage and colonic irrigation—the Tweedy, Rotunda, or Dublin treatment of eclampsia.

Nurse's Responsibilities in Eclampsia. The nurse's responsibilities in the management of a case of eclampsia are serious. Some of them have already been mentioned in the discussion of treatment. They may be enumerated as follows.

1. Protect patient from self-injury. Never leave the patient unless relief is actually at the bedside. Restrain any movements which might prove to be harmful, but do this gently in order to conserve patient's strength. Canvas sides to the bed, as well as pads at the head and the foot of the bed, are helpful. A rubber or padded mouth-gag to be inserted between the upper and the lower teeth at the outset of a convulsion must always be within easy reach. Never give an eclamptic patient fluids by mouth unless you are certain that she is fully conscious.

2. Protect patient from extraneous stimuli. The room should be darkened except for a small table lamp so shaded that none of the light falls on the patient. For catherization, rectal instillations and the doc-

tor's examinations, use a flashlight, directed well away from the patient's face. Slamming of doors, clanking of pans and jarring of the bed must be avoided. Absolutely necessary conversation with doctors should be in the lowest tones possible.

3. Watch for signs of labor. In eclampsia this may proceed with few external signs, and occasionally such a patient gives birth beneath the sheets before anyone knows that the process is under way. Be suspicious when the patient grunts or groans or moves about at regular intervals— every 5 minutes or so. If this occurs, feel the consistency of the uterus, watch for "show," and report your observations to the doctor.

4. Keep careful record of fluid intake and output.

5. Keep careful record of duration of each convulsion, depth and duration of coma, whether patient responds to her name, etc.; note also character of respiration, whether stertorous, gurgling, etc.

CHRONIC HYPERTENSIVE VASCULAR DISEASE. Hyperemesis, preeclampsia and eclampsia have been discussed in some detail because the nurse's role in the management of these three conditions is extremely important. In the hypertensive vascular disease, the responsibilities of the nurse, although substantial from the viewpoint of nursing care, are lighter in nature.

As the name indicates, this disease is a chronic disorder of the vascular system associated with high blood pressure. In other words, these patients have a tendency to have hypertension whether pregnant or not. Not infrequently the kidneys are also affected, with the result that albumi-

nuria may be present as well as diminution in the excretory power of the kidneys. The age of these patients is usually in the thirties or late twenties; most of them are multiparae with a number of children. The course of pregnancy in these chronic hypertensive women is often troublesome, the blood pressure showing a tendency to reach higher and higher levels as the last three months of pregnancy are reached. In general, the outlook for the baby is poor. The fetus often dies *in utero*. Following delivery, there may be a slight recession in the blood pressure, but it usually remains at a figure only slightly below that observed during pregnancy. Each subsequent pregnancy adds its increment to the hypertension and, as a rule, the exacerbation in blood pressure occurs earlier and earlier in each succeeding pregnancy.

Aside from the high blood pressure, the signs and symptoms of hypertensive vascular disease may be surprisingly few. Headache is rather common, but even this complaint may be absent. The doctor's examination of the retina very often shows a narrowing of the arterioles, indicative of the fact that there is a generalized sclerosis of the small arterioles throughout the body.

In patients with chronic hypertensive vascular disease, we cannot prevent the occurrence of hypertension, because they already had hypertension when conception took place. They already had the sclerosed, inelastic arterioles mentioned above, and it is understandable that the 50 per cent increase in minute output of the heart which pregnancy imposes (p. 141) will place a severe burden on such a vascular system. In the face of this chronic process and this burden imposed by pregnancy, very little can be done in such cases to relieve the hypertension. But the patient can be aided by helping her to prevent pregnancy. Hence, the problem is largely one of preventive medicine, in the sense that pregnancies should either be avoided altogether or limited.

Decision as to the best way of managing a case of hypertensive vascular disease will be made by the doctor after taking into consideration a number of circumstances, such as the severity of the hypertensive process, the number of children in the family, the duration of the pregnancy when first seen, etc. If the process is mild, the pregnancy may be allowed to continue with the patient under close observation for signs of impending trouble. On the other hand, if the process is very severe it may be necessary to interrupt the pregnancy in order to save the mother's life. In most cases in this group, the doctor will wish to prevent further pregnancies and will recommend either ligation of the fallopian tubes or the use of some method of contraception.

HEMORRHAGIC COMPLICATIONS

By far the most common cause of bleeding in pregnancy is abortion. Other important causes are ectopic pregnancy, placenta previa, and premature separation of the normally implanted placenta (abruptio placentae).

Abortion. DEFINITION. Abortion is the termination of pregnancy before the fetus is viable (28 weeks), that is, before it is capable of extra-uterine existence. Since some 97 per cent of

all abortions occur during the first five months of pregnancy, when there is no hope whatsoever of the fetus' survival, abortions in general constitute a group which the nurse will have no difficulty in recognizing.

Premature labor is the termination of pregnancy after the fetus is viable but before it is full term. By general consensus, a full-term fetus is regarded as one which weighs 2,500 Gm. (5½ lbs.) or more.

In occasional cases termination of pregnancy near the seventh month may raise the question as to whether the case is to be classified as one of abortion or of premature labor. This question may be answered differently in different hospitals, but, in general, a birth is regarded as an abortion if the fetus weighs under 1,000 Gm. (2 lbs., 3 oz.). A fetus weighing 1,000 Gm. has a gestational age of about 28 weeks. This does not mean that a fetus weighing under 1,000 Gm. has no chance of survival; it simply means that, in order for the fetus to have an appreciable chance, it must have attained that weight. Modern improvements in caring for premature infants make it possible occasionally for fetuses weighing only 800 to 900 Gm. (1 lb., 13 oz. to 2 lbs.) to survive. If a fetus weighing less than 1,000 Gm. does survive, it is termed a premature infant and not an abortion. Many hospitals set a fetal weight of 1,500 Gm., instead of 1,000, as the borderline between abortion and premature birth.

TERMINOLOGY OF ABORTION. The term abortion, as employed by physicians and nurses, includes all varieties of termination of pregnancy prior to viability—both cases in which the process started of its own accord (spontaneous) and cases in which it was artificially induced. The laity, however, are inclined to associate the word "abortion" with instances in which criminal interference with

In medical parlance the word "miscarriage" is used only occasionally, and, when employed, it may be taken as synonymous with "abortion," but a few doctors prefer to

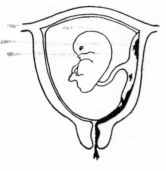

Threatened

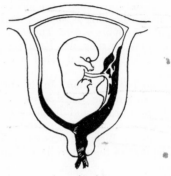

Inevitable

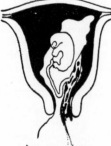

Incomplete

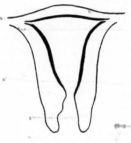

Complete

Fig. 134. Stages of abortion. (Cooke, Willard R.: Essentials of Gynecology, Philadelphia, Lippincott)

pregnancy has been perpetrated, and to them, therefore, the term often carries a definite stigma. They employ the word *"miscarriage"* to designate spontaneous abortion, and the nurse will do well, in discussing the matter with patients or relatives, to use that term.

restrict its use to the termination of pregnancy in the second trimester, that is, to late abortions.

Threatened Abortion. An abortion is regarded as threatened if a patient in early pregnancy has vaginal bleeding or spotting; this may or may not be associated with mild cramps. The cervix is closed. The process has presumably started but may abate under suitable treatment (Fig. 134).

Inevitable Abortion. Inevitable abortion is so called because the process has gone so far that termination of the pregnancy cannot be prevented. Bleeding is copious, and the pains are more severe. The membranes may or may not have ruptured, and the cervical canal is dilating.

Incomplete Abortion. In incomplete abortion the fetus is passed, but the membranes and the placenta, either entire or in part, are retained in the uterus. Bleeding persists until the contents of the uterus have been passed.

Complete Abortion. Complete abortion is the expulsion of the entire product of conception.

Missed Abortion. In a missed abortion the fetus dies in the uterus, but, instead of being expelled, it is retained indefinitely. The term is generally restricted to cases in which 2 months or more elapse between fetal death and expulsion. During this period the fetus undergoes marked degenerative changes. Of these, maceration, or a general softening, is the most common. Occasionally it dries up into a leatherlike structure (mummification) and very rarely it becomes converted into stony material (lithopedion formation). Symptoms, except for amenorrhea, are usually lacking, but occasionally such patients complain of malaise, headache, anorexia and a peculiar taste in the mouth.

Habitual Abortion. By this term is meant a condition in which abortion occurs in successive pregnancies (3 or more) and at about the same stage

of gestation. This is a most distressing condition, some women having 6 or 8 spontaneous abortions. Although the condition is unsatisfactory to treat, modern hormonal preparations, notably progesterone (p. 63), are helpful in some cases.

Criminal Abortion. Criminal abortion means the instrumental induction of abortion without medical and legal justification. Since these operations always are performed secretly, accurate figures concerning their frequency are difficult to secure, but the very minimum estimate is 100,-000 annually in the United States, while some authorities put the figure at over half a million a year. This means that each year in this country between 100,000 and 500,000 potential lives are destroyed simply for "convenience," a frightful wastage of human life and a sorry reflection on our civilization. Quite apart from this destruction of fetal life, criminal abortion is one of the most common causes of maternal death. Unless the mother's health is at stake, no reputable physician will induce an abortion, for it constitutes murder. Consequently, these clandestine operations usually are performed by hands which are not only unskilled but unclean. As a result, fatal infections are common. Of those who survive many are left invalids, others permanently sterile. Most cases of so-called "infected abortion" are of this origin.

Every year huge quantities of castor oil, quinine and other "powerful" drugs are sold for the express purpose of interrupting early pregnancy. As a rule, these concoctions merely produce nausea and vomiting, while pregnancy is not interrupted. Certain of the patent medicines sold for this purpose, however, contain ingredients which act with such violence that hemorrhages into the bowel and the kidneys sometimes ensue with results that may be exceedingly grave. The reputation of these drugs rests on the circumstance that the menstrual interval in the same woman often varies widely; a woman who has been accustomed to menstruate every 28 days may occasionally experience a 35-day cycle without apparent cause or detriment to health. If, in such a long cycle, when she thinks herself 5 or 6 days "overdue," she takes one of these medicines and starts menstruating the next day, the drug is naturally acclaimed as the benefactor. It is obvious that the same end would have been attained had she done nothing. At the present writing there is no drug known to the medical profession which will produce abortion in the human being, whether given by mouth or hypodermically.

Therapeutic Abortion. Therapeutic abortion means the instrumental induction of abortion by a physician because of some grave maternal disease which would make continuation of the pregnancy extremely hazardous. As a rule, one or more physicians are called into consultation to make certain that the procedure is absolutely necessary. Modern methods of prenatal care are making the necessity for therapeutic abortion relatively rare. The nurse must recall, moreover, that the Roman Catholic Church forbids the procedure, and that it may not be performed in hospitals of that faith.

CLINICAL PICTURE. About 75 per cent of all spontaneous abortions occur during the second and the

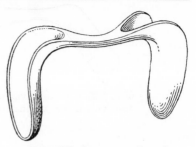

FIG. 135. Sims speculum for inserting into the vaginal canal so as to expose the cervix to view.

third months of pregnancy, that is, before the twelfth week. The condition is very common; it is estimated that about 1 pregnancy in every 10 terminates in spontaneous abortion. Almost invariably the first symptom is bleeding due to the separation of the fertilized ovum from its uterine attachment. The bleeding is often slight at the beginning and may persist for days before uterine cramps occur; or, the bleeding may be followed at once by cramps. Occasionally the bleeding is torrential in nature, leaving the patient in shock. The uterine contractions bring about softening and dilatation of the cervix and expel the products of conception either completely or incompletely.

CAUSES. What causes all these spontaneous abortions—so tragic and shattering to so many women? Is Mother Nature actually so cruel to our mothers as these figures would suggest? If the evidence is reviewed with some perspective and with full fairness to all concerned, it is the inevitable conclusion that most of these abortions, far from being tragedies, are blessings in disguise, for

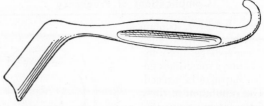

FIG. 136. Schroeder vaginal retractor for drawing back the vulval or vaginal walls during an operation.

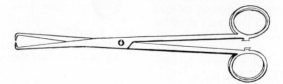

FIG. 137. Bullet forceps used in grasping the lips of the cervix.

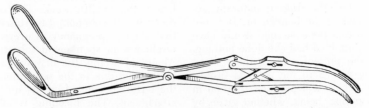

FIG. 138. Modified Goodell-Ellinger dilator used for enlarging the canal of the cervix.

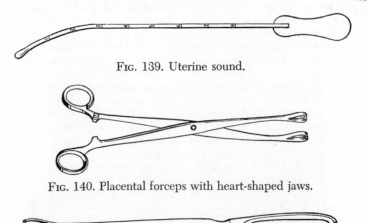

FIG. 139. Uterine sound.

FIG. 140. Placental forceps with heart-shaped jaws.

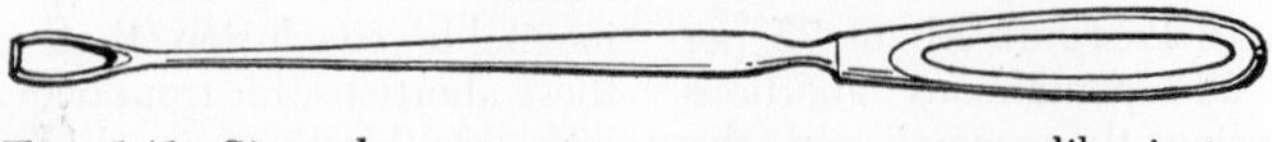

FIG. 141. Sims sharp curette, a scraper or spoonlike instrument for removing matter from the walls of the uterus.

they are Nature's beneficent way of extinguishing embryos which are imperfect. Indeed, careful microscopic study of the material passed in these cases shows that the commonest cause of spontaneous abortion is an inherent defect in the product of conception. This defect may express itself in an abnormal embryo, in an abnormal *trophoblast* (p. 76), or in both abnormalities. In early abortions, 80 per cent are associated with some defect of the embryo or trophoblast which is either incompatible with life or would result in a grossly deformed child. The incidence of abnormalities passed after the second

month is somewhat lower, but not less than 50 per cent. Whether the germ plasm of the spermatozoon or the ovum is at fault in these cases it is usually difficult, if not impossible, to say. Abortions of this sort are obviously unpreventable and, although bitterly disappointing to the parents, serve a useful purpose.

Although many spontaneous abortions are due to causes other than defects in the product of conception, little is known about these causes. Severe acute infections, such as pneumonia and typhoid fever, often lead to abortion. Heart failure is another etiologic factor. Occasion-

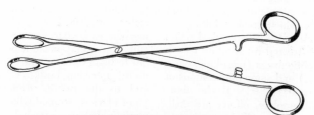

FIG. 142. Sponge holder.

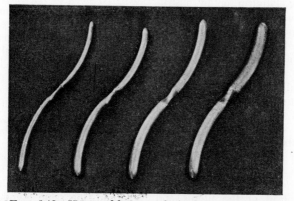

FIG. 143. Hegar dilators, of graduated diameters from 5 to 12 mm. Larger sizes are also used.

ally, malposition of the uterus, notably retroposition, produces the accident. Many women tend to explain miscarriage on the grounds of injury of one type or another, or excessive activity. Different women exhibit the greatest variation in this respect. In some the pregnancy may go blithely on despite falls from second-story windows and automobile accidents so severe as to fracture the pelvis. In others a trivial fall or merely overfatigue seems to contribute at least to abortion. Since there is no way of telling who is susceptible and who is not, it would seem prudent for every expectant mother to follow the dictates of common sense and avoid long automobile trips, lifting heavy weights, and any form of activity which involves jolting.

TREATMENT. Threatened abortion usually is treated by absolute rest in bed, narcotic drugs (morphine, paregoric, etc.) and some preparations of progesterone (p. 62). If the abortion is incomplete, efforts are ordinarily made to aid the uterus in emptying its contents either by administering Pituitrin or by instrumental removal of the retained products of conception, particularly if no evidence of infection exists. Active bleeding may make this urgently necessary. The instruments commonly used in completing an incomplete abortion are shown in Figs. 135 to 143. If evidence of infection is present (fever, foul discharge or suspicious history of criminal abortion), the doctor may prefer to withhold any invasion of the uterine cavity, lest it disseminate bacteria into the venous sinuses of the uterus and thence into the general circulation.

On the other hand, bleeding and certain other circumstances may make removal of the uterine contents desirable despite the presence of infection. Complete abortion requires exactly the same care as that given during the postpartum period. As already indicated, habitual abortion may be helped by endocrine therapy as well as by meticulous attention to general hygiene, rest, vitamin requirements, etc.

NURSE'S RESPONSIBILITIES IN ABORTION CASES. The nurse will be consulted as a trusted confidante on countless aspects of reproduction. In regard to criminal abortion, she can have only one attitude, namely, to regard it as the murder of a potential human being and also as a procedure which kills thousands of mothers each year. Occasionally, circumstances may make it possible for her to be of definite educational help on this question, both to her patients and to the public. From another point of view, women who have had a criminal abortion recently or whose history is suspicious (the majority deny it) must be regarded as potentially infected and put under strict isolation in order to prevent spread of the infection to other patients.

Bleeding in the first half of pregnancy, no matter how slight, always must be considered as threatened abortion. The patient must be put to bed and the doctor notified. If the bleeding is so copious as to be alarming, raise the foot of the bed (shock position) and apply hot-water bottles while awaiting the doctor's arrival. In preparing a patient for instrumental completion of an incomplete abortion, the same aseptic regimen is carried out as for full-term deliv-

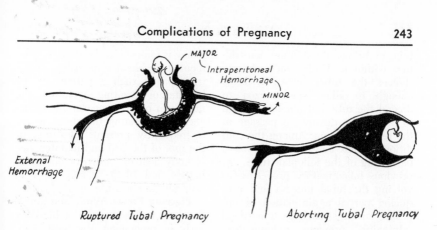

FIG. 144. (*Left*) Rupture of tubal pregnancy into peritoneal cavity. (*Right*) Tubal abortion. (Cooke, Willard R.: Essentials of Gynecology, Philadelphia, Lippincott)

ery (p. 325). Moreover, the nurse never must forget that all material passed by the patient, including blood clots, should be saved. The doctor will wish to examine these, to make sure that all the product of conception has been passed, and, in addition, to ascertain, if possible, the cause of the abortion (defective germ plasma, etc.).

Ectopic Pregnancy. About once in every 300 pregnancies the fertilized ovum, instead of traversing the length of the fallopian tube to reach the uterine cavity, becomes implanted within the wall of the fallopian tube. This condition is known as "ectopic pregnancy" (literally, a pregnancy which is out of place), or as "tubal pregnancy" or "extra-uterine pregnancy." Since the wall of the tube is not sufficiently elastic to allow the fertilized ovum to grow and develop there, rupture of the tubal wall is the inevitable result. Rupture most frequently occurs into the tubal lumen with the passage of the products of conception, together with

much blood, out the fimbriated end of the tube and into the peritoneal cavity—so-called "tubal abortion." Or, rupture may occur through the peritoneal surface of the tube directly into the peritoneal cavity; and, again, there is an outpouring of blood into the abdomen from vessels at the site of rupture. In either case, rupture usually occurs between the second and the fourth months.

Occasionally an ectopic pregnancy may develop in that portion of the tube which passes through the uterine wall, a type known as "interstitial pregnancy." In very, very rare instances, the product of conception, after rupturing through the tubal wall, may implant itself on the peritoneum and develop to full term in the peritoneal cavity. This extraordinary occurrence is known as "abdominal pregnancy." Surprisingly enough, quite a few living infants have been delivered in such cases by means of abdominal incision.

Ectopic pregnancy may be due to any condition which narrows the tube or brings about some constriction within it. Under such circumstances the tubal lumen is large enough to allow spermatozoa to ascend the tube but not big enough to permit the downward passage of the fertilized ovum. Among the conditions which may produce such a narrowing of the fallopian tube are: previous inflammatory processes involving the tubal mucosa and producing partial agglutination of opposing surfaces, such as gonorrheal salpingitis; previous inflammatory processes of the external peritoneal surfaces of the tube causing kinking, such as puerperal and postabortal infections; and developmental defects resulting in a general narrowing of the tubes.

In cases of ectopic gestation the woman exhibits the usual early symptoms of pregnancy and, as a rule, regards herself as being normally pregnant. After missing one or two periods, however, she suddenly experiences pain which is knifelike in nature and often of extreme severity, in one of the lower quadrants. This is usually associated with very slight vaginal bleeding, commonly referred to as "spotting." Depending on the amount of blood which has escaped into the peritoneal cavity, she may or may not undergo a fainting attack and show symptoms of shock.

Ectopic pregnancy is a grave complication of pregnancy and in about one case in 30 proves to be fatal. Moreover, if a woman has had one ectopic pregnancy and subsequently becomes pregnant, she is more likely than the average woman to have another such accident.

The treatment of ectopic pregnancy is removal of the tube, supplemented by blood transfusion. While transporting such a patient to the hospital or awaiting operation, the nurse can be of immeasurable assistance in combating the shock which is frequently present. Elevation of the foot of the bed and maintenance of body heat by means of hot-water bottles and blankets may help to save the patient's life.

Placenta Previa. While abortion is the most frequent cause of bleeding early in pregnancy, the most common cause during the later months is placenta previa. In this condition the placenta is attached to the lower uterine segment (instead of high up in the uterus as usual) and either wholly or in part covers the region of the cervix. There are four types, differentiated according to the degree to which the condition is present:

1. *Total placenta previa,* in which the placenta completely covers the internal os.

2. *Partial placenta previa,* in which the placenta partially covers the internal os.

3. *Marginal placenta previa,* in which only the edge of the placenta reaches the edge of the internal os.

4. *Low insertion of placenta,* in which the placenta encroaches upon the region of internal os, so that it can be reached by the physician on digital exploration about the cervix but is not actually in contact with the os.

Painless vaginal bleeding during the second half of pregnancy is the main symptom of placenta previa. The bleeding usually occurs after the seventh month. It may begin as mere "spotting" and increase or it may

PLATE 6

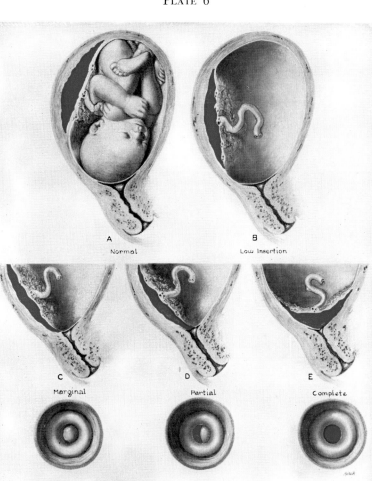

The three types of placenta previa (showing position at the internal os) (C, D and E) contrasted with normal placental insertion (A). Below, the placenta as felt by the physician on vaginal examination in marginal, partial and complete placenta previa.

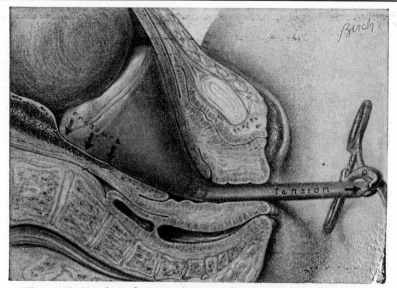

Fig. 145. Voorhees bag in place in placenta previa, showing the principle involved in treating placenta previa per vaginum, namely, exertion of pressure on placenta and lower uterine segment.

start with profuse hemorrhages. The patient may awaken in the middle of the night to find herself in a pool of blood. The bleeding is caused by separation of the placenta as the result of changes which take place in the lower uterine segment during the later months. This separation opens up the underlying blood sinuses of the uterus from which the bleeding occurs.

Fortunately, placenta previa is not a very common condition, occurring about once in every 400 or 500 pregnancies. It occurs much more frequently in multiparae than in primigravidae. Placenta previa always must be regarded as a grave complication of pregnancy. Until recent years it showed a maternal mortality of approximately 10 per cent. Modern methods of treatment, plus the more liberal use of blood transfusion, have reduced this figure considerably. The outlook for the baby is always dubious, not only because the placental separation interferes with the infant's oxygen supply but also because many of these babies are very premature when delivery must necessarily take place.

TREATMENT. There are two main forms of treatment: (1) pressure therapy exerted *per vaginum* and (2) cesarean section. The principle underlying the first of these is to compress the bleeding sinuses by exerting pressure on them and the overlying placenta. Depending on the nature of the case, the physician

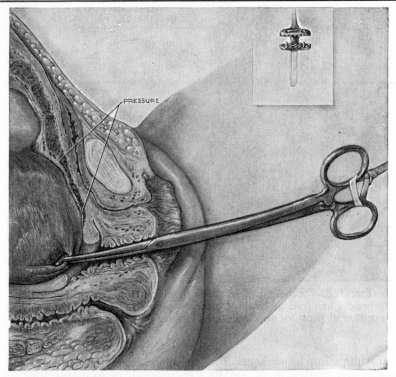

Fig. 146. Willett's forceps in place, showing another method of exerting pressure of baby's head on placenta and the lower uterine segment in placenta previa. Insert shows front view of forceps' tip.

may choose to do this in one of four ways: (1) rupture of the membranes, which allows the head to gravitate downward and exert a certain amount of pressure on the placenta and the lower uterine segment; (2) application of Willett's forceps to the scalp with traction (Fig. 146); (3) insertion of a bag; or (4) Braxton Hicks' version, by which the fetus is turned and a leg brought down so that a thigh and a buttock of the fetus compress the lower segment. In addition to checking hemorrhage by pressure effects, these four measures serve to dilate the cervix and to hasten the moment when delivery can be effected. The other main form of treatment, cesarean section, has been used more and more in recent years, particularly in the severe forms of the complication, such as complete and partial placenta previa. As in other hemorrhage complications of pregnancy, blood transfusion plays an important—often a life-saving—role in the management of these cases.

Bleeding, shock and infection are the main dangers. Before the arrival of the doctor, the nurse should keep a solicitous eye on the amount of bleeding and the pulse rate and watch for signs of oncoming shock (pallor, increased pulse rate, cold extremities, etc.). Should the bleeding be profuse, elevation of the foot of the bed and application of external heat may forestall shock. If the diagnosis is not clear, the nurse may be asked to watch the patient for amount of bleeding. Under such circumstances, the patient should be instructed to report feeling the escape of fluid from the vulva. The nurse, in turn, should inspect the pad or bed frequently for hemorrhage.

One of the important facts about placenta previa to keep in mind is that a vaginal or rectal examination may precipitate severe hemorrhage. Therefore, such procedures are regularly performed in the delivery or operating room where everything is set up for the immediate carrying out of any procedure which may be necessary for treatment, from insertion of a bag to cesarean section. This is usually referred to as the "double setup" (i.e., a setup for both vaginal and abdominal delivery).

Many patients with placenta previa later develop puerperal infection. This is understandable when one recalls that the open venous sinuses, low down about the cervix, are particularly accessible to infection and toxic conditions due to any bacteria which might have been introduced into the vagina. Hemorrhage, moreover, lowers the patient's resistance to infection. It is essential, therefore, that meticulous attention be given to antiseptic and aseptic

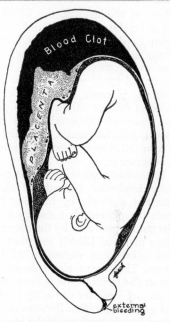

FIG. 147. Premature separation of placenta with large blood clot between placenta and uterine wall.

precautions in the handling of these cases.

Premature Separation of the Normally Implanted Placenta. As the name indicates, this is the separation, partial or complete, of a normally located placenta, occurring either in the later months of pregnancy or at the beginning of labor. Synonymous are "abruptio placentae" (meaning that the placenta is torn from its bed), "accidental hemorrhage" and "ablatio placentae" (*ablatio* means removal). Bleeding may be apparent or concealed, or both. In other words, if a separation occurs at the margin, the blood is apt to lift the membranes and trickle down to the cervical os and thus escape externally. If the placenta begins to separate centrally, a huge amount of blood may be stored behind the placenta before any of it becomes evident. Although the precise cause of the condition is not known, it is frequently encountered in association with cases of toxemia of pregnancy.

Premature separation of the normally implanted placenta is characterized not only by bleeding beneath the placenta but also by pain. The pain is produced by the accumulation of blood behind the placenta with subsequent distention of the uterus. The uterus also enlarges in size as the result of the accumulated blood and becomes distinctly tender and exceedingly firm. Because of the almost woody hardness of the uterine walls, fetal parts may be difficult to determine. Shock is often out of proportion to blood loss, as manifested by a rapid pulse, dyspnea, yawning, restlessness, pallor, syncope and cold, clammy perspiration.

Clear-cut examples of this complication occur much less frequently than placenta previa and are uncommon. However, the condition constitutes one of the gravest accidents which can befall a pregnant woman, and it has been estimated that from 10 to 25 per cent of the affected mothers and almost all the babies die. Treatment consists either in cesarean section or in rupturing the membranes and applying a tight binder. Transcending all else in importance is therapy of the shock which is almost invariably present— measures similar to those used in placenta previa.

Mistaken Diagnosis of Hemorrhage. A false alarm concerning hemorrhage is sometimes due to a normal "show" at the beginning of labor. It simply means that dilatation of the cervix has begun, causing slight bleeding. No treatment is required. However, the nurse should reassure the patient and watch to determine whether or not the bleeding which is present is more than the normal show.

Hydatidiform Mole. Hydatidiform mole is a cystic degeneration of the chorion. The villi become transparent vesicles containing clear, viscid fluid. They have a "grapelike" appearance, and are arranged in clusters involving all or part of the decidual lining of the uterus. It is a rather rare condition, occurring about once in every 2,000 pregnancies. It may be benign or malignant. The uterus enlarges rapidly, and profuse hemorrhage may occur in which these cystic particles may be evident in the vaginal discharge. The treatment consists in emptying the uterus by dilatation of the cervix and digitally extracting the contents. There is always great danger of injury to the uterine wall, which is weakened and is of a spongy consistency due to the growth of the mole (Fig. 148). Some doctors advise hysterectomy.

BLOOD GROUPS AND THE RH FACTOR

Following the 1900 discovery of four main types of human blood, now arbitrarily called A, B, AB and O types or groups, it was observed that the red cells of certain individuals became clumped (agglutinated) or dissolved (lysed) when transfused into certain other individ-

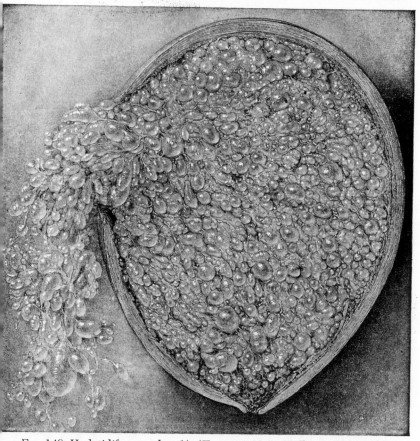

Fig. 148. Hydatidiform mole ×½. (Eastman, N. J.: Williams Obstetrics, New York, Appleton-Century)

uals, thus preventing any advantage from the transfusion and even causing injurious or toxic effects due to the "clash" of incompatible substances. In general,* an O person's blood may be given with safety to any one of the other three types. Therefore, O individuals are often

* Important exceptions in O and other persons are concerned with the Rh situation, discussed later in this section.

called "universal donors." Strangely enough, an O individual is least able to receive blood from the other three types; if transfusion is necessary, he should be given O blood. Any person of the other three blood types is preferably transfused with O type blood or with blood of his own type; that is, A with A type, B with B type, and AB with AB type. Thousands of tests show that about 40 per cent of

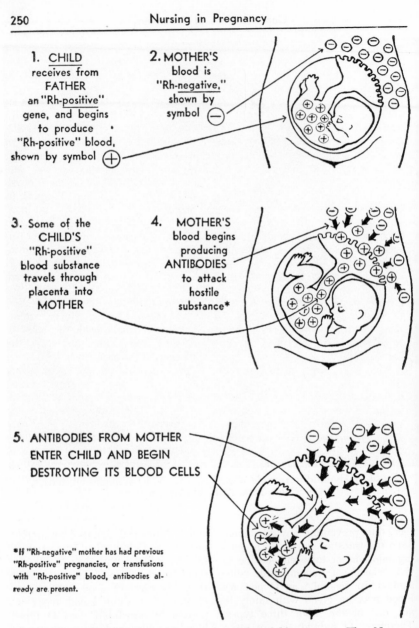

1. CHILD receives from FATHER an "Rh-positive" gene, and begins to produce "Rh-positive" blood, shown by symbol ⊕

2. MOTHER'S blood is "Rh-negative," shown by symbol ⊖

3. Some of the CHILD'S "Rh-positive" blood substance travels through placenta into MOTHER

4. MOTHER'S blood begins producing ANTIBODIES to attack hostile substance*

5. ANTIBODIES FROM MOTHER ENTER CHILD AND BEGIN DESTROYING ITS BLOOD CELLS

*If "Rh-negative" mother has had previous "Rh-positive" pregnancies, or transfusions with "Rh-positive" blood, antibodies already are present.

FIG. 149. Effect of the Rh factor. (Scheinfeld, Amran: The New You and Heredity, Philadelphia, Lippincott)

our population are O type and about 40 per cent are A type.

These blood groups are not related to racial differences. All four types have been reported in all known nationalities, though they differ in proportions. In the United States the average for whites is roughly 45 per cent O and 40 per cent A, but in the American Indians about 75 per cent are of O type and 25 per cent the A type.

It was once thought that blood from one member of a family would be compatible with that of any other member, but blood types may differ greatly within a given family. It is possible for a child born to an O and an AB parent to have O, A, B or AB blood. If the child had O blood it might receive transfusions from the O parent but not from his AB parent. However, his O blood could be transfused with safety to either his O or his AB parent.

The Rh Factor. Even carefully matched blood, e.g., A to A, or universal O to one of the other three types, has not always been free from undesirable effects. It is now known that there are several blood types in addition to the four A, B, AB and O types. The most important of the recently discovered types depends upon the presence or the absence of an Rh substance or factor, named for the first two letters of the rhesus monkey in which it was observed in 1940. The blood of about 85 per cent of our white population and slightly more of our Negro population contains this Rh factor. Therefore, such persons are said to be Rh positive (Rh +); persons lacking in Rh are termed Rh negative (Rh −). Since such a high percentage of persons

are Rh positive, difficulties following transfusions are relatively infrequent in ordinary transfusions, but they may become a serious hazard in pregnancy.

There are two pregnancy situations in which differences in the Rh condition may affect the developing fetus. They occur almost entirely in Rh-negative pregnant women: (1) if they have previously had one or more transfusions of Rh-positive blood or (2) if the other parent of the developing fetus is Rh positive.

Rh and Transfusions. Transfusion of an Rh-negative person with Rh-positive blood is attended with danger, as was shown in World War II experiences, when many Rh-negative men received blood from Rh-positive donors. Chills, fever and ever graver effects often resulted, due to the formation of antagonistic or anti-Rh-positive substances received by the Rh-negative person.

The greatest danger lies in giving Rh-positive blood (male or female) to an Rh-negative woman; although the anti-Rh-positive substance (or antibodies) form slowly, they may be retained for years. This Rh blood difference has caused more cases of erythroblastosis in newborn infants than the mating of an Rh-positive father and an Rh-negative mother. Today it is recognized that only in the most extreme emergency should a woman be given blood transfusions without previous testing for Rh types, even though 6 out of 7 persons are Rh positive in type and presumably have compatible Rh blood. Incompatible transfusions may show up years later in erythroblastosis infants and then interdict any future pregnancies.

Rh Differences in Mates. Since at least six sevenths of all persons, male or female, are Rh positive, Rh incompatibility is not as frequent as one might at first suppose. Even when an Rh-positive male parent mates with an Rh-negative female, there may be no erythroblastosis in the offspring, for about half of the male spermatozoa are Rh negative, and the rest are Rh positive (heterozygous), and no difficulty occurs if the fetus has Rh-negative inheritance from both parents. The danger is much greater when all the spermatozoa are Rh positive (homozygous), for the fetus will inherit the Rh-positive factor against which the mother produces antisubstances which (as in the transfusion of incompatible Rh-positive blood to Rh-negative mothers) may lead to the destruction of the Rh-positive blood cells of the fetus. The danger to the fetus is increased with the ability of the mother's antisubstances to pass through the placenta.

In Rh differences in mates, as well as in blood transfusions, the reactions of the Rh-negative mother are slow, and one or even two normal births may occur before erythroblastosis occurs. Once it occurs, all later pregnancies are risky, and future pregnancies should not be undertaken.

Prevention of Erythroblastosis. As already indicated, this condition may be prevented by proper checks of the Rh type of the women patients and any blood donors from whom they receive blood. In pregnancy the mother's Rh type must be determined early. If she is negative, the father's Rh type should be determined and rechecked, in case he is

Rh negative, for even then some of his spermatozoa may be Rh positive as already stated. During pregnancy the mother's blood should be checked monthly, to see if her antisubstances are increasing, indicating harmful reactions against Rh positive. This is done very simply by adding any known Rh blood (male or female) to a specimen of the mother's blood liquid or plasma and noting whether the Rh-positive red cells agglutinate or dissolve. With such checks marriage between an Rh-positive male and an Rh-negative woman may be perfectly safe, unless earlier Rh-positive blood transfusions complicate the situation. Even then some degree of control is possible.

If such antisubstances increase markedly, predelivery preparations should be made. The child may be delivered prematurely (induced labor or cesarean operation), and a supply of Rh-negative blood should be available for treating the infant, if born alive.

Records of Blood Types. Members of our military forces, patients preparing for operations, and pregnant mothers should have their blood types determined in case blood transfusion is needed. The same precautions should be taken for anemic and other hospital patients. Even when the records are determined they are not always available, e.g., in traffic accidents or when the individual is in a distant town. The tags furnished to military personnel could well give way to such procedures as tattooing on the lower trunk, both front and back, showing the 4-group and the Rh type of all individuals whose types have been determined.

DISEASES AND PREGNANCY

In pregnancy every effort should be made to improve the general physical condition of the mother and to decrease any attendant strain and depletion of her energy due to illness.

Any disease which affects health adds unnecessary complications in pregnancy; e.g., a streptococcic sore throat may lead to puerperal fever.

A number of general physiologic conditions are aggravated by pregnancy or not infrequently develop in that period. Anemia, insomnia, nosebleed and unusual heart manifestations often occur. These conditions and thyroid disturbances, abnormal (high or low) blood pressure, diabetes and nephritis or other types of kidney disease should be checked early in pregnancy and preferably beforehand; they are really part of the general health control of any individual. In addition to these and other pregnancy conditions already mentioned, physiologic conditions in relation to pregnancy are discussed briefly in the following pages.

GENERAL PHYSIOLOGIC DISTURBANCES

Anemia. During pregnancy the blood is more dilute (p. 141). Because of this hydremia, hemoglobin estimations in gestation are likely to be lower than ordinarily considered normal—usually between 75 and 85 per cent. This is not a true anemia, since the total amount of hemoglobin in the body remains the same, and sometimes the condition is referred to as the "pseudo-anemia of pregnancy."

As the result of a number of factors, the hemoglobin levels fall below 7 per cent in about 10 per cent of pregnant women. Most of these cases represent a true anemia due to iron deficiency. The need of the fetus and the growing uterus for iron, inadequate iron intake in the diet, and a low hemoglobin level at the start of pregnancy combine to bring about this anemic state. It is encountered more commonly in Negro women than in white women.

The symptoms are few, but some of these patients complain of becoming tired easily; many are pale; and in a few the pulse rate is fast. Because of this rather frequent occurrence of anemia in pregnancy hemoglobin determinations are a routine part of prenatal care. The treatment consists in an iron-rich diet (emphasis on liver, meat, eggs, spinach, etc.) supplemented by the administration of some iron compound such as ferrous sulfate. In extreme cases, blood transfusions may be necessary.

Cardiac Complications. Heart affections, especially those of the mitral valve, may be greatly aggravated by pregnancy, and often their fatal termination is hastened from this cause.

If the patient has placed herself under medical care at the beginning of gestation, and if the physician has made a proper and thorough examination of all her organs at that time, he will be in a position to administer promptly such treatment as may be necessary. In this day of heart specialists, the specialist and the obstetrician must work hand in hand; and each, in his own province, is of the greatest help to the other. It is also absolutely essential to have close co-operation between the patient and the physician. In this situation the nurse may play an important part—by helping the patient to understand and to observe with care the primary principles of prenatal care.

In heart complications, alcohol, tea, coffee and all undue excitement must be avoided during pregnancy. The intestinal tract and the kidneys need particular attention. Rest probably will accomplish more than any other single measure, and the amount of rest needed will naturally vary with each individual, some patients having to be kept at rest a great part of the time. The great majority, however, may safely indulge in moderate activity, and all should be in the fresh air as much as possible. Upper respiratory infections play great havoc in patients with heart disease and they may even precipitate heart failure; accordingly, the nurse should advise all such patients to take special precautions against catching cold—that is, they should avoid large gatherings and people known to have sore throats, colds, etc. All of these safeguards will be advised by the physician, but the nurse may aid greatly in helping the patient to carry out his instructions.

If, in any case, it seems to her that the heart probably is affected, she should report the matter at once to the doctor; for, fortunately, much can now be done to aid heart cases. In the past many such patients have had their pregnancies terminated by the induction of abortion, but today many a mild heart case is carried to a happy completion by providing thorough medical supervision and careful nursing during pregnancy and labor. However, these successes should not lead us to forget that, if not adequately cared for, even mild affections of the heart as well as the severe types result in definite invalidism or even death.

Diabetes. The diabetic woman who becomes pregnant requires meticulous supervision, and the nurse can be of much help in such cases by stressing the extreme importance of rigid adherence to diet and regular visits to the physician. The younger the patient when diabetes manifests itself, the more severe the disease is likely to be. A patient who cooperates and in whom the diabetes has been and is easily controlled is more likely to have a successful pregnancy than one who is difficult to control. During pregnancy the patient should be observed carefully, with special reference to control of diet to prevent undue weight gain. She probably should have salt restricted from the beginning, and in addition the protein intake should be increased. Careful checking of the diabetes is essential at frequent intervals; the patient should be under the care of an internist who is thoroughly competent in the management. Diabetic patients are more apt to have complications. They are inclined to produce large babies and to suffer from toxemias of pregnancy. The last trimester is the most trying time, and during this stage the patient should be watched for early signs of toxemia. Patients with this disease should be acquainted with the fact that they may have diabetic children.

Urinary-tract infection, or inflammation of the ureter and the pelvis of the kidney, is not uncommon during pregnancy. It seldom occurs earlier than the fourth month, and occasionally an acute attack of great severity occurs in the puerperium, in which case care will be required to distinguish it from puerperal infection. It is due to several causes, each of which may aggravate the condition: improper intestinal elimination, an increase of colon bacilli, pressure from the gravid uterus upon the ureter at the pelvic brim, leading to retention of urine above the line of pressure, and certain displacements of the bladder due to pregnancy itself. The symptoms may be gradual and slight, or quite acute in their onset, with chills and high temperature, 103° or 104° F. The patient often complains of frequency of urination, pain in the kidney region and malaise. In the acute form suddenly the patient is seized with acute abdominal pain, sometimes attended with chills or shivering; and after a few hours the abdomen may become distended, and vomiting may occur. The pain, diffused at first, usually localizes in the right side. It is necessary for the nurse to secure definite instructions from the physician concerning the treatment; but rest, forced fluids and a bland, non-irritating diet (chiefly milk) may be advised in the interim. Heat over the kidneys will relieve pain.

DRUGS. The main aim of treatment in urinary-tract infection is to rid the urine and the urinary tract of bacteria. During recent years the treatment of infections of the urinary tract has been revolutionized by the introduction of the sulfonamide group of drugs. The drug most frequently used is sulfadiazine, the usual dosage being 4 Gm. (60 gr.) for the first day and 2 Gm. (30 gr.) daily for the next five or six days. This is usually accompanied by sodium bicarbonate, 4 Gm. (60 gr.) daily, and the fluid intake is maintained between 2,500 and 3,000 cc. The doctor will follow the results of treatment not only by means of the temperature chart but also by thorough and repeated examinations of the urine. These examinations will entail both a microscopic study of the number of pus cells present and a survey of the bacteria yielded on culture. Accordingly, the nurse will be asked to secure frequent catheterized urine specimens. Follow-up of these cases is highly important and must be carried out not only during the remainder of pregnancy but for several months after delivery, until it is certain that the urine is sterile and x-ray studies of the kidney reveal a normal state.

Insomnia. Sleeplessness often proves to be troublesome during pregnancy and is best relieved by strict hygienic methods: open-air exercise, diversion, and massage supplemented by alcohol rubbing after the patient has retired for the night. If possible, the sleeping-room should be large and well ventilated and so situated that the patient will not be subjected to any disturbing influences. Often a cup of hot milk with an added pinch of salt, with or without a cracker, taken just before going to bed, may produce sleep. If these measures do not enable her to secure a proper amount of natural and refreshing sleep, the physician should be consulted; doubtless he will order a sedative. Insomnia may precede more serious complications.

Palpitation of the Heart; Syncope or Fainting. These conditions may be associated with, and due to, some definite organic disease or may be merely a neurotic manifestation. These symptoms usually occur in the early part of a first pregnancy, especially when the patient is in a hot, crowded and badly ventilated room. The nurse may meet the emergency by placing the patient flat on her back in a well-ventilated place, loosening the clothes, applying cold water to the forehead and the wrists, and providing the patient with smelling salts or aromatic spirits of ammonia. In ordinary palpitation some doctors recommend quiet, normal activity—moving around easily, drinking a glass of warm water—to start again the normal body rhythms. A glass of water may be all that is necessary. The condition should be reported to the physician.

Ptyalism. While this is one of the rarer complications of pregnancy, it is one which is most annoying to the patient and very stubborn in resisting treatment. It is due entirely to altered innervation, or changes in nerve control, and is characterized by an enormously increased secretion of the salivary glands. Women at times have been known to discharge as much as 2 quarts of saliva daily from this cause. This complication, if it occurs at all, usually appears in the early months of pregnancy and lasts a considerable time, but fortunately it is inclined to cease spontaneously. It is seen in highly nervous women of low vitality and is likely to cause great mental depression and interfere with nutrition.

The treatment should be relegated to the physician. It consists in building up the general health with iron and arsenic and in the use of astrin-

gent mouthwashes accompanied by medications, such as bromides or chloral, or injections of atropine. Any treatment may seem to be inadequate, and the condition is most disagreeable.

Nosebleed occasionally occurs late in pregnancy or early in labor and is due to the existing hydremic condition of the blood, coupled with a congested state of the nasal mucosa. It is seldom troublesome but, in certain rare cases, it proves to be very intractable and may persist until the patient loses an alarming quantity of blood. Such cases are, of course, very unusual; but the possibility of their occurrence should be kept in mind, and any profuse hemorrhage from the nose should be reported to the physician.

Communicable Diseases and Pregnancy

Certain communicable diseases have no proved specific ill effect on the mother or the baby, but, if possible, any communicable disease should be avoided during pregnancy, for even mild diseases add strain at this difficult time. The old idea that tuberculosis improves the physical status of a pregnant mother has no foundation (p. 258).

With communicable diseases two types of effects may occur: (1) on the mother and (2) on the fetus. The diseases which often have serious effects on the infant are discussed under the section Disorders of the Newborn, page 504. Among those directly affecting the mother are the following:

The Common Cold. The susceptibility to the common cold is apparently greater during pregnancy. Prompt medical attention is usually desirable because the early symptoms often resemble those of measles, influenza and other diseases affecting the upper respiratory tract. Advances in antibiotics, such as aureomycin, suggest that they should be used in preference to the various antihistamin drugs obtainable without a prescription. Rest in bed helps the individual and aids in checking the spread of the disease.

Pneumonia. Pneumonia which often follows the common cold frequently leads to abortion or premature labor. The pneumonia organisms, especially streptococci, may infect the uterus, causing puerperal infections. Prompt use of penicillin and other antibiotics, such as aureomycin, is most helpful.

Influenza. Serious complications may follow influenza, especially in the pneumonic type in which pregnancy is sometimes interrupted. Sulfa drugs and such antibiotics as penicillin are usually given to help control the influenza virus and any accompanying bacteria.

Measles. Ill effects are not commonly noted in pregnancy, but pregnant mothers are said to be more likely to have premature births. No other definite effects are reported, although eruptions have been noted on infants at birth.

German Measles. Rubella or German measles is caused by a virus—distinct from the virus of measles (rubeola) which is present in nose and throat discharges. Complications may be lacking or mild, except for the unborn baby of a pregnant mother with German measles. There are no antiserums against German measles, although globulin is considered by some to be a wise precaution for pregnant mothers. (See p. 519.) This disease seems to produce the most serious effects on the fetus if it occurs in the first trimester of pregnancy.

Typhoid Fever. Typhoid fever which is now relatively rare in this country, may cause serious complications in pregnancy, resulting in abortion, prematurity and infant mortality. Immunization, although generally successful, is not advisable during pregnancy, especially during the first half, as it leads to violent reactions, including abortions.

Brucellosis (Undulant Fever), Malta Fever. These debilitating diseases in humans are contracted mainly from unpasteurized milk. The bacteria have been found in the human placenta, but abortion in humans is very infrequently traced to this organism, although brucella bacteria do cause abortion in cattle. Good results have been attained with aureomycin and also with combined streptomycin-sulfadiazine.

Scarlet Fever. There seems to be greater susceptibility to scarlet fever (with the typical rash or without a rash as in septic sore throat) during the puerperium. If the cause is a streptococcus, as generally stated, the risk of developing puerperal fever is clear. Some authors state, however, that there is some degree of immunity during pregnancy; but sometimes abortion is caused by scarlet fever contracted during early pregnancy. Gamma globulin, sulfadiazine and penicillin are all reported favorably.

Erysipelas. This disease, usually caused by streptococci, may be very serious at any time, but in pregnant women there is the danger of developing puerperal fever. Care must be taken to avoid transferring streptococci from any local lesion to the genital area. Strict isolation is essential. Appropriate drugs (penicillin, sulfa drugs, etc.) should be used and if necessary continued through the puerperium. Streptococcus antitoxin may be used with the selected drug. The streptococci may pass through the placenta and cause the death of the fetus.

Smallpox. Cases of abortion and prematurity increase with the severity of the attack, especially with the hemorrhagic type. As in measles smallpox may be transmitted through the placenta, for eruptions may be present in live births.

Malaria. Malaria organisms have been found in the blood of the cord and the fetus; they are frequently found in the placenta, although no ill effects have been noted on the infants. Quinine or the newer related drugs should be administered to women with malaria history to prevent recrudescence during pregnancy and the puerperium. The decrease in malaria reported (1951) by the Communicable Disease Center of the U. S. Public Health Service makes malaria much less important as a complication of pregnancy.

Tuberculosis. The average case of tuberculosis in itself has only a slight effect on the course of pregnancy, since it rarely predisposes to abortion, premature labor or even stillbirth. (Fortunately, the disease is seldom acquired congenitally, although a small number of authentic cases have been reported in which, in addition to a tuberculous condition of the placenta, tubercle bacilli were found in the cord blood, together with tuberculous lesions in the baby.) Medical opinions differ, and some authorities think that this disease becomes aggravated by pregnancy and that only an arrested case should consider becoming pregnant. Pregnancy is undertaken with some risk, for while a tuberculous lesion may remain latent for an indefinite time, provided that the natural resistance is not overtaxed, it must be noted that pregnancy is one of the factors often responsible for overtaxing the resistance sufficiently to convert a latent, inactive lesion into an active one. Proper hygiene, nutrition and excellent surroundings so as to conserve health in every possible way will do much to prevent activity in a latent focus. Other authorities deny that the tuberculosis is necessarily aggravated by pregnancy, basing this belief on statistics of large series of tuberculous patients who have progressed satisfactorily in pregnancy.

The symptoms of tuberculosis in pregnancy do not differ materially from those that accompany the disease in other conditions. During the early months of gestation, the characteristic anemia and general malnutrition of tuberculosis are usually pronounced, but in the latter months there is often considerable improvement. Too often, however, this is followed by a rapid decline after delivery.

Treatment will depend upon the type of involvement as well as upon the particular stage of pregnancy. Prophylactic treatment is most important, since it offers most chance of success. The patient must be given every medical and hygienic advantage, wholesome food (milk is of very great value), fresh air and sunshine and absolute rest. Any cough or rapid loss of weight should be reported. It is not uncommon for the physician to interrupt the pregnancy; and when a tuberculous patient is allowed to go to term, the labor is made as easy as possible to conserve her strength. Under no circumstances should a tuberculous woman be allowed to nurse her baby, for the baby's sake as well as for her own. Months of careful follow-up treatment will be necessary in order to give a reasonably hopeful prognosis. The patient should not consider becoming pregnant again until a sufficient time has elapsed to establish a reasonable certainty that her disease has been arrested.

It is in the group in which tuberculosis is unsuspected that tragedies occur, many of which could be avoided. Therefore, a complete medical history always should be taken. Exposure to tuberculosis in the family, a history of hemoptysis, pleurisy, or fistula in ano, and a cough or loss of weight over a period of time suggest strongly the presence of possible tuberculosis. These danger signals are of the utmost value, and if heeded will often enable the physician to recognize tuberculosis symptoms developing during pregnancy which he might otherwise attribute to the pregnancy itself.

Examinations of the chest (x-ray) and sputum (microscopic) should be prenatal routine. The newer antibiotics (streptomycin, hydrostreptomycin, neomycin) should be available if need is indicated. There may be undue alarm due to confusion of tuberculosis with the milder disease, histoplasmosis, unless expert testing (skin and sputum) facilities are available.

Poliomyelitis. Poliomyelitis generally does not complicate pregnancy or delivery, except in the very unusual cases where respiratory paralysis develops; in these rare cases cesarean section has given satisfactory results. Fortunately, the fetus rarely contracts the disease. Of about 80 cases reported during pregnancy less than one fifth occurred in the first trimester. A milder form of infection of poliomyelitis is attributed to a different virus, the Coxsackie virus, which has less paralysis but is often unrecognized.

Gonorrhea should be studied by the student nurse with the other infectious diseases; but, because of the consequences of gonorrheal infection to the mother at the time of labor and during the puerperium, as well as the risk of permanent injury to the baby's eyes at the time of birth, this disease is of special concern to the obstetric nurse.

The disease is due to a micro-organism, known commonly as the gonococcus organism (*Micrococcus gonorrhoeae* or *Neisseria gonorrhoeae*). It may affect any mucous membrane, e.g., that of the eye, but usually attacks the mucosa of the genital tract, particularly the opening of the bladder and the crypts around the cervix, causing a catarrhal discharge of pus. It is called a venereal disease simply because the usual mode of transfer of this infection is by sexual intercourse. The infection often extends into the uterus and tubes, causing a very serious localized peritonitis, and may cause sterility by a mechanical blocking of the tubes. Gonorrhea is not commonly considered a fatal disease, in the sense that a high proportion of the cases terminate in death, but in the list of diseases causing chronic ill health, especially in the female sex, gonorrhea is most important.

Gonorrhea does not greatly modify the course of pregnancy, and its existence is often unsuspected by the patient. The vaginal discharge may increase, as it normally does during pregnancy, and, with the local congestion of the venous system, the patient may have some irritation in the vulvar region. Pregnancy may act as a barrier to the ascent of the gonococcus, and thus the fetus may be protected during development. The patient may abort, but more commonly she carries the baby to full term and delivers normally. However, after delivery conditions are quite different. Even when a patient has had a normal labor, the cervix is dilated, and the minute tears and abrasions offer many avenues for the spread of the infection, and the lochial discharge makes an ideal culture medium for the bacteria. This condition may lead to the development of a form of puerperal fever.

During the prenatal period, if a patient complains of a profuse discharge accompanied by urinary manifestations, such as burning and frequency of urination, it should be reported to the physician so that he may take a vaginal, cervical or urethral smear to be able to make a diagnosis and follow it with penicillin treatment, which yields dramatic results in this disease. Cure may be effected by a single muscular injection of suitable dosage of penicillin in at least 90 per cent of the cases. In chronic cases one or two repeated doses or the administration of another drug (aureomycin) may be necessary.

Gonorrhea is not hereditary, but, if a woman is infected at the time of her confinement, the organism may get into the baby's eyes and cause blindness. This infection of the eyes is called ophthalmia neonatorum. The prophylactic treatment of the baby's eyes at this time never should be neglected (Fig. 154).

Syphilis. The study of infant mortality rates shows that as a result of syphilis a considerable number of infants are stillborn, die in the early months of life or, if they live, are infected. Like gonorrhea, this venereal disease is best studied with the other infectious diseases, but because of its definite relation to the life and the health of mothers and babies a few facts are mentioned here.

DEFINITION. Syphilis may be defined as an infectious systemic disease which runs a prolonged course and, during this course, it may, at one time or another, attack nearly every part of the body. Many women do not know that they or their children are infected; therefore, they seek no advice. In many patients, even with no history of infection or any manifestations of the disease, the first intimation of the existence of syphilis is a positive Wassermann (or other blood test) reaction or the birth of a premature or macerated fetus. Although macerated fetuses may be produced in consequence of nephritis, tuberculosis of the mother, premature loosening of the placenta or strangling by the umbilical cord, the suspicion of syphilis arises in every instance. Unlike the effects of gonorrhea, syphilis does not cause sterility.

Syphilis and Pregnancy.*

Causal Organism. Syphilis is a specific infectious disease caused by a spirochete, *Spirochaeta pallida* or *Treponema pallidum,* discovered by Schaudinn and Hoffmann in 1905.

Types of Syphilis. Syphilis in any individual may be acquired or congenital. The acquired form is usually transmitted by sexual intercourse; however, other forms of personal contact may transmit the infection, such as kissing, an examination of the patient by a contaminated physician and the nursing of the newborn by an infected person.

Congenital syphilis is a term applied to syphilis transmitted to the child before birth. An infected mother may transmit syphilis to the fetus through the placenta. Such transfer may occur from mothers whether they were syphilitic at the time of conception or whether they acquired syphilis during early pregnancy.

In this discussion of syphilis and pregnancy, we may focus our attention on three points: (1) the detection of syphilis in the pregnant mother; (2) the treatment of such infected mothers; and (3) the prompt detection of syphilis in the baby after birth.

Diagnosis of Syphilis in Pregnant Mothers: Clinical Symptoms. In syphilis there is usually a primary lesion or hard chancre located where there was a defect in the surface epithelium, allowing the entrance of the spirochete. In women, the initial lesion of syphilis is less easily observed than in men, and, unless seen on the vulva, is usually unnoticed. In a large proportion of recently infected women, no evidence of a scar of a chancre of the genitals may be seen. The secondary manifestations, likewise, are often unnoticed. The skin eruptions are mild and dis-

* By William T. Daily, M.D., Department of Obstetrics and Gynecology, The Long Island College Hospital, Brooklyn, N. Y.

appear rather rapidly. On the other hand, the presence of condylomata lata may cause the patient to consult her physician.

Previous Pregnancy History. The history of previous pregnancies is most significant in indicating syphilis in the mother. In a series of pregnant syphilitic women studied, a large proportion of pregnancies failed to go to term, ending in a miscarriage, in a premature, a fullterm stillbirth, or in the birth of a syphilitic infant. Abortion in the first trimester of pregnancy is noted but slightly more frequently than in ordinary pregnancy; on the other hand, interruption of pregnancy during the fifth, sixth or seventh month is common.

Blood Tests. Blood tests constitute a third method of detecting syphilis. The importance of blood tests is evident when we realize that syphilis complicating pregnancy in a primigravida is seldom recognized until the damage is done, unless the practice of making routine serologic tests is followed. The advantage of this third method of detecting syphilis is shown by the fact that out of 144 pregnant women thus shown to have syphilis, only six gave evidence of a primary lesion, and the history and physical examination were suggestive of syphilis in but 34 patients in the series. Without the blood tests, over 100 of these mothers would have failed to receive the necessary treatment.

The tests devised by Wassermann, Kahn, Kline, Mazzini and the U. S. Public Health Service test V.D.R.L. are the ones now most frequently used in this country. If the blood test is found to be positive or questionable, the test is repeated to make sure that any possible laboratory error is eliminated. Should a test be strongly positive, treatment is inaugurated, even though there were no other indications of syphilis (lesions, pregnancy history). Treatment is also given to all patients with a definite pregnancy history indicating syphi-

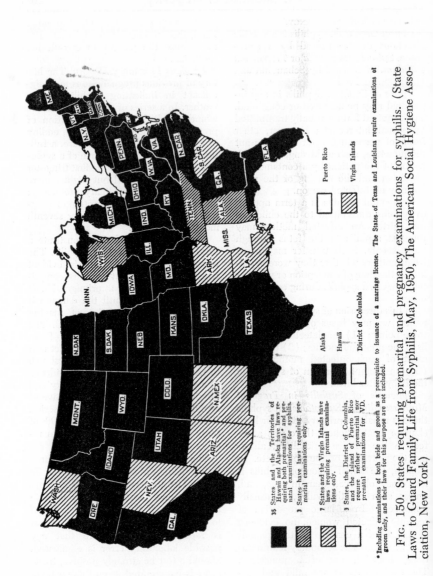

FIG. 150. States requiring premarital and pregnancy examinations for syphilis. (State Laws to Guard Family Life from Syphilis, May, 1950, The American Social Hygiene Association, New York)

35 States and the Territories of Hawaii and Alaska have laws requiring both premarital* and prenatal examinations for syphilis.

3 States have laws requiring premarital examinations only.

7 States and the Virgin Islands have laws requiring prenatal examinations only.

3 States, the District of Columbia, and the Island of Puerto Rico require neither premarital nor prenatal examinations for VD.

Alaska

Hawaii

District of Columbia

Puerto Rico

Virgin Islands

The States of Texas and Louisiana require examinations of

*Including examinations of both bride and groom as a prerequisite to issuance of a marriage license. The States of Texas and Louisiana require examinations of groom only, and their laws for this purpose are not included.

lis, even though the blood test may be but mildly positive or negative.

Provocative Test. When a suspicious history is accompanied by a negative or questionable blood test, a provocative injection of 0.3 gram of neosalvarsan in 10 cc. of freshly distilled water is given intravenously; blood is then taken for (Wassermann) tests one, four and eight days subsequently. If after this provocative treatment the blood test is strongly positive, the patient is given the routine antiluetic treatment. The value of such provocative treatment is shown by a recent case which revealed syphilis in the mother and so led to the discovery of syphilis in her husband and her two children, in none of whom the disease had been suspected.

Treatment of Syphilitic Mothers. 1. With Neosalvarsan. Three-tenths gram of neosalvarsan in 10 cc. of freshly distilled water is injected into the basilic or cephalic vein. If this is well tolerated, the dose is increased to 0.6 gram and is repeated weekly. In addition, 1 cc. of 10% bismuth salicylate in oil is given intramuscularly into the buttocks two days before each intravenous injection of the arsenical. In our treatment there are no so-called "courses," nor are there rest periods. The treatment with both bismuth and neosalvarsan, accordingly, is repeated at weekly intervals continuously from the time of the first injection until the child is delivered.

Prior to each neosalvarsan injection, the blood pressure is taken and the urine examined for albumin. If any evidence of toxemia is present, the arsenical is withheld until all toxic signs have disappeared. In case of doubt regarding a toxic condition, the treatment is not given. That the use of this drug is not without danger is shown by the fact that deaths from arsenical poisoning are not uncommon. When, however, the responsibility for the treatment of pregnancy syphilis is taken over by a member of the obstetrical staff, and the patients are treated in the prenatal clinic, repetition of these unfortunate arsenical accidents may be prevented.

During pregnancy, treatment is given primarily in the interest of the child, and, fortunately, the chance of obtaining a good result in this respect is excellent. All who are experienced in the use of arsphenamine for this purpose agree that comparatively few injections have a most marked effect upon fetal syphilis. This drug, accordingly, has proved itself to be a worthy adversary of the arch-destroyer of fetal life. How these remarkably good results are obtained has not been explained, aside from the observation that relatively large amounts of arsenic have been recovered from meconium, proving that arsenicals pass through the placenta and reach the unborn child. For some unexplained reason, their potency as spirocheticides seems to be much greater in fetal than in mature tissues, as is shown by the fact that even though the blood test may continue to be positive in a well-treated mother, her child often is born free from syphilis.

Naturally, the earlier in pregnancy that treatment is inaugurated the better will be the results for both the mother and the child. Our aim should be to secure a negative blood test as soon as possible. Treatment should start immediately after the diagnosis is made, in the hope that this desired effect may be obtained. The fear that arsphenamine might cause a miscarriage formerly led many conscientious physicians to avoid its use during pregnancy. However, those who had the courage to treat vigorously all cases of pregnancy syphilis soon found that it was the disease and not the treatment that causes these interruptions of gestation. Pregnancy, therefore, is not a contraindication but a strong indication for the vigorous use of arsenicals in the fight against congenital syphilis.

Even though circumstances prevent early treatment, the use of arsphenamine as late as the third trimester often is productive of extraordinary results. Inadequate as the treatment may be at this late date, stillbirths frequently are thus prevented, syphilis in the surviving children usually is rendered less innocuous and more easily controllable, and, occasionally, a child is born without any evidence of the disease.

Tests for Syphilis in the Newborn. The newborn baby should be tested for the presence of syphilis. Several types of tests are used to determine the condition of the infant.

1. The cord blood test should be made on every suspicious or treated case. However, this test is not wholly reliable; but a positive cord blood test indicates the need for close follow-up and frequent examinations.

2. The placenta may furnish suspicion, if not evidence, of pathologic changes. The normal placenta at full term weighs about 500 Gm. Normally, the relative weight of the baby to placenta is about 6:1. The placenta of syphilitic infection is larger, heavier and paler than normal. Since a premature placenta is relatively heavier than a placenta at term, and because many syphilitic babies are born prematurely, this may account for the too common opinion regarding the great size and weight of a syphilitic placenta. Histologically, the chorionic villi are greatly enlarged; they show diminished branching and they are more club-shaped. On cross section, the vessels are seen to be diminished in number and stenosed or obliterated by endo-arteritic changes. The stroma is more granular, and the stroma cells lose their normal stellate appearance. The villi, due to their greater size or thickness, approach each other, reducing the intervillous spaces. Syphilis of the placenta is not a common lesion, and many hesitate to make a positive diagnosis unless the spirochete is seen in microscopic darkfield examination.

3. The umbilical cord vein, in an area near the placenta, may be scraped and studied for spirochetes under a darkfield examination.

4. An x-ray examination of the long bones, especially the lower and upper ends of the femur, upper fibula and tibia, and the upper humerus and lower radius, is most valuable in determining the syphilitic condition of the infant. The usual lesion is an epiphysitis.

5. Blood tests may also be used. The newborn baby of a treated mother should be referred to a pediatrician familiar with the treatment of syphilis in the newborn about the sixth week after birth, for repeated serologic and x-ray examinations.

Conclusion. Syphilis of the newborn is preventable, and, if a child is delivered with the infection or succumbs to its virulence, either before delivery or neonatally, two and only two persons are largely responsible: first, the mother for her failure to be examined early in her pregnancy, and, secondly, the physician (or clinic) whom she consults, if he neglects to take routine serologic tests and which, if positive, he fails to treat intensively.

2. With Penicillin. The present-day treatment of syphilis in pregnancy consists in the intensive administration of penicillin as soon as the disease is recognized. The earlier in pregnancy therapy is started, the better are the results. Patients are hospitalized for this purpose, and 30,000 units of penicillin are administered intramuscularly every three hours until from approximately 4,-000,000 to 6,000,000 units have been given. It is well established that this dosage is several times that necessary to protect the baby from syphilis, and it is believed to be enough to cure the mother also; but it is quite possible that further experience will result in a still higher dosage in order to make certain of permanent maternal cure. A simple calculation will show that the period required for the administration of this quantity of penicillin at the rate mentioned is between 16 and 24 days. This has posed a difficult problem in regard to hospitalization for these patients but it has been met in many cities by special treatment centers.

Penicillin, with rare exceptions, has been free from serious toxic effects. The frequent injection schedules have now been replaced by schedules permitting 1, 2 or 3 injections a week for from 1 to 4 weeks. This relatively short treatment period with its freedom from severe toxic reactions has a great advantage over the previously accepted 1 to 2 years of arsenical and bismuth therapy. However, for patients who do not tolerate penicillin, massive arsenotherapy is the treatment of choice. Penicillin also possesses the ability of being filtered through the placenta and consequently can act as a very potent agent in the treatment of congenital syphilis in utero. Unfortunately, failures do occur as the result of relapse or reinfection, and this accounts for most of the rare instances of congenital syphilis resulting from treated mothers.

SUGGESTED READING

Adair, F. L.: Maternal Care and Complications, Chicago, Univ. Chicago Press, 1937.

Bowden, Anita E., and Gould, George: Summary of State Legislation Requiring Premarital and Prenatal Examinations for Venereal Disease, New York, American Social Hygiene Association, 1949. (Being revised, due 1952.)

Bunim, Joseph J., and Appel, S. Baer: Pregnancy and rheumatic heart disease, J.A.M.A. 142:90, 1950.

Bysshe, Stanley M.: Premature separation of the normally implanted placenta, Am. J. Obst. & Gynec. 62:38, 1951.

Chen, Calvin H., Dienst, Robert B., and Greenblatt, Robert B.: Aureomycin in treatment of gonorrhea, J.A.M.A. 143:724, 1950.

Cosgrove, S. A., and Chesley, L. C.: Management and treatment of the late toxemias of pregnancy, Am. J. Obst. & Gynec. 51:67, 1946.

Curtis, Arthur C., et al.: Penicillin treatment of syphilis, J.A.M.A. 145:1223, 1951.

Douglass, Louis H., and Hoopes, Lorman L.: The cardiac patient in pregnancy, Am. J. Obst. & Gynec. 61:373, 1951.

Eastman, N. J.: Diabetes mellitus and pregnancy. A review, Obst. & Gynec. Survey 1:3, 1946.

Eastman, N. J., and Whitridge, J. W., Jr.: The prevention of toxemia in pregnancy, J.A.M.A. 120:729, 1942.

Fox, Max J., and Belfus, Frank H.: Poliomyelitis in pregnancy, Am. J. Obst. & Gynec. 59:1134, 1950.

Fox, Max J., and Bortin, M. M.: Rubella in pregnancy causing malformations in the newborn, J.A.M.A. 130:568-569, 1946.

Given, William P., Douglas, R. Gordon, and Tolstoi, Edward: Pregnancy and diabetes, Am. J. Obst. & Gynec. 59:729, 1950.

Gordon, Dan M.: Routine examination of the ocular fundi in management of toxemias of pregnancy, J.A.M.A. 146:810, 1951.

Greenhill, J. P., and Loeff, H. L.: Heart disease in pregnancy, Today's Health 29:18, 1951.

Hall, Robert E., and Tillman, Alvin J. B.: Diabetes in pregnancy, Am. J. Obst. & Gynec. 61:1107, 1951.

Johnson, Herman W.: The management of placenta previa, Am. J. Obst. & Gynec. 59:1236, 1950.

Kitchen, D. K., et al.: Placental transmission of penicillin following single injections of procaine penicillin G in oil with 2 per cent aluminum monostearate (300,000 units). Antibiotics and Chemotherapy 1:110, 1951.

Kotila, G.: Discomforts of pregnancy, Am. J. Nursing 42:359, 1942.

McElin, Thomas W., Faber, John E., Randall, Lawrence M.: True toxemia of pregnancy occurring before the third trimester, Am. J. Obst. & Gynec. 61:379, 1951.

Pearse, Harry A., and Ott, Harold A.: Hospital control of sterilization and therapeutic abortion, Am. J. Obst. & Gynec. 60:285, 1950.

Pillsbury, M. E., and Sachs, Elizabeth: Nursing Care of Communicable Diseases, ed. 7, Philadelphia, Lippincott, 1952.

Potter, Edith L.: Rh. Its Relation to Congenital Hemolytic Disease and to Intragroup Transfusion Reactions, Chicago, Yr. Bk. Pub., 1947.

Rolf, Bruce B.: The obstetrician's responsibility to the Rh-negative patient, Am. J. Obst. & Gynec. 61: 139, 1951.

Rosenthal, H., Stern, F., and Rosenthal, J.: Diabetic Care in Pictures, Philadelphia, Lippincott, 1946.

Simpson, G. A., and Long, A. C.: Pregnancy and pulmonary tuberculosis, Am. J. Obst. & Gynec. 59: 505, 1950.

Speiser, Mortimer D.: Modern therapy of syphilis in the pregnant woman, M. Clin. North America 35:631, 1951.

State Laws to protect family health. A summary of state legislation requiring premarital and prenatal examination for venereal diseases, 1935-1949.

Stevenson, Charles S., et al.: Treatment of thyroid in pregnancy with chloramphenicol, J.A.M.A. 146: 1190, 1951.

Stromme, W. B., and Kuder, K.: Heart disease in pregnancy, Am. J. Obst. & Gynec. 52:264, 1946.

Sullivan, Charles L.: The use of Prostigmin in heartburn of pregnancy, Am. J. Obst. & Gynec. 60: 205, 1950.

Taussig, F. J.: Abortion, cause, prevention, treatment, Am. J. Nursing 39:857, 1939.

Thomas, Evan W.: Syphilis: Its Course and Management, New York, Macmillan, 1949.

Tietze, Christopher, Guttmacher, Alan F., Rubin, Samuel: Unintentional abortion, J.A.M.A. 142:1348, 1950.

Wammock, Virgene S., et al.: Penicillin therapy of the syphilitic pregnant woman, Am. J. Obst. & Gynec. 59:806, 1950.

Wiley, Harold M.: Etiology and treatment of heartburn, Am. J. Obst. & Gynec. 51:221, 1946.

Wolf, A. M., et al.: Clinical study of prevention of erythroblastosis with Rh Hapten, J.A.M.A. 144:88, 1950.

A climate room for research on eclampsia, Trained Nurse & Hospital Review 123:2, 1949.

11

The Mental Hygiene of Pregnancy

Leo Kanner, M.D.

Director, Children's Psychiatric Service, the Johns Hopkins Hospital, Baltimore, Md. Associate Professor of Psychiatry, the Johns Hopkins University School of Medicine.

INTRODUCTION

Human pregnancy is a biologic event and an emotional experience. It begins with the relationship between two people and ushers in a new relationship between them and their offspring. The nature of the biologic event depends on anatomic and physiologic conditions; the nature of the emotional experience is determined by the mother's attitude toward herself, her husband and her child. The physical hygiene of pregnancy is directed primarily toward the mother's body; the mental hygiene of pregnancy addresses itself to her as a thinking, feeling and behaving individual.

It is true of all branches of medicine that a physician's or nurse's attention should not be limited exclusively and impersonally to the functions and the ailments of the patient's body. The need for sympathy and understanding has been emphasized since the days of Hippocrates. The combination of pro-

267

fessional competence and humane interest in the patient has been rightly extolled as the ideal attribute of persons who make themselves responsible for the health of human beings.

The nature of childbearing is such that medical contacts with the parturient mother extend over a period of approximately a whole year. For nearly 12 months, the obstetrician and the obstetric nurse take over the guidance of an adult woman, supervise her nutrition, regulate her activities, answer her questions, clear up her puzzlements, advise her about the handling of the baby when it comes, and generally chart her conduct during the 24 hours of the day. This offers ample opportunity to become acquainted with the mother's personality, the circumstances of her environment, her attitudes and opinions, her outlook on life and the degree of her emotional stability. It is not too difficult to sense and spot genuine happiness over the pregnancy, resentful rebellion against it, stunned acceptance of the conception as an unexpected decree of destiny, or disturbing apprehension regarding the outcome.

The present can be rarely understood without reference to the past. Obstetrics cannot possibly dispense with a thoroughgoing evaluation of the patient's past history. Verbal reports, clinical examination and laboratory tests are indispensable as a preparation for the adequate physical hygiene of pregnancy. Needed information is thus obtained about factors of pelvic formation, miscarriages and stillbirths, cardiac illness, tuberculosis, syphilis and other conditions which existed before the recent conception and may complicate the course of events and influence the direction of obstetric procedure.

Analogously, a true appreciation of mental health during pregnancy can be obtained only by the ability to trace the mother's present attitudes to those personal experiences which have helped to shape them. In one sense, it is relatively easy to become familiar with such experiences and their effects, because no special or elaborate equipment is required. In another sense, such a study is extremely difficult and complex. Few people are inclined to disclose their most intimate feelings unless they are reasonably assured that the listener has the maturity, the tactfulness and the honest desire to understand, to guard confidences and to alleviate perplexities and anxieties.

THE MOTHER'S ATTITUDE TOWARD HER PREGNANCY

Under ordinary circumstances, the discovery of a woman's pregnancy is a happening which is welcome to her and to her husband. It is a source of rejoicing or at least of tranquil acceptance. The temporary discomforts, restrictions and changes of appearance which go with gravidity are awaited and borne with good nature. Even if there is some fear of the delivery, it is richly counterbalanced by the wish to have the baby, the gentleness of husband, relatives and friends, the full confidence in the physician and the nurse, the knowledge of good health and of satisfactory progress of the pregnancy and the ever-shortening distance from the moment of childbirth.

Such an attitude of positive and gratifying anticipation of motherhood, which is the essence of good mental hygiene, is usually predictable because it is based on a definite constellation of fortunate factors.

1. The mother herself has had a happy childhood and thereby has come to think of a family with children as something desirable and enjoyable. Her vision of a family unit is one of reciprocal satisfactions. Having experienced the benefits of parental fondness, she is prepared to give affection as she has received it.

2. The mother is secure in her relationship with her husband. The child comes to her as the result of intimacy with a man whom she loves and of whose love she is certain. She has no doubt about the safe and unperturbed continuity of her marriage.

3. The mother is not harassed by the drudgeries and the worries which arise from material insecurities, such as the husband's unemployment or protracted hospitalization, poor housing conditions or severe illness of one of her children.

Luckily, this combination of circumstances prevails often enough to deserve being regarded as the average, ordinary mental state of a mother at the onset of pregnancy. If it exists, her medical guides may look forward with a feeling of relief to the likelihood of freedom from untoward psychologic complications. There is ground for the same sense of relief as that which obtains when, at the end of a thorough physical examination, the findings warrant a favorable prediction of the course of the biologic process.

But departures from these healthy preliminary conditions are not at all uncommon. They can and should be studied, diagnosed and treated with the same care, knowledge and interest as are the major and minor deviations from bodily health and comfort. The principal directions of an unwholesome maternal attitude toward pregnancy present themselves to the knowing observer in the form of two disturbing psychologic complexes: (1) fear of the delivery and of the fate of the child to be delivered; and (2) rejection of the child to be delivered.

FEAR

Helene Deutsch, whose work on the psychology of women has received great acclaim, wrote in the volume devoted to motherhood: "That great power in human psychic life, *fear*, whatever its nature, certainly has a considerable influence on the emotional course of pregnancy."

A pregnant woman may be beset by two types of fearful anticipations, which often run concurrently: (1) fear for herself; and (2) fear for the baby.

The Mother's Fear for Herself. Every expectant mother knows that there will be pain, hospitalization or at least confinement in bed, perhaps the administration of an anesthetic, and a revolutionary physical change at the end of the pregnancy road. The whole procedure of childbirth, however normal it may turn out to be, must impress her as a sort of surgical intervention to which she will have to submit and from which there is no possible escape. There is hardly a human being who is entirely devoid of fear of an operation. The astounding progress of medicine and preventive hygiene has greatly reduced the actual dangers; also it has reduced, but not entirely eliminated, the dread. Statistics have shown a marked decline in maternal mortality, but this fact does not remove from the individual woman the anxiously perplexing question: What if it gets *me?* In the not too distant past many more women have lost their lives in pregnancy, labor and soon after birth than it is pleasant to contemplate. Even though conditions have improved tremendously and there is good reason for the expectation of further improvement, the public is still held in awe by the experiences gathered in centuries. Pregnant women's fear of death is therefore understandable and not at all unusual. It has been emphasized by every author who has ever written about the mental hygiene of pregnancy.

There are many possible reactions to fear; some of them are flight, shrinking, avoidance of danger, stupefied inactivity, panic and bravery. No soldier, not even the most courageous, has ever gone into battle without being afraid; when we speak of "fearlessness" on such occasions, we do not refer to absence of fear but the conquest of fear. The conquest is successful if it is prompted and aided by a consistent motive. A pregnant woman is not unlike a soldier with regard to her attitude toward anticipated dangers. When there is an eager desire for a child, when security has been built up by the same kind of confidence in the people important to the mother which brave soldiers have in their commanders and buddies, then the motive is strong enough to conquer

fear to the point that it is not even realized. The more the motive has been weakened by anxiety, insecurity and unhappiness, the less strength will the mother have to subdue her fear of childbirth, the more will the manifestations of her dread come to the fore.

The Mother's Fear for the Child. Pregnancy is in many respects a journey into the unknown. There are justified uncertainties about the expected baby's gender, appearance and general endowment. Uncertainty is a breeder of fear, particularly if previous experiences and orientations have tended to select some special areas of apprehension. Nobody can prophesy the future destiny of a human embryo even with approximate definiteness. But a mother to whom life has been good, who is thrilled by the prospect of having a child, who has fortified herself with a reasonable degree of optimism in all other respects, does not go around imagining all or any of the possible misfortunes which may befall her child. If, however, there is a background of anxiety, then the memory of dire happenings, pseudoscientific notions and folk beliefs may contrive to introduce torturing visions of impending disaster. There are three types of maternal fears for the baby which occur with special frequency.

1. Fear of losing the baby is apt to arise if the pregnancy has been preceded by spontaneous abortions, miscarriages or stillbirths; if previous pregnancies have been, or the present gestation is, accompanied by pathologic complications; or if these things have happened to relatives or close friends.

2. Fear of heredity is based on the

layman's vague and frequently distorted interpretations of the results of scientific research. No real scholar has ever claimed that a child's personality development is merely an inherited repetition of some progenitor's antics, that traits are handed down as trinkets are, or that statistics can be applied to individuals. But this is exactly what "heredity" means to many people. As a result, anxious parents consult their respective genealogic trees and, finding an uncongenial ancestor hanging from one of the branches, worry themselves sick in the expectation of similar propensities in the baby-to-come. It can be said with considerable assurance that fear of heredity has caused at least as much mental anguish as heredity itself ever did.

3. Superstitious fears are found not only among the lowly and ignorant; they sometimes seem to be too powerful to be squelched even by a college diploma. The idea of mysterious prenatal influences which are said to "mark the baby" is still prevalent in many quarters. The notion is still abroad that a mother's experiences during her pregnancy will in some fashion shape the baby's fate. If she looks wistfully at a handsome child, the beauty will communicate itself to the embryo in her womb. She must be careful to keep her glances off ugliness and misshapen features or her baby may grow up to be ugly and misshapen.

The well-educated young wife of an army officer once related the agonies which she had suffered because on a railroad trip she found herself sitting opposite a Chinese girl. For several months she feared that, as a result, her expected baby might turn out to be a Mongolian idiot! She did not dare tell anybody about her apprehension, knowing that she would be ridiculed as superstitious. She was greatly relieved when she learned that she had given birth to a normal infant; but this relief was preceded by months of unnecessary misery.

REJECTION

Not all children arrive in this world because they have been wanted by their parents. The number of unplanned and unwanted pregnancies in our civilization is truly appalling. Statistics cannot possibly reach the annual total of illegally induced abortions because every effort is made by the participants to keep them under the cover of secrecy. The unquestionably high figure is augmented by numerous unskillful attempts which do not succeed in destroying the child, who therefore comes into existence as an "unsuccessful abortion." This is a tragic state of affairs, both because of the interference with human life and because of the circumstances and the mental attitudes leading to the interference.

However, rejection of the pregnancy does not always end in the drastic ejection of the embryo from the uterus and from life. It often expresses itself more or less subtly in the parental attitude toward the unwanted pregnancy. It is not too unusual to hear rejecting mothers speak of the conception as an "accident" and describe their feelings at the time of the discovery as a "shock."

Maternal rejection therefore results in one of three clearly circumscribed reactions: (1) illegal abortion, (2) unsuccessful attempt at abortion, (3) a nonaccepting attitude toward the pregnancy.

It is not easy for the average healthy person to comprehend the fact of a woman's repudiation of her own offspring. Maternal rejection is indeed a very complex phenomenon anchored deeply in the mother's personality and relationships formed over a long period of time. What seems to be solely a matter of her feelings limited to *bearing and borne* has its origins in her own childhood and adolescence, her sexual orientation, her way of facing and adjusting to life in general. Of course, nurses cannot be expected to undertake the specifically psychiatric task of delving into the details or even the essentials of every pregnant woman's life history and its meaning to her. Nevertheless, there are several typical situations, ascertainable without too much difficulty, which play a prominent part in the immediate etiology of maternal rejection.

Socially unsanctioned, "illegitimate" conception is one of the most easily recognized sources of maternal resentment. The child so borne may unfortunately learn that he will be a permanent reminder of his mother's misstep, will either precipitate a "forced marriage" or be a hindrance in the consideration of future matrimonial aspirations, will raise the difficult problem of support, may estrange her from her relatives and friends and may thoroughly alter her status in society. All this naturally makes for an unhappy state of mind. Nevertheless, illegitimate pregnancy is not always synonymous with rejection. In our Negro population, in

which wide circles have a tolerant attitude toward babies born out of wedlock, such pregnancies are often accepted by the mothers with far greater ease than is generally the case.

Unplanned, "accidental" pregnancies are often resented because of economic distress. There already are too many mouths to be fed out of a meager budget. The mother already has her hands full cooking, cleaning, laundering and taking care of her older children. Under such circumstances, the newcomer may be viewed chiefly as an added expense and burden. The husband's displeasure with the addition to the family may further aggravate the resentment.

The mother's feelings about her husband and her marital happiness determine to a considerable extent the degree of her acceptance or rejection of her pregnancy. If dissensions and incompatibilities have led to disillusionment and raised the specter of eventual dissolution of the marriage, it is extremely difficult to look forward to the birth of a child with unmixed pleasure and equanimity. This is equally true of pregnancies which, though planned and premeditated, have been entered into with ulterior motives in which the genuine desire for a child figures much less than the purpose which his existence is intended to serve. Children are sometimes conceived as part of a scheme to keep the husband (or wife), to appeal to the marital partner's sense of responsibility, to satisfy the family's clamor for an heir to the name. If the mother finds that the disclosure of her pregnancy has not reduced her husband's alcoholism, gallivanting, lack of ambition or indifference toward her, then the child's coming has failed to accomplish the major purpose for which it was designed and therefore is resented as a bad investment.

Our culture has departed healthily and progressively from the idea that childbearing is a woman's only function and fulfillment. Women have embarked fruitfully on many occupations which had not been open to them previously. Many women come to matrimony and motherhood from the ranks of stenographers, salesgirls, nurses, teachers, factory workers, entertainers and waitresses. Some continue working while married until some time during the first pregnancy. Few people realize that the transition from a busy vocational life, from participation in group activities (office, store, hospital, school, factory, restaurant, etc.), and from a variety of interests and associations to quiet domesticity, change and narrowing of duties, and limitation of contacts with people, calls for major adjustments of routine and attitudes. Stable mothers, happily married, have gained a great deal from their jobs, which had given them an opportunity for personal enrichment, the satisfaction of having had a fling at life before their domestication, and practice in dealing with human beings. The new experience of pregnancy is enjoyed because the mother obtains a richer biologic and psychologic gratification from motherhood than she has obtained from her job, because she wants a child or children from the man whom she loves.

However, if the marriage turns out to be emotionally and economi-cally disappointing, often there is a compensatory toying with the idea of returning to the former occupation and associates. Then comes the first pregnancy, which is either "accidental" or desired as a means of cementing a brittle husband-wife relationship and giving to the mother a new content in life. With it, however, comes a realization of finality. The child's expected arrival is looked upon with mixed feelings as a trap and a promise of something more precious than a job. This constant swaying between acceptance and rejection creates many quandaries which complicate the mother's attitude toward her pregnancy. I have heard a sizable number of mothers report how, under such conditions, they had felt "trapped," "hemmed in," "confined," or "cooped up" during pregnancy and how, in their night dreams and daydreams, they were not pregnant and were happily back at their jobs.

Though matrimonial unhappiness is one of the outstanding immediate factors in the etiology of maternal rejection, there are many other elements which color the picture in individual instances. A few specific examples may suffice.

Mrs. A. conceived immediately after marriage. A vivacious friend of hers, whose defiance of local bigotry had caused the neighbors' tongues to click for years, had given premature birth to a child seven months after her wedding; the whole community had raised suspicious eyebrows and cast aspersions. Mrs. A., who was pathetically dependent on the opinions of other people, lived throughout her pregnancy in dread that her child might come prematurely and arouse similar suspicions. She began to resent her pregnancy as coming "too soon." The combination of fear and rejection created an urgent psychiatric problem, caused her to attempt an abortion, and almost wrecked the marriage.

Mrs. B. avowedly did not want children. Her husband likewise did not wish to "be bothered." They got along well for ten years. Their relatives and friends did not approve of their childlessness. They pointed out that, being people of wealth and standing, it was their "duty" to have children. They finally yielded when Mrs. B. decided that, having reached her thirties, she should "hurry up" if she was to have any children at all. But once pregnant, she felt very bad and hated the child from the moment she discovered her pregnancy. She hated her advisers and blamed her husband for submitting to their dictates.

Mrs. C. was kept despotically under the thumb of her domineering mother, who consented to her marriage at 19 years on the condition that, being "too young," she promise not to have any children for several years. Mrs. C. was in love with her husband, who was anxious to become a father before his anticipated departure for the Pacific combat zone. When Mrs. C.'s mother learned about the pregnancy, she reproached her daughter, kept reminding her of the broken pledge, and finally refused to speak to her for several weeks. Matters were aggravated by the fact that, after the husband's departure, Mrs. C. was enticed by her mother to live in her house. Worried about her husband, made to feel guilty by her mother who ascribed recurrent headaches to her daughter's "disobedience," Mrs. C. was driven to despair. She came to accept her mother's endlessly repeated verdict that she should not have become pregnant so soon and looked on her pregnancy as an irreparable mistake destined to be a permanent reminder of her filial disloyalty.

EFFECT OF FEAR AND REJECTION

Fear and rejection, the principal obstacles in the path of good mental health in pregnancy, may be damaging in a variety of ways. An attitude of dread of the things to come and a revulsion against that which has become inevitable are obviously not conducive to comfort and composure.

However, it should be pointed out from the start that mild fear and resentment which are not too deeply rooted in the mother's personality can often be handled by her satisfactorily, without too much interference with her equanimity. She is ready to seek and accept from her physician or nurse enlightenment with regard to her apprehensive puzzlements. She is able to overcome the first "shock" of the discovery of her pregnancy and to adjust to, or at least compromise with, the new situation.

A different picture obtains when strong emotional conflicts are at play, when the mother is the victim of powerful unconscious crosscurrents, and when the pregnancy is complicated by fundamental personality difficulties.

It is well known that psychologic distress has marked effects on one's ordinary physiologic functions. Everybody is familiar with headache, stomach ache and backache which obtrude themselves as "body protests" against emotional conflicts, even though no organic pathology can be demonstrated in the head, the stomach or the back.

Pregnancy is accompanied by a number of physical discomforts on a biologic basis. Nausea and vomiting are among the most frequent and most disturbing. Certainly enough momentous changes are taking place in the mother's somatic condition to explain nausea as a physiologic by-product of the pregnancy. Nevertheless, there are several features which have convinced obstetricians that emotional influences play a significant part in the picture.

1. Nausea, with or without vomiting, is not universal. It has been estimated that in about one third of all pregnancies it is either absent or so mild and fleeting that it constitutes no problem. This has rightly raised the question why identical bodily processes cause severe vomiting in one woman and barely a trace of nausea in another. The search for an answer to this question has led to the observation that the mother's personality and attitudes could be correlated with the degree of severity of the vomiting.

2. This assumption was strengthened by the fact that emotional factors were found to alleviate or aggravate the nausea. There were many instances during the war in which the husband's furlough put a stop to an expectant woman's nausea. A young, "accidentally" impregnated primipara became nauseated as soon as she had discovered the fact. Her husband had a poorly paid job at the time; her nausea was very disturbing for several weeks and ceased abruptly when her husband was offered a well-paying position.

3. The milder forms of nausea are usually restricted to the early part of pregnancy. This indicates that nausea has a tendency to fade away when there has been a psychologic as well as somatic adjustment to the condition.

4. Excessive or pernicious vomiting seems to respond to psychotherapeutic measures at least as well as to other efforts.

Aside from nausea and vomiting, pregnancy is by its very nature associated with other discomforts, which stable mothers take in their stride. Fear-ridden and rejecting mothers tend to be disturbed by them to a much greater extent. When the pregnancy as such is resented, the necessary changes of routine, the temporary limitation of social activities or the disruption of employment are equally unwelcome. This attitude often results in poor co-operation with the regimen which has been mapped out by the physician and the nurse. Individual behavior differs in accordance with personalities.

One woman will not only follow recommendations anxiously but be exasperating in her demands for the constant and undivided attention of the nurse, her husband, her relatives and everybody else. Her self-spoiling, forever-complaining and dissatisfied demeanor will calculate to surround her with people expected to cater to her hypochondriac whining or nagging. It is possible, though not certain, that some pregnant women's peculiar appetite for strange and not easily obtainable food items may have an unconscious basis in this type of self-indulgence.

Other women may go out of their way to disregard recommendations. They may continue scrubbing floors, rushing up and down the stairs or—in socially different settings—riding on horseback beyond the time when such strenuous activities are permissible. Their poor mental hygiene may cause them to neglect the essentials of physical hygiene. This devil-may-care or leave-me-alone attitude sometimes poses major problems to the obstetric nurse.

THE MOTHER'S ATTITUDE TOWARD LABOR

Dershimer has called attention to the great facility of childbirth among primitive peoples. Many ethnologists were amazed at the easy labor in civilizations less complex than our own. Deutsch wrote: "In some tribes, the whole confinement period is a matter of minutes. The young mother immediately bathes herself and the newborn infant in the nearest river and returns to her interrupted work as though nothing had happened. If a woman is suddenly seized with labor pains while traveling on land or by water, she resumes her journey immediately after delivery and continues on her way until she reaches her destination."

From this one might—a little too hastily, perhaps—infer that such bliss can be bought for the price of ignorance only. For it is true that primitive woman has not had the day of delivery calculated and marked for her on the calendar; she has not been enlightened about the process of parturition; and she has utter faith in the protective magic of her amulets. But this is not the whole story by far. There are many other primitive tribes, equally untutored, in which there is considerable agitation, kindled by all sorts of rituals, in connection with childbirth. Furthermore, precipitate deliveries occur in our culture as well as in any other. The psychology of labor and delivery is not too well known as yet to afford satisfactory explanations for differences in duration, intensity of pain and psychosomatic relationships in different cultures.

We are on safer ground when we consider differences among individual women in our own midst. We can understand that a stable, well-adjusted mother accepts the confinement as a hoped-for climax, at the end of which comes the coveted reward—the baby. The pain is felt as strongly by her as by any other woman in labor but is tolerated with a determination which keeps the goal in mind. It is recognized as a transition, demanded by Nature, to something that has been eagerly desired. There may be fear similar to that which is felt immediately before a surgical operation. But a stable person, though afraid, submits to the operation because she keeps in mind the goal of relief from the illness which has necessitated the surgeon's intervention. To a woman in good mental health, labor represents not only a first step toward the full restoration of her usual physical adequacy but also the welcome realization of imminent fulfillment.

But long-term anxiety reinforced by rejection makes labor appear as something like the painful signing of a contract into which a person has been pushed against her will. Or, if the analogy of an operation may again be resumed, delivery under those circumstances may be compared with a major surgical procedure from which the patient, instead of looking forward to relief, expects lifelong suffering and unpleasantness. Such an attitude rarely appears in undisguised form. No mother can afford to admit even to herself that she does not want her child. The closer the baby's arrival is at hand, the less can the mother's conscience allow her to wish the baby out of the way. There is no such thing as a "maternal instinct," but there is definitely a need for protection against the "unnatural" feelings of rejection. This protection is supplied by an unconscious mechanism called *ambivalence*.

Ambivalence is a fundamental human trait which makes it possible to love and hate the same person simultaneously, to want and not to want a child at the same time. When love and desire predominate, as they do in emotionally healthy mothers, any coexisting negative feelings are weak and negligible and hardly ever come to the surface. But when there is resentment and rejection, the mother has the face-saving need for strengthening and emphasizing whatever positive feelings she has for the baby. The matrimonially unhappy mother discovers that the child, conceived against her wishes, will after all be everything that is left to her to live for. She begins to feel guilty about ever having felt an aversion toward the pregnancy and is determined to make up for this when the child arrives.

All these sentiments and attitudes, some of which are intricately embedded in the mother's unconscious,

are a significant part of her mental status during labor. It has been said that they may even influence the vigor of uterine contractions but this, though quite possible, still remains to be demonstrated.

Some obstetricians, realizing the role of fear in labor, have tried to devise methods intended to alleviate the fear. In England, Read, convinced that much of the labor pain is attributable to tension produced by fear, worked out an obstetric regimen intended to keep the mother free from fear and pain by appropriate instruction, preparation and assistance. He described his method in a book entitled *Childbirth Without Fear*. Though in individual cases this may prove to be a helpful contribution to obstetric technic, Read did not pay sufficient attention to the basic mechanisms of the emotional conflicts which are at the bottom of a mother's tensions and fears.

THE MOTHER'S ATTITUDE TOWARD THE NEWBORN

People differ in their attitudes even toward inanimate possessions. One woman will treat her new set of furniture casually. Another will keep dusting and polishing it almost incessantly. A third will have spots and scratches on it in no time. Casualness, obsessiveness and negligence are expressions of personality and, when present, are applied to all phases of living.

A new baby certainly means much more than a new set of furniture. A woman's whole biography, the sum total of her philosophy of life, the background of her attitudes and relationships, her past and her vision of the future are reflected in her mode of adjustment to motherhood and to the newborn. Furthermore, a baby is, unlike a set of furniture, sensitive to the manner in which he is treated. The realization of an infant's responsiveness to affection or lack of affection has been one of the most significant discoveries made by students of human development. Many people are still skeptical when they are confronted with evidences of this discovery. Are not proper nutrition and physical hygiene all that a baby needs? What can he possibly know of his mother's worries or satisfactions? Indeed, he "knows" nothing about them. But he "senses" and responds to a tense or relaxed attitude, a personal or impersonal approach, genuine acceptance or dutiful subjection to regulations.

A series of studies in the past decade brought clinical proof of these observations. Babies reared for the first two or three years in orphanages under ideal hygienic and nutritional conditions, but without attention to their emotional needs, were found to be severely damaged psychologically. The emotional deprivations had lasting results which showed themselves in behavior deviations, character defects and intellectual deficit. By contrast, control groups reared in foster homes during early infancy achieved a much more satisfactory life adjustment and did far better in intelligence and personality tests.

An infant's need for maternal affection is now recognized as an undisputed scientific fact, as is the need for food and shelter. A loved child is a happy and secure child. An unloved child is unhappy, insecure and riddled with anxieties.

Rejected children are unloved children. A rejecting attitude is apt to push the mother into one of several sets of practices which are harmful to the child's mental hygiene as well as her own. There are, in our civilization, three principal types of maternal behavior in response to the rejection of her baby: open hostility and neglect, perfectionism and overprotection.

1. **Open hostility and neglect.** Abandonment and desertion are the extreme forms of such behavior. They are, in a sense, postpartum "abortions"; the baby is tossed out of its mother's existence. But the tossing is sometimes done in a much subtler and more refined form which, though sanctioned by convention, still deprives the baby of a mother. There is no fondling and cuddling. The bottle takes the place of the breast. The mother returns as soon as possible to her work or social functions and leaves the care of her child to relatives or governesses. I have known working mothers who went to see their boarded babies once a week, mainly in order to pay for the board. I have known socialite mothers who had their babies brought to them for a few minutes' inspection "by appointment."

2. **Perfectionism.** Ambivalence plays an important part after childbirth, as it has played during pregnancy and labor. The inability to accept a child is coupled with a desire for the ability to accept him. The rejecting mother, justifying her feelings on the basis of the child's imperfections (no "perfect" human has ever existed), goes out of her way

to assure the child's acceptability by trying to make him perfect. These are usually mothers who have long had a tendency to obsessive perfectionism, who scrub (or have the maid scrub) the floor until it sparkles, who live by the clock and make a fetish of orderliness and regularity. The baby must be made to fit into this scheme. All sorts of books on child rearing and child psychology are consulted and all but memorized. The advice of doctors and nurses is taken and carried out far too literally. If the baby does not comply with the desired ideal of perfection, the impatient mother resorts to coercion. Psychiatrists have learned that many difficulties of personality development have their origin in forced feeding and coercive bowel training in early infancy. Force and restraint lead to meek submission, listless withdrawal or rebellious negativism. All of these reactions are signs of frustration of a child who, being human, cannot live up to the demanded standards of perfection.

3. **Overprotection.** Some mothers cannot stand the thought that they have resented the pregnancy and the baby's coming. The mother's unsolved conflicts over her own unhappy childhood, matrimonial disillusionment, or disrupted career are, after all, not the poor baby's fault. There is a feeling of remorse about the rejection. This feeling is compensated and overcompensated by a determination to sacrifice everything to the baby, to center on him all attention and energy every moment of the day. The child is wrapped in a heavy blanket of overprotection and oversolicitude.

Overprotection is not always the result of rejection. A woman who has lost one or more children through miscarriage, stillbirth or illness, a mother of an only child incapable of having more children because of hysterectomy, a woman whose child has come to her after a long period of childlessness may come to feel that she must be perpetually on guard lest something disastrous befall the child. Her overprotection of the baby is not an expiation for a rejecting attitude but an overdose of mothering and, figuratively speaking, the constant pulling at an uncut umbilical cord.

Regardless of the psychologic origin of maternal overprotection, the result is unmerciful "spoiling" of the child. While the neglected or coerced child lives in an emotional refrigerator, the overprotected child lives in a heated oven in which mother love becomes smother love. Maturation and gradual emancipation are made impossible; whenever the child attempts to make use of his newly acquired abilities, he is pushed back into the oven. The mother is alarmed if he cries or if he does not cry, if he wants more food or less food than she believes that he should have, if his stools are softer or harder than she thinks they should be.

Neglect, perfectionism and overprotection are poor substitutes for genuine, natural maternal affection. They indicate emotional difficulties in the mother and create profound emotional difficulties in the infant. A sustained atmosphere of warmth, equally removed from refrigerator and oven, is a sign of good mental health of the parent and the safest guarantee of an infant's wholesome personality development.

THE PSYCHOSES OF PREGNANCY

In rare instances, the mother's emotional conflicts have been so deeply intrenched that they cannot be solved by neurotic mechanisms. The ordinary psychopathologic escapes and defenses, such as neglect, perfectionism and overprotection, are insufficient to keep the mother's personality functioning, even though the function be inadequate. The unconscious conflicts then become so overwhelmingly powerful that a major psychosis results. Estimates about the frequency of psychoses of pregnancy vary widely; they range from one in 400 pregnancies to one in 1,000 pregnancies.

Puerperal psychoses, with very few exceptions, have their onset after the birth of the child, usually between the first and the fourteenth day following the delivery. Apparently, even though there may have been symptoms of emotional discomfort during the period of gestation, the psychotic break does not come until the process of childbirth has been completed. It is then that the need for new adaptations which confront the mother finds her pathetically unprepared. Psychoses occur in primiparae and multiparae with almost the same frequency. Acute psychotic episodes have been known to repeat themselves in subsequent pregnancies.

There is no specific puerperal psychosis. Its general nature and symptoms may vary considerably. It usually takes the form of one of the two principal types: schizophrenia or manic-depressive psychosis. Recent studies have made it certain beyond question that neither mode of mental collapse is brought about by the pregnancy as such. Childbirth is a strong precipitating factor rather than the actual cause. It is mainly the agent which, shortly after the baby's arrival, tends to disintegrate a personality structure which has long been held together rather loosely and falls apart under the impact of the incisive psychobiologic experience of parturition. Toxic and infectious elements undoubtedly contribute to and hasten the process of disorganization.

The onset is characterized by a noticeable change of general demeanor. Sleeplessness, irritability, anxiety, excessive sadness or excitement, talkativeness, suspiciousness, preoccupation with trivialities, and tense agitation should make one very cautious and mindful of psychotic developments. Once the clinical features have established themselves, their recognition presents no difficulty even to a lay person. Regardless of the type of the psychotic condition, antagonism toward the husband, hostility to the baby and concern over sexual matters are encountered with great frequency. The pathologic attitude toward the child may express itself in a variety of ways. The mother develops an amnesia for the birth of her child; she refuses to believe that the baby is her own; she has the delusional conviction that the baby is dead; she shrinks from contact with the baby because of the tormenting apprehension that she may harm him; she even may actually attempt to kill the baby.

Whenever there is the slightest suspicion of psychotic development, the nurse should immediately inform the physician in charge of the patient. He, in turn, will make immediate provisions for psychiatric care.

THE NURSE'S CONTRIBUTION TO THE MENTAL HYGIENE OF PREGNANCY

Psychiatry has gained important insights into the psychology and the psychopathology of pregnant women. In the great majority of instances psychiatrists are not, and need not be, consulted. This does not mean, however, that in our day and age every pregnant woman should not receive the benefits of existing knowledge. All branches of medicine are now availing themselves of the modern achievements of psychiatry and mental hygiene. Obstetricians, dealing as they do with women who are pregnant, guiding them for a period of almost a whole year, perceiving the great variety of marital and parent-child relationships, have been especially alert in this respect. If proof of this were necessary, one could point to Menninger's questionnaire, the answers to which bespeak great interest and understanding, and to Baker's work, which was carried out at the invitation and under the auspices of the Obstetrical Clinic of the Johns Hopkins Hospital.

The psychiatrically oriented and informed obstetrician and obstetric nurse are the ideal mental hygienists of pregnancy. The nurse, without being a psychiatrist, can contribute a lion's share to the emotional well-being of the mother and to the baby's wholesome start in life. For this purpose, she needs three major attributes: (1) the ability to understand; (2) the ability to listen; (3) the ability to guide.

The Ability to Understand. Adequate information is one of the first prerequisites. As everywhere else in science, there are a few basic facts which must be learned before any sort of understanding can be reached. Furthermore, a nurse needs this knowledge not only for the sake of her own enlightenment; she also needs it in order to be able to impart it to her patients. Hall and Mohr recorded the types of questions which expectant mothers ask of their mentors in the course of pregnancy. The most frequently recurring questions were about physical care during pregnancy, the initial needs of the child, heredity and "marking." Some of these questions indicate in themselves the presence of quandaries and apprehensions and a desire for clarification.

The Ability to Listen. Patient, sympathetic listening is one of the greatest assets of anyone who tries to help human beings. People who have problems appreciate nothing more than an opportunity to pour out their troubles. The very act of verbalizing one's perplexities, of trying to hold them before oneself, of setting them forth before someone else, often affords great relief and helps the complainant to gain a better perspective regarding her complaints. There is nothing more frustrating than the experience of a patient who is anxious to talk herself out and is shut off with a remark, however well meant, such as: "Oh, forget it," "Now, don't let that worry you," or "This is just your imagination." It is far more helpful to encourage the speaker by asking interestedly: "What makes you feel that way?", or "Why does this bother you?"

The Ability to Guide. There is a great difference between guidance and direction. Inexperienced, insecure or tactless people often have a tendency to parade their authority and their better knowledge. Advice is given in terms of: "Do as I tell you," and "Take it or leave it." Such an approach does not invite willing co-operation. Patients want to be guided, not bullied. Guidance includes readiness to explain one's directions and to make them acceptable. The aim is voluntary compliance through insight, not blind obedience through intimidation.

Understanding, listening and guidance are the cornerstones of the nurse's positive contribution to the mental hygiene of pregnancy. Without them, mothers will shy away from an otherwise most efficient nurse. They will, and should, shrink back if, having reached out for psychologic help, they find that their plea is not recognized or is handled clumsily.

The first contact between the expectant mother and the obstetric nurse should be made an occasion for the establishment of a cordial mutual relationship. In this first interview, the pregnant woman should be helped to feel that she has acquired a sympathetic friend to whom she can talk about herself without hesitation. If there is economic distress, the nurse ought to be sufficiently familiar with the communal resources to be able to advise the family about possibilities of applying for and obtaining the necessary financial assistance.

The expectant mother's fears about herself and the baby-to-come should not be dismissed lightly with some indifferent phrase. When the mother has been allowed to reveal the nature and, as far as she can, the sources of her apprehension, she can be reassured by the nurse's explanations based on her better knowledge of the facts. Superstitious fears can thus be dispelled; erroneous notions about heredity and prenatal influences can thus be corrected. There will always be a greater or lesser degree of anxiety about the delivery, especially in primiparae and in mothers whose earlier pregnancy or pregnancies have been aggravated by unpleasant complications. In such instances, no amount of reasoning or disputing will succeed in removing the residual fear but the mother can be helped to accept and adjust to the fear, much as a brave soldier accepts and adjusts to the fear of impending battle. She will be helped particularly by being allowed to live a normal and active life as long as this is possible. Activity is the best prophylaxis against brooding. Though a reasonable amount of rest is needed and highly desirable, modern obstetricians are rightly not in favor of inactivity and inertia during pregnancy. Eastman, discussing "The abuse of rest in obstetrics," wrote: "In whatever class of society, unoccupied life is not conducive to the health of the expectant mother." In view of the experiences with employed pregnant women in both world wars in this country and in England, Eastman felt that "it seems to have been clearly established that it is just as safe, with certain reservations, for pregnant women to work in industrial plants as it is for them to work at home."

The nurse often has an opportunity to contribute to the mental hygiene of the expected baby's older sibling. Profound jealousies among brothers and sisters are created sometimes by the improper preparation of a child for the arrival of a new baby. The existing child, who has had all the attention of his parents, suddenly and unexpectedly finds that an unannounced intruder is occupying his place and, by the very nature of things, seems to be monopolizing his mother's time. Prudishness or ignorance of the possible effects keeps many parents from introducing the new situation to the child gradually and in a manner which would help him to welcome, instead of jealously resenting, the new baby. The nurse can enlighten the family about the best means to prepare the child and bring home to them an understanding of his emotional needs for continued attention and show of affection.

There is little that a nurse can do about the fundamental mechanisms of maternal rejection. Rejection, as we have seen, involves deep-rooted unconscious conflicts which cannot be solved on a conscious level. Nevertheless, even then it helps the mother if she can voice her feelings in the presence of an understanding listener who, by her sympathetic attitude, can at least relieve her of some of her guilty feeling and anxiety. Besides, as Menninger stated, many "prospective parents can accept consciously an unwanted pregnancy with few, if any, manifestations of rejection," especially if they have a chance to discuss their failings with someone who has insight into their emotional attitudes.

Even though the basic background of rejection is beyond the nurse's scope, she can do much to alleviate some of its most disturbing effects, namely, those of perfectionistic coerciveness and overprotection. In fact, she can be a key figure in the task of parent education.

We have but recently emerged from an era in which physicians and psychologists alike not only sanctioned parental perfectionism but imposed on mothers rigid rules and regulations which invited obsessiveness. Even then, the average mother, using common sense, did not allow herself to become a mechanized robot to whom the rules were more important than the baby. But insecure mothers, unable to rely on their own resources, inclined to punctiliousness, binding themselves to thou-shalts and thou-shalt-nots, developed a habit of rearing their children "by the book." The psychologic school of behaviorism preached the gospel of impersonal "conditioning." Earlier pediatrics tried to cultivate addiction to the clock, a prescribed number of ounces, standard weight charts, and calculation of calories. She was considered a good mother who never departed an iota from all these commandments. The sooner and the more persistently she started with toilet training, the higher was her efficiency rating in the eyes of her environment.

The past two decades witnessed a wholesome rebellion against this enthrallment of mother and child. The discovery—or rediscovery—of the character-shaping value of maternal warmth, affection, naturalness and personal handling of the baby initiated a trend toward recognition of "the rights of infants." A baby is no longer regarded as something like a machine to be oiled, cleaned, purged of refuse and immobilized by the clock. He is looked upon as a human being on the way to form relationships with other human beings, relationships which depend on the attitudes of the people closest to him as much as the health of his body depends on proper nutrition, shelter and cleanliness.

This by no means indicates an abandonment of principles and rules based on such principles, but it does indicate an abandonment of obsessive enslavement to rules. It introduces the emphasis on *enjoyment* of the baby whose care is made a pleasure rather than a succession of chores. It was found that, unless there are physical obstacles, breast feeding makes for a happier contact between mother and child than bottle feeding. It was learned that patient and not too precocious bowel training is far better for the mental hygiene of the child than coercive bowel training. It has been established that occasional picking up and fondling, far from resulting in the dreaded "spoiling," builds in the child a sense of security and of being accepted and loved.

A mother who had reared two children well found herself "accidentally" pregnant again. The discovery was a "shock" to her. Remembering that her two children occasionally refused their spinach and sometimes did not obey her promptly, she made up her mind to rear her third child "scientifically." She lived up to every rule. The child was kept in her crib, was never picked up except to have the diapers changed. Nutrition, ventilation and everything else pertaining to physical welfare were perfect. Yet the baby, who was well endowed, failed to relate herself to her environment. She lived "in a world of her own." When I saw her at the age of five years, she was completely withdrawn and, in her schizophrenic aloneness, gave the impression of an idiotic child. This girl, who had been reared "perfectly," became a tragic victim of this type of perfection.

An obstetric nurse could have saved this child by helping the mother to recognize the grave hazards of impersonal perfectionism. Pregnancy and puerperium are the best time for implanting healthy methods of child rearing. It cannot be emphasized strongly enough that the obstetric nurse, in conjunction with the obstetrician, can do more than any other group of professional people to engender wholesome attitudes in parents toward their children. The work can then be taken up by pediatricians. Psychiatrists are not called into play until something has gone wrong. It is their job to study the causes of the damage and to communicate these causes to the natural mental hygienists of childhood—obstetricians, pediatricians and public health nurses.

SUMMARY

The mental hygiene of pregnancy, extending over a period of almost a year, is concerned with the emotional health of the expectant mother, the baby-to-come and sometimes the children already present. The mother's fear for herself and the baby and a rejecting attitude toward pregnancy and the child are the most powerful obstacles to emotional well-being. Rejection can manifest itself through neglect, perfectionistic coercion or overprotection. The public health nurse can do much to prevent mental difficulties by her understanding, ability to listen and tactful guidance, by dispelling pseudoscientific and superstitious fears and, above all, by helping the mother to institute adequate methods of child rearing. Such an orientation places the nurse in the front line of mental hygiene.

SUGGESTED READING

Anderson, Camilla: Emotional Hygiene, Philadelphia, Lippincott, 1948.

Caner, Colket G.: It's How You Take It, New York, Coward-McCann, 1946.

Cohen, L. H.: Psychiatric aspects of childbearing, Yale J. Biol. & Med. 16:77, 1943.

Dershimer, F.: The influence of mental attitudes in childbearing, Am. J. Obst. & Gynec. 31:444, 1936.

Deutsch, H.: Psychology of Women, Vol. II: Motherhood, New York, Grune & Stratton, 1945.

Eastman, N. J.: The abuse of rest in obstetrics, J.A.M.A. 125:1077, 1944.

Fries, M.: Mental hygiene in pregnancy, delivery and the puerperium, Ment. Hyg. 25:221, 1941.

Jacobson, Edmund: You Must Relax, Garden City, N. Y., Blue Ribbon Books, 1946.

Kanner, Leo: In Defense of Mothers, New York, Dodd, 1945.

Kartchner, Fred D.: A study of the emotional reactions during labor, Am. J. Obst. & Gynec. 60:19, 1950.

Menninger, W. C.: The emotional factors in pregnancy, Bull. Menninger Clin. 7:15, 1943.

Parks, John: Emotional reactions to pregnancy, Am. J. Obst. & Gynec. 62:339, 1951.

Read, G. D.: Childbirth Without Fear, New York, Harper, 1944.

Thompson, L. J.: Attitudes of primiparae as observed in a prenatal clinic, Ment. Hyg. 26:243, 1942.

12

Preparations for Labor and Delivery

PRELIMINARY PLANS

Parents, today, will need little argument to convince them that the mother should have supervision by a competent obstetrician throughout pregnancy. This care is the mother's first obligation to herself and her baby. She will desire to acquire the knowledge concerning the kind of care that will be most beneficial to her and her baby, for ignorance and disregard of scientific truths regarding this care are often followed by tragedy. She will expect to follow the obviously reasonable suggestions in order to have a normal pregnancy. The advice, the care and the watchfulness of the obstetrician may be depended upon to avert and combat complications, should they arise; but to assure the best results the mother also must observe the details of physical and mental hygiene, as well as follow the obstetrician's advice during the whole period of pregnancy.

HOSPITAL VS. HOME CARE

Some patients prefer to be delivered in a hospital because of the many advantages. To the average woman who desires both comfort and a feeling of safety, hospital care appeals very strongly. It provides for every emergency and obviates all interruptions to the domestic routine, except that due to a temporary absence from the home.

As the first labor is usually longer and more difficult than later ones, and as the percentage of patients showing lacerations and demanding operative deliveries is greater among primiparae, they should be encour-

286

aged to be delivered in hospitals whenever possible. Any patient who has definite abnormal symptoms or complications should also be taken care of in the hospital.

The final decision is determined by hospital facilities, the normalcy of the patient and the home conditions.

bilities of the home. During the last weeks of pregnancy, a definite arrangement should be made so that the patient is not left alone or, at least, has someone to call upon to take her to the hospital when labor begins. Labor is too involved to be complicated by unnecessary worry.

HOSPITAL DELIVERY

In selecting a hospital, it should be one that is recognized by the American Medical Association. No doubt, the obstetrician will have proposed this idea. It may be not only interesting but also reassuring for both the patient and her husband to visit the hospital before making her hospital plans. A mental picture of where she is to go when labor begins may relieve mental tension and help to allay fears. When the obstetrician, the patient and the husband have decided upon a hospital delivery, there will be many arrangements and details to be discussed with the doctor and the nurse. If the patient is going through the experience of a first pregnancy and labor, the anticipation of going to the hospital may be rather terrifying. If the obstetrician and the nurse will outline both the symptoms of the onset of labor and the hospital admission routine, it will do much to stimulate the patient's confidence and allay her fears. These symptoms should be explained to the husband also. It should be suggested to the patient that even though first labors are longer, it will be safer for her to go to the hospital when labor first begins. If there are children, provision will have to be made in advance for their care, as well as plans for the other responsi-

HOME DELIVERY

Even though, at the present time, 85.6 per cent of the mothers are delivered in hospitals, there are still about 14.4 per cent of the deliveries at home. In cities 94 per cent of the deliveries occur in hospitals, and in rural areas, 73.4 per cent. In 1948 there were approximately 600,000 deliveries that occurred in the home. Therefore, the nurse should acquaint herself with the knowledge of how a home delivery is conducted. In an emergency, too, the nurse may need this knowledge and experience. The nurse midwife training centers, such as The Frontier Nursing Service of Kentucky, The Maternity Center Association of New York, and the Catholic Maternity Institute of New Mexico, today offer training for the practical application of a home delivery service. Only a few visiting nurse services offer this experience.

If a home delivery is preferred, the decision is based on the normalcy of the patient, accessibility of the obstetrician, facilities at home and available care. Adequate preparations should be made by the parents. Preparations for a home delivery should be begun early in pregnancy, because the patient will feel less able to expend her energy during the last two months. Then, too, the possibility of a premature labor must be kept

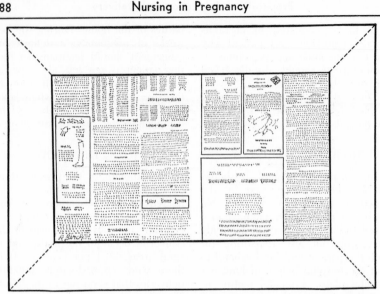

Fig. 151. Newspaper pad made of 12 thickness of newspaper sewed together at the outer edges and covered with unbleached muslin. The muslin covers are mitered at the corners so that they may be removed, laundered and used again.

in mind. The preparations consist of those articles needed for the mother's care and the care of the baby at the time of delivery.

Today, in many parts of the country, the public health nurse visits the patient in her home during the prenatal period. The nurse aids the patient in carrying out the advice of the doctor and reports her findings to the doctor. When there is a home delivery service, these same nurses may attend the delivery with the doctor. If the service of a private nurse is desired, it is well to ask the obstetrician's advice in choosing the nurse.

In homes of small means, economy is often of vital importance. The nurse can be most helpful here by her ability to improvise, for it is possible to do excellent work with a small amount of equipment. All patients will appreciate such help, for having a baby always involves unusual expense.

Many obstetricians give their patients a list of the supplies they need for delivery, but where the matter is left to the parents and the nurse, the following suggestions may be helpful. Even when the mother has been able to avail herself of the opportunity of attending a Mothers' Club and obtaining suggestions, she may desire to discuss some of them, along with personal problems, with the obstetrician and the nurse.

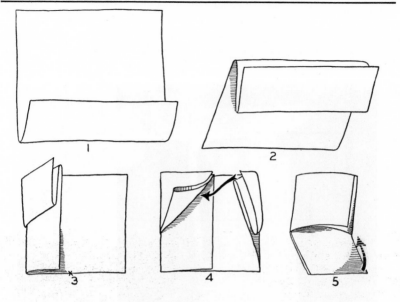

FIG. 152. Steps in making a newspaper bag. These are useful receptacles for waste material. May be made in small and large sizes. (Fig. 363.)

SUPPLIES FOR THE MOTHER

The supplies suggested are listed in a form which makes it convenient to check.

Nightgowns
Bed jackets, kimono, slippers, toilet articles
Blankets
Chest blanket
Towels—bath and face
Washcloths
Pillow cases
Sheets. It is a good idea to have an old sheet that may be used by the nurse for draping the patient at the time of delivery.
Waterproof material—large enough to cover the mattress

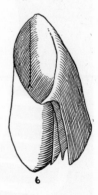

Six newspaper pads. These bed pads are made from 12 thicknesses of newspaper opened to full size (sewed together at the edges) and covered with freshly laundered old or new muslin. The corners may be mitered, so that the cover may be removed and laundered when necessary and fresh newspaper in-

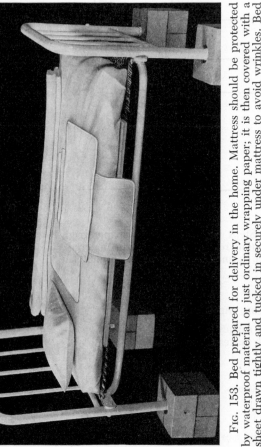

FIG. 153. Bed prepared for delivery in the home. Mattress should be protected by waterproof material or just ordinary wrapping paper; it is then covered with a sheet drawn tightly and tucked in securely under mattress to avoid wrinkles. Bed pads are used for extra protection for the mother and the bed. If the top covers are "fanned" to the far side of the bed they may be more easily kept out of the way. A table leaf or other available board should be slipped under mattress to prevent it from sagging. Blocks to elevate bed help to make care given by doctor, nurse and those attending the mother less difficult.

serted. Underpads and large-size paper diapers may also be purchased for this purpose.

Newspapers. A supply should be saved for the many uses to which they may be put at this time, for newspapers save washing of sheets, pads, etc.

Newspaper bags. The large newspaper bag is especially useful at the time of delivery (Fig. 363).

Three dozen safety pins

Three T-binders or sanitary belts

Three or four abdominal binders (if the doctor wishes the patient to wear them). Abdominal binders may be made of unbleached muslin wide enough and long enough to fit the patient, allowing a lap of about 6 to 8 inches. They should be about 18 inches wide, and the material may be of two thicknesses. If they are washed and ironed beforehand, they are more comfortable. Wide Ace bandages or knit binders may be purchased Fig. 250).

Three or four breast supports. These may be the regular brassières the patient usually wears or they may be Ace bandages, 10 inches wide, or terry-cloth breast supports.

One pair of white stockings—may be an inexpensive variety

Four to six dozen sanitary pads. The absorbent sanitary pads may be purchased, or they may be made of freshly laundered material, folded and ironed, ready for use.

One pound of sterile cotton, in original package, unopened

Hot-water bag, with flannel cover— a combination hot-water bag and fountain syringe may be useful.

One bed pan

Three basins: one for the doctor to use for his hands, one for sponging the patient's genitals (preparation for delivery), and one to receive the placenta

Large pail (diaper pail)

Two kettles (one may be a teakettle): one for cooled boiled water and one for boiling water

Ladle or dipper

One pitcher or Mason jar with cover

Medicine dropper

One bent glass drinking tube (not necessary but convenient)

Disinfectant that the doctor advises

White petroleum jelly

One new nail brush and an orange stick

Board for placing under mattress of delivery bed (table leaf or ironing board)

Blocks to raise bed to convenient height (Fig. 153)

Flashlight

Obstetric leggings. In order to subject the patient to the least possible exposure and chilling during delivery, these may be made of an old pair of pajamas cut in half. The nurse may tie a strip of bandage above each knee, thus keeping any fullness out of the way. The result is an obstetric suit much like the maternity stockings. Knee caps may be used for delivery and post-parturition care (Fig. 258).

Four pieces of cord tie, bobbin or narrow tape, 10 inches long, with knots tied in the ends. (The knots prevent the operator's fingers from slipping when tying the cord.)

Two cord dressings and bands

Scissors

Mineral oil

HOME PREPARATIONS

In preparing for a home delivery, the nurse should explain and demonstrate to the patient how to prepare the articles that are to be used during delivery.

Sheets (for the bed and for draping)

Towels

Bed pads and perineal pads (home-made variety)

These articles should be washed with soap and water, dried in the sun if possible, ironed, and folded so that the ironed surfaces are folded upon each other. The ironed surface should be used for the field of delivery. These articles should be put away in a pillow case or wrapped in a piece of ironed paper. The other articles needed at the time of delivery should be laid aside ready for use.

If it seems necessary to have sterile supplies, it may be possible to have the package autoclaved at a local hospital. It is possible to sterilize dressings, etc., in the oven at home, but this is a most difficult procedure and more often with unsatisfactory results. The important factor to be achieved in a home delivery is cleanliness. Soap and water, sunshine and the hot iron have proved effective. On the whole, only a few articles must be sterile. The more simple and carefully prepared the preparations are, the more efficient will be the results. For the supplies prepared by the mother, the emphasis should be on cleanliness rather than sterilization.

Room for Delivery

Deciding on the room in which the patient is to be delivered is one of the "preparations." It should be the room in which the patient will be most comfortable. Many mothers during this period have to assume certain responsibilities for the management of the household, so it means much to be where the household affairs can be directed with the least exertion.

Ideally, it should be a room that is light, airy, quiet, cheerful and comfortable, conveniently near a bathroom and with an adjoining room for the nurse and baby. The room furnishings should be simple, so that they are easy to keep clean, as cleanliness is one of the first essentials of good obstetric care. The bed should be so placed that the light is convenient either day or night. Ample light is a necessity.

The nurse may help select the room, but the choice is limited or even fixed by the possibilities of the house. Naturally, the nurse will avoid putting the family to any unnecessary inconvenience, but always her first thought must be in the interest of her patient.

The nurse should make sure that the room has not been occupied recently by a patient suffering from any contagious, infectious, or suppurative disease. In such cases, another room should be chosen even though less convenient. If, for any reason, it is impossible to make use of another room, the infected one should be thoroughly disinfected in accordance with the rules of the local Board of Health, with which every nurse should be familiar.

In any event, the room should be cleaned thoroughly, and all unnecessary furniture removed, only enough being left to make the room comfortable and cheerful. Rugs can be removed temporarily without causing dust and confusion. The obstetrician will need a plain table or a substitute. The nurse will need a table or chair for supplies, unless perhaps the corner of the chest may be used. A card table may be very practical. The patient may be much interested and assist the nurse in planning beforehand the arrangement of light, furniture and supplies (Figs. 204 and 205).

PREPARATION OF THE DELIVERY BED

The mother's bed should be comfortable. The springs should be in good condition, and the mattress firm. A single bed is preferable to the wider or double bed because it is easier for the obstetrician and the nurse to care for the patient. If the bed is low, it may be raised to a more convenient height by using blocks. The bed should be so arranged that after the labor the patient may be made clean and comfortable without too much disturbance. The best way to accomplish this is first to prepare the bed as it is to be after delivery and then to add the necessary preparations for the labor and delivery.

The mattress should be supported by means of boards placed between it and the springs, so that it will be perfectly firm and level and not sag. Table leaves, ironing board, or plain board may be used for this purpose. Such supports should lie crosswise under the mattress at a point directly under the patient's buttocks and should be removed at the conclusion of delivery. A firm, flat mattress prevents the blood and the discharges from collecting in a pool under the patient's back.

The mattress should be covered with a piece of waterproof material, if available; if not, brown paper, newspaper or water repellent paper may be used. Over this covering, a white sheet should be placed and tucked in securely along the edges. The top sheet, the blanket and the spread should be fanned to the far side of the bed, where they will be convenient to cover the patient immediately after delivery. Newspaper or moistureproof pads afford excellent protection and are so arranged that they protect the bed at the time of delivery, and a fresh one is left under the patient after delivery (Fig. 153).

If these preparations are first demonstrated and their uses explained to the patient and her husband, they may be more interested in making adequate preparations and having them ready at the time of labor.

THE PHYSICIAN'S EQUIPMENT

The physician will in all probability have all the other supplies needed, such as follow:

Instruments
Sutures
Medications
Packing
Gloves
Gown

If an anesthetic is to be given, the nurse may improvise a cone. A very good cone may be made either from a sieve or from a newspaper and a towel (Fig. 159).

THE NURSE'S SUPPLIES

The nurse should have in her equipment the following supplies:

Hypodermic syringes, with large and small needles (always sharp)
Thumb forceps
Blunt scissors
Artery clamps
Cord ties
Cord dressing
Prophylactic for baby's eyes

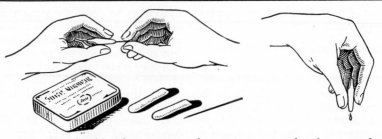

Fig. 154. (*Left*) Silver nitrate solution 1 per cent for the care of the eyes of newborn babies; needle puncture of wax ampule. (*Right*) Showing how to manipulate the ampule in administering the drug. (Eli Lilly and Company)

FINAL PREPARATIONS FOR DELIVERY

A description of the onset of labor will have been given to the patient by her doctor. He will also have directed her when to go to the hospital, if she is to have her baby there, or when to notify the doctor and the nurse if it is to be a home delivery. If the nurse is an hourly nurse or one from a nursing organization, the nurse and the physician will be called at the same time; if a private nurse has been engaged, in all probability she will be with the patient before this time.

A few preparations cannot be made until labor begins, such as boiling two kettles of water (for ten minutes) in two covered vessels and setting one aside to cool. It is a good idea to also boil a ladle or dipper in one kettle and leave it, with the handle exposed, in the kettle that is set aside to cool.

The bed should be prepared and the delivery supplies arranged. The patient should then take a warm sponge bath (this is invigorating as well as soothing) and comb her hair.

She should then put on sufficient warm clothing to avoid becoming chilled, if she is to remain out of bed. She may put on the white stockings at this time and wear them whether she is lying down or is up and about.

In the baby's bed should be placed a hot-water bottle, a complete set of clothes, and a receiving blanket. (The blanket may be one of the flannel squares or an old piece of blanket with a diaper arranged in it.) A sterile cord dressing, binder, cord tape, prophylactic for the baby's eyes, and the oil for anointing the baby (with provision for heating it) should also be in readiness (Fig. 204).

The nurse should see that the provisions for lighting the room at night are ample, and that the room is warm and as comfortable as possible (without drafts, etc.). Another of her responsibilities is to encourage the patient to take light nourishment and to get as much rest and relaxation as possible between pains.

If the obstetrician so advises, the nurse should give the patient a hot soapsuds enema. This will empty the lower bowel, reduce the pressure against the baby and also render delivery more cleanly. The patient should be advised to urinate at short intervals; this also helps to reduce the pressure.

If the physician wishes, the hair about the vulva may be closely clipped, or the parts shaved, after protecting the vaginal opening with a cotton ball, as used in preparing for a vaginal examination. This procedure is part of the ordinary routine in hospitals, but occasionally the obstetrician prefers to have the area neither shaved nor clipped.

Unless delivery is imminent, it is best to wait until the arrival of the doctor before proceeding with the cleansing of the external genitals.

SUGGESTED READING

Children's Bureau Publication: Number 260, Manual for Teaching Midwives.

Mississippi State Board of Health: Manual for Midwives, 1939.

Morlock, Maud: Homemaker service to mothers at the time of con-finement, Pub. Health Nursing 42:282, 1950.

The Mother: Policies and Practices in Home Delivery Service 2:18-20, 1942.

Read, G. D.: Childbirth Without Fear, New York, Harper, 1944.

CONFERENCE MATERIAL

1. What opportunities are available for teaching in the prenatal clinic while the patients are waiting their "turn" for examination?

2. How would you arrange for the placing of children during the time the patient is in the hospital? What organizations would you contact? When investigating the various shelters, what health items would you keep in mind when placing little girls?

3. For the antepartal patient who never has had any hospital experience, how would you introduce her to the antepartum clinic and prepare her for the complete physical examination?

4. How would you stimulate the father's interest in helping with the preparations for the new baby and the care of both the mother and the baby after delivery?

5. In discussing antepartal care with parents, how would you explain the relationship of diet to the baby's development from the time of conception until his birth?

6. In regard to the danger signals of pregnancy, how could you present these to a nervous, apprehensive patient without creating undue alarm?

7. What are the reasons for stressing the importance of completing the preparations for delivery (home or hospital) by the seventh month of pregnancy?

8. What sources would you consult to find out which states in the United States require premarital and antepartal examinations for syphilis?

9. What type of referral system is used when it is necessary for the patient to consult other services or organizations?

Situation Questions

Read through the entire question and place your answers in the parentheses.

1. Below are some signs, symptoms and conditions commonly associated with pregnancy. Check in the appropriate columns those which the patient might notice and describe in the prenatal clinic and those which the physician would observe in arriving at a positive diagnosis of pregnancy.

	Column I Patient's signs 3 mos.	Column II Positive signs 3 mos.	Column III Patient's signs 6 mos.	Column IV Positive signs 6 mos.
A. Amenorrhea				
B. Blueing of vagina				
C. Enlargement and tenderness of breasts				
D. Enlargement of tubercles of Montgomery				
E. Enlargement of uterus				
F. Frequent micturition				
G. Goodell's sign				
H. Hearing fetal heart sounds				
I. Morning nausea and vomiting				
J. Movement of the fetus				
K. Palpation of outline of uterus				
L. Pigmentation of skin of abdomen				
M. Primary areola darkened				
N. Positive Aschheim-Zondek test				
O. Positive Friedman's test				
P. Varicosities of the vulva				
Q. Roentgenogram				

2. A. In pregnancy, morning sickness is most common during which of the following periods?
    1. First month
    2. First 6 weeks
    3. Sixth to twelfth week
    4. First 4 months

5. Eighth to sixteenth week   (_____)

B. A nurse should suggest to the patient who complains of morning sickness that she might overcome this discomfort by using remedies to help:

1. Emptying the stomach.
2. Washing the stomach.
3. Eating 6 small meals instead of 3 per day.
4. Digestion of fats.   (_____)

3. A pregnant woman seen for the first time in the prenatal clinic has a hemoglobin of 70 per cent. The nurse should understand that this condition is:

A. A true anemia.
B. Caused by increased blood volume.
C. Dangerous to baby's development.
D. Predisposing to postpartum hemorrhage.   (_____)

4. The nurse in the obstetrician's office should instruct the patient regarding the collection of the specimen for the Aschheim-Zondek test by telling the patient to:

A. Save the first voided specimen in the morning.
B. Withhold fluid intake during the night and bring in the first voided specimen in the morning.
C. Report to the laboratory in the morning for a blood specimen.
D. Take a warm voided specimen to the laboratory.   (_____)

5. Though the pregnant woman is usually advised to include a quart of milk in her diet daily, which of the following, if any, would justify the omission of milk?

A. Milk makes her constipated.
B. She is gaining weight too rapidly.
C. She is not gaining fast enough and needs more concentrated foods.
D. Milk causes a feeling of fullness, decreasing her appetite for other foods.
E. Milk causes heartburn.
F. None of the above; milk should not be omitted.   (_____)

6. The most essential foods in a 2,500-calorie diet for a pregnant woman are:

A. High in carbohydrate, low in protein.
B. High in protein, low in carbohydrate.
C. High in protein, low in fat.
D. High in fat, low in protein.   (_____)

7. The nurse in the prenatal clinic will encourage the pregnant woman to see her dentist at the earliest convenience because:

A. Each baby causes the mother to lose one tooth.
B. Bone development of the baby requires calcium.
C. Foci of infection should be removed early in pregnancy.
D. The increased carbohydrate needed in pregnancy is detrimental to sound teeth.   (_____)

8. What instruction should the clinic patient be given concerning the care of her breasts during pregnancy?

A. A brassière should:
1. Not be worn.
2. Be worn snugly enough to support and lift up the breasts.
3. Be worn snugly enough to press the breasts flat against the chest wall.
4. Be worn snugly enough to apply constant firm pressure toward the midline. (_____)

B. Special care of the nipples should begin:
1. As early as pregnancy is confirmed.
2. Between the third and fourth month.
3. Between the sixth and seventh month.
4. At the beginning of the ninth month. (_____)

9. The exercises developed by Dr. Thoms at Yale included in the program of "Natural Childbirth":

A. Have as the central purpose:
1. Teaching the patient how to relax.
2. Informing the patient of physiologic changes of pregnancy.
3. Developing intra-abdominal space for uterine enlargement.
(_____)

B. In addition to the exercises given prenatally, the pregnant patient needs during labor:
1. Sympathetic care
2. Heavy sedation
3. Understanding of the progress of labor (_____)

C. Which week of pregnancy should the nurse teach these exercises in the prenatal clinic?
1. Sixth
2. Tenth
3. Fourteenth
4. Thirty-sixth (_____)

10. A. If the pregnant woman complained of painful, swollen veins in the legs, the nurse would understand that the condition would be likely to be due to:
1. Infection of the blood-vessel wall.
2. Toxins accumulating in the blood.
3. Pressure against the abdominal veins in the pelvis.
4. Pressure directly against the walls of the veins.
5. Force of gravity. (_____)

B. To remedy this condition, the nurse would expect that the patient would be advised that she should:
1. Refrain from wearing restricting clothing around the legs or the abdomen.
2. Refrain from wearing a corset.
3. Lie down each day for an hour's rest.

4. Apply an Ace bandage, starting above the source of obstruction.

(_____)

11. The nurse teaching parent classes should stress the importance of which one of the following?

A. Husbands doing the housework for their wives during the period of pregnancy.

B. The idea of sharing responsibility in parenthood.

C. The causes of invalidism during pregnancy.

D. The moral responsibility of being parents.   (_____)

12. If a woman 6 months pregnant asked if she should or should not wear a corset, in your opinion the patient should be advised:

A. To avoid wearing any corset.

B. To adjust her regular corset loosely.

C. To wear a corset that will keep the uterus from rising too high in the abdomen.

D. To wear a corset that will firmly support the lower portion of the abdomen and back.

E. To wear a corset that will not disclose her condition.   (_____)

13. The reason that pregnant women are warned against wearing high-heeled shoes from the seventh to the ninth month is:

A. To avoid additional backstrain.

B. To increase venous pressure in the legs.

C. To allow freer movement in taking daily exercises.

D. To dress themselves according to current styles.   (_____)

14. The industrial nurse would recommend that a pregnant employee who operates a hand machine be granted leave for a period of:

A. 2 months

B. 4 months

C. 6 months

D. 8 months   (_____)

15. The clinic nurse would expect the pregnant patient to be advised to get in touch with her doctor *immediately* as soon as she observed which of the following?

A. Abdominal pain

B. Bleeding with bright blood

C. Blood-streaked mucus

D. Chills and fever

E. Constipation

F. Enlargement of mammary glands

G. Dyspnea in last trimester

H. Headache, severe continuous

I. Heartburn

J. Interference with breathing

K. Morning nausea

L. Puffiness of fingers, eyes

M. Rhythmic contractions of muscles of uterus.

N. Scanty urine
O. Spots before the eyes
P. Sudden flow of water from the vagina
Q. Swelling of ankles, legs
R. Vaginal discharge, mucoid
S. Varicosities of legs
T. Vomiting, persistent   (_____)

16. The pregnant patient who has a history of heart disease:

A. Should cause the nurse to anticipate which of the following signs and symptoms?

    1. Dyspnea
    2. Slow pulse rate
    3. Decrease in blood pressure
    4. Hemorrhage   (_____)

B. The reasons for the above are:

    1. Increased need for oxygen intake.
    2. Increased blood volume.
    3. Toxic damage to heart muscle.
    4. Failure of kidneys to excrete.   (_____)

17. A pregnant woman was brought into the hospital with hypertensive disease. The nurse would understand that this disease might also be associated with kidney disease because at this time:

A. The conditions were present previously but aggravated by the added strain of pregnancy.

B. Pregnancy might cause previously normal kidneys to become damaged because of added strain.

C. Pregnancy could cause kidney damage because of excess poisons which are irritating fetal waste products that must be excreted.
                    (_____)

18. A message reached the emergency ward that a physician was bringing in a patient with a ruptured fallopian tube.

A. For which of the following should the nurse make preparations?

    1. Immediate induced labor
    2. Vaginal packing
    3. Complete hysterectomy
    4. Laparotomy
    5. Application of ice and pressure to the abdomen   (_____)

B. This condition results when:

    1. Conception takes place in one of the tubes.
    2. Conception takes place in the abdominal cavity.
    3. There is an abnormally rapid growth of the embryo.
    4. There is an attachment and development of embryo within the tube.
                    (_____)

C. One of the most characteristic signs of this condition is:

    1. Chadwick's sign

  2. Hegar's sign
  3. Bathroom sign
  4. Crede's sign   (_____)
 D. To what extent would the patient have pain?
  1. Not at all
  2. Slight
  3. Intense   (_____)
 E. To what extent would the patient manifest symptoms of shock?
  1. Not at all
  2. Slight
  3. Profound   (_____)
19. One of the best known methods of prevent of erythroblastosis is:
A. Early determination of Rh factor of parents.
B. Transfusing the mother during pregnancy.
C. Transfusing all Rh-negative fathers.
D. Transfusing all Rh-negative babies.   (_____)

Note: The key to the correct answers to these questions is given on pages 643 and 644.

UNIT THREE

NURSING DURING LABOR AND DELIVERY

ORIENTATION

ORIENTATION

The subject of labor deals with a period which is the "crisis" of all maternity care. To attempt to understand this phenomenon and to have some appreciation of its immediate reactions involves not only the knowledge of the subjects discussed in the previous chapters, but also some medical and surgical experience. During this transition period, the nurse must try to understand the mental as well as the physical adjustments which the patient is trying to make. Labor is a crisis of extraordinary importance. No one really knows what problems the patient may have in addition to her delivery. In any case, labor is supreme in importance. It is one experience which must be "faced." There can be no postponing or evading "the issue." There is also another aspect to be considered, and that is that the outcome of the delivery may determine the future health of the mother or the baby or both. These situations for the nurse are different from any other in her hospital experience, because she is sharing so intimately various emotional reactions—they may be joy and excitement or they may be depression and tragedy.

13

Phenomena of Labor

DEFINITIONS

By labor is meant the series of processes by which the products of conception are expelled from the mother's body. Childbirth, travail, accouchement, confinement—all are names for the same process. The word "delivery" refers, as a rule, to the actual birth of the baby.

PREMONITORY SIGNS OF LABOR

During the last few weeks of pregnancy, a number of changes indicate that the time of labor is approaching. Particularly in primigravidae lightening occurs about 10 to 14 days before delivery. This alteration is brought about by a settling of the fetus into the brim of the pelvis, often to the level of the ischial spines. This may occur at any time during the last four weeks, but occasionally does not eventuate until labor has actually begun. Lightening may take place suddenly, so that the expectant mother arises one morning entirely relieved of the abdominal tightness and diaphragmatic pressure she had experienced previously. But the relief in one direction is often followed by signs of greater pressure below, particularly shooting pains down the legs, an increase in the amount of vaginal discharge, and greater frequency of urination due to pressure on the bladder. In patients who have had previous children, lightening occasionally takes place during the last week or ten days of pregnancy but is more likely to occur after labor begins.

For a varying period before the

establishment of true labor pains, the patients will often suffer from so-called "false pains," and the nurse should be able to distinguish between them and effective uterine contractions. False pains may begin as early as three or four weeks before the termination of pregnancy. They are merely an exaggeration of the intermittent uterine contractions which have occurred throughout the entire period of gestation but are now accompanied by pain. They occur at decidedly irregular intervals, are confined chiefly to the lower part of the abdomen and the groin, and rarely extend around to the back. These pains are short and ineffectual, unlike true labor. Another sign of impending labor is pink "show." After the discharge of the mucous plug which has filled the cervical canal during pregnancy, the pressure of the descending presenting part of the fetus causes the minute capillaries in the mucous membrane of the cervix to rupture. This blood is mixed with mucus and therefore has the pink tinge. The nurse should understand that pink show is simply the appearance of a small amount of blood-tinged mucus, and that any substantial discharge of blood should be reported to the physician.

Occasionally, rupture of the membranes is the first indication of approaching labor. It used to be thought that this was a grave sign, heralding a long and difficult labor, but present-day statistics show that this is not true, and that rupture of the membranes is often followed by labors which are even shorter than the average. Nevertheless, the doctor should be notified at once; under these circumstances, he will usually advise the patient to enter the hospital immediately, or if she expects to be delivered at home, to go to bed and remain in a recumbent position. After the rupture of the membranes there is always the possibility of a prolapsed cord (Fig. 217).

CAUSE OF THE ONSET OF LABOR

Regardless of species, whether the fetus weighs 2 Gm. at the end of a 21-day pregnancy, as in the mouse, or whether it weighs 200 pounds at the end of a 640-day pregnancy, as in the elephant, labor regularly begins at the right time for that particular species: namely, when the fetus is mature enough to cope with extra-uterine conditions, but not yet large enough to cause mechanical difficulties in labor. The process responsible for this beautifully synchronized and salutary achievement is obscure. Nevertheless, countless theories have been advanced to explain the phenomenon. Among them may be mentioned increased irritability of the uterus as the result of greater distention, growing distention of the lower uterine structures with pressure on the surrounding nerves, and the influences of hormones.

UTERINE CONTRACTIONS

In all languages, the word for the uterine contractions of labor means the same: namely, "pain." Alone among normal physiologic muscular contractions, moreover, those of labor are painful. The duration of these contractions ranges from 45 seconds to 1 minute and a quarter, averaging about 1 minute. Each contraction presents three phases: a period during which the intensity of the contraction increases (increment), a period during which the contraction is at its height (acme), and a period of diminishing intensity (decrement). The increment, or crescendo phase, is longer than the other two combined. The contractions of the uterus during labor are intermittent, with periods of relaxation between, resembling in this respect the systole and the diastole of the heart. The interval between contractions diminishes gradually from about 10 minutes early in labor to about 1 or 2 minutes in the second stage. These periods of relaxation not only provide rest for the uterine muscles and for the mother but are essential for the welfare of the fetus, since unremitting contractions may so interfere with placental functions as to produce fetal distress as a result of lack of oxygen. Another characteristic of labor pains is that they are quite involuntary, their action being not only independent of the mother's will, but of extra-uterine nervous control. In other words, uterine action in labor, like that of the heart, is under control of nerves located within the organ itself. Today, when "natural childbirth" is being publicized, it is believed that the manifestations of suffering are more often influenced by mental and emotional reactions than by the physical condition.

THE THREE STAGES OF LABOR

The process of labor is divided, for convenience of description into three distinct stages.

The first stage of labor, or the dilating stage, begins with the first true labor pain and ends with the complete dilatation of the cervix.

The second stage of labor, or the stage of expulsion, begins with the complete dilatation of the cervix and ends with the delivery of the baby.

The third stage of labor, or the placental stage, begins with the delivery of the baby and terminates with the birth of the placenta.

THE FIRST STAGE OF LABOR

In the beginning of the first stage, the pains are short, slight, are 10 or 15 minutes or more apart, and may not cause the patient any particular discomfort. She may be walking about, and between pains is generally quite comfortable. Early in the first stage, the pain is usually located in the small of the back, but as time goes on it sweeps around girdlelike to the anterior part of the abdomen. The pains recur at shortening intervals, become stronger and last longer. Indeed, the pains which precede and accompany full dilatation are often of excruciating severity. At this time, furthermore, there is usually a marked increase in the amount of show due to rupture of capillary vessels in the cervix and the lower uterine segment. The average duration of the first stage in primigravida is 16 hours; in multiparae, 11 hours or less.

As the result of the uterine contractions, two all-important changes are wrought in the cervix during the first stage of labor—*effacement* and *dilatation*.

Effacement is the shortening of the cervical canal from a structure 1 or

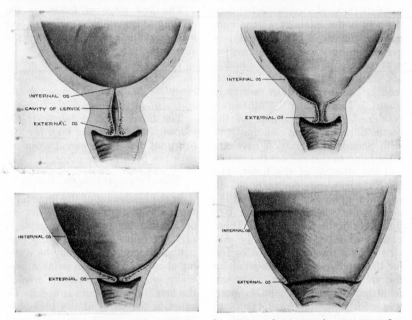

Fig. 155. Cervix in primagravida. (*Top, left*) At beginning of labor; no effacement or dilatation. (*Top, right*) About one half effaced, but no dilatation. (*Bottom, left*) Completely effaced, but no dilatation. (*Bottom, right*) Complete dilatation (Bumm).

2 cm. in length to one in which no canal at all exists, but merely a circular orifice with almost paper-thin edges. As may be seen in Figure 155, the edges of the internal os are drawn several centimeters upward, so that the former cervical mucosa becomes part of the lower uterine segment and lies parallel with and contiguous to the chorion membrane. Effacement may be compared with a funneling process in which the whole length of a moldable tube (the cervical canal) is converted into a very obtruse, flaring funnel, with only a small circular orifice for an outlet. In primigravidae, effacement is usually complete before dilatation begins, but in multiparae it is rarely complete, dilatation proceeding, as a rule, with rather thick cervical edges. Synonymous with effacement are the terms "obliteration" and "taking up" of the cervix.

Dilatation of the Cervix. By this is meant the enlargement of the external os from an orifice a few millimeters in size to an aperture large enough to permit the passage of the fetus—that is, to one with a diameter of about 10 cm. When dilatation has reached this figure, it is said to be complete. Although the forces concerned in dilatation are not well understood, several factors appear to be involved. In the first place, the muscle fibers about the cervix are so arranged that they pull upon its edges and tend to draw it open. In the second place, the uterine contractions make pressure on the bag of waters and this, in turn, burrows into the cervix in pouchlike fashion, exerting a dilating action (Fig. 85). This is usually called the hydrostatic pressure of the bag of waters. In the absence of the bag of waters, the pressure of the presenting part against the cervix and the lower uterine segment has a similar effect.

It should be noted that the dilatation of the cervix in the first stage of labor is solely the result of uterine contractions, which are involuntary. In other words, there is nothing that the mother can do, such as bearing down, which will help the slightest in expediting this period of labor. Indeed, bearing-down efforts at this stage serve only to exhaust the mother.

The Second Stage of Labor

The pains are now severe and long, lasting from 50 to 100 seconds and occurring at intervals of 2 or 3 minutes. Rupture of the membranes usually occurs during this stage of labor by a gush of amniotic fluid from the vagina. Sometimes, however, they rupture during the first stage and occasionally, as already indicated, before labor begins. In rare instances, the membranes fail to rupture, and the baby is born with the intact amniotic sac surrounding it. Obviously, in such cases the mem-

branes must be artificially ruptured at once, for otherwise the infant will drown. In some rare cases the baby is born in a "caul," which is a piece of the amnion which sometimes envelops the baby's head. Such a birth is supposed to endow the baby with a "sixth sense."

During this stage, as if by reflex action, the muscles of the abdomen are brought into play; and when the pains are in progress the patient will strain, or "bear down" with all her strength so that her face becomes flushed and the large vesels in her neck are distended. As a result of this exertion she may perspire profusely. During this stage the patient directs all her energy toward expelling the contents of the uterus.

Toward the end of the second stage, when the head is well down in the vagina, its pressure often causes small particles of fecal material to be expelled from the rectum at the occurrence of each pain. This condition must receive careful attention in order to avoid infection. As the head descends still farther, the perineal region begins to bulge, and the skin over it becomes tense and glistening. At the same time, the anus becomes patulous and everted.

The pains now occur very rapidly, with scarcely any interval between. As the head becomes visible, the vulva are stretched more and more and finally encircle the largest diameter of the baby's head. This encirclement of the largest diameter of the baby's head by the vulvar ring is known as "crowning." The doctor now supports the tissues surrounding the perineum and delivers the head between pains. One or two more pains are normally enough to effect the birth of the baby.

Whereas in the first stage of labor the forces are limited to uterine action, during the second stage two

conversely, bearing-down efforts in the absence of uterine contractions are futile. As explained in Chapter 15, "Conduct of Normal Labor," these facts have most important practical implications.

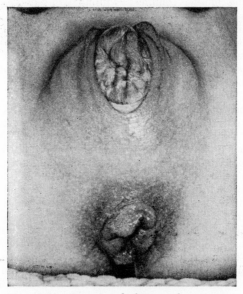

Fig. 156. Extreme bulging of perineum showing patulous and everted anus.

forces are essential, namely, uterine contractions and intra-abdominal pressure, the latter being brought about by the bearing-down efforts of the mother. The force exerted by the mother's bearing down is the same as that used in forcing an evacuation of the bowels. Both forces are essential to the successful spontaneous outcome of the second stage of labor, for uterine contractions without bearing-down efforts are of little avail in expelling the infant, while

In its passage through the birth canal, the body of the fetus undergoes certain positional changes designed to present the smallest possible diameters to the pelvic passageway, so that it will encounter as little resistance as possible. This adaptation of the baby to the birth canal, as descent takes place, involves the four processes called flexion, internal rotation, extension and external rotation (Plate 7).

PLATE 7

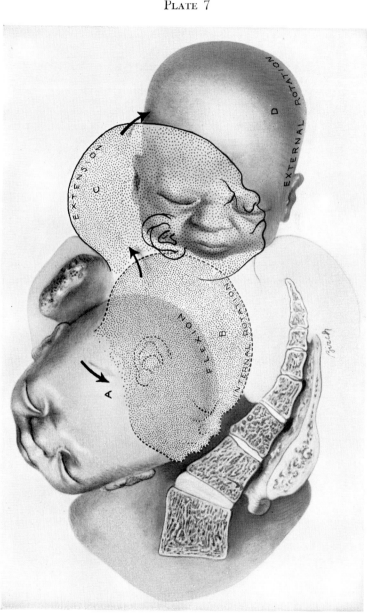

L.O.A. Positional changes of head in passing through birth canal.

PLATE 8

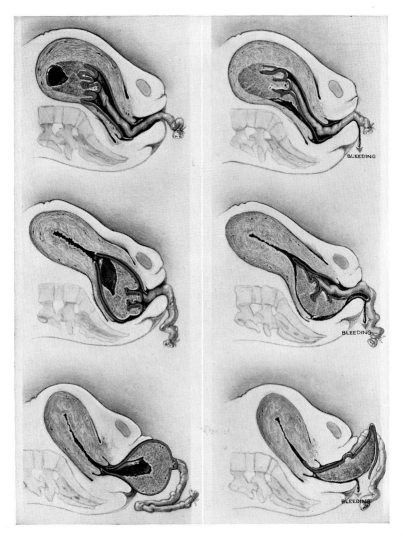

Successive stages of extrusion of placenta: (*left*) by Schultze's mechanism; (*right*) by Duncan's mechanism.

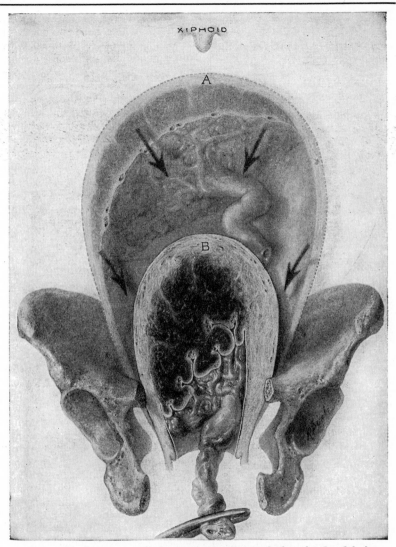

Fig. 157. (A) Area of placental attachment before birth of baby. (B) Greatly reduced area of placental attachment after birth of baby. Note folding or festooning of placenta brought about by the reduced area of attachment. (Coccyx and pubic bones cut away for clarity.)

SUMMARY OF MECHANISM OF LABOR

FIRST STAGE—DILATING STAGE

Definition. Period from first true labor pain to complete dilatation of cervix.

What Is Accomplished? Effacement and dilatation of cervix.

Forces Involved. Uterine contractions.

SECOND STAGE— EXPULSIVE STAGE

Definition. Period from complete dilatation of cervix to birth of baby.

What Is Accomplished? Expulsion of baby from birth canal —facilitated by certain positional changes of fetus: flexion, internal rotation, extension, external rotation.

Forces Involved. Uterine contractions plus intra-abdominal pressure.

THIRD STAGE— PLACENTAL STAGE

Definition. Period from birth of baby to birth of placenta.

What Is Accomplished? (a) Separation of placenta; (b) expulsion of placenta.

Forces Involved. (a) Uterine contraction; (b) intra-abdominal pressure or external pressure exerted by attendant on fundus.

Flexion. Very early in the process of descent the head becomes so flexed that the chin is in contact with the sternum and, as a consequence, the very smallest anteroposterior diameter (the suboccipitobregmatic plane) is presented to the pelvis.

Internal Rotation. As seen in Chapter 2, the head enters the pelvis in the transverse or diagonal position. When it reaches the pelvic floor, the occiput is rotated anteriorly and comes to lie beneath the symphysis pubis. In other words, the sagittal suture is now in the anteroposterior diameter of the outlet (Fig. 10).

Extension. After the occiput emerges from the pelvis, the nape of the neck becomes arrested beneath the pubic arch and acts as a pivotal point for the rest of the head. Extension of the head now ensues, and with it the frontal portion of the head, the face and the chin are born (Fig. 181).

External Rotation. After the birth of the head, it remains in the anteroposterior position only a very short time and shortly will be seen to turn to one or another side of its own accord. This is known as external rotation, and is due to the fact that the shoulders of the baby, having entered the pelvis in the transverse position, undergo internal rotation to the anteroposterior position as did the head; this brings about a corresponding rotation of the head which is now on the outside. The shoulders are born in a manner somewhat similar to that of the head. The anterior shoulder begins to emerge first from the pelvis, but becomes arrested beneath the pubic arch and acts as a pivotal point for the other or posterior shoulder, which is born by a lateral flexion of the body.

The average duration of the second stage of labor in primigravidae is an hour and and a half, and in multiparae about 30 minutes.

THE THIRD STAGE OF LABOR

The third stage of labor is made up of two phases, namely, *the phase of placental separation* and *the phase of placenta expulsion.*

Placental Separation. After the birth of the baby, the uterus contracts down on its diminishing content and consequently the area of placental attachment is greatly reduced. The great disproportion between the reduced size of the placental site and that of the placenta brings about a folding or festooning of the maternal surface of the placenta; with this process separation takes place. Meanwhile, bleeding takes place within these placental folds, and this expedites separation of the organ. The placenta now sinks into the lower uterine segment or upper vagina as an unattached body.

Placental Expulsion. Occasionally, actual expulsion of the placenta may be brought about by bearing-down efforts on the part of the mother, but in modern obstetrics it is usually effected through gentle pressure on the uterine fundus by the physician. The extrusion of the placenta may take place by one of two mechanisms: (1) It may become turned inside out within the vagina and be born like an inverted umbrella with the glistening fetal surfaces presenting. This is known as Schultze's mechanism, and occurs in about 80 per cent of cases. (2) On the other hand, it may become somewhat rolled up in the vagina with the maternal surface outermost, and be born edgewise. The latter is known as Duncan's mechanism, and is seen in about 20 per cent of deliveries. It is believed that the Schultze's mechanism signifies that the placenta has become detached first at its center, and usually a collection of blood and clots is found in the sac of membranes. The Duncan mechanism, on the other hand, suggests that the placenta has separated first at its edges, and it is in this type that bleeding usually occurs at the time of separation.

The contraction of the uterus following delivery serves not only to produce placental separation but to control uterine hemorrhage. As the result of this contraction of the uterine muscle fibers, the countless blood vessels within their interstices are clamped shut. Even then, a certain amount of blood loss in the third stage is unavoidable, the average being about 300 cc. It is one of the aims of the conduct of labor to reduce this bleeding to a very minimum.

SUGGESTED READING

Caldwell, W. E., Moloy, H. C., and D'Esopo, D. A.: A roentgenologic study of the mechanism of the engagement of the fetal head, Am. J. Obst. & Gynec. **28**:824, 1934.

——: The role of the lower uterine soft parts in labor, Am. J. Obst. & Gynec. **37**:618, 1939.

Danforth, D. N., and Ivy, A. C.: A consideration of the cause of the onset of labor: Collective Review, Internat. Abstr. Surg. **69**:351, 1939; in Surg., Gynec. & Obst. (Oct.) 1939.

Hamilton, B. G.: The preliminary stage of labor, Am. J. Obst. & Gynec. **35**:477, 1938.

Javert, Carl T., and Hardy, James D.: Measurement of pain intensity in labor and its physiologic, neurologic, and pharmacologic implications, Am. J. Obst. & Gynec. **60**: 552, 1950.

King, A. G.: Newer concepts of dry labor, J.A.M.A. **114**:238, 1940.

14

Anesthesia and Analgesia in Labor

TYPES OF PAIN RELIEF

Pain relief in labor may be of two main types: (1) *obstetric anesthesia* and (2) *obstetric analgesia.*

By obstetric anesthesia is meant the administration of certain drugs at the time of delivery for the purpose of rendering the birth of the baby painless; it is employed chiefly in operative deliveries and is the same as surgical anesthesia.

By obstetric analgesia is meant the administration of certain drugs during the first and the second stages for the purpose of lessening the suffering caused by the labor pains prior to the actual birth of the baby.

Certain drugs may be used both as anesthetic and as analgesic agents, but in that event the dosage and the method of administration are quite different in the two types of pain relief.

METHODS OF ANESTHESIA

The most commonly employed methods of obstetric anesthesia are: *inhalation* of ether, nitrous oxide, chloroform, cyclopropane, or ethylene; *spinal* anesthesia, produced by introducing a solution of procaine (Novocain) or similar drug into the lower spinal canal, thereby abolishing sensation below the level of the umbilicus; *caudal* anesthesia, produced by introducing a solution of procaine into the caudal space (in the sacrum), thereby producing an effect similar to that of spinal anesthesia; *intravenous* anesthesia, in which an anesthetic, such as Pentothal Sodium, is introduced directly into the bloodstream by needle; and *local infiltration* anesthesia, in which the tissues concerned are injected with a solution of procaine, thereby deadening sensation in that particu-

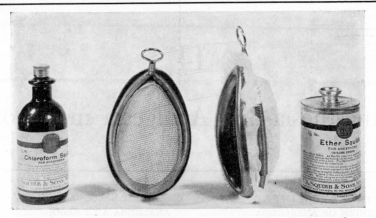

Fig. 158. Outfit for the administration of chloroform or ether. Flow from bottle or can may be regulated by patented screw tops. The mask is covered with four thicknesses of gauze.

lar area. Inhalation and intravenous anesthesia, of course, produce unconsciousness; in spinal, caudal and local infiltration the patient is awake, but sensation has been abolished in the areas concerned.

METHODS OF ANALGESIA

The most commonly employed methods of obstetric analgesia are: momentary inhalation of chloroform, nitrous oxide or ether with each pain ("analgesia à la reine"); administration of morphine or Demerol; administration of certain amnesic drugs, notably, barbiturate compounds, paraldehyde and scopolamine; and continuous caudal analgesia.

Unless the nurse has had special training in a school of anesthesia, she should not be expected to assume the responsibility of administering complete obstetric anesthesia. In an emergency, however, the nurse may proceed with the anesthesia (almost

always ether) under the physician's direction. On the other hand, it is very often the nurse's responsibility to administer and supervise obstetric analgesia; and with these methods, their technics and dangers, she must be intimately familiar.

OBSTETRIC ANESTHESIA

Ether Anesthesia

The patient lies flat on her back with no pillow under her head. False teeth, chewing gum, or any other foreign object must be removed from the mouth because these may be swallowed or aspirated when the patient loses consciousness. Her face should be anointed with petrolatum to prevent irritation of the skin by the ether; and a towel is placed over the eyes for the same purpose. The reason for this should be explained to the patient. Towels and an emesis basin must be within easy reach, as

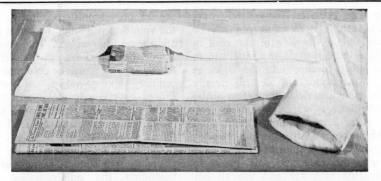

Fig. 159. Improvised cone (showing steps in making) for giving anesthesia.

vomiting is likely to occur during inhalation of the drug. The use of ether near an open fireplace or flame is dangerous because of the explosion hazard.

The usual type of mask employed is shown in Figure 158. In the emergency cases that may fall to the nurse, an improvised "cone" made of folded newspapers covered with a towel or muslin may be employed. It can be put together with safety pins or needle and thread, and the towel or muslin should cover it inside as well as out. It should be of such a size that it will fit snugly over the patient's mouth and nose, and its depth should be from 6 to 7 inches. A piece of absorbent cotton or crumpled gauze about the size of a lemon should be placed inside the cone, care being taken that it is wedged securely in the inhaler with a sufficient space between it and the patient's face to allow free evaporization of the ether. A bent safety pin is put through the cap of the ether can to make a dropper, or a small V-shaped incision is made lengthwise in the cork which comes with the

ether can; a wick of gauze an inch or so long is inserted into the crevice made, and when the cork and the gauze wick are inserted in the can, the ether will drop off the gauze wick.

During the entire period of anesthesia, the neck must be extended and the lower jaw held up by pressure against the mandible to prevent interference with respiration. The ether mask or cone is placed over the patient's nose and mouth, at a short distance away from her face to avoid the choking sensation caused by the drug.

As soon as the patient's throat and lungs have become accustomed to the irritating action of the vapor of the anesthetic, the cone is to be brought gradually toward her face, until it fits snugly.

The gauze or cotton inside the cone should be kept saturated with the drug, and for this purpose about a dram of ether must be poured into it every 2 or 3 minutes. In doing this the bottle or can is uncorked, the cone is removed for an instant only, as the fresh ether is added, and it is then replaced immediately over the face. A large safety pin may be wedged at the side of the cork in the ether can to allow a small stream of ether to flow into the cone. A few inspirations of air will usually be enough to delay the action of the anesthetic.

After 5 or 10 minutes, and often when the patient seems to be passing quietly into a state of unconsciousness, she may suddenly begin to struggle violently and use all her strength to tear the cone from her face and get off the table or out of bed. This is due to the primary exhilarating effect of the drug and is a condition to be watched for in every case. The patient is then partly anesthetized, as will be evident from her incoherent speech and unnatural behavior; and she must be securely held by assistants and fresh ether given freely until she becomes quiet again.

The essential point in controlling the struggling of a partially anesthetized patient consists in keeping her legs and arms extended at full length, so that she cannot get a "purchase" on anything. Her arms must be held straight out at her sides, so that she cannot bend her elbows; and sufficient downward pressure must be exerted just above her knees to prevent her from drawing up her legs.

At about this time the patient will often begin to vomit; and at the first sign of retching her head should be turned to one side to allow the vomitus to escape from her mouth and prevent its possible entrance into the larynx. As this is done, the lower jaw should be drawn upward and forward; and fresh ether should be administered freely, for the vomiting will stop as soon as the anesthesia is complete. The mouth should be wiped frequently with a towel, or with gauze or cotton in an ordinary sponge-holder; and care should be taken to make sure that the tongue is still well forward and has not fallen back and occluded the throat.

Complete anesthesia will be attained in from 10 to 20 minutes after beginning the administration of ether, and it is maintained by adding about a dram of ether to the cone every 4 or 5 minutes.

During ether narcosis, the patient's face should be slightly flushed, but never pale or cyanotic; her respiration should be deep, possibly stertorous, but never irregular; and her pulse should be full, of good quality, fairly rapid, but never intermittent.

The nurse should not only watch the respiratory movements of the chest and the abdomen, but she should make sure that respiration is properly carried on by noting that ether vapor actually escapes through the cone with each expiratory act.

As the patient's wrist is not usually within the reach of the anesthetist, the pulse may be taken at other points: at the facial artery as it passes under the edge of the mandible at about the middle of the lower jaw; at the temporal artery, just in front of the ear; or at the posterior temporal artery, directly above the ear at the margin of the hairy scalp. When there is any doubt as to the character of the pulse taken at these points, it should always be counted at the wrist as well.

In the majority of cases in which

the administration of ether will fall to the nurse, the physician will first anesthetize the patient himself, and whenever the nurse is in the slightest doubt as to the subsequent condition of the patient under operation, she should call upon the physician for assistance or advice without delay. A nurse should grasp every opportunity to perfect herself in the knowledge of anesthesia; if she has a rural practice such knowledge is a rich possession.

OBSTETRIC ANALGESIA

Analgesia à la Reine

In 1853, when Queen Victoria's seventh child was born, she was given momentary inhalations of chloroform with each labor pain. It proved to be a highly efficacious means of pain relief, and since that time the method has been known as "Queen's anesthesia" or *anesthesia à la reine*. Actually, the procedure does not produce complete anesthesia but simply diminishes the intensity of the pain and may best be regarded as a form of analgesia. Although chloroform, the original drug employed, is still widely used for this purpose, similar results may be achieved with nitrous oxide or ether.

Analgesia with Chloroform. Chloroform à la reine may be begun toward the end of the first stage and may be continued throughout the second stage. Before beginning its administration, the patient's face should be anointed with petrolatum, as previously described, and the eyes shielded with a towel. As soon as the patient feels that a pain is coming on, or better, when the nurse feels the

uterus begin to harden, the nurse pours from 10 to 15 drops of chloroform on the mask and, holding this 2 or 3 inches above the patient's nose, instructs her to breathe normally. If the pain lasts longer than a minute, a few more drops may be added. At the end of the contraction, the mask is removed, and the same procedure is repeated with each pain. When the baby's head is about to pass through the vulva, the mask can be lowered somewhat and the chloroform given more continuously; however, even then, the mask always should be held a finger's breadth away from the face and the drug should not be administered for longer than 2 or 3 minutes. Under no circumstances should towels be placed around the mask when giving chloroform since an ample admixture of air is essential to safety. Nor should the mask be held very close to the patient's face if she is breathing deeply.

In many respects, chloroform is ideal for this form of analgesia. It is pleasant to take, rapid in action and in recovery, and rarely gives rise to nausea. For the mother, on the other hand, it may be dangerous unless handled with care. It must never be "pushed"—that is, anesthetic action must never be hastened by pouring the chloroform on rapidly or by lowering the mask to the face. Nor should it be continued to the point of complete anesthesia since the prolonged administration of chloroform anesthesia (for the repair of laceration, for instance) may give rise to liver damage. For the latter reason, chloroform is used less frequently than formerly. Even in giving chloroform à la reine the following danger signals should be watched for: pallor;

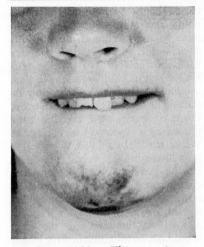

Fig. 160. This patient chipped off her right front tooth and bruised her chin when under analgesia with amnesic drugs, as the result of throwing herself against a radiator near the bed. Such patients must never be left for a second.

shallow, jerky respirations; weak pulse; cyanosis, and deep, stertorous respiration (the last a sign that complete anesthesia has been produced). If any of these develop, the mask should be removed at once and the doctor notified.

Analgesia with Nitrous Oxide. This is almost always administered by the doctor or by a specially trained nurse anesthetist. It is very rapid in action and recovery, efficacious, and, when given momentarily with each pain, is safe for both mother and infant. It is expensive, however, and requires a somewhat complicated apparatus.

Some obstetricians today use one or another of the small portable gas machines for the self-administration of analgesia. The mask through which the patient receives the gas is equipped with a long spring release. As long as the patient squeezes this with her hand, she receives the gas mixture, but when her hold weakens (as the result of anesthetic action), she receives nothing but air. The nurse may be asked to supervise one of these machines, but always it must be done under the physician's direction.

Analgesia with Ether. Ether may be used in a manner similar to chloroform for the production of analgesia à la reine. The method of administration differs somewhat in that more ether is necessary, and the mask must be held against the face. Ether is a safer anesthetic than chloroform, but it is slower in action and recovery is less rapid.

Morphine

Of all analgesic agents used in labor, morphine is probably the most widely employed. Administered hypodermically in doses of ¼ gr. (16 mg.) or ⅙ gr. (10 mg.), it promptly relieves the severity of the pains, and the effect lasts, as a rule, for about 4 hours. Moreover, its hypnotic action often produces sleep between pains. Nevertheless, its disadvantages are several. First, it sometimes stops labor altogether for several hours. Second, if given within 4 hours prior to delivery, the baby at birth may be slow to breathe. However, given in the mid-part of a long labor, it is a most valuable drug, since it affords a means of giving the patient a much-needed rest.

DEMEROL

Demerol is a synthetic compound which resembles morphine in its analgesic properties and atropine in its antispasmodic effects. Hence, in labor it not only relieves pain but is believed to exert also a relaxing effect on the cervix and so expedite dilatation. It is usually administered intramuscularly in dosages of 100 mg., with repetition of the dosage in an hour or two, perhaps. A moderate sedative effect is produced, the patient usually sleeping between pains but awakening when spoken to. Demerol, used alone, does not cause excitement or disorientation, but rather a mental state of well-being. The effect of Demerol on the respiratory center is decidedly less depressing than morphine and, in the opinion of many authorities, no harmful effect on the respiration of the infant at birth is observed.

Demerol alone produces analgesia but not amnesia. If amnesia also is desired, scopolamine or barbiturates are used in conjunction with it. Like morphine, Demerol is included under the Harrison Act, and its distribution and sale are governed by the regulations of the Federal Bureau of Narcotics.

AMNESIC DRUGS

An amnesic drug, it will be recalled, is one which obliterates memory of whatever events occur when under its influence. The aim in giving such a drug is not so much actual pain relief as it is forgetfulness, or amnesia (Greek for "without memory"). Thus, a woman under its influence may shriek, make grimaces, and show other evidence of pain, but upon awakening from the drug will remember nothing about her labor and will vow that she experienced no discomfort whatsoever. In hospital practice, this is perhaps the most successful and most widely used form of analgesia.

The most important thing for the nurse to know about these amnesic drugs is that the patient becomes very groggy and irrational under their influence and may injure herself if left alone. The restlessness which this medication sometimes produces, particularly during pains, adds to the likelihood of self-injury. Figure 160 illustrates the results of an accident which occurred when the patient was under this type of analgesia. Not only may the woman throw herself out of bed or against a wall, but she may vomit, and, unless the patient's head is turned quickly to the side, she may aspirate the vomitus. Again, let it be emphasized, patients under the influence of amnesic drugs must never be left alone, even for a second.

Another important fact about this form of analgesia is that the baby's respiration at birth may be somewhat sluggish. Therefore, facilities for resuscitation must be made ready. Nevertheless, statistics indicate that the results for these babies are as good as for babies whose mothers received no analgesia.

"Twilight Sleep." The first medication used to produce amnesia in labor was a combination of morphine and scopolamine. Introduced in Germany during the early years of this century, this method met with wide acclaim in the United States about 1915 under the name of "twilight sleep." A moderate initial dose of morphine (⅙ to ¼ gr.; i.e., 10 to 16 mgm.), followed by small doses of scopolamine (1/200 to 1/150 gr.; i.e., 0.3 to 0.4 mgm.), is still used with satisfaction in many hospitals.

Barbiturates. Since about 1934, derivatives of barbituric acid, usually in combination with scopolamine, have become increasingly popular for obstetric analgesia. Some of the more commonly employed are Nembutal (Pentobarbital Sodium), Amytal Sodium and Seconal Sodium. These three drugs are very similar in their action, but Amytal Sodium is likely to be the choice of the doctor when labor gives prospects of being prolonged, because its effect is more enduring than the other two. As an example of the technic commonly employed in barbiturate analgesia, the following program is the one carried out at the Johns Hopkins Hospital when this form of pain relief is desired.

> When labor is definitely established.
> Amytal Sodium 0.4 Gm. *or* Nembutal 0.3 Gm. *or*
> Seconal Sodium 0.3 Gm. with
> Scopolamine .0004 Gm. (1/150 gr.)
> In one hour.
> Scopolamine .0003 Gm. (1/200 gr.)
> In one hour.
> Scopolamine .0002 Gm. (1/300 gr.)
> Repeat scopolamine .0002 Gm. (1/300 gr.) whenever patient begins to talk coherently.

The room should be darkened, and quiet maintained. The patient should not be restrained except to prevent self-injury.

Paraldehyde. This pungent-smelling liquid enjoys favor with many obstetricians as an analgesic and amnesic agent. It may be administered in several ways: by rectum, by mouth in the form of capsules and by mouth as an elixir. One leading obstetrician mixes it with port wine and water to disguise the taste. The effect is similar to that produced by the barbiturate-scopolamine program described above. When paraldehyde is given by rectum, the initial dose is about 20 cc. usually mixed with 45 cc. of olive oil; this is repeated from time to time as necessary and is often supplemented by other drugs.

CAUDAL ANALGESIA

Continuous Caudal Anesthesia. At the lower end of the sacrum and on its posterior surface, there is an opening resulting from the nonclosure of the laminae of the last sacral vertebra. It is screened by a thin layer of fibrous tissue. This opening is called the sacral hiatus and leads to a space within the sacrum known as the caudal canal, or caudal space. This space is really the lowermost extent of the bony spinal canal. Through it a rich network of sacral nerves passes downward after they have emerged from the dural sac a few inches above. The dural sac separates the caudal canal below from the spinal cord and its surrounding spinal fluid.

By filling the caudal canal with a suitable anesthetic solution, pain sense in the sacral nerves is abolished, and anesthesia of the pelvic region is produced. This is called caudal anesthesia. In continuous caudal analgesia a pliable needle with rubber tube attached is inserted through the sacral hiatus and into the caudal space and left there throughout labor. The space is then kept continuously filled with anesthetic solution. If the procedure is successful, the patient experiences no pain in labor whatsoever and is conscious neither of uterine contractions nor of perineal distention.

Continuous caudal analgesia was introduced in the autumn of 1942 by Dr. Robert A. Hingson and Dr. Waldo B. Edwards, of Staten Island, N. Y. It was received with wide acclaim, and at the present writing is being employed in many hospitals.

Spinal Anesthesia. Spinal anesthesia, as used in obstetrics, falls into two major divisions. The first is a semiterminal type of anesthesia which is employed for the latter part of labor and delivery and is provided by low dosage of a hyperbaric or isobaric solution. The second is a terminal type and is administered either by the single dosage method or the continuous technic; its largest field of employment in cesarean section. Although minute doses of spinal anesthesia can be given to provide pain relief throughout labor, this technic is difficult and, by and large, unsatisfactory. Too often labor is stopped by spinal anesthesia.

Low-Dosage Hyperbaric Spinal (Saddle Block). This form of anesthesia is one of the most popular in the United States today. Nearly all the local anesthesia agents have been used in saddle-block anesthesia. By the addition of glucose to the solution of Nupercaine or other anesthetic agent, localization and concentration of the drug in the conus of the dural sac are facilitated. Inasmuch as this anesthetic is of short duration, it is necessary to time its administration properly, and delivery should be anticipated within an hour or so following the onset of anesthesia.

Bilateral Paravertebral Lumbar Sympathetic Block. This is a new method of obstetric analgesia; it is a continuous conduction anesthesia obtained by injecting the drug bilaterally into the sympathetic lumbar chain (instead of directly into the spine) in the region of the first lumbar vertebral body located along its lateral anterior surface. It is being employed in several hospitals with good results.

SUGGESTED READING

Cartwright, Earle W.: Choice of anesthesia for normal delivery, J.A.M.A. 145:1111, 1951.

Greenhill, J. P.: Anesthesia in obstetrics, Am. J. Obst. & Gynec. 54:74, 1947.

Lull, C. B., and Hingson, R. A.: Control of Pain in Childbirth, ed. 2, Philadelphia, Lippincott, 1948.

Lund, Curtis J.: Choices of analgesics during the first stage of labor, J.A.M.A. 145:1114, 1951.

Read, G. D.: Childbirth Without Fear, New York, Harper, 1944.

Reich, Arthur M.: Paravertebral lumbar sympathetic block in labor, Am. J. Obst. & Gynec. 61:1263, 1951.

Whitacre, R. J., and Cressman, P. G.: Choices of anesthesia for operative vaginal and abdominal delivery, J.A.M.A. 145:1118, 1951.

15

Conduct of Normal Labor

HOSPITAL DELIVERY
    ADMISSION PROCEDURES
    IS THE PATIENT IN LABOR?
    ATTITUDE TOWARD THE PATIENT
    EXAMINATIONS IN LABOR
    CONDUCT OF THE FIRST STAGE
    NURSE'S DUTIES
    CONDUCT OF THE SECOND STAGE
    NURSE'S DUTIES

CONDUCT OF THE THIRD STAGE
    NURSE'S DUTIES
    IMMEDIATE CARE OF BABY
DELIVERY IN THE HOME
    PROCEDURES CONDUCTED BY THE
      PHYSICIAN
    PREPARATION OF SOLUTIONS AND
      INSTRUMENTS
EMERGENCY DELIVERY BY THE NURSE
NATURAL CHILDBIRTH PROGRAM

HOSPITAL DELIVERY

ADMISSION PROCEDURES

The preparation for a hospital delivery will of necessity vary, since every hospital has its own admission procedure. Usually, the patient has visited her doctor or attended the hospital prenatal clinic at stated intervals during her pregnancy, and has been instructed by the doctor or the nurse concerning her admission when labor begins. It is well for the nurse to find out during the prenatal period if these instructions are clearly understood by the patient. If this is the patient's first hospital experience, it will be much easier for her if she has been told about the necessary preliminary procedures, such as the bath, the vaginal preparations, the examination by the doctor, and why these details are necessary. She should also be advised to come to the hospital at the onset of labor, for after labor progresses these activities are more difficult to carry out and are much more distressing to the patient.

In most hospitals, after greeting the patient the nurse ascertains her condition, that is, the frequency of her pains, their duration, their intensity, the amount of show, and

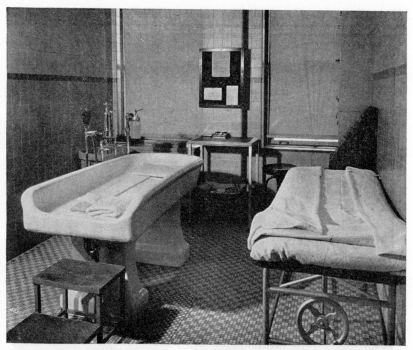

FIG. 161. Admission bath. (Margaret Hague Maternity Hospital, Jersey City, N. J.)

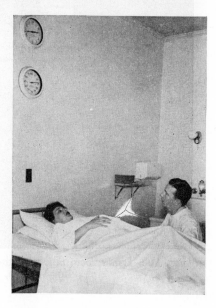

FIG. 162. Labor room where the husband may stay with his wife during labor. With the wall clock the husband can observe the duration and the interval of the contractions. Also he can help to allay fears and give her comfort during this period. The patient not only derives confidence from having her husband share this experience with her, but with the present shortage of nurses this may be a real aid. (Chicago Lying-In Hospital)

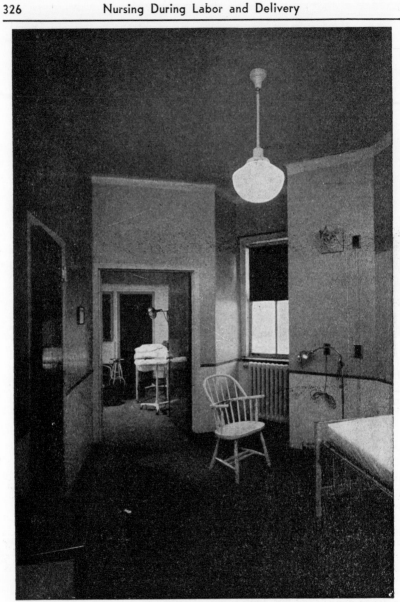

Fig. 163. Labor room adjoining the delivery room. (Sloane Hospital for Women, New York)

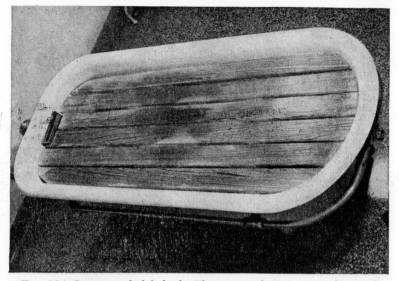

Fɪɢ. 164. Improvised slab bath. The patient lies on a sturdy wooden removable platform which rests on metal supports which have been installed by a plumber in the side walls of an ordinary bathtub. The planks have been smoothly sandpapered and are one half inch apart. A rubber pillow is used, and a rubber mattress may be placed under the patient if desired. A spray bath is given, the water running out the usual waste pipe. Such a bath has been used successfully at the Johns Hopkins Hospital for over ten years.

whether the membranes have ruptured or are intact. The nurse then reports these findings to the doctor. While waiting for the physician, the nurse will take the temperature, pulse and respiration and in some hospitals the blood-pressure reading and the fetal heart count, and will then prepare the patient for an examination which may include one by rectum. If the patient is in labor and is to be admitted, the doctor probably will order such procedures as the collection of a urine specimen, a soap-and-water enema, shaving and cleansing of the vulva, and a bath.

Patients in labor are never allowed to use the toilet because it is important that the physician should have available for examination not only the urine specimen, but whatever material may be passed per vagina.

Vulvar and Perineal Preparation. The aim in shaving and washing the vulva should be to cleanse and disinfect the immediate area about the vagina but to allow nothing to enter. First, the patient is draped and placed on a bed pan or douche pan with her legs flexed. A sponge soaked with an antiseptic solution, or simply a dry sponge, is usually placed just

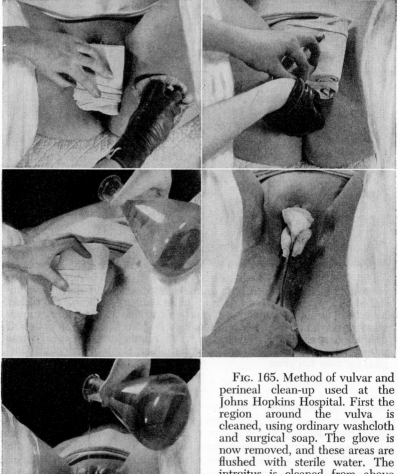

FIG. 165. Method of vulvar and perineal clean-up used at the Johns Hopkins Hospital. First the region around the vulva is cleaned, using ordinary washcloth and surgical soap. The glove is now removed, and these areas are flushed with sterile water. The introitus is cleaned from above downward with surgical soap on a sponge stick. Only one thorough stroke downward is used at a time and then repeated with another sponge. The introitus is then flushed with bichloride of mercury solution.

within the introitus prior to any lathering and shaving of the part. This prevents contaminated fluids from entering the vagina. In some hospitals, the pubic and vulvar hair are lathered prior to shaving, but in others a dry shave is employed. An ordinary safety razor is used, the direction of the stroke being from above downward, care being taken not to get any hair and soap into the introitus.

Since a tub bath might permit infected bath water to gain access to the vagina, a tub bath is never given at this time, just as it is forbidden in the last months of pregnancy. The type of bath used, when it is deemed desirable, will depend to some extent upon the set-up of the hospital. The types usually given are the spray, the shower and the sponge bath. As shown in Figure 164, an ordinary bathtub can easily be converted into a satisfactory slab bath.

While washing the genitals, the nurse again holds a sponge in the introitus to prevent wash water from running into the vagina; as shown in Figure 165, a dry towel pressed against the vulva serves the same purpose. The strokes must be from above downward and away from the opening. Special attention should be paid to separating the vulvar folds and to the removal of such smegma as may have accumulated around the base of the clitoris and in the folds of the labia minora. In washing the region around the anus, it must be remembered that a sponge which has passed over that region must not be returned near the vulvar orifice, but must be discarded immediately. The solutions used in cleansing the genitals will vary in different hos-

pitals, but sterile water with soap, followed by flushing with sterile water, is probably the most commonly employed technic. After the vulva has been cleansed, the labia are separated gently, and the introitus is flushed with an antiseptic solution, usually a bichloride of mercury solution. The patient is instructed not to touch the genitals (lest she infect herself), is dressed in a hospital gown and is taken to the labor room.

The nurse must understand, particularly in reading the present chapter, that many details may be accomplished equally well in a number of ways. Very few hospitals employ precisely the same technic in preparing a patient for delivery, and in some the procedures used may seem quite different from those with which the nurse is familiar. Actually, the differences are in details only, the objectives sought being the same everywhere, namely, asepsis and antisepsis.

In many hospitals the simple cleansing described above is all that is used at the time of admission, being repeated immediately prior to delivery. In other institutions some such technic is followed immediately by the application of an antiseptic solution to the vulva, the pubis and the perineum. This is usually applied by means of a spray. There are a large number of such antiseptic preparations in use, each with a trade name given to it by the manufacturer (Mercurochrome, Metaphen, Zephiran, Mercressin, for instance). They are colored solutions, so that it is easy to make sure that all the areas sprayed are actually covered. In still other hospitals, instillation into the vagina of some antiseptic preparation is added to the above procedures. As an example of this technic, the routine at the Methodist Hospital, Brooklyn, N. Y., is as follows.

ROUTINE OF METHODIST HOSPITAL,
BROOKLYN, N. Y.

Preparation of Patient on Admission.
Shave the pubic hair and cleanse the

or if the instillation is done when the cervix is fully dilated and retracted past the presenting part, it is evident that it is impossible to instill the vagina properly. This is the reason why we insist that the instillation be started as near the beginning of labor as possible. Two small sponges, held one on each labium, will keep the gloved hand from slipping; and as the syringe is withdrawn and the excess fluid starts to escape, it

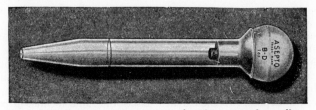

FIG. 166. Mayes asepto syringe for the vaginal instillation of mercurochrome (Becton-Dickinson Company)

perineum and the surrounding field with green soap and water, making sure that all the sebaceous material is removed from around the clitoris and the labial folds.

Spray the external genitalia and the surrounding area with a 2 per cent aqueous solution of Mercurochrome.

The asepto vaginal syringe that we use should have an outside diameter of ⅞ inches and a barrel 7 inches long with a circular mark which indicates a capacity of three drams. The syringe should be filled with Mercurochrome to this point. Then, separating the labia, pass the point of the syringe along the vaginal floor until it reaches the vault of the vagina. After the syringe is inserted properly, the labia should be held together around the syringe with the thumb and the fingers of the gloved hand. This keeps the fluid from leaking when the bulb is pressed, causes the fluid to enter the vagina under slight pressure and ensures its coming in contact with the entire vaginal mucosa. If the labia are not held closely together,

may be collected in the syringe by releasing the bulb. Any fluid not taken up by the syringe is absorbed by the sponges. If the labia are not held closely together around the syringe, the barrel of the syringe tends to keep the Mercurochrome in the vagina, but in spite of this, a large part of the fluid may escape without ballooning the vaginal vault.

A thick pad placed under the patient will absorb the spill from the vagina and protect the bed linen.

Care of the Perineum During Labor.
The perineum should be cleansed thoroughly, using three or more moist, not wet, sterile sponges; and the spraying and the instillation are repeated every 12 hours. It is very important to keep the dried blood and mucus from collecting on the perineum.

Vaginal Examination. The perineum should be cleansed thoroughly with three or more moist sponges, discarding each sponge as soon as it comes in contact with the anal region; dry and then spray the perineum with 2 per cent acetone-alcohol solution of Mercurochrome. Separate the labia with the gloved hand, insert two fingers into the vagina, depress the pelvic floor and put two drams of aqueous or, better still, a 2 per cent solution of Mercurochrome in glycerine into the vagina from a small asepto syringe. (The glycerine in the solution acts as a lubricant and should be used not only for vaginal examinations but also for the delivery.) (If the Mercurochrome is used carelessly a large amount may be wasted. The cost of the Mercurochrome should not be more than 5 or 10 cents per patient.) Separating and withdrawing the fingers will allow the Mercurochrome to reach the upper part of the vagina. It is better that no vaginal examination be done until the patient has been instilled for one hour.

Preparation for Delivery. Cleanse the perineum with three or more sterile moist sponges, removing all dried blood and mucus, then dry with a sterile towel. Green soap may be used but it is incompatible with some antiseptics. Spray the perineum and the surrounding area with a 2 per cent acetone-alcohol solution of Mercurochrome. (Antiseptic solutions may be applied to the perineum and the surrounding area either with a sponge stick saturated with the antiseptic or with a DeVilbiss atomizer No. 120. In the delivery and the operating rooms we use an electric pump, which also has a suction attachment, for spraying the solution, either to the perineum or to the abdomen before an operation. The atomizer is much more economical than the sponge stick, which wastes a considerable amount of the solution.) The spraying should be done systematically, by beginning over the pubes and moving the atomizer back and forth over the field as the bulb is pressed, until the whole area is covered. Never use the acetone-alcohol solution for the instillations.

As soon as the perineum is sprayed the patient is draped, and the vagina is instilled with a 2 per cent solution of Mercurochrome in glycerine. This is done as already described, but the solution should be worked well into the vaginal folds and around the presenting part. The instillation is generally repeated before the delivery is undertaken, and, if the delivery is prolonged or if a forceps is to be applied, more Mercurochrome should be used in the vagina. If the perineum becomes soiled with feces, it should be cleaned with a moist sponge, more Mercurochrome instilled or the perineum sprayed.

Postpartum Care. The perineum is sprayed at least once daily with the aqueous solution of Mercurochrome, and the vagina should be instilled daily with the same solution for 4 or 5 days following delivery. This prevents the development of a foul lochia, will aid in clearing up a previous vaginitis and will hasten the healing of any laceration of the cervix or perineum. These instillations should be done with the small asepto vaginal syringe.

Is the Patient in Labor?

Since the nurse is with the patient more constantly than the doctor, she will be expected to report on the general character of the labor pains, the appearance of show and any other symptoms. First comes the question—Is the patient actually in labor? While this is occasionally a difficult problem to settle, usually a decision can be reached on the grounds of the following differential points between true and false labor:

TRUE LABOR

Pains
  Occur at regular intervals
  Intervals gradually shorten
  Intensity gradually increases
  Located chiefly in back
  Intensified by walking
Show is usually present
Cervix becomes effaced and dilated

FALSE LABOR

Pains
  Occur at irregular intervals
  Intervals remain long
  Intensity remains same
  Located chiefly in abdomen
  Walking has no effect; often relieves
No show
Cervix usually uneffaced and closed

ATTITUDE TOWARD THE PATIENT

For many a young patient in labor, admission to a maternity hospital marks her first acquaintance with hospitals, as well as with the world of nurses and doctors. The immediate reaction may be one of strangeness, loneliness and homesickness. Moreover, not a few of these young patients enter labor thoroughly afraid of the whole process. Accordingly, it is one of the first duties of the nurse to encourage and reassure her patient. Her suffering never should be minimized, but attention should be directed to the fact that progress is being made, that this is the usual procedure, and that her co-operation at this time will be a great help. At the same time, the nurse should be a vigilant watcher for any sign or symptom which may point to abnormal developments. For instance, an increase in pulse rate or a rise in temperature, excessive bleeding, changes in the character of the uterine contractions, rupture of the membranes, passage of meconium or alterations in the fetal heart sounds are changes which the physician must know at once. The nurse, accordingly, is counted upon to be the zealous guardian of both the mental and the physical welfare of the patient in labor.

EXAMINATIONS IN LABOR

General. The pulse, respiration and temperature are taken. This is repeated every 4 hours. In cases in which there is fever or in which labor has lasted more than 24 hours, it is desirable to repeat these observations every 2 hours. The blood pressure is recorded by either the doctor or the nurse and is repeated every 6 hours or so; in cases of toxemia of pregnancy, this is done more frequently. A complete examination of the heart and the lungs is carried out by the physician to make certain that there are no conditions present which might contraindicate the type of analgesia or anesthesia to be used.

Abdominal. The abdominal examination is similar to that carried out in the prenatal period, comprising estimation of fetal size and position and listening to the fetal heart sounds.

The behavior of the fetal heart sounds in labor is of great importance, and this examination is carried out at least every 3 hours during the first stage, while during the second stage it should be done every 5 or 10 minutes. It will be recalled that the rate of the fetal heart ranges between 120 and 160, averaging about 140. After a contraction, it normally becomes much slower than usual and may range between 90 and 100. Provided that the baby is in good condition, it will return rapidly to its previous rate, usually within 15 or 20 seconds. On the other hand, if the baby is in distress, either because of the lack of oxygen or due to an abnormal degree of pressure exerted on its head or cord, the fetal heart rate is constantly slow,

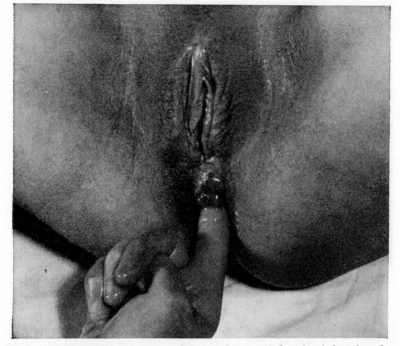

Fig. 167. Rectal examination, showing flexion of thumb of the gloved hand to prevent contamination of the vulva.

often as low as 80 per minute or below. Occasionally, this slow rate is accompanied by irregularity and sometimes by the passage of meconium—signs indicative of fetal distress.

Rectal. In modern obstetrics, the majority of the examinations during labor are abdominal and rectal only —not vaginal. Rectal examinations are much safer than vaginal examinations, since they avoid the risk of carrying pathogenic bacteria from the introitus and the lower vagina to the region of the cervix and the lower uterine segment. In making a rectal examination the index finger

is used, the hand being covered by a clean but not necessarily sterile rubber glove. As shown in Figures 168 and 169, the thumb should be fixed into the palm of the hand, because otherwise it may enter the vagina and cause infection. The finger is then anointed liberally with a lubricating jelly and introduced slowly into the rectum. The cervical opening usually can be felt as a depression surrounded by a circular ridge. The degree of dilatation and the amount of effacement are noted. Very often the membranes can be felt bulging into the cervix, particularly during a pain. The level of the fetal head is

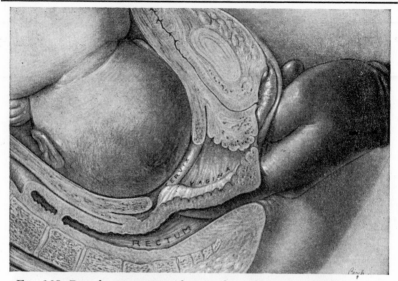

Fig. 168. Rectal examination, showing how the examining finger palpates the cervix and the head through the rectovaginal septum.

now ascertained and correlated with the level of the head as being a certain number of centimeters above or below the ischial spines.

Vaginal. Preparation for vaginal examination should be identical with that used for delivery, that is, full vulvar and perineal preparation. The physician scrubs his hands, as for an operation, and dons sterile gloves. Before introducing his fingers into the vagina, he takes care to separate the vulva widely in order to minimize possible contamination of his examining fingers by the structures of the introitus. Vaginal examination is more reliable than rectal, since the cervix, the fontanels, etc., can be palpated directly with no intervening rectovaginal septum to interfere with tactile sense. However, since vaginal examinations carry with them a

greater possibility of infection, ordinarily they are employed only when rectal examination is unsatisfactory or when the physician suspects that it is not yielding complete information.

CONDUCT OF THE FIRST STAGE

The first stage of labor (dilating stage) begins with the first symptoms of true labor and ends with the complete dilatation of the cervix. The physician examines the patient early in labor and sees her from time to time throughout the first stage but is rarely in constant attendance at this time. In normal labor his examinations (fetal heart, rectal) will show that the baby is in good condition, and that steady progress is being made. The rate of progress, furthermore, will often give some indication as to when delivery is to be expected. Since the physician is usually unable to be with the patient constantly during this stage, he must rely on the nurse not only to safeguard the welfare of mother and fetus but also to notify him whenever delivery seems to be imminent.

Nurse's Duties in the First Stage. In most hospitals the respective duties of the doctor and the nurse are definitely outlined. Generally, the main duties of the nurse in the first stage of labor are as follows.

1. *Encourage the Patient.* As already emphasized, an attitude toward the patient in which are combined cheerfulness, sympathy and encouragement is all-important. Most patients tolerate their pains much better if they can be told that progress is being made or that they are showing great courage.

2. *Observe the Character of the*

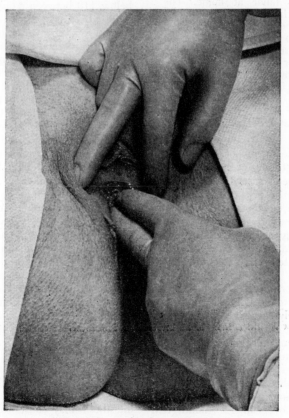

FIG. 169. Vaginal examination.

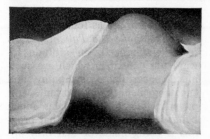

Fig. 170. The patient shown
in this photograph (J. H. H.
217811) was sent into the
hospital after 3 days of ineffectual labor at home. The
cervix had been fully dilated,
it is believed, for 24 hours;
yet no progress was made.
The tremendously distended
bladder is plainly seen in
the photograph. Catheterization yielded 1,000 cc. of
urine. Following this, the
baby's head descended at
once, and delivery was easy.

Pains. The frequency, the duration
and the intensity of the pains should
be watched closely and recorded.
The presence of show in substantial
amounts (blood-stained mucus, *not*
actual bleeding!) suggests that rather
rapid progress may be taking place
and should be reported, particularly
if associated with frequent severe
pains.

3. *Record the Pulse, Temperature
and Respiration.* The pulse in normal
labor rarely exceeds 100 and is usually in the seventies or the eighties.
A persistent pulse rate over 100 suggests exhaustion or dehydration and
should be reported. The temperature
in labor should be normal, and the
doctor should be notified of any
elevation over 99° F. (mouth temperature). These observations are
usually made every 4 hours, more
frequently if there is an elevation. A
chill in the first stage (fortunately
rare) may be a serious omen; it demands report at once. The respiration should be in the lower twenties.

4. *Observe the Fetal Heart Rate.*
In some hospitals, this is done by the
nurse; in others, by the intern or the
physician in charge. As already explained, the rate is normally between
120 and 160 per minute, except immediately after a pain, when it slows.
Any continued slowing of the rate
below 110 between pains should be
reported. Passage of meconium-
stained fluid in a vertex presentation
also suggests fetal distress.

5. *Urge the Patient to Void Frequently.* A full bladder may be a
serious impediment to labor. Accordingly, the patient should be asked to
void every 3 or 4 hours; if she is unable to do so and if the distended
bladder can be palpated above the
symphysis, the doctor should be informed. Not infrequently he will
order catheterization in such cases.
Various technics are used, all designed at maintaining strict asepsis.
One technic showing the use of
sterile tisssue forceps to hold the
catheter is shown in Figure 171.

6. *Watch the Fluid and Food Intake.* The practice here varies greatly
among different doctors and in different institutions. Therefore, the
wishes of the doctor in charge should
be ascertained before proceeding.
In general, it is customary to urge
the patient to take water and liquid
diet unless delivery is likely within
4 hours. If the patient takes fluid or
food shortly before delivery, the
anesthesia may cause vomiting and
consequent difficulties. On the other

hand, in a prolonged labor it is most important to maintain adequate fluid and caloric intake in order to forestall dehydration and exhaustion. In some cases, the physician may find it necessary to supplement oral intake by the intravenous administration of glucose solutions.

7. *DO NOT Urge the Patient to Bear Down.* Since during the first stage of labor the uterine contractions are involuntary and uncontrolled by the patient, it is futile for her to "bear down," because this only leads to exhaustion.

8. *Watch for Signs of the Second Stage.* These signs are as follows. (a) The patient begins to bear down of her own accord; this is caused by a reflex when the head begins to press on the perineal floor. (b) There is a sudden increase in show; sometimes there may be slight actual bleeding. (c) The patient thinks that she needs to evacuate; this symptom is also due to pressure of the head on the perineal floor and consequently against the rectum. (d) The membranes rupture with

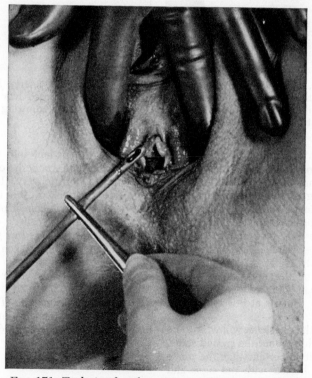

Fig. 171. Technic of catheterization, showing use of 6-inch sterile tissue forceps to insert catheter.

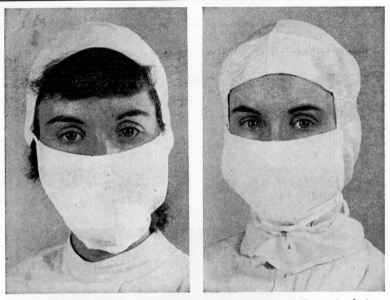

Fig. 172. (*Left*) *Incorrect* method of wearing cap. Bacteria, hairs and other infectious particles can readily fall from exposed hair and contaminate sterile fields. (*Right*) *Correct* method of adjusting cap so that *all* hair is covered.

discharge of amniotic fluid. This, of course, may take place at any time but occurs most frequently at the beginning of the second stage. (e) The perineum begins to bulge and the anal orifice to dilate. This is a late sign, but if a, b, c and d occur, it should be watched for with every pain. Only rectal or vaginal examination (or the appearance of the head) can definitely confirm the suspicion. Emesis at this time is not unusual.

Since the physician will wish to be present throughout the second stage, it is most important that the nurse acquaint herself with the signs and symptoms of this period of labor. It is also important from the viewpoint of getting the patient into the delivery room and properly cleansed and draped for delivery. If these signs are overlooked, the delivery may occur without benefit of attention (colloquially called B.O.A., "born on arrival"). In general, primiparae should be taken to the delivery room when fully dilated and multiparae when 7 or 8 cm. dilated.

9. *Assist with Analgesia* (*Pain Relief*). This is extremely important and has been considered in detail in Chapter 14.

CONDUCT OF THE SECOND STAGE

The second stage of labor (expulsion stage) begins with the com-

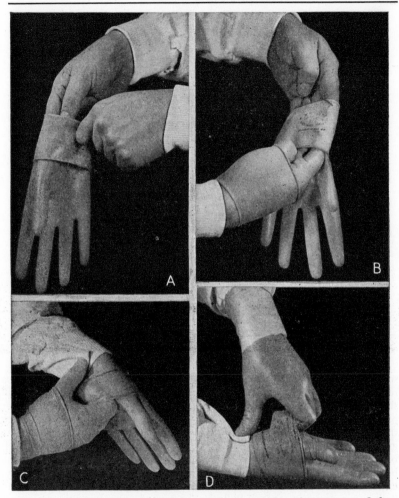

Fig. 173. Method of putting on sterile gloves so that the exterior of the glove never is touched by the ungloved hand.

plete dilatation of the cervix and ends with delivery of the baby. Except in emergencies, the physician is in attendance throughout the second and the third stages and will take complete charge. During this period, he may want the patient to exert her abdominal forces and "bear down"; and frequently the nurse will be asked to "coach" and encourage the patient in this procedure. In some hospitals, straps are placed in the patient's hands—straps firmly attached to the delivery table and

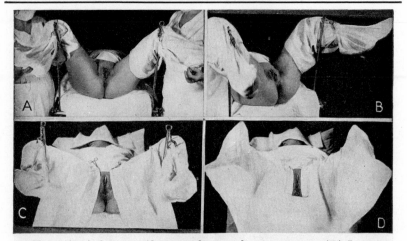

Fig. 174. (A) Raising legs simultaneously into stirrups. (B) Legs in stirrups. These are rods with heel stirrups; many hospitals, however, prefer aluminum knee crutches, as shown in Fig. 195. The patient's buttocks must be brought well down on the delivery table so that they protrude a few inches over the edge. (C) Three sterile towels have been applied. (D) Draping completed by covering sterile towels with sterile delivery sheet. The sheet contains "pillow-case-like" inserts to encase legs and stirrups in addition to aperture for delivery.

so adjusted in length that she can reach them comfortably. Her legs should be half flexed so that she can push with them against the floor of the table. Instructions should be given the patient to take a deep breath as soon as her next pain begins and, with her breath held, to exert downward pressure exactly as if she were straining at stool. Pulling on the straps at this time is a helpful adjunct. The effort should be as long and sustained as possible, since short "grunty" endeavors are of little avail. Usually, these bearing-down efforts are rewarded by increased bulging of the perineum, that is, by further descent of the head. The patient should be informed of

such progress, for encouragement is all-important. The physician will listen to the fetal heart sounds after each pain, or at least every 5 minutes or so.

When the physician deems birth to be imminent, he will ask the nurse to prepare the patient for delivery. In hospital practice, the latter may be carried out in the lithotomy position, but may be effected with the patient in the prone position with the knees drawn up slightly and separated. In either event, the nurse again carries out the cleansing of the vulva and the surrounding area as previously described; then the physician, who meanwhile has scrubbed his hands and donned

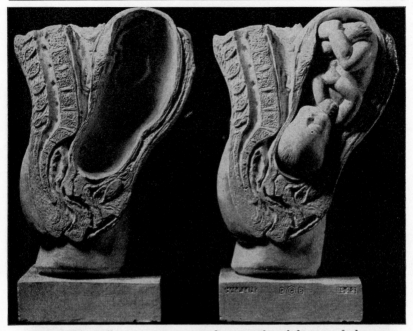

FIG. 175. Full-term pregnancy, showing the abdomen of the patient in the standing position. (Dickinson-Belskie models, Cleveland Health Museum, Cleveland)

sterile gown and gloves, drapes the patient with towels and sheets appropriate for the purpose (Fig. 174).

Of prime importance in the conduct of the second stage are strict asepsis and antisepsis. To this end, everyone in the delivery room must wear cap and mask; those actually concerned in carrying out the delivery are in sterile attire. The physician will employ sponges (as a rule soaked with antiseptic solution) to remove any fecal material which may escape from the rectum. As soon as the head distends the perineum to a diameter of 6 or 8 cm., the physician will often place a towel over the rectum and exert forward pressure on the chin of the baby's head while the other hand exerts downward pressure on the occiput. This is called Ritgen's maneuver, and allows the physician to control the egress of the head; it also favors flexion so that the head is born with the smallest diameter presenting. The head is usually delivered between pains, and as slowly as possible. All these measures (control of head by Ritgen's maneuver, flexion, and slow delivery between pains) help to prevent lacerations. If a tear seems inevitable, an incision which is called an episiotomy may be made in the

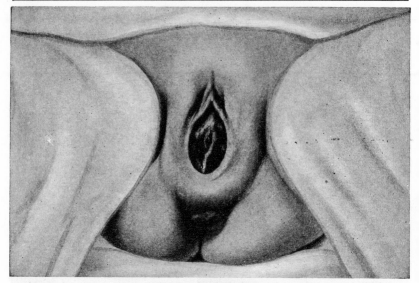

Fig. 176. First appearance of the baby's head at the outlet. (After Bumm; Robert L. Dickinson, M.D.)

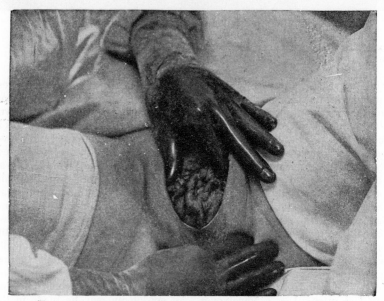

Fig. 177. Preserving the perineum from tearing (Shears).

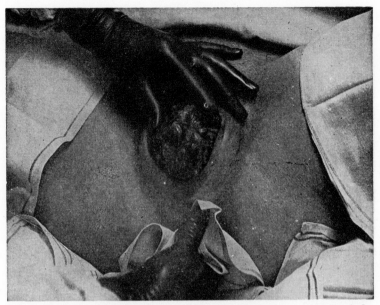

Fig. 178. Preserving the perineum during advanced crowning of the head (Shears).

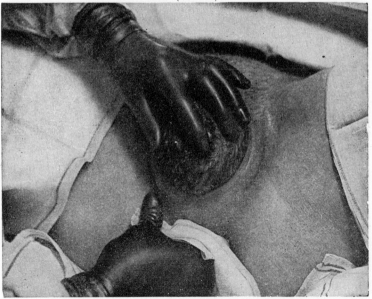

Fig. 179. The same case, farther advanced. It is becoming necessary to use the full hand in retarding the progress of the head as it crowns the perineum (Shears).

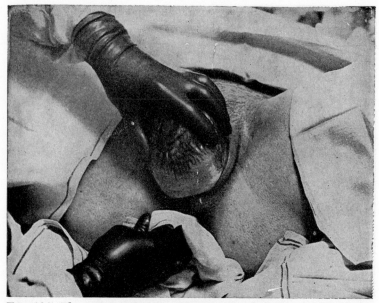

FIG. 180. The same case again. Emergence of the forehead and the face. No perineal tear visible as yet (Shears).

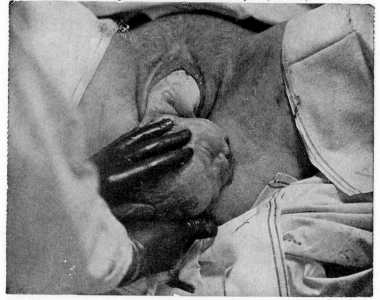

FIG. 181. The same case continued. Delivery of the anterior shoulder. Note the congestion of the baby's face (Shears).

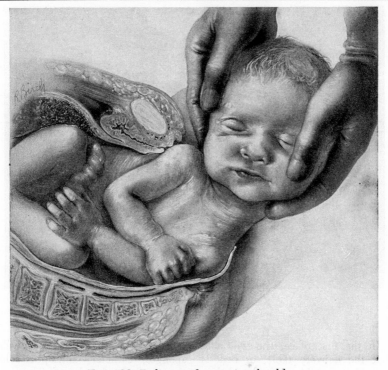

Fig. 182. Delivery of posterior shoulder.

perineum by the physician (see p. 395). As shown in Figures 181 and 182, the posterior shoulder usually is delivered first, and then the remainder of the body follows without particular mechanism. The exact time of the baby's birth should be noted.

Nurse's Duties in the Second Stage. Good obstetric care during the second stage of labor demands the closest teamwork between physician and nurse. By previous understanding, or more often by established hospital routine, both physician and nurse have their own responsibilities in the delivery room,

and, if the best interests of the patient are to be served, the duties of each must be carried out smoothly and efficiently. The main duties of the nurse are as follows.

1. *Preparation of the Delivery Room.* There are no two hospitals in which the set-up of a delivery room is precisely the same, and this is is one phase of the nurse's work which she must learn almost wholly from actual observation and experience in her own institution. Nevertheless, she can obtain an idea of the main equipment used from Figures 195-197.

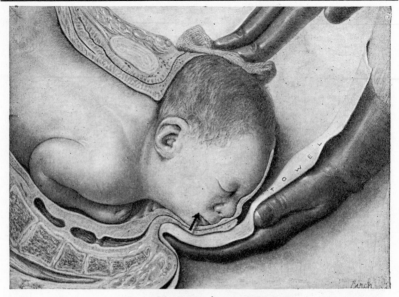

FIG. 183. Ritgen's maneuver.

In the first place, she will note that the delivery table, or bed, is actually two tables joined together. This permits the patient to lie in the prone position until it is desired to put her legs up into stirrups, that is, put her in the lithotomy position; the smaller section of the delivery table is then detached and rolled away, giving ready access to the perineal region. Or, if it is desired to deliver the patient in the prone position, the detachable portion of the table can be allowed to remain in place. The delivery table thus differs decidedly from an operating table.

The table opposite the foot of the delivery bed contains the principal sterile supplies and instruments needed for normal delivery, includ-ing, among other articles, towels, sponges, catheter, antiseptic solutions and the "cord set." The cord set is a group of instruments used for clamping and cutting the umbilical cord: namely, 2 hemostats, a pair of scissors, and a cord tie. More instruments are often included because it is so often necessary for the physician to repair lacerations or an episiotomy incision (p. 395). Additional instruments frequently included are: 6 hemostats, 4 Allis clamps, 2 mousetooth tissue forceps, 2 sponge sticks, 2 vaginal retractors, 2 tenaculae, 2 needle holders, assorted needles and a pair of obstetric forceps.

2. *Coaching the Patient to Bear Down.* This should be done only at the physician's request, since in certain cases it is undesirable.

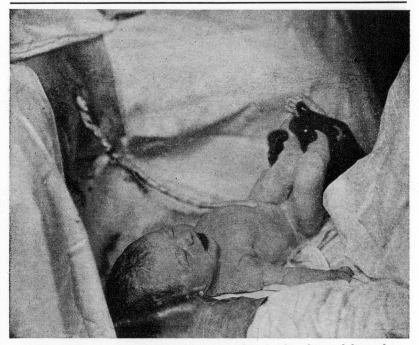

Fig. 184. This shows the baby just after he has been delivered. He is lying very comfortably on the doctor's lap. The baby's head is well supported, and there is no traction on the cord, which is still attached to the placenta. The doctor is now ready for the instruments for clamping and tying the cord. (Maternity Hospital, Western Reserve University Hospitals, Cleveland)

3. *Catheterization.* After the patient has been prepared for delivery, catheterization, if done, is carried out by the physician, but prior to that time it is performed by the nurse at the physician's request. Sometimes it is difficult to catheterize a patient in the second stage of labor, since the baby's head may compress the urethra. If the catheter does not pass easily it is best to inform the doctor; force should never be employed.

4. *Relieving Muscular Cramps.* Cramps in the leg are common in the second stage because of pressure exerted by the baby's head on certain nerves in the pelvis. These are relieved by changing the position of the leg (as illustrated in Fig. 129), forcing the foot upward with pressure on the knee, until the cramp subsides. These cramps cause excruciating pain and must never be ignored.

5. *Preparing the Patient for Delivery.* In putting the legs of the pa-

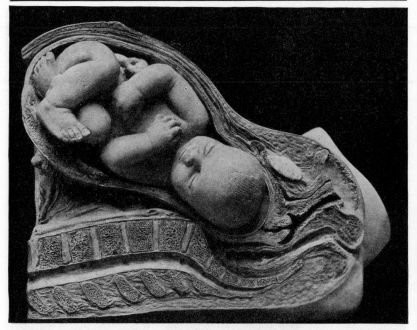

Fig. 185. Before labor. (The following series of pictures are repro-
ductions of the models made by Robert L. Dickinson, M.D., and
Abram Belskie, Sculptor. These pictures were reproduced for teaching purposes in the *Birth Atlas* published by Maternity Center Association, New York. For the student nurse they more clearly depict
the mechanism of labor and delivery.)

tient up into stirrups, care should be
used not to separate the legs too
widely or to have one leg higher
than the other. Both legs should be
raised and lowered at the same time,
with a nurse holding each. Failure to
observe these instructions may result
in straining the ligaments of the pelvis, with consequent discomfort in
the puerperium.

6. *Asepsis.* Masking must include
both nose and mouth. Caps should
be so adjusted as to keep *all* hair
covered. Persons with colds or those

who have had recent respiratory infections should not be permitted in
the delivery room. If the nurse scrubs
to assist the doctor, the strictest
aseptic technic must be observed.
Scrubbing the hands should be
started sufficiently early so that full
time may be allotted, as well as to
immersing the hands and the forearms in antiseptic solutions. Figure
173 shows the correct method of
donning gloves so that the exterior
of the glove never is touched by the
ungloved hand. Even after scrubbing

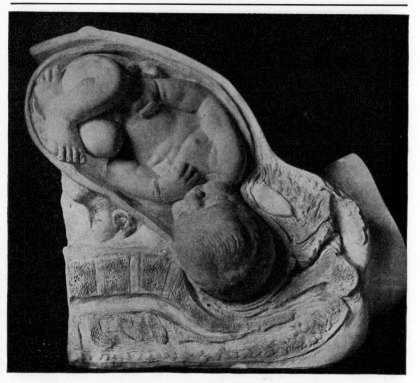

Fig. 186. Cervix dilating. With each rhythmic contraction and as dilatation takes place the baby advances along the birth canal.

and immersing the hands in antiseptic solution they are not considered sterile.

7. *Anesthesia.* Nurses are sometimes called upon to administer anesthesia for delivery. This is discussed on pages 319 and 320.

CONDUCT OF THE THIRD STAGE

The third stage of labor (placental stage) begins after the delivery of the baby and terminates with the birth of the placenta. Immediately after delivery of the infant, the height of the uterine fundus and its consistency are ascertained. The physician may do this by palpating the uterus through a sterile towel placed on the lower abdomen, but it is a duty which is often delegated to the nurse, at least while the physician is engaged in clamping and cutting the umbilical cord. So long as the uterus remains hard and there is no bleeding, the policy is ordinarily one of watchful waiting until

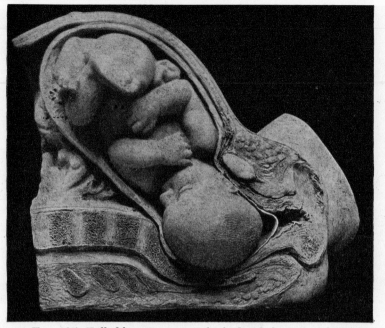

Fig. 187. Full dilatation: cervix high, head deep in pelvis.

the placenta is separated; no massage whatsoever is practiced, the hand simply resting on the fundus to make certain that the organ does not balloon out with blood. Since attempts to deliver the placenta prior to its separation from the uterine wall are not only futile but may be dangerous, it is most important that the signs of placental separation be well understood. The signs which suggest that the placenta has separated are as follows.

1. The uterus rises upward in the abdomen; this is due to the fact that the placenta, having been separated, passes downward into the lower uterine segment and vagina, where its bulk pushes the uterus upward.

2. The umbilical cord protrudes 3 or more inches farther out of the vagina, indicating that the placenta also has descended.

3. The uterus assumes a globular shape and becomes, as a rule, more firm.

4. A sudden gush of blood often occurs.

These signs are sometimes apparent within a minute or so after delivery of the infant, usually within 5 minutes. When the placenta has certainly separated, the physician first ascertains that the uterus is firmly contracted. He may then ask the patient, if not anesthetized, to "bear down," and the intra-abdomi-

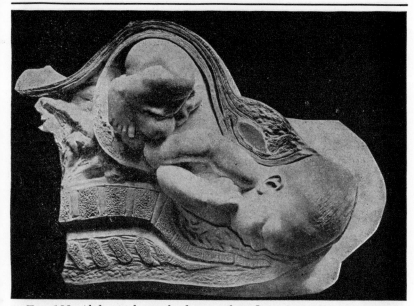

Fig. 188. Abdominal muscle drive, pelvic floor thin. "Caput" or top of baby's head showing.

nal pressure so produced may be adequate to expel the placenta. If this fails or if it is not practicable because of anesthesia, the physician, again having made certain that the uterus is hard, exerts gentle pressure downward with his hand on the fundus and, employing the placenta as a piston, simply moves the placenta out of the vagina. This procedure, known as placental "expression," must be done gently and without squeezing. It never should be attempted unless the uterus is hard, otherwise the organ may be turned inside-out. This is one of the gravest complications of obstetrics and is known as "inversion" of the uterus (p. 391). Pituitary extract and/or ergonovine may be administered to increase uterine contraction and thereby minimize bleeding. These agents never are given before the placenta has been delivered because of the possibility that the uterus may contract, thereby causing retention of the placenta, another serious complication. The physician carries out a careful inspection of the placenta to make sure that it is intact; if a piece is left in the uterus, it may cause subsequent hemorrhage. The uterus is now held, usually by the nurse, for one hour to make sure that it does not relapse and balloon with blood. Constant massage of the uterus during this period is unnecessary and undesirable, but if the

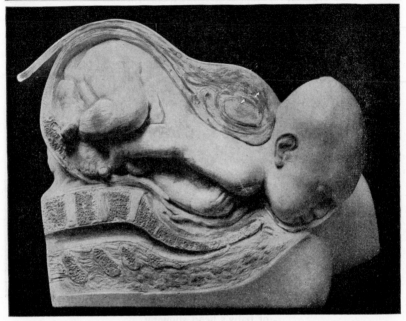

Fig. 189. Head turns upward; pelvic floor retreats.

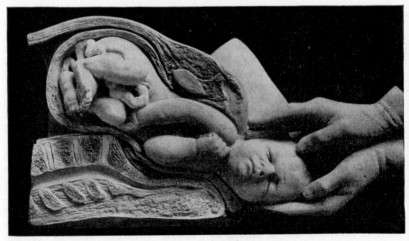

Fig. 190. Birth of shoulders: rotation.

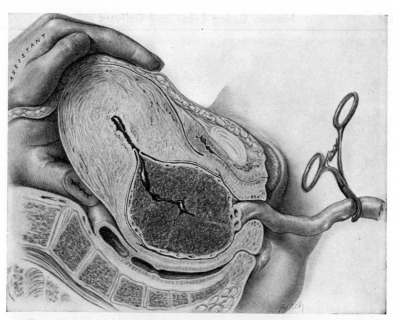

FIG. 191. Expression of placenta by nurse assisting physician. The *uterus must be hard* if this is attempted. Note that the uterus is not squeezed.

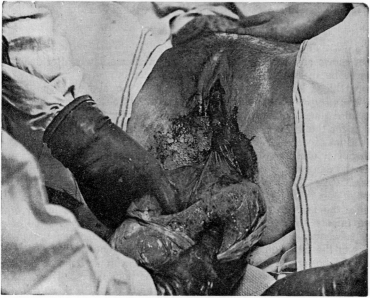

FIG. 192. Delivery of membranes by gentle traction (Shears).

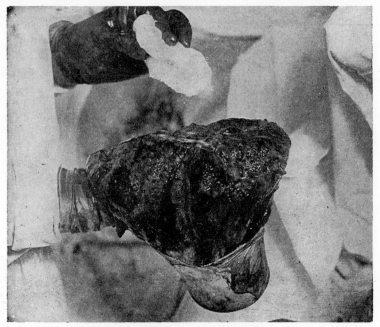

Fig. 193. Inspecting the placenta (Shears).

organ shows any tendency to relax, it must be massaged vigorously to prevent blood loss.

Nurse's Duties in the Third Stage. The third stage of labor is a critical period for the mother and baby, as well as an exceedingly busy one for both doctor and nurse. The mother faces the danger of hemorrhage and shock, while the baby is passing through the most hazardous period of life, the first 15 minutes, when more infants succumb than during any subsequent time. The main duties of the nurse during the third stage of labor are as follows.

1. To palpate and guard the uterus (upon the request of the phy-sician) immediately after delivery of the infant.

2. If the above responsibility is entrusted to the nurse, she should watch for the signs of placental sepa-ration and report such to the physi-cian.

3. To watch the mother's pulse and color for signs of impending shock (rapid, weak pulse; pallor, cold perspiration).

4. To carry out (upon the request of the physician) expression of pla-centa. This is done sometimes by the nurse, sometimes by the doctor.

5. To keep her hand on the uterus for one hour after delivery, massag-ing the fundus if it relaxes.

6. Upon the physician's order, to administer pituitary extract (one ampule) intramuscularly, and ergonovine (0.2 mg.—that is, 1/320 gr.) intramuscularly or orally.

7. To inspect the baby frequently to make sure that it is breathing normally, has a good color and is not bleeding from the cord.

8. Finally, after the third stage has been completed and when so instructed by the physician, to replace the lower end of the table, to lower the patient's legs from the stirrups (being careful not to strain ligaments), to apply sterile perineal pads and to cover the patient with sheet and blanket.

IMMEDIATE CARE OF THE BABY

As soon as the head of the baby is born, the physician passes his finger up above the occiput to feel whether the cord is about the baby's neck; if so, the loop is gently pulled down and slipped over the baby's head to prevent pressure on the cord from the baby's shoulder thereby interfering with his oxygen supply. In rare cases, the cord may have to

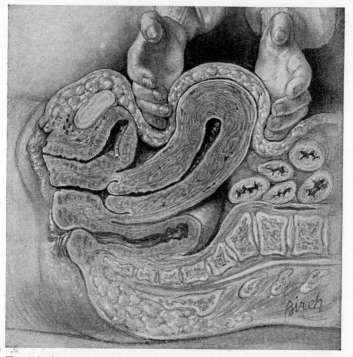

FIG. 194. Proper method of grasping fundus of uterus during first hour after delivery to guard against relaxation and hemorrhage.

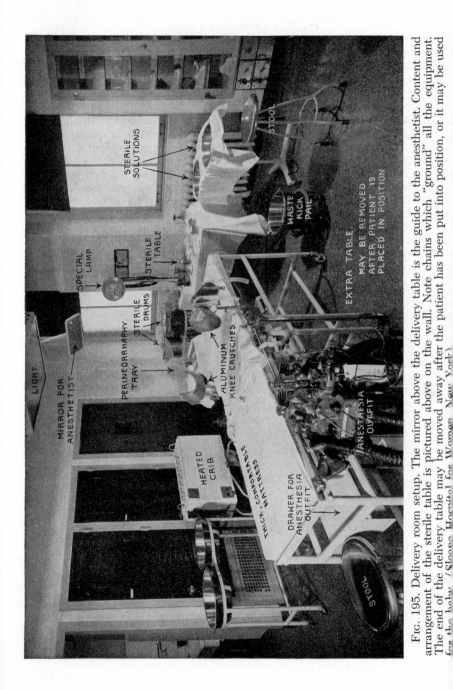

Fig. 195. Delivery room setup. The mirror above the delivery table is the guide to the anesthetist. Content and arrangement of the sterile table is pictured above on the wall. Note chains which "ground" all the equipment. The end of the delivery table may be moved away after the patient has been put into position, or it may be used for the baby. (Sloane Hospital for Women, New York.)

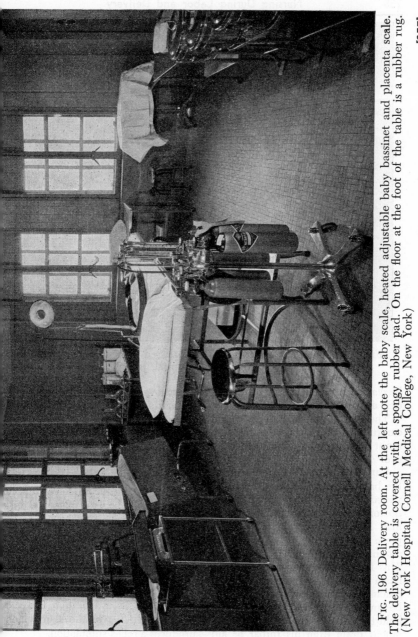

Fig. 196. Delivery room. At the left note the baby scale, heated adjustable baby bassinet and placenta scale. The delivery table is covered with a spongy rubber pad. On the floor at the foot of the table is a rubber rug. (New York Hospital, Cornell Medical College, New York)

[357]

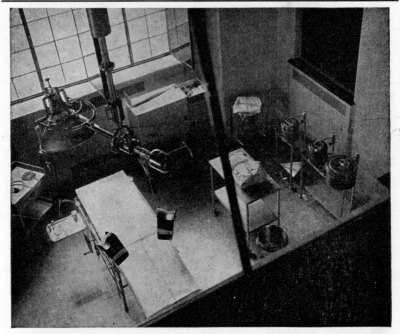

Fig. 197. Delivery room from the glassed-in observation gallery. (Margaret Hague Maternity Hospital, Jersey City, N. J.)

be clamped and cut before the shoulders are delivered.

The baby's eyes should be wiped carefully at this time, a separate moist pledget being used for each eye.

Care Following Birth. As soon as the baby is born, the nose should be wiped and any fluid removed. If the doctor wishes, the back of the mouth may be wiped very gently with a piece of wet gauze or cotton wound around the end of the little finger. This is to be done before the baby has a chance to gasp and inhale the mucus. Sometimes, if there seems to be much mucus, the physician will hold the baby by his feet and let the mucus drain from his throat or aid

its removal by passing his thumb and finger along the course of the trachea toward the mouth.

The baby may not "cry" at once, but he usually gasps or cries after the mucus has been removed, as he now needs oxygen by way of the lungs, since the accustomed supply was cut off when the placental circulation stopped. If crying has to be stimulated, it is usually done by rubbing the baby's back carefully, by tapping gently on the bottom of his feet or by dropping a drop of alcohol on his chest and gently blowing it to hasten its evaporation and the resulting chilling of the skin which produces a reflex stimulation.

Care of the Cord. As soon as the baby has cried vigorously and expanded the lungs, the pulsation in the cord will begin to fail, and the physician will then clamp or tie the cord. The cord is usually tied about one inch from the umbilicus, a sufficient length to allow a second ligature if there is any subsequent bleeding. A second ligature is then put on the maternal end to prevent leakage. There are several types of umbilical clamps, such as the Kane and the Ziegler. With this type there is a more rapid dehydration of the stump tissue, and the cord separates in less time. The possibility of hemorrhage is also minimized. The cord is cut with sterile scissors and wiped carefully to see that there is no bleeding, thus indicating that the ligature is secure. After the cord has been ligated and cut, a sterile pad of gauze (plain or filimated) is applied. This dressing is a 4-inch square with a hole in the center through which the stump protrudes. The corners are folded over the stump, and then the straight binder is applied as a bandage. This dressing must be inspected frequently to note any signs of bleeding (Fig. 282).

In some hospitals no dressing is applied; in others the binder and the dressing are removed at the end of 48 hours. The cord is left dangling, and it apparently dries and separates more quickly than when kept covered. There is less irritation of the abdomen and the back, which some-

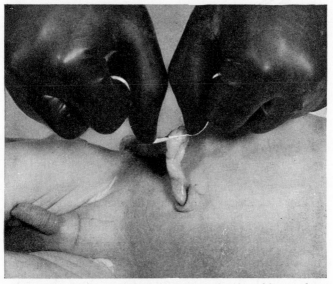

Fig. 198. Tying umbilical cord. Note that knuckles are kept together. This gives a better controlled tie and is a safeguard against jerking and tearing the cord in case one hand should slip.

times results from the moist binder. Some pediatricians think that the abdominal muscles become stronger by not being bound. This method apparently has been very satisfactory.

There always should be at hand a warm blanket to wrap around the baby; for it must be remembered that any room is much cooler than the temperature of the mother's body, and the baby never should be exposed to chilling.

Care of the Eyes. At this time, the baby's eyes should receive prophylactic treatment, which, according to the present laws of 44 states, is the instillation of one drop of silver nitrate (1 per cent solution) or argyrol (15 per cent), in each eye. If silver nitrate solution is used it usually is followed by a gentle flushing with a 2 per cent warm boric-acid solution or sterile water. Physiologic saline is contraindicated because the

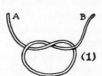 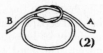

Fig. 199. Square knot: first and second steps in tying.

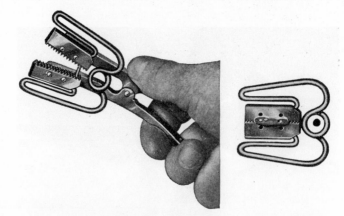

Fig. 200. Ziegler cord clamp. As soon as the cord has ceased pulsating, it is clamped with two artery forceps from 4 to 6 inches from the umbilicus and cut between them. When the baby is ready for the cord dressing, the clamp is held open with the retractor by one hand while the cord stump is pulled through the opening with an artery forceps in the other hand. The clamp is applied to the stump close to the skin of the abdomen (being careful not to include any of the skin). The excess stump is then trimmed to within about one-quarter inch of the clamp. (Clinical Supplies, Inc., Pittsburgh, Pa.)

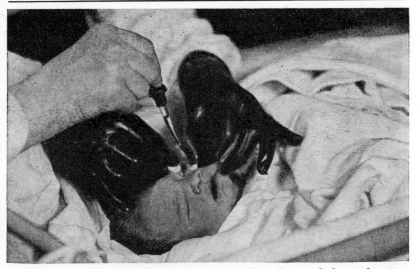

FIG. 201. This shows the method of instilling the prophylactic drops in the baby's eyes soon after birth (now required by law in 44 states of the United States). The eyes are first cleansed with sterile wet gauze or cotton, and the lids very gently separated to prevent pressure on the eyeball or the face. Note that the baby is very carefully wrapped in blankets. (Maternity Hospital, Western Reserve University Hospitals, Cleveland)

chloride reacts with the silver to form an insoluble precipitate which renders inert any soluble silver which has not combined with the chlorides in the lacrimal secretion. Instilling drops in the baby's eyes is more easily accomplished if the nurse shades the baby's eyes from the light while putting the drop first in one eye, allowing time for the baby to recover from the shock, the cold and the smarting before she again shades the eyes and puts the drop in the other eye. One of the best methods is to draw down the lower lid gently and carefully drop the solution in the conjunctival sac, using great care not to drop it on the cornea. This

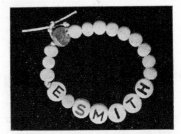

FIG. 202. Identification method, using strand of beads. If surname is at all common use initial of mother's first name also, as shown above. The beads must be sealed around baby's ankle before he leaves the delivery room.

Birth Certificate

This Certifies that _____ was born in

_____
Hospital   City   State

on the _____ day of _____ A. D. 19 _____ at _____ M

_____
ATTENDING PHYSICIAN

In Witness Whereof this Hospital has caused this Certificate to be signed by its duly authorized officer.

SUPERINTENDENT

FATHER'S NAME
ADDRESS
BIRTHPLACE   DATE
MOTHER'S MAIDEN NAME
BIRTHPLACE   DATE

MOTHER'S RIGHT THUMB PRINT

BABY'S HAND OR FOOT PRINT   No. _____

FAUROT INKLESS SYSTEM, N. Y. C.-PATENTED   FORM 105

Fig. 203. Sample form of the Birth Certificate (pink or blue border) including a space for the baby's palm prints and the mother's thumb prints, for permanent identification. Some hospitals use the footprints only. Inkless kits are used in many institutions. (Faurot Inc., New York)

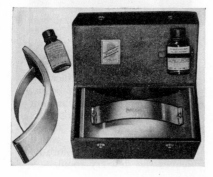

saves the awkward and irritating manipulation of the baby's eyelids. The nurse must take especial precautions against allowing any contamination of the eyes and against dropping any silver solution upon the face. This drug administration is a very important feature in the care of the baby at this time, as silver nitrate or argyrol protects the baby's eyes against ophthalmia neonatorum (p. 513).

Recent research has resulted in the adoption of penicillin by many doctors as prophylaxis for the baby's eyes. The methods used have been intramuscular injections and the local instillation of an aqueous solution or ointment. At present the most practical and effectual is the ointment preparation. It is easy to instil into the conjunctival sac and it is economical, the cost being about the same as that of the silver nitrate ampules. The recommendation is made that, where necessary, statutes and board of health regulations be changed to permit in hospital practice the instillation of penicillin ointment when the doctor prefers it as a prophylaxis against ophthalmia neonatorum.

Identification Methods. Some method of identification of the newborn is applied before the cord is cut or before the baby is removed from the delivery room. However, before this is done, it is important that the mucus be cleared from the baby's mouth and nose, and that respiration be established. There are several satisfactory methods in use. Some hospitals use the linen tapes marked with the mother's name and hospital number, fastening one to the baby's wrist or ankle and the other to the mother's. The identification beads are made up with the mother's surname and initials and sealed with a lead bead. This bracelet or anklet is applied before the baby leaves the delivery room (Fig. 202). The pliable plastic bracelet or anklet has space for the mother's name and initials as well as a permanent lock which has to be cut to be removed. They are made in color to identify sex.

The palmprint and footprint method of identification consists of a stainless procedure made on chemically treated sensitized paper used in the birth certificate. It is designed to take the palmprints or footprints of the baby and the thumbprint of the mother at the time of delivery and may be repeated at the time of discharge from the hospital. It is a simple, quick and permanent method.

The Pond method of permanent identification of the newborn follows.*

The possibility of "mixing" infants in maternity hospitals in the present-day trend of mass hospitalization of obstetric cases is a menace which all hospitals try to avoid. Many methods have been devised to prevent mixed identity of infants, and one method—that of footprints—which was introduced shortly after the First World War, became very popular almost to the point of being a fad. These prints have almost universally been merely smudge prints made for the purpose of recording the wrinkles in the sole of the foot. Too often they have been hastily made by inexperienced pupil nurses or interns without any real knowledge of what they were doing or why they were doing it. Only in very few instances has there been any thought of cleaning the feet to remove the vernix caseosa prior to printing, and the result has been that seldom are any papillary ridges ever discernible in any of the prints. As long as wrinkles are changeable and papillary ridges are permanent, no print is worth the time it takes to make it if only wrinkles and no ridges are recorded.

There has been much doubt in the minds of many who employ the footprint method as to its real value even for the duration of hospitalization, but they have felt that it was of definite psychologic value in reassuring the patients with regard to the possibility of their offspring being mixed, so they have continued to use it. Another reason for the continued use of the footprint method is that no one, prior to 1932, had devised a better one.

* Positive and Permanent Identification of the New Born by Means of Palm Prints, by Gilbert Palmer Pond, M.D., West Suburban Hospital, Oak Park, Ill.

It is rather a treacherous thing to continue to fool the public with a method that is admittedly not what it is represented to be. Some day a set of hastily made smudge prints will be offered in court as a proof of identity in an alleged mix-up of babies. When such a case does occur, the courts will not approve of the psychology of deceiving the parents of a newborn babe with a false sense of security, and newspaper publicity will cause a reaction which will seriously injure not only the hospital in question but all the hospitals in the country.

The author believes that the hospital's responsibility does not rest solely in giving a mother her own child and proving the identity in an immediate disputed case, but that the hospital is essentially an institution for public benefit, with that benefit paid for by the public, either by fees for services rendered or by charitable contributions, and that if a hospital takes prints of infants born under its roof for the protection of its reputation and to protect itself against litigation, those prints should be available, within reason, to the public in a form allowing ready reference even over a period of many years.

With this in mind, the author devised a means of identification of newborn infants that would not only create a positive and permanent record of every child, but one which would lend itself to classification, such as the fingerprint method.

The advantages of a positive and permanent method of infant identification are very definite and comprehensive and at a glance indicate the far-reaching effect. If the proposed palmprint method were universally adopted:

It would provide an incontrovertible proof of birth for life of the individual, and all persons would carry the proof of birth and their identity with them at all times in the prints of their palms.

It would protect parents, babies, and hospitals against the possible mixing of newborn infants.

It would provide means of identifying abandoned children and foundlings and would help to lessen abandonment.

It would provide a means of identifying returned kidnaped children, either dead or alive, regardless of time.

It would provide a means of identifying unclaimed children after major disasters, such as earthquakes, floods, fire, etc.

It would provide identification of all unknown dead after a generation of prints were on file.

It would preserve the identity of all children during the first few years of life when the possible loss of identity is greatest.

It would provide a record of relationship between the infant and its mother.

It would disprove false claims of parenthood of a given infant.

It would disprove false claims of identity in claims for insurance, legacies, etc.

It would be as acceptable in court as a proof of identity as fingerprints are today.

It would seldom be used for criminal identification because palmprints are almost never found as clues, therefore there would be no odium in the popular mind such as is attached to fingerprints.

It would, in short, provide a "birth certificate" par excellence.

Supervision of Baby in Delivery Room. After caring for the baby, the nurse will return to assist the physician, but from time to time, as opportunities offer, she should glance at the baby to make sure that he is breathing properly, that the mouth and the nose are free from mucus, and that there is no bleeding from the cord. If the infant is well wrapped and in a warm place, he needs no further attention until the placenta has been delivered and the mother made clean and comfortable.

Baptism of Baby. If there is any probability that the baby may not live, the question of baptism should be considered in cases where the religion of the family is Catholic. This is an essential duty and means a great deal to the families concerned, and thoughtfulness in this matter will never be forgotten by them.

The following simple instructions were given by the late Rev. Paul L. Blakely, S.J., Ph.D.

The Catholic Church teaches that in case of emergency, anyone may and should baptize. What is necessary is to make the intention of doing what the Church wishes to do and then to pour the water on the child (the head by preference) saying at the same time, "I baptize thee in the name of the Father and of the Son and of the Holy Ghost." The water may be warmed if necessary but it must be pure water and care should be taken to make it flow. If there is any doubt whether the child is alive or dead, it should be baptized, but conditionally; i.e., "If thou art alive, I baptize thee," etc.

DELIVERY IN THE HOME

When plans have been made during the prenatal period for home delivery, it may be conducted with very little inconvenience and confusion. During the prenatal period, the patient and her husband will have prepared the needed supplies. They have been instructed concerning the symptoms of labor and when to call the doctor and the nurse. Many doctors wish to be with the patient from the onset of labor; however, this will have been arranged beforehand, and if the nurse's arrival precedes that of the doctor, she will make her observations of the patient's condition and proceed accordingly.

If time allows, the patient should have the routine preparation for delivery. The patient probably will have taken a warm sponge bath. According to the doctor's specific orders a low soapsuds enema should be given to empty the lower intestine in order to make more room in the pelvis for the descending head and to prevent fecal discharge during delivery. The external genitals are to be cleansed with special care, and the vulva clipped or shaved. The former practice of keeping a perineal or vulva pad on the patient while in labor has been largely discarded because of the danger of carrying infection, notably the colon bacillus, into the parturient canal from the anal region. The nurse will be familiar with the physician's technic.

During the first stage of labor, the patient usually is allowed to be up and about, therefore she should be dressed in stockings, slippers, nightclothes, and dressing gown. From the beginning of the true labor, the patient should use a commode or bed pan, as it may not be wise for her to go to the toilet. During the latter part of the first stage and the first part of the second stage, the patient has an almost constant desire to empty her bowels, because of pressure made upon the rectum by the descending presenting part. This condition should be explained by the nurse, so that the patient may not exert herself unnecessarily. After each bowel movement or urination, the external genitals should be sponged with the antiseptic solution ordered by the doctor.

The nurse should endeavor to make this trying ordeal as light as possible by reassuring the patient in every way. The patient is to be dissuaded from attempting to help herself by voluntary straining of the abdominal muscles, for such efforts only exhaust or deplete her strength. It is important to conserve the patient's energy during the first stage by urging her to rest. The doctor may suggest that liquids be given freely and that some light refreshment be offered, such as tea and toast or crackers (if delivery isn't imminent).

If the membranes rupture in the first stage, the danger of prolapse of the cord must be kept in mind, and the physician should be notified immediately. This should be done, however, without alarming the patient, especially if it is her first labor, as the incident is apt to cause her great alarm. She should be informed in advance of the nature of the watery discharge and should be assured that it is a perfectly natural phenomenon. If her clothing has become soiled with amniotic fluid, it should be replaced.

As soon as it is apparent that the patient is in or near the second stage of labor, she should be put to bed, for at this time the os uteri is, of course, fully dilated, and if she is allowed to remain on her feet precipitate delivery may occur.

The room should be warm (70° to 72° F), well lighted and well ventilated; hot and cold sterile water and provision for boiling the physician's instruments must be provided; and the needed supplies described in Chapter 12 should be arranged in a convenient manner and place.

The nurse should have ready, if possible, on the arrival of the physician, hot water, soap, a nail brush and an orange stick for the scrubbing of his hands, antiseptic solution, according to the physician's orders. As many physicians do not include an apron or gown in their personal equipment, the nurse should have in readiness a small clean sheet, which can be pinned first around his neck and again lower down about the waist, thus making a fairly good substitute for an operating gown.

PROCEDURES CONDUCTED BY THE PHYSICIAN

After the arrival of the physician he will take charge of the further management of the case, and, if the patient is still up and about, the doctor will decide when she should go to bed.

If the case is at all advanced, the physician will wish to make a vaginal or rectal examination at once in order to determine the amount of dilation of the cervix and inform himself as to the progress the patient has made. While he is disinfecting his hands, the nurse will prepare the patient for examination.

Rectal Examination. The patient should lie on her back with her knees flexed, lying on the side of the bed which is most convenient for the doctor (right or left hand used in examination). The nurse should drape the patient so that she is well protected, but with the perineal region exposed. Any other detail of preparation will be suggested by the doctor. He will use a rubber glove or finger cot and lubricant.

Vaginal Examination. Some physicians prefer to make the examination with the patient lying on her back, across the bed, the buttocks resting on the edge and the feet supported by two chairs. A pillow may be placed under the patient's head for comfort.

This method is preferred by some doctors to examining the patient on the side of the bed, as it is less awkward and permits a fuller and more thorough exploration of the pelvic cavity.

The patient is draped in the same manner as for the rectal examination, but the preparation of the perineal area will be according to the wishes of the physician. The technic for local preparation of the patient for vaginal examination varies, but if the nurse always regards the perineal region as a site for an operation and proceeds accordingly, with the least expenditure of time and the least possible disturbance to the patient, it will not be so difficult to carry out the physician's detailed orders. Everything that is used for the patient at this time must be surgically clean, and great care must be taken so that no soap or solution enters the vaginal opening.

A simple preparation is to drape the patient as described and proceed as follows: Place the patient on a bed pan, or improvised Kelly pad, and with warm soap solution scrub the inside of the thighs and the groin, then the lower part of the abdomen and the top of the pubes, and following this across the buttocks and the anus. A fresh cotton pledget should be used for each part. After protecting the vaginal opening with a cotton ball or vulvar pad, thoroughly wash between the folds of the labia, always stroking from above downward and never using the same pledget twice. This area is then rinsed with antiseptic solution or with sterile water. The nurse should remember that the cleansing solution is primarily the soap and the warm water and should not place too much confidence in the properties of the antiseptic solution. The vulva is then covered with a sterile towel or perineal pad and is ready for the vaginal examination. If this procedure is done a short time before the patient is delivered, this preparation will not have to be repeated.

Preparation of Solutions and Instruments

The nurse should see that fresh solutions for the hands are always ready and at a proper temperature (100° F.), that soiled sponges are removed at once, that scissors and tape for tying the umbilical cord and wipes for the baby's eyes are ready (the sterile package not necessarily open); and that a warm woolen blanket is provided to wrap around the baby as soon as he is born.

All the instruments required are usually provided by the physician, and on his arrival he will hand over to the nurse whatever he thinks he may need for the particular case. These are to be boiled for 10 minutes, so that they will be ready. In normal labors the only instruments that are needed are a cord set (two clamps, scissors, forceps), a cord tie and dressing, and a catheter.

The baby's bed should be arranged with a hot-water bottle (or substitute), and a set of clothes should be ready and warm. Other articles for the baby's care should be arranged conveniently. Any emergency material, such as a tub (should the baby

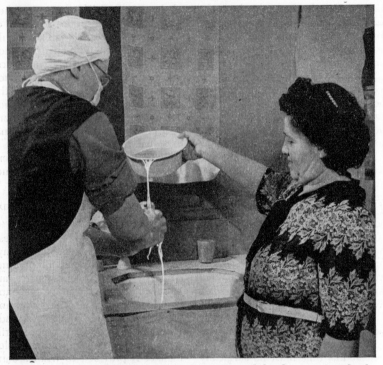

Fig. 206. Grandmother pours the water while the nurse-midwife scrubs for the delivery. Where running water is not available, a satisfactory substitute is employed. (Catholic Maternity Institute, Santa Fe, N. Mex.)

need to be resuscitated) or hypodermic equipment, and the basin to be used to receive the placenta should be prepared.

EMERGENCY DELIVERY BY THE NURSE

In certain cases, the nurse will find it necessary to manage the entire labor herself, either because of precipitate delivery or through delay in securing the services of a physician.

It is needless to say that such emergency cases progress rapidly, and that almost before any careful preparations can be made the pains are recurring with such frequency and severity that the patient must be put to bed and given the undivided attention of the nurse.

If time permits much can be done for the comfort of the patient: holding her hands at the height of the pains and in the intervals between them; and rubbing her back and legs, which often become lame and cramped. Bathing her face and

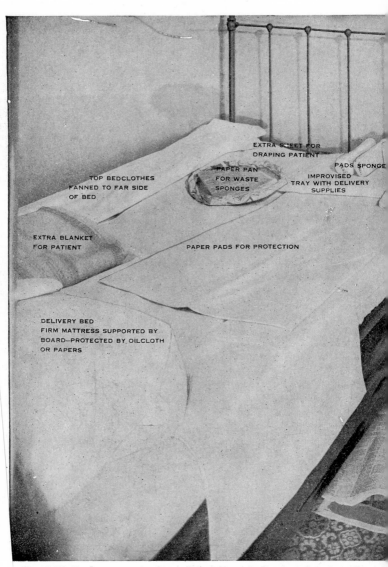

TOP BEDCLOTHES FANNED TO FAR SIDE OF BED

EXTRA SHEET FOR DRAPING PATIENT

PADS SPONGE

PAPER PAN FOR WASTE SPONGES

IMPROVISED TRAY WITH DELIVERY SUPPLIES

EXTRA BLANKET FOR PATIENT

PAPER PADS FOR PROTECTION

DELIVERY BED FIRM MATTRESS SUPPORTED BY BOARD—PROTECTED BY OILCLOTH OR PAPERS

FIG. 205. Bedroom setup for a delivery in the home. For the purpose... pillow for the patient is at the foot end of the bed (lower left-hand co... Picture taken for Louise Zabriskie)

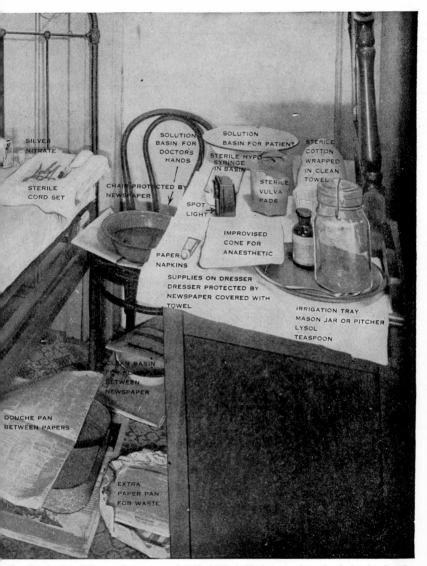

of clarity, the delivery supplies are arranged at the head end of the bed. The
ner of picture). At the time of the delivery, the douche pan is under the bed.

hands, changing her position and keeping the wrinkles out of the bed will also do much to keep the patient feeling fresh. Many women like to have something to pull on as the pains occur; and there is no objection to fastening a twisted sheet to the foot of the bed, with which the patient can brace herself, as it were, when her suffering is most severe.

It seldom happens that the nurse and her patient are entirely alone; usually the husband, some relative or friend can be called upon to prepare some sort of antiseptic solution and place it on a chair or a table by the side of the patient for the nurse's hands. The wipes for the infant's eyes can also be ready; and, as there is never any special hurry about tying and cutting the umbilical cord, there is usually time for the scissors and tape to be boiled. Time may be saved by using only enough water to cover the instruments. The pan may be covered with another pan, thus sterilizing both. In emergency cases, when there has been no previous preparation, an ordinary pair of scissors and a piece of new white cotton twine may be boiled and used for tying and cutting the cord.

If the patient is fully dressed, as may be the case in precipitate delivery, the nurse should do what she can to protect the patient's clothing and the bedding. The procedure is, of course, essentially the same as when the physician is present; but since the nurse's share is wholly different, it may help her to have the steps described, in order to aid her in assuming the responsibility until she is relieved.

Delivery of the Head Between Pains. As the head distends the peri-neum, the nurse must watch it carefully and prevent undue stretching of the parts by holding it back at the acme of each pain. This interference with the descent of the head to prevent its sudden expulsion through the vulva and consequent laceration of the tissues may be kept up until the parts are stretched to their utmost capacity. The essential points are (1) to delay the descent of the head and (2) to prevent the sudden delivery of the baby's head, for it is often this sudden expulsion that results in tearing the perineum. If possible, the baby's head should be delivered between pains. If at any time feces are expelled, such material should be deftly wiped away with fresh sponges, and the disinfecting solution used skillfully to prevent contaminating her gloves. Every precaution should be taken to avoid any chance of an infection from the feces, e.g., by the colon bacillus.

Rupture of the Membranes. If the membranes have not ruptured, they may remain intact until they appear at the vulva. If they protrude, they usually rupture with the next pain, or soon. The patient should be informed of the nature and the harmlessness of the discharge of waters which is about to occur. A towel should be placed against the vulva to receive the gush of waters and to hold back the presenting part.

Precautions Concerning the Cord. As soon as the head is born, the nurse should feel about the neck for the umbilical cord, and if it is found, it should be drawn gently to one side until it can be slipped over the head. No force should be used in this manipulation of the cord, for fear of traction on the umbilicus and the placenta.

Immediate Care of the Infant's Face. The mouth, the eyes, the nose and the throat of the infant are now to be cleansed carefully from blood and mucus, as described previously. The baby's head should be so supported that he will be protected from the blood and the liquor amnii which may have been expelled.

Delivery of the Shoulders. There is no occasion whatever for haste in the delivery of the body. In another moment the uterus will again contract, and the body of the baby will be expelled.

When the shoulders appear, there is no harm in passing a finger, which has been carefully rinsed in the antiseptic solution, into the axilla and gently extracting the posterior arm. The body will now follow very easily and quickly. The exact time of the baby's birth should be noted. If the baby does not cry voluntarily, he may be made to cry by gently rubbing his back or by snapping one's fingers on the bottoms of his feet. If there seems to be mucus, the baby should be held by his heels so that the mucus may drain from his mouth; care must be taken that no traction is exerted on the umbilical cord. The baby should be laid on his right side in a sterile or clean towel to cover the cord and should be covered with a warm woolen blanket.

Observation of the Fundus. The instant the baby is born, the nurse, or one of those present in the room, should place a hand on the patient's abdomen and grasp the fundus, particularly if there is the slightest tendency toward relaxation of the uterine muscles, or if the pulse or other symptoms indicate possible hemorrhage even though no bleeding is visible.

Care of the Cord. The umbilical cord may be tied according to the previous description, or it may be clamped and left for the doctor to tie when he arrives. It is a good plan to tie a tape around the cord, close to the vulva, to serve as a guide in measuring the descent of the placenta. As the after-birth is forced out of the uterus the cord will also escape from the vagina, and the progress of this expulsion can be estimated by watching this third ligature, which at the beginning was made as close to the vulva as possible

The ligature should be tied with a "square knot" (Fig. 199), for the ordinary, or so-called "Granny," knot will almost surely slip, after a short time, no matter how tightly it may have been drawn when it was applied. The characteristic feature of the "square knot" lies in the fact that both ends pass under the same side of the loop. A hemorrhage from the cord is a very serious condition, for even if it does not cause death, it seriously depletes the baby. Consequently, the nurse who intends to practice obstetrics should make it a point to perfect herself in the method of tying a square knot and avoid the possibility of any such accident.

Secondary hemorrhage from the cord may occur in feeble or premature babies; the tendency to bleeding is very great; and they must always be watched with the utmost care. As many of the precipitate deliveries which will fall to the care of the nurse may be cases of premature birth, she must be extremely careful about tying the cord securely and must inspect it for hemorrhage at frequent intervals, tying it a second, or even a third time, if necessary.

The Delivery of the Placenta. After the delivery of the baby, the nurse will direct her attention to the third stage of labor, the delivery of the placenta. There need not be the slightest haste about the delivery of the placenta, and while it is usually expelled in from 15 to 30 minutes after the birth of the baby, no harm will result if it is delayed for an hour or more, provided that there is no excessive bleeding. It is to be remembered that the uterus is resting during this period, and that when its muscular fibers have recovered from the exhaustion of labor, they will contract firmly and expel the after-birth. Under no circumstances should traction be made on the cord in an effort to extract the placenta from the vagina, for this probably will result in tearing the cord from its attachment. If the placenta has not completely separated there is also danger of everting the uterus.

In the majority of cases, after a reasonable period of time, the patient will have another "labor pain," and the placenta will appear at the vulva. It should be received into a sterile bowl or basin held for this purpose, and the string of membranes that trails behind should be extracted with the utmost gentleness and deliberation to prevent the detachment of any tag-ends or fragments. All that is necessary is to extract the membranes from the vagina slowly and carefully, taking plenty of time and using no force.

The placenta is saved until the arrival of the physician, in order that he may inspect it and make sure that it is intact and has been completely expelled.

Care of the Fundus. The fundus should be held for one hour after delivery. As the nurse is very busy at this time, it is advisable that she show some member of the family how to hold the fundus. However, the nurse should assume the responsibility of observing the fundus at intervals.

NATURAL CHILDBIRTH PROGRAM

Dr. Herbert Thoms says, "The natural childbirth program is the physical and psychological preparation of the expectant mother so that childbirth will be anticipated and experienced, not in terms of pain and distress, but with real satisfaction and joy. It is a program of care and attention during the birth process itself that will enable her to participate in the event without marked discomfort. A mother giving birth should know that she is doing something wonderful; she need not feel that something terrible is being done to her."

The patients who have been interested in the education and training for natural childbirth and where sincere efforts have been made to eliminate fear and tension during labor, the results have been (in most cases) satisfactory. If the utmost cooperation is to be expected from the patient she must have learned the physical processes of labor (prenatal classes) and the controlled breathing and relaxation exercises. These exercises aim to increase the tone and the control of the abdominal, back and pelvic muscles. The aim of the natural childbirth program is for a minimum of discomfort at the time of labor and delivery, not necessarily painless. The possible need of anesthetics and drugs, which has been explained previously, are used when indicated.

SUGGESTED READING

Burnett, Elizabeth: An effective use of on-call time, Pub. Health Nursing (reprint), Oct., 1943.

Dieckmann, W. J., et al.: The placental stage and postpartum hemorrhage, Am. J. Obst. & Gynec. 54:415, 1947.

Gold, Edwin M., et al.: Principles for improving patient care in the hospital labor and delivery suite, J.A.M.A. 146:1459, 1951.

Goodrich, Frederick W., Jr.: Natural Childbirth, New York, Prentice-Hall, 1950.

Heardman, Helen: A Way to Natural Childbirth, Baltimore, Williams & Wilkins, 1948.

Hogan, Aileen: Bomb born babies, Pub. Health Nursing 43:383, 1951.

Knowlton, Wilson W.: The elements of a safe delivery, The Mother 7:7, 1945.

Martin, M.: A normal mother and baby, Am. J. Nursing 39:1144, 1939.

Mayes, Harry W.: Vaginal antisepsis during labor, New York State J. Med. 43:1518-1520, 1943.

Olson, Ruth M., and Clifford, Martha L.: Nursing techniques in maternity hospitals, Am. J. Pub. Health 35:1199, 1945.

Owen, Ruth E., and Denman, Lucille G.: Experiences in childbirth, Am. J. Nursing 51:26, 1951.

Ratcliff, J. D.: Birth, New York, Dodd, 1951.

Read, Grantly Dick: Childbirth Without Fear, New York, Harper, 1944.

Roth, Lawrence G.: Natural childbirth in a general hospital, Am. J. Obst. & Gynec. 61:167, 1951.

Summers, Vanda: Saddle bag with log cabin technique, Frontier Nursing Service, Inc. 17: (reprint), 1941.

Thoms, Herbert: Training for Childbirth, New York, McGraw-Hill, 1950.

Thoms and Roth: Understanding Natural Childbirth, New York, McGraw-Hill, 1950.

16

Complications of Labor

MECHANICAL DYSTOCIA

Occasionally the nurse will see cases in which hours and hours of labor pass without progress and in which even a day or two may transpire without the birth of the baby. In such instances, obviously there is something wrong with the mechanics or "machinery" of labor. In other words, these are cases of dystocia (difficult labor) in which the mechanics of the process are at fault— cases of mechanical dystocia. But what precisely *is* wrong?

Reduced to its simplest constituents, the process of labor resolves itself into the propulsion by certain *forces* of an irregular object (the baby or *passenger*) through the birth canal (the *passage*). There are only three factors involved in labor,

therefore—the forces, the passenger and the passage. When, despite many hours of labor, the baby fails to come, one of these three factors or some combination of them must be at fault.

Let us make this clear by a homely example. If a person were trying to force his foot into a boot and was unable to do so, what could be the causes of his failure? First, he might not be pushing hard enough. (Forces at fault.) Second, he might not be holding his foot in the correct position; the foot cannot be jammed in any way but must be flexed sharply so that the smallest diameters present themselves. (Faulty position.) Third, the boot may be too small or (what amounts to the same thing) the foot may be too big. (Disproportion between size of foot and boot.)

373

Likewise, when Nature tries to propel a baby through the birth canal and fails to do so, there can be only three causes of the failure—the same three. The forces are inadequate (uterine inertia); or the position of the infant is at fault; or there is disproportion between the size of the infant and that of the birth canal.

UTERINE INERTIA

In some cases, from the very beginning of labor, the pains are weak, irregular, brief in duration, and ineffectual. Even after 12 or 15 hours the pains are still 8 or 10 minutes apart, last only 20 or 30 seconds and are of weak intensity. This matter of the intensity of labor pains is something with which the nurse must familiarize herself in order that she may report intelligently about such cases. At the height of an excellent uterine contraction it is impossible to indent the uterine wall with one's finger-tips. With a fairly good pain it may be possible to cause some slight indentation, but if the uterine wall can be indented easily at the height of a pain, it is a poor one. In evaluating the intensity of a labor pain, reliance should be placed on this tactile examination and not on the amount of complaining done by the patient.

Primary Uterine Inertia. When pains are poor from the very onset of labor, the condition is known as primary uterine inertia. The cause is unknown. The essence of the treatment is to give the patient more time, a program which calls for much patience and waiting on the part of everyone concerned. The nurse can be very helpful in encouraging the patient and in keeping up her morale

during the long hours. Fluids should be offered to the patient frequently, and unless delivery seems imminent, liquid diet should be given at frequent intervals in order to maintain strength. Hot soapsuds enemas probably will be ordered from time to time in the hope of stimulating more effectual uterine contractions. In certain cases (in some it may be dangerous) the doctor may ask that the patient be allowed to walk about in the belief that this may favor descent of the head, which in turn will exert greater pressure on the lower uterine segment and thereby stimulate stronger pains. In very stubborn cases some doctors may order extremely minute doses of pituitary extract intramuscularly (one-half to one minim). However, unless used with the utmost caution and in very small doses, the employment of pituitary extract in labor is fraught with dangerous possibilities—tetanic contraction of the uterus with asphyxiation of the fetus and even rupture of the uterus. The majority of doctors, consequently, are opposed to its use prior to the birth of the baby.

Secondary Uterine Inertia. In another group of cases, the pains are excellent for the first 10 or 15 hours of labor, then become gradually weaker, irregular and far apart. There is often an associated quickening of the pulse rate. This condition is called secondary uterine inertia because it is secondary to (that is, caused by) exhaustion. The treatment is rest and fluids. This is usually accomplished by giving a hypodermic of morphine plus the administration of from 500 to 700 cc.

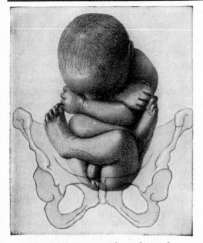

FIG. 207. Complete breech.

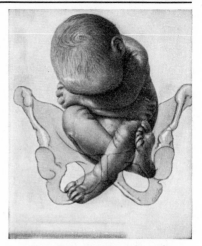

FIG. 208. Footling breech.

of glucose solution (usually 10 per cent) intravenously. The morphine, as a rule, stops the pains altogether for a few hours and gives the patient a much-needed sleep. Upon awakening, the pains are likely to return to their original vigor, and the remainder of labor progress without difficulty.

In such patients who have been in labor for more than 24 hours, whether from uterine inertia or other causes, bacteria are likely to ascend into the uterus and give rise to infection. This is known as *intrapartum infection* and is a serious complication. It is signalized by a rise in temperature, often in association with a chill. Because of this danger, it is customary to take temperatures every two hours in patients whose labors have lasted more than 24 hours. Even an elevation of half a degree should be reported at once to the doctor. Intrapartum infection

is much more likely to occur if the membranes have been ruptured for a long time.

ABNORMAL FETAL POSITIONS

Breech presentations are those in which the breech instead of the vertex presents at the pelvic brim. They occur in about 3 per cent of all term deliveries. In breech cases, the infant often passes meconium from its rectum during the course of labor; and if, after the membranes are ruptured and the liquor amnii has escaped, the nurse finds a black, tar-colored discharge coming from the patient's vagina, she may very properly suppose that the case is one of breech presentation.

Breech presentations are classified as follows:

1. *Complete,* when the feet and the legs are flexed on the thighs, and the thighs are flexed on the abdo-

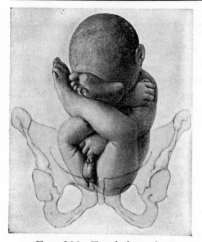

FIG. 209. Frank breech.

men, so that the buttocks and the feet present.

2. _Footling_, when one or both feet present through the cervix.

3. _Frank_, when the legs are extended and lie against the abdomen and the chest with the feet meeting the shoulders, and the buttocks present.

With strong pains, particularly in multiparae, breech cases may be delivered spontaneously, or at least with very little aid by the attendant. The breech is pushed through the vulva as the result of the mother's bearing-down efforts and rises upward in front of the symphysis pubis. With the emergence of the trunk, the legs descend, the attendant simply receiving them and steadying the breech. With further bearing-down efforts, the shoulders are expelled; then, as the attendant holds up the body, the head is extruded with the face directed back at the perineum.

However, in the majority of breech cases, especially in primigravidae, it is necessary for the doctor to give more aid than is indicated above, and, as a rule, this amounts to extraction of the shoulders and the head after the umbilicus has appeared.

Occasionally, cases of precipitate breech delivery may fall to the care of the nurse. These cases are uncommon and, when they do occur, seldom give rise to difficulty because the very fact that they are precipitate presupposes a small baby, excellent expulsive forces and a capacious birth canal. As the breech emerges, it is received and is steadied with a sterile towel and sterile hands, and the patient is urged to bear down strongly. This will usually effect delivery of the shoulders in cases of this sort, but if it does not, the arm which is the more posterior is drawn out of the vagina by passing the first and the middle fingers over the infant's shoulder, down the arm to the elbow, and then drawing the forearm and the hand across the face and the chest and out. The other arm is delivered in the same way; and then to favor the birth of the head, the body of the baby is raised upward in a vertical position. If there is any great delay, the nurse may pass her two fingers into the baby's mouth, with the trunk resting on the palm of the same hand and the legs straddling her forearm. Then, with the other hand, upward and outward traction is made on the shoulders while firm downward pressure is made by an assistant on the lower abdominal wall.

The great danger in breech delivery is to the baby as the result of the trauma which it may sustain in delivery. In footling presentations,

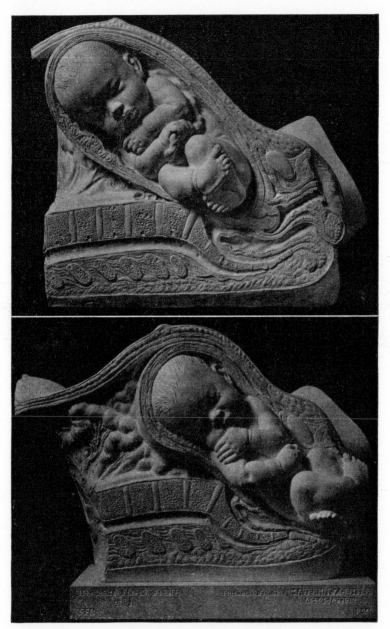

Fig. 210, A and B. Delivery in footling breech presentation. (Fig. 210 A to F from the Dickinson-Belskie Breech Delivery Series, sculptured for the Maternity Center Association, New York)

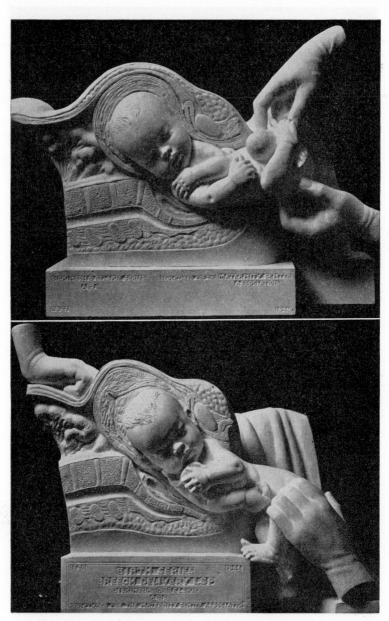

FIG. 210, C and D. Delivery in footling breech presentation.

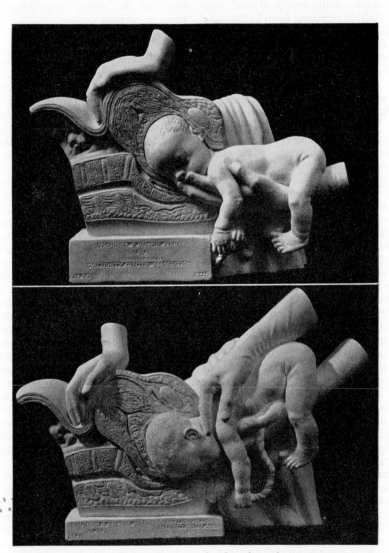

Fig. 210, E and F. Delivery in footling breech presentation.

prolapse of the umbilical cord (see p. 390) is common. Even in the most skilled hands and considering only full-term infants, about one breech infant in 15 succumbs as the result of delivery. The danger to the mother is not appreciably greater than in vertex deliveries, but lacerations of the birth canal are more frequent.

Transverse, Face and Brow Presentations. In transverse or shoulder presentations, the infant lies crosswise in the uterus instead of longitudinally (Fig. 70). This complication occurs about once in every 200 cases and is seen most often in multiparae. Not infrequently an arm prolapses into the vagina, making the problem of delivery even more difficult. The doctor usually will turn the baby in these cases, bringing a foot or both feet into the vagina, an operation known as "version" (p. 401). Transverse presentation is a serious complication, occasionally causes rupture of the uterus (p. 388), and carries a much greater risk to the baby than either vertex or breech presentations.

Face presentations are also seen about once in every 200 cases. They usually terminate spontaneously, the face coming through the vulva with the chin anterior. As edema of the scalp is common in vertex presentations (caput succedaneum) so in face presentations the presenting part, the face, becomes greatly swollen and purplish. This disappears within a few days. Brow presentations are even more rare and are much more difficult to deliver because the largest diameter of the fetal head, the occipitomental, presents. They frequently convert themselves into face or occipital presenta-

tions; or the doctor may convert them or perform version.

DISPROPORTION

Contracted Pelvis. Disproportion between the size of the infant and that of the birth canal (commonly spoken of simply as "disproportion") is caused most frequently by contracted pelvis. The pelvis may be contracted at either the inlet or the outlet. Inlet contraction is most often due to *rickets,* a fact indicating how much good may be accomplished by the prevention of rickets in infants and children through the routine administration of cod-liver oil or some vitamin D preparation. Contracted pelvis due to rickets is much more common in the colored race than in the white. In outlet contraction, the angle formed by the pubic rami is narrow, and the ischial tuberosities are close together; it thus resembles a male pelvis in so far as the outlet is concerned. This type of pelvic contraction occurs with equal frequency in the white and the Negro races, but its cause is not known. It is not only likely to hinder the egress of the baby at the outlet but may be responsible for deep lacerations, since the narrow pubic rami tend to push the infant's head posteriorly in the direction of the rectum.

One of the main functions of prenatal care is to detect pelvic contraction during pregnancy so that long before labor begins—some intelligent decision can be reached about how best to deliver the baby. Of course, in such a case, as shown in Figure 213, cesarean section is obligatory. But all gradations of contracted pelvis are encountered, and, depending on the size of the baby and other

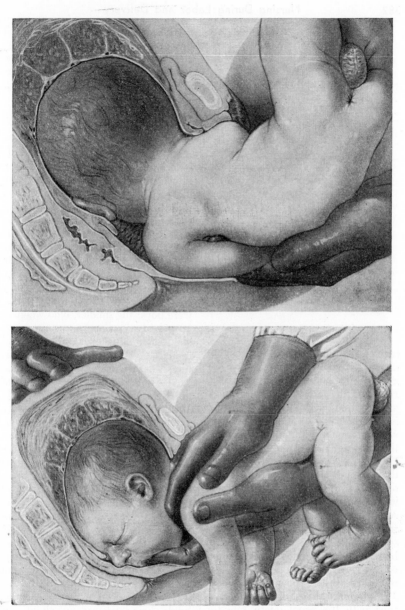

FIG. 211. (*Top*) Extraction of posterior shoulder in breech delivery. (*Bottom*) Extraction of head in breech delivery (Mauriceau maneuver).

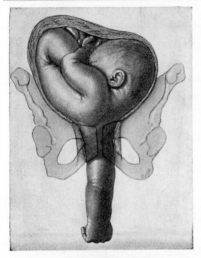

Fig. 212. Transverse or shoulder presentation with prolapse of arm.

factors, many patients with moderate degrees of the condition can be delivered vaginally without difficulty. In doubtful cases, the doctor may give the patient a "trial labor," that is, 6 or 12 hours of labor to ascertain whether or not, with adequate pains, the head will pass through the pelvis.

2 **Oversize Baby.** Excessive size of the infant is not commonly a cause of serious dystocia unless the fetus weighs over 4,500 Gm. (10 pounds). About one infant in a hundred will fall in this class. The trauma associated with the passage of such huge babies through the birth canal causes a decided increase in fetal mortality; this has been estimated as 15 per cent (almost 1 in 6) in contrast with the usual death rate for normal-size babies of 4 per cent. Uterine inertia is frequent in labors with excessive-size infants, and, at the time of delivery, the shoulders may give great difficulty. Even though these babies are born alive, they often do poorly in the first few days because of cerebral hemorrhage, and must be watched closely for signs of that condition (p. 511).

One of the common causes of excessive-size infants is diabetes. Large babies are also more commonly seen in older multiparae and after prolonged pregnancies; the majority of such infants are boys.

Despite tales to the contrary, tremendously large babies—weighing over 13 pounds—are extremely rare and almost all are born dead. In 50,000 deliveries at the Johns Hopkins Hospital, there have been only two such cases. Both these babies were boys: the smaller, who weighed 13 pounds, 7 ounces, was the ninth child of a 34-year-old negress; and the larger, 14 pounds, 4 ounces, was the seventh child of a white woman aged 44. The largest infant born at the New York Lying-In Hospital in 100,000 cases weighed 15 pounds. While there may be rare exceptions, most stories one hears of babies weighing over 15 pounds at birth are the result of either gross exaggeration or incorrect scales.

Hydrocephalus. Hydrocephalus, or an excessive accumulation of cerebrospinal fluid in the ventricles of the brain with consequent enlargement of the cranium, is encountered in one fetus in 2,000, approximately, and accounts for some 12 per cent of all malformations at birth. Associated defects are common, spina bifida being present in about one third of the cases. Varying degrees of cranial enlargement are produced,

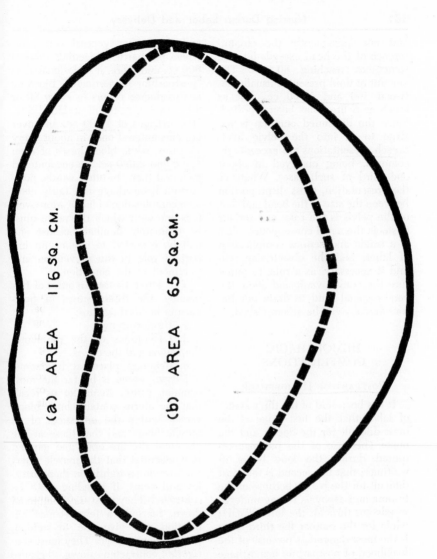

FIG. 213. Areas (actual size) of normal pelvic inlet (a) and contracted inlet (b). The extreme degree of pelvic contraction shown in (b) occurred in a 26-year-old colored woman who had had severe rickets in infancy. This might have been prevented by giving cod-liver oil in infancy and childhood. (J. H. H. 283193.)

and not infrequently the circumference of the head exceeds 50 cm., sometimes reaching 80 cm. The amount of fluid present is usually between 500 and 1,500 cc., but as much as 5 liters has been reported. Since the distended cranium is too large to fit into the pelvic inlet, breech presentations are exceedingly common, being observed in about one third of such cases. Whatever the presentation, gross disproportion between the size of the head and that of the pelvis is the rule, and serious dystocia the usual consequence. This is a tragic and serious complication of labor, and the obstetrician will find it necessary, as a rule, to puncture the cranial vault and allow the cerebrospinal fluid to drain out before delivery can be accomplished.

HEMORRHAGIC COMPLICATIONS

Postpartum Hemorrhage

It has been said of the three stages of labor that the first stage is the most difficult for the doctor and the nurse (because of the patience required during the long hours of waiting); that the second is the most difficult for the baby (because of the trauma and asphyxia it may undergo in passing through the birth canal); while for the mother the third stage is the most dangerous because of the likelihood of postpartum hemorrhage and shock.

Definition and Incidence. The average blood loss postpartum is about 300 cc. The term "postpartum hemorrhage," as ordinarily used, does not refer to bleeding of this magnitude, but only to excessive blood loss;

and, by rather general consensus, when postpartum bleeding reaches 600 cc. and more, it is designated as "postpartum hemorrhage." Bleeding of this degree occurs in every 20 or 30 cases despite the most skilled care. Hemorrhages of 1,000 cc. and over are encountered once in about every 75 cases, while blood losses of even 1,500 and 2,000 cc. are encountered now and then. In other words, postpartum hemorrhage is a fairly common complication of labor. Moreover, it is one with which the nurse must be intimately familiar because she will be expected to assume an important role in the prevention and treatment of the condition.

The Three Causes. In order of frequency, the three causes of postpartum hemorrhage are:

1. Uterine atony.
2. Lacerations of the perineum, the vagina and the cervix.
3. Retained placental fragments.

Uterine atony is by far the most common cause. Again let us recall that the uterus contains huge blood vessels within the interstices of its muscle fibers and that those at the placental site are open and gaping. It is essential that the muscle fibers contract down tightly on these arteries and veins, if bleeding is to be controlled. They must *stay* contracted down, for only a few seconds' relaxation will give rise to sudden, profuse hemorrhage. They must stay *tightly* contracted down, because continuous, slight relaxation gives rise to continuous oozing of blood, one of the most treacherous forms of postpartum hemorrhage.

Lacerations of the perineum, the vagina and the cervix are naturally more common after operative delivery. Tears of the cervix are particularly likely to cause serious hemorrhage. Bright red arterial bleeding in the presence of a hard, firmly contracted uterus (no uterine atony) suggests hemorrhage from a cervical laceration. The doctor will establish the diagnosis by actual inspection of the cervix (retractors are necessary) and, after locating the source of bleeding, will repair the laceration.

Retained Placental Fragments. Small, partially separated fragments of placenta may cause postpartum hemorrhage by interfering with proper uterine contraction. Careful inspection of the placenta to determine whether a piece is missing will rule out or confirm the diagnosis; the treatment, obviously, is to remove the placental fragment. This is an uncommon cause of postpartum hemorrhage, but occasionally the nurse will encounter cases in which profuse bleeding occurs suddenly a week or more after delivery. These late hemorrhages are usually designated by the term "puerperal hemorrhage." They are almost always caused by a retained placental fragment.

Predisposing Factors. There are certain factors which predispose to postpartum hemorrhage so that, to a certain extent, it may be anticipated in advance. Among these, one of the most important is the size of the baby. With a 9-pound baby, the chances of postpartum hemorrhage are five times as great as they are with a 5-pound infant. Excessive bleeding is twice as common in twin pregnancy. Hydramnios (excessive amount of amniotic fluid) is another predisposing factor. Other conditions in which postpartum hemorrhage is extremely frequent are premature separation of the placenta and the placenta previa. Finally, operative delivery, particularly if a prolonged general anesthetic has been given, greatly increases the likelihood of this complication.

Clinical Picture. Excessive bleeding may occur prior to the birth of the placenta, but it is seen more commonly thereafter. Although it is occasionally torrential in character, the most common type is a continuous trickle—minute by minute. These small constant trickles are not alarming in appearance, consequently no one may become alarmed and no one may do anything. This is what makes this type of hemorrhage so treacherous. This fact has been emphasized particularly by Doctor Beecham, of Philadelphia, in his survey of 52 deaths from postpartum hemorrhage which occurred in that city. The average interval between delivery and death in this series was 5 hours and 20 minutes. Only 6 patients, 11.5 per cent, died within 2 hours of delivery, and none in less than 1½ hours. In other words, there would have been ample time for intensive treatment in any of these cases, had the attendant known how much blood was being lost.

Treatment. The first and most important thing to do is to grasp the uterus and massage it vigorously. This must be continued until the uterus assumes a woody hardness; if the slightest relaxation occurs, the massage must be re-instituted. In many cases, the uterus stays contracted most of the time but occasionally relaxes; it is therefore obligatory to keep a hand on the fundus

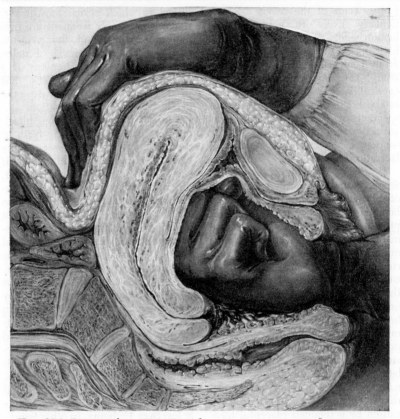

Fig. 214. Bimanual compression of uterus in treatment of postpartum hemorrhage.

constantly for a full hour after bleeding has subsided. Even then the danger is not over since relaxation sometimes occurs two or more hours after delivery; in these cases, the uterus may balloon with blood with very little escaping externally. Accordingly, the size and the consistency of the uterus should be checked frequently until several hours have elapsed. The nurse must

make absolutely certain that she is actually massaging the uterus. Frequently, these big, boggy, relaxed uteri are difficult to outline through the abdominal wall, and it may be necessary to push the hand well posteriorly to the region of the sacral promontory to reach it. The very fact that the uterus is hard to identify usually means that it is relaxed. If the nurse is not sure that she is

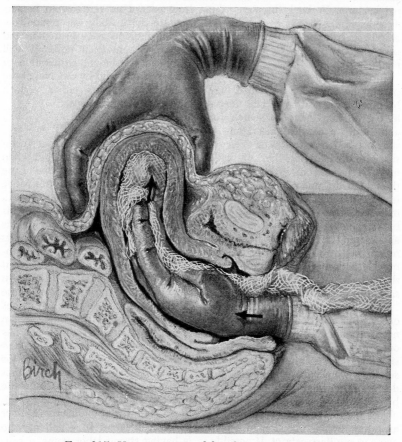

Fig. 215. Uterus tamponed by the manual method.

feeling the uterus, she should inform the doctor at once.

If the bleeding occurs prior to delivery of the placenta, the physician may find it necessary to extract the placenta manually. (Change of gloves as well as gown may be called for.) Oxytocics will invariably be requested—ergonovine or pituitary extract intramuscularly, or both. One or another of these may be given by the doctor intravenously. If these measures fail to stop the bleeding, the doctor probably will either pack the uterus or carry out bimanual compression of the organ. The latter provides the most efficient means of massaging the uterus as well as compression. Packing may be done either manually or by means of the Holmes packer; this instrument prevents contamination of the gauze by vaginal bacteria. If shock threatens, the Trendelenburg position should be employed, external heat applied, and preparations for blood transfusion made.

In the handling of a case of postpartum hemorrhage, the nurse may be taxed to her utmost. The doctor in charge may have to search for and suture a cervical laceration or start a blood transfusion or even resuscitate the baby; another physician may be needed to give the anesthesia. To the nurse, or nurses, will usually fall the important tasks of massaging the uterus, giving oxytocics, helping with the transfusion and keeping an eye on the baby. The nurse must be prepared to act quickly and efficiently if the lives of these bleeding mothers are to be saved.

If postpartum hemorrhage should occur after the doctor has left, the nurse should grasp the uterus at once, press out as much blood as possible, and begin vigorous massage, sending word, of course, to the doctor. If massage fails to stop the bleeding, the doctor usually will not object if the nurse gives the patient an intramuscular injection of ergonovine or pituitary extract. If possible, this arrangement should be understood beforehand.

Late Postpartum Hemorrhage. Occasionally postpartum hemorrhage may occur later than the first day following delivery. These late postpartum hemorrhages may take place any time between the second and twenty-eighth day, are usually sudden in onset and may be so massive as to produce shock; they are due almost always to retained placental

fragments. Late postpartum hemorrhage is fortunately uncommon, occurring perhaps once in a thousand cases. The physician probably will carry out instrumental dilatation of the cervix followed by removal of the placental fragments either with a curette or ovum forceps.

RUPTURE OF UTERUS

Rupture of the uterus is fortunately a rare complication, but when it does occur it constitutes one of the gravest accidents in obstetrics, since almost all of the babies and about a third of the mothers are lost. In this condition, the uterus simply bursts because the strain placed upon its musculature is more than it can withstand. It may occur in pregnancy but is more frequent in labor. In modern obstetrics, the most common cause is rupture of the scar of a previous cesarean section. Accordingly, when observing labor in a patient who has had a previous cesarean section, the possibility of this accident always should be borne in mind. Other causes are disproportion, traumatic delivery, such as version and extraction, and the injudicious use of pituitrin in labor. In a patient who is having strong labor pains, a sudden tremendously severe, lancinating pain followed by complete cessation of regular pains suggests rupture of the uterus; due to the outpouring of blood into the abdominal cavity, signs of shock are a frequent but not invariable accompaniment. As soon as the diagnosis of rupture of the uterus is made, rapid preparations for an abdominal operation should be made, since hysterectomy is the usual treatment.

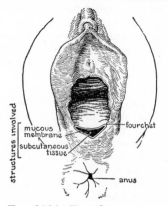

Fig. 216A. First-degree tear.

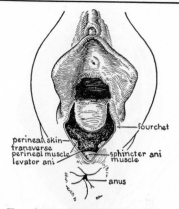

Fig. 216B. Second-degree tear.

ACCIDENTAL
COMPLICATIONS

LACERATIONS OF PERINEUM

Lacerations have already been referred to as a cause of postpartum
hemorrhage. In addition, perineal
tears may do great damage in destroying the integrity of the perineum and in weakening the supports
of the uterus, the bladder and the
rectum. Unless these lacerations are
repaired properly, the resultant
weakness, as the years go by, may
cause prolapse of the uterus (called
by the laity "falling of the womb"),
cystocele (a pouching downward of
the bladder), or rectocele (a pouching forward of the rectum). These
conditions, which originate from
perineal lacerations at childbirth,
give rise to many discomforts and
often necessitate operative treatment.

Perineal lacerations, or tears, are
usually classified in three degrees.

First-degree tears are those which
involve the fourchet, the perineal

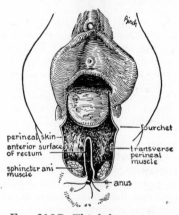

Fig. 216C. Third-degree tear.

skin and the vaginal mucous membrane without involving any of the
muscles.

Second-degree tears are those
which involve (in addition to skin
and mucous membrane) the muscles
of the perineal body but not the
rectal sphincter (sphincter ani muscle). These tears usually extend upward on one or both sides of the

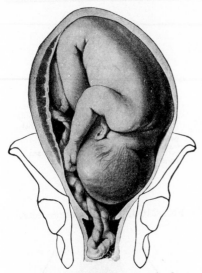

FIG. 217. Prolapse of the umbilical cord (Bumm). As the head comes down, the compression of the cord between the fetal skull and the pelvic brim will shut off its circulation completely.

vagina, making a triangular injury.

Third-degree tears are those which extend completely through the skin, the mucous membrane, the perineal body *and* the sphincter ani muscle. This type is often referred to as a complete tear. Not infrequently, these third-degree lacerations extend a certain distance up the anterior wall of the rectum.

The causes of perineal lacerations are rapid and sudden expulsion of the head (particularly when it "pops" out); excessive size of the infant; difficult forceps deliveries and breech extractions; outlet contraction of the pelvis, forcing the head posteriorly; and very friable maternal tissues. The majority are unavoidable even

in the most skilled hands. First- and second-degree lacerations are extremely common in primiparae, and for this reason episiotomy (p. 395) is widely employed. Third-degree lacerations are fortunately uncommon, occuring only once in every 200 cases or so. Unless properly repaired, they may result in loss of bowel control. All three types of tears are sutured carefully by the obstetrician immediately after delivery; when this is done, the perineal structures are returned approximately to their former condition.

PROLAPSE OF UMBILICAL CORD

In the course of labor, the cord prolapses in front of the presenting part about once in every 400 cases. It is a grave complication for the fetus, since the cord is then compressed between the head and the bony pelvis, and the fetal circulation shut off. The accident is usually due to premature rupture of the membranes when the head, the breech or the shoulder is not sufficiently down in the pelvis to prevent the cord from being washed past it in the sudden gush of amniotic fluid. After the membranes rupture, the cord comes down, and it may be either a concealed or an apparent prolapse. In the latter instance, the diagnosis is made when the cord is seen; but when the cord is not visible, the correct diagnosis will not be made unless the patient is examined and the cord is felt, or examination of the fetal heart reveals distress due to pressure on the cord. This is why many doctors make it a routine to listen to the fetal heart sounds immediately after the membranes rupture.

If the nurse is alone with the patient, she should send immediately for the physician and then attempt to relieve the pressure on the cord by elevating the patient's hips, thus allowing the head to gravitate away from the pelvis. This takes place in either the "knee-chest position" (Fig. 252) or the Trendelenburg position. In the home, the latter is arranged by slipping the back of a straight-backed chair, covered with a flat pillow, under the buttocks and the shoulders, with the knees down over the rungs of the chair. In putting the patient in such positions, her hips must be kept raised above the level of her shoulders. If the patient is unable to remain in either of these positions very long, she may be put in the elevated Sims' position, that is, on her side with the hips elevated by pillows in order to raise the hips higher than the thorax. Any change in position must be carried out slowly!

If the doctor is expected to arrive on the scene within the next 15 minutes, this is all that the nurse should do. If he can be reached by telephone in this period, instructions about further therapy should be sought. If no medical advice can be obtained at the end of 15 minutes, the nurse should wash the cord with a soapy antiseptic solution and, with the patient in the knee-chest or Trendelenburg position, replace it in the vagina, using a plug of sterile cotton to keep it there. In handling the cord, great care must be exercised not to compress it.

INVERSION OF UTERUS

Inversion of the uterus is a rare and highly fatal accident of labor in which, after the birth of the baby, the uterus turns inside out. Shock is profound, in many cases causing the death of the mother. This rare complication is mentioned here only to stress the two common causes: (1) pulling on the umbilical cord and (2) trying to express the placenta when the uterus is relaxed. In the former case, the traction on the attached placenta simply pulls the uterus inside out, while in the latter, the hand pushes the relaxed muscular sac inside out. The umbilical cord never should be pulled on, and the uterus never should be pushed upon unless it is firmly contracted.

MULTIPLE PREGNANCY

When two or more embryos develop in the uterus at the same time, the condition is known as multiple pregnancy. Twins occur once in 92 births, approximately; triplets once in 9,400 births; and quadruplets once in 620,000. Over 30 cases of quintuplets have been recorded, but with two notable exceptions, none of these infants has survived more than a few weeks. The familiar one, of course, is the Dionne quintuplets, and the fact that all five of these little girls are now alive is one of the miracles of modern times. Heredity plays an important causative role in twin pregnancy, and if there are twins in the family of either the expectant mother or her husband, the likelihood of twins is greater.

Twins may be of two kinds: identical and nonidentical. Identical twins *are* identical because they come from a single egg; hence they are called "single-ovum twins." Fertilization takes place in the usual way, by a

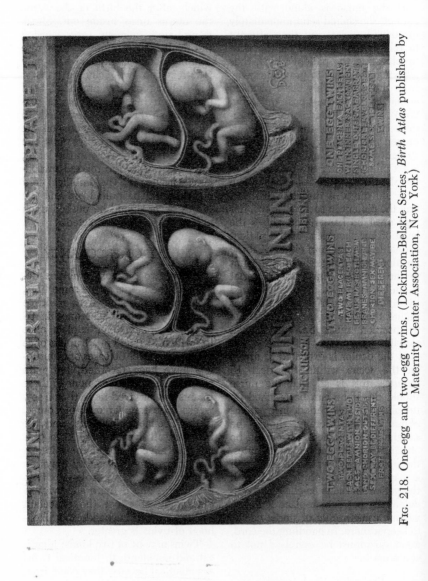

Fig. 218. One-egg and two-egg twins. (Dickinson-Belskie Series, *Birth Atlas* published by Maternity Center Association, New York)

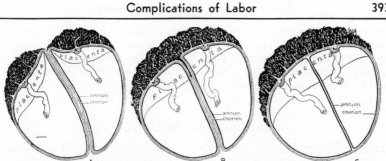

Fig. 219. Single- and double-ovum twin differences. A and B, double-ovum twins; there are two chorions; in B the two placentas have fused. C, single-ovum twins; there is only one chorion and one placenta.

single spermatozoon, but then, very early in the ovum's development, it divides into two identical parts instead of continuing as a single individual. Such twins are always of the same sex and, as we have implied, show close physical and mental resemblances. Nonidentical twins come from the fertilization of two ova by two spermatozoa and are therefore known as "double-ovum twins." Such twins, according to chance, may be of the same sex or of opposite sexes; and the likelihood of their resembling each other is no greater than that of any brother and sister.

Single-ovum twins have one placenta and one chorion, but there are normally two amnions and two umbilical cords. In double-ovum twins, each fetus has its own chorion, amnion, cord and placenta, but the placentas may be partially fused. These double-ovum twins are much the more common of the two types, making up about 85 per cent of all twins.

In the majority of instances (but not all) it is possible for the physi-

cian to make a diagnosis of twins by abdominal examination during the last few months; in doubtful cases, a roentgenogram may be necessary to settle the question.

Twins are likely to be born about two weeks before the calculated date of delivery. Even though pregnancy goes to full term, twins are usually smaller than single infants by nearly one pound; however, the outlook for such babies, provided that the pregnancy continues into the last month, is almost as good as that for single infants.

The patient with a multiple pregnancy faces greater discomforts and greater hazards than does a woman with a single pregnancy. The latter weeks of a twin pregnancy are likely to be associated with heaviness of the lower abdomen, back pains and swelling of the feet and ankles. Moreover, there are two serious complications which such patients are particularly prone to develop: toxemia and postpartum hemorrhage. Eclampsia is four times more common in twin pregnancy. Therefore, the prenatal course of these patients should be followed with especial care for signs of beginning toxemia. Postpartum hemorrhage is twice as common in twin pregnancy. Mechanical difficulties in labor are less frequent than might be expected. Uterine inertia, however, is encountered rather often. Not infrequently, the physician has to rupture the membranes of the second twin and occasionally deliver it by version and extraction.

SUGGESTED READING

Bradley, Chester D.: Retained placenta, Am. J. Obst. & Gynec. **59:**141, 1950.

Brandeberry, Keith R., and Kistner, Robert W.: Prolapse of the umbilical cord, Am. J. Obst. & Gynec. **61:**356, 1951.

Cole, J. T.: Method of treating massive obstetric hemorrhage, J.A.M.A. **135:**142-144, 1947.

Gordon, C. A.: Hemorrhage as the most frequent cause of maternal death. An analysis of the puerperal deaths in Brooklyn, 1944, Am. J. Surg. **70:**277, 1945.

Gusberg, S. B.: Prolapse of the umbilical cord, Am. J. Obst. & Gynec. **52:**826-829, 1946.

Guttmacher, A. F.: An analysis of 521 cases of twin pregnancy: (1) differences in single and double ovum twinning, Am. J. Obst. & Gynec. **34:**76, 1937.

——: An analysis of 473 cases of twin pregnancy: (2) hazards of pregnancy itself, Am. J. Obst. & Gynec. **38:**277, 1939.

Macklin, Madge T.: The Use of monozygous and dizygous twins in the study of human heredity, Am. J. Obst. & Gynec. **59:**359, 1950.

Moore, W. T., and Steptoe, P. P., Jr.: The experience of the Johns Hopkins Hospital with breech presentation, South. M. J. **36:**295, 1943.

Potter, Edith L.: Fundamentals of Human Reproduction, New York, McGraw-Hill, 1948.

17

Operative Obstetrics

EPISIOTOMY AND REPAIR OF LACER-
ATIONS
FORCEPS
VERSION

CESAREAN SECTION
DESTRUCTIVE OPERATIONS
INDUCTION OF LABOR

Although the nurse will rarely be called upon to perform obstetric operations, she will be a much more intelligent and understanding assistant to the obstetrician if she knows why the more common operations are done and how they are carried out. The only operative procedure of major importance which the nurse may be obliged to perform in emergencies is breech extraction. This has been discussed on page 375 in connection with the management of breech delivery.

EPISIOTOMY AND THE REPAIR OF LACERATIONS

If, as the head distends the vulva, a laceration seems to be inevitable, the obstetrician may choose to incise the perineum rather than allow that structure to sustain a traumatic tear. This operation is called "episiotomy" and serves several purposes:

1. It substitutes a straight, clean-cut surgical incision for the ragged, contused laceration which is otherwise likely to ensue; such an incision is easier to repair and heals better than a tear.
2. The direction of the episiotomy can be controlled, whereas a tear may extend in any direction, sometimes involving the anal sphincter and the rectum.
3. It spares the baby's head the necessity of serving as a battering ram against perineal obstruction; if prolonged, this "pounding" of the infant's head against the perineum may cause brain injury.
4. The operation shortens the duration of the second stage.

In view of these several advantages of episiotomy, many obstetricians employ it routinely in primigravidae, particularly before forceps delivery. The incision is made with blunt-pointed straight scissors about

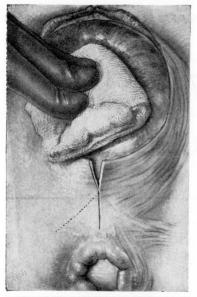

FIG. 220. Episiotomy. Showing lines of incision for median and mediolateral episiotomy.

(Technic employed at the Johns Hopkins Hospital. Many other methods are equally satisfactory.)

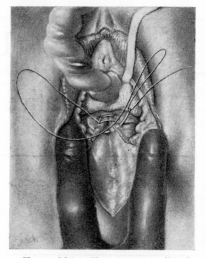

FIG. 221. Episiotomy. "Tail-sponge" in vagina to occlude bleeding, continuous suture in vaginal mucosa.

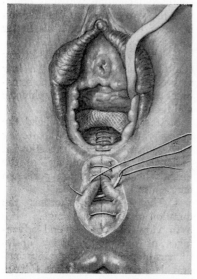

FIG. 222. Episiotomy. After the levator ani muscle has been united by two or more sutures (shown tied and cut), the fascia covering the muscle is sutured. Note the "tail-sponge."

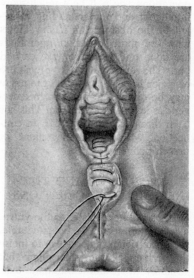

FIG. 223. Episiotomy. After suturing to the lowermost angle of the fascia, the round needle is replaced by cutting needle and the running suture continued upward in subcuticular fascia.

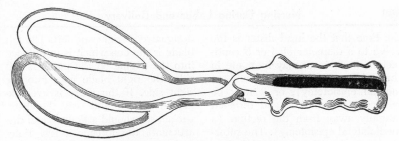

FIG. 224. Simpson forceps.

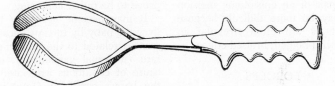

FIG. 225. Tucker McLane forceps.

A

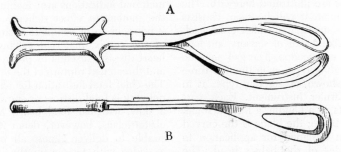

B

FIG. 226. Kielland forceps. (A) Front view; (B) side view.

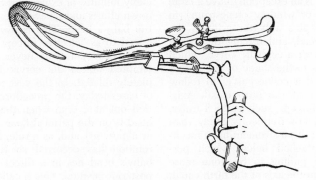

FIG. 227. Tarnier axis-traction forceps.

the time that the head distends the vulva to a diameter of 4 or 5 centimeters. Such a cut may be made in the midline of the perineum (a median episiotomy), or it may be begun in the midline and directed laterally away from the rectum (a mediolateral episiotomy). The suturing of spontaneous perineal lacerations is similar to that illustrating the repair of an episiotomy incision but may be more difficult because such tears are often irregular in shape with ragged, bruised edges.

FORCEPS

The common types of obstetric forceps are illustrated herewith. The instrument, it will be seen, consists of two steel parts which cross each other like a pair of scissors and lock at the intersection. The lock may be of a sliding type, as in the first three types shown, or a screw type, as in the Tarnier instrument. Each part consists of a handle, a lock, a shank and a blade; the blade is the curved portion designed for application to the sides of the baby's head. The blades of most forceps (the Tucker McLane is an exception) have a large opening or window (fenestrum) in them to give a better grip on the baby's head, and usually they have two curves: a cephalic curve, which conforms to the shape of the baby's head, and a pelvic curve, to follow the curve of the birth canal. Axis-traction forceps, such as the Tarnier, are used less frequently today than formerly; this instrument has a mechanism attached below which permits the pulling to be done more directly in the axis of the birth canal.

The two blades of the forceps are designated as right and left. The left blade is the one which is introduced into the vagina on the patient's left side; the right blade goes into the right side. If the nurse is ever expected to scrub and assist the obstetrician, she should articulate and disarticulate the forceps a few times and make sure that she knows which blade is which. Otherwise, this may prove to be rather confusing.

It may become necessary to deliver the baby by forceps because of reasons related to the mother's welfare (maternal indications), or because of conditions associated with the baby's condition (fetal indications). Among the more common maternal indications are: inability of the mother to effect delivery after 2 hours or so of complete dilatation of the cervix, maternal exhaustion, heart disease, toxemia of pregnancy, and threatened rupture of the uterus. The chief fetal indication for forceps delivery is fetal distress as shown by a slow, irregular fetal heart. Many obstetricians, however, deem it desirable to deliver almost all primigravidae with forceps in the belief that the operation spares the mother many minutes of exhausting bearing-down efforts and relieves pressure on the baby's head. This is usually referred to as "elective forceps."

Forceps operations never are attempted unless the cervix is completely dilated. In the vast majority of cases today, the procedure is carried out at a time when the baby's head is on the perineal floor (visible or almost so) and, as a rule, internal rotation has occurred so that the baby's head lies in a direct anteroposterior position. This is called "low forceps," sometimes "outlet forceps."

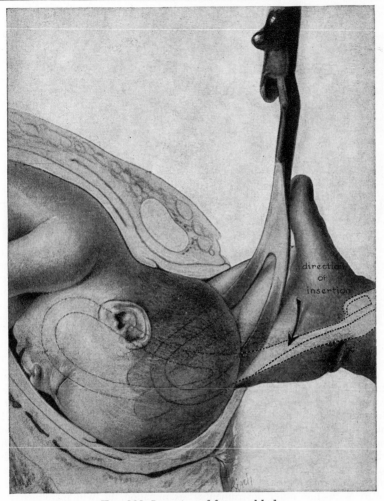

FIG. 228. Insertion of forceps blade.

When the head is higher in the pelvis, with its lowermost point near the level of the ischial spines, the operation is called *"mid-forceps."* If the head has not yet engaged, the procedure is known as *"high for-*ceps."* High-forceps delivery is an exceedingly difficult and dangerous operation for both mother and baby and is rarely done. The obstetrician will inform the nurse of the type of instrument he wishes to use. Boiling

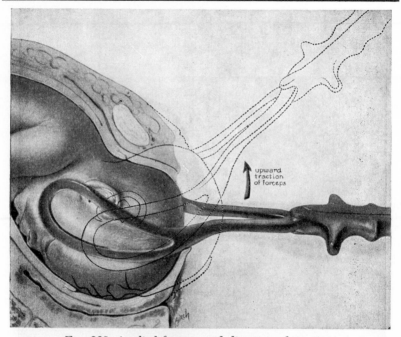

Fig. 229. Applied forceps and direction of traction.

is the usual type of sterilization employed, but in many hospitals several pairs of the generally approved Simpson forceps, each encased in suitable wrappings, are dry sterilized and kept in the delivery room for immediate use. If the latter procedure is not done, most obstetricians will request that a pair of forceps be boiled with the other instruments prepared for delivery in case they should be necessary in an emergency. The other instruments needed for a forceps delivery are the same as those required for a spontaneous delivery plus those necessary for repair work; these are listed on page 346.

Complete anesthesia is necessary, but in low-forceps deliveries it may be light, and in many institutions this type of operation is performed successfully under local infiltration anesthesia. The patient is placed in the lithotomy position and prepared and draped in the usual fashion. The obstetrician will first catheterize the patient. After checking the exact position of the baby's head by vaginal examination, he will introduce two or more fingers of his right hand into the left side of the vagina; these fingers will guide the left blade into place and at the same time protect the maternal soft parts (vagina, cervix) from injury. Taking the left blade of the forceps in his left hand, he introduces it into the left side of the vagina, gently insinuating it

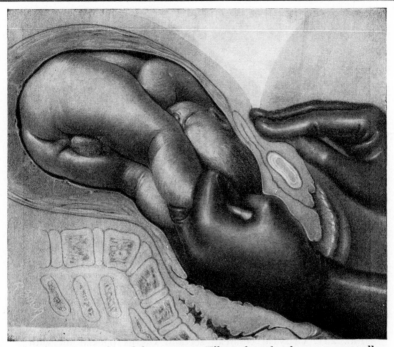

Fig. 230. Internal podalic version. Elbow length gloves are usually worn for this operation.

between the baby's head and the fingers of his right hand. The same procedure is carried out on the right side, and then the blades are articulated. Traction is not continuous but intermittent; and between traction, the obstetrician will partially disarticulate the blades in order to release pressure on the baby's head. Episiotomy is almost routine nowadays in these cases.

VERSION

Version consists of turning the baby in the uterus from an undesirable into a desirable position.

There are three types of version: external, internal and Braxton-Hicks.

External version is an operation designed to change a breech presentation into a vertex presentation by external manipulation of the fetus through the abdominal and the uterine walls. It is attempted in the hope of averting the difficulties of a subsequent breech delivery. Obstetricians find the procedure most successful when done about a month before full term; it often fails, however, either because it proves to be impossible to turn the fetus around or because the fetus returns to its original position within a few hours.

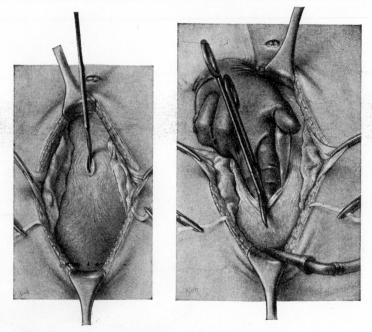

Fig. 231. Classical cesarean section. Uterus packed off with
warm, moist gauze pads. Start of incision with knife.
Fig. 232. Classical cesarean section. Continuation of incision
with bandage scissors.

Some obstetricians disapprove of it
altogether.

Internal version, sometimes called
internal podalic version, is an operation designed to change whatever
presentation may exist into a breech
presentation. With cervical dilatation
complete, the whole hand of the
operator is introduced high into the
uterus, one or both feet are grasped
and pulled downward in the direction of the birth canal. With his external hand the obstetrician may expedite the turning by pushing the
head upward. The version usually is
followed by breech extraction (p.

375). Internal version finds its greatest usefulness in transverse presentation and in cases of multiple pregnancy in which the birth of the second twin is retarded.

Braxton-Hicks Version. In this procedure, two fingers are introduced
into a partially dilated cervix and,
after manipulating the fetus to effect
turning, one leg is drawn through
the cervix. The operation is not designed to bring about immediate delivery and never is followed at once
by extraction. Its purposes are either
to compress the lower uterine segment with the infant's buttock (see

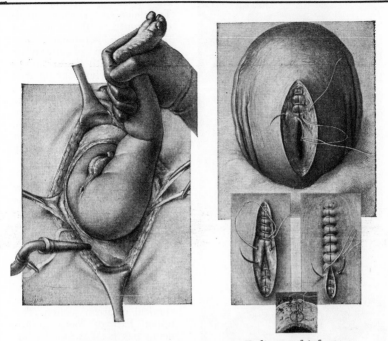

Fig. 233. Classical cesarean section. Delivery of infant.
Fig. 234. Classical cesarean section. Method of suturing uterus.

placenta previa, p. 244), or to stretch the cervix with the infant's thigh so that labor may be initiated.

CESAREAN SECTION

Cesarean section is the removal of the infant from the uterus through an incision made in the abdominal wall and the uterus. The main indications for cesarean section fall into five groups: (1) Disproportion between the size of the fetus and that of the bony birth canal, that is, contracted pelvis (p. 380), tumor blocking birth canal, etc. (2) Certain cases in which the patient has had a previous cesarean section, the operation being done because of fear that the uterine scar will rupture in labor. (3) Certain cases of very severe toxemia of pregnancy, but rarely in eclampsia. (4) Certain cases of placenta previa and premature separation of the normally implanted placenta. (5) Miscellaneous complications.

There are four main types of cesarean section:

Classical Cesarean Section. The incision is made directly into the wall of the body of the uterus; the baby and the placenta are extracted, and the incision is closed by three layers of catgut sutures. As a rule, classical cesarean section is employed only in

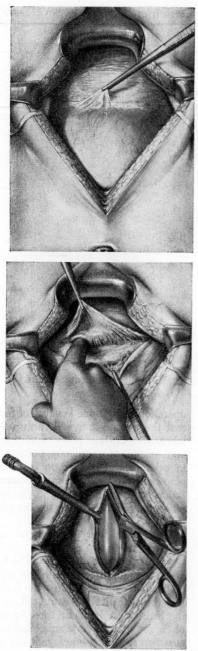

FIG. 235 (*Top*). Low cervical cesarean section. High Trendelenburg position, bladder empty, with catheter in place. The peritoneum over lower portion of uterus is picked up with tissue forceps to determine how far up it is loosely attached to uterus. A transverse incision of the peritoneum, slightly concave downward, is to be made about 1 inch below the point where the peritoneum is firmly attached to the uterus.

FIG. 236 (*Center*). Low cervical cesarean section. The lower edge of the incised peritoneum is picked up by the tissue forceps and gently stripped off the underlying uterine segment by finger dissection.

FIG. 237 (*Bottom*). Low cervical cesarean section. The upper flap of loose peritoneum has been stripped from the underlying muscle by finger dissection and is held back by a retractor. A small incision with a scalpel is made at the upper end of the lower uterine segment and carried downward with bandage scissors.

those cases in which the operation is done prior to the onset of labor. At this time, the uterine contents are sterile, but after 6 or more hours of labor, particularly if the membranes have been ruptured, bacteria ascend from the vagina into the uterus and are potential sources of infection. When done after the patient has been in labor many hours, this type of operation is considered dangerous because of the ease with which infectious material, during the puer-

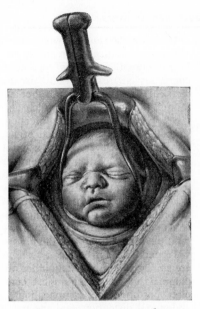

FIG. 238. Low cervical cesarean section. Extraction of baby with forceps. Pituitary extract (1 cc.) intramuscularly is usually given as soon as the head is delivered.

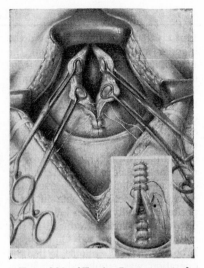

FIG. 239 (*Top*). Low cervical cesarean section. After delivery of baby and placenta, edges of the lower segment incision are grasped with ring forceps and sutured.

FIG. 240 (*Bottom*). Low cervical cesarean section. After upper peritoneal flap is pulled down over the uterine wound and sutured, the lower flap is pulled upward and sutured with running suture.

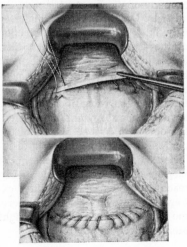

perium, may escape directly through the uterine wound into the peritoneal cavity. When any type of cesarean section is done prior to the onset of labor, as the result of a prearranged plan, it is known as "elective" cesarean section. (As with "elective low forceps," the obstetrician is not forced to perform the operation but elects to do it as the best procedure for mother and baby.)

Low Cervical Cesarean Section. (Synonyms: two-flap cesarean section; laparotrachelotomy.) The initial incision (the abdomen having been opened) is made transversely across the uterine peritoneum where it is attached loosely just above the bladder. Two flaps of peritoneum are thus created. The lower flap and the bladder are now dissected off the uterus, and the uterine muscle is incised either longitudinally or transversely. The baby is ordinarily delivered head first, usually with forceps. After the placenta has been extracted and the uterine incision sutured, the lower flap is imbricated over the upper. This two-flap arrangement seals off the uterine incision and is believed to prevent the egress of infectious lochia into the peritoneal cavity. When low cervical cesarean was first introduced in this country by Dr. Alfred C. Beck, of Brooklyn, N. Y., about 1919, the operation was employed chiefly on patients who had been in labor for a number of hours, and it is undoubtedly safer than the classical procedure in such cases. But it has other advantages, and many obstetricians today prefer it in elective cases as well.

Extraperitoneal Cesarean Section. There are two extraperitoneal operations, one devised by Dr. W. Latsko, formerly of Vienna, Austria, and the other by Dr. E. G. Waters, of Jersey City, N. J. By appropriate dissection of the tissues around the bladder, access to the lower uterine segment is secured without entering the peritoneal cavity. The baby is delivered through a transverse incision in the lower uterine segment. Since the entire operation is done outside of the peritoneal cavity, neither spill of infected amniotic fluid nor subsequent seepage of pus from the uterus can reach the peritoneal surfaces. An extraperitoneal operation is, therefore, the safest type in cases of outright uterine infection.

Cesarean Section — Hysterectomy. (Synonyms: radical cesarean section; Porro operation.) This operation comprises cesarean section (usually classical) followed by removal of the uterus. It is a procedure which also gives protection against infection, since it removes the infected organ. Obviously, however, it is a most undesirable operation in younger women, and obstetricians try to avoid it whenever possible. It may become necessary, however, in certain cases of premature separation of the placenta and in patients who have multiple fibroid tumors of the uterus.

Preparations for cesarean sections are similar to those for any other abdominal operation. The most common postoperative complication is abdominal distention, and the nurse must watch for this and report it at once. The obstetrician will direct the treatment, which probably will include enemas, insertion of a rectal tube, and frequent turning of the patient from side to side. Today in some hospitals patients delivered by cesarean section are allowed early ambulation (12 to 72 hours following operation), depending on the routine advised by the obstetrician.

It is well to remember that the patient who has had a cesarean section has had both an abdominal operation and a delivery. She will suffer from the discomforts of both. In addition to the abdominal and intestinal distress to be expected, she may have "after-pains," engorgement of the breasts, and the emotional reactions which accompany a normal delivery. It may be difficult to nurse the baby, but an effort should be made to encourage breast feeding, both because the baby needs breast milk and because the maternal processes need this stimulation.

It is important that satisfactory intestinal elimination be established before any solid food is given or any increase in diet is made. The patient needs fluids, but the increase will depend upon the presence of nausea and vomiting and her elimination. Any other care will be similar to that given to any operative or postpartum patient.

DESTRUCTIVE OPERATIONS

Destructive operations (designed for the most part to reduce the size of the baby's head and thus expedite delivery) are rarely done in modern obstetrics; and with the possible exception of hydrocephalic infants, they are never performed on a living child. Even in large maternity hospitals several years may pass without a single destructive operation. This salutary state of affairs is attributable in part to the widespread extension of prenatal care, in part to better management of women in labor, and in part to the recent perfection of the extraperitoneal cesarean section which makes it reasonably safe to effect abdominal delivery even in neglected cases. In the event a destructive operation is necessary, the obstetrician will choose the necessary instruments.

INDUCTION OF LABOR

By the induction of labor is meant the artificial bringing on of labor after the period of viability. This may be attempted by medication, by instrumental means, or by a combination of both methods. Toxemia of pregnancy is the most frequent reason for the procedure, since in this disorder continuation of pregnancy is often fraught with considerable danger to both mother and infant. Labor is also induced occasionally in patients who have gone beyond their calculated date of confinement and whose babies are large.

Medicinal Induction. This is not an operation but is considered here because many obstetricians employ it as a preliminary step to instrumental induction. It consists in the administration of one or two ounces of castor oil followed by the administration of a hot soapsuds enema as soon as the castor oil has acted. It is believed that the intestinal peristalsis produced by the cathartic is somehow transferred to the uterus with the consequent initiation of uterine contractions. Some obstetricians may supplement the above procedure with small doses of quinine sulfate, while others may follow it with minute injections of pituitary extract, but many prefer to limit medicinal induction simply to the castor oil and the enema. Whether or not quinine and pituitary extract are included, medicinal attempts to induce labor fail in over half the cases. As a preliminary to operative induction, however, they seem to sensitize the uterus and make it more responsive to the instrumental methods described below.

Artificial Rupture of the Membranes. This is today the most common method of inducing labor. It is accomplished after placing the patient in the lithotomy position and carrying out full antiseptic preparation of the vulva as for delivery. The

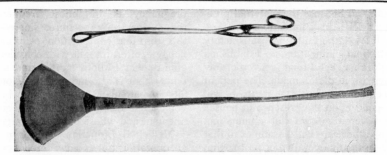

FIG. 241. Voorhees bag (made in three sizes) for dilation of the cervix. The bag is rolled up and held in a sponge forceps when inserted.

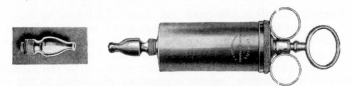

FIG. 242. Metal syringe used to fill Voorhees bag after it has been inserted. (Becton-Dickinson Company)

first two fingers of one hand are inserted into the cervix until the membranes are encountered. The cervix is stretched gently, and the membranes are stripped from the region of the internal os. A long hook, similar to one blade of a disarticulated vulsellum tenaculum, is inserted into the vagina, and the membranes are simply hooked and torn by the tip of the sharp instrument. As much fluid as possible is allowed to drain. Anesthesia is seldom necessary in multiparae, occasionally in primigravidae. As noted above, it is common practice to precede the actual puncture of the membranes with castor oil and a hot enema. Provided that the patient is near term, with other conditions favorable, artificial

rupture of the membranes will almost always initiate labor within a few hours.

Bag Induction. There are several other methods of inducing labor which may be chosen by the obstetrician under special circumstances. Thus, labor is sometimes induced by means of a rubber bag distended with water. These bags are of several types, the one commonly used being the Voorhees bag. All varieties come in sets of various sizes, and the largest that can be inserted is passed into the cervix and slowly distended with water, using a glass or metal syringe. The water should be warm (110° F.) and always must be sterilized by boiling, so that if the bag bursts it will not lead to in-

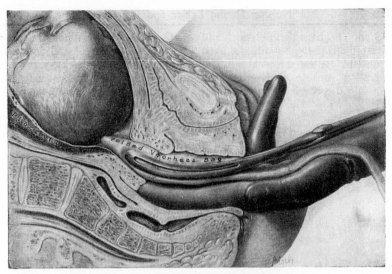

FIG. 243. Insertion of Voorhees bag.

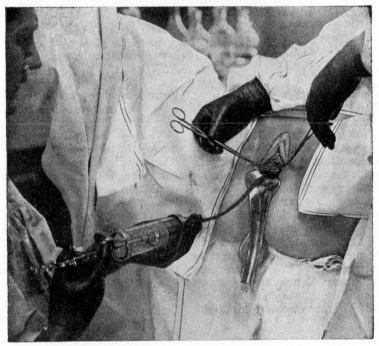

FIG. 244. Method of inflating bag (Shears).

fection. The bags themselves should be sterilized. Before sterilizing, each bag should be tested for leakage. The operation consists of inserting the bag into the cervix by means of an

Other Methods. When the pregnancy is between 20 and 28 weeks duration, Braxton-Hicks version is often the method of choice for the induction of labor. Packing the cervix

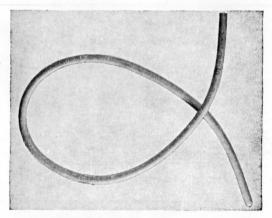

Fig. 245. Solid rubber bougie, 18 inches long, for inducing labor. The entire piece of tubing is inserted. (Bellevue Hospital, New York)

ordinary sponge-holder. The bag should be rolled or folded as compactly as possible, so that there are no rough surfaces, and held securely between the blades of the sponge-holder. It is then introduced well within the cervix and distended with water or some antiseptic solution.

Bougie Induction. Occasionally, labor is induced by introducing a bougie into the uterus. This is introduced between the membranes and the uterine wall where it acts as an irritating foreign body, and initiates contractions. Bougies are used much less frequently today than formerly. and the lower uterine segment with

gauze is another procedure which is used occasionally to induce labor.

So far as the nurse is concerned, these obstetric operations do not differ greatly from any other surgical operations. The direction of these operations is entirely the responsibility of the physician, and the nurse's share consists of these three responsibilities: (1) having everything in readiness beforehand, (2) giving reassuring advice to the patient and her family and (3) making sure that no opportunity is lost in rendering all possible assistance to the doctor.

SUGGESTED READING

Brierton, John F.: Rupture of the pregnant uterus, Am. J. Obst. & Gynec. 59:113, 1950.

Broomes, E. L. C.: Full term abdominal pregnancy with the delivery of a living child, J.A.M.A. 145:399, 1951.

Cosgrove, Robert A.: Management of pregnancy and delivery following cesarean section, J.A.M.A. 145:884, 1951.

Cosgrove, S. A., and Waters, E. G.: Cesarean section. An evaluation of extraperitoneal cesarean section, Am. J. Obst. & Gynec. 52:237-247, 1946.

Douglas, R. Gordon, and Landesman, Robert: Recent trends in cesarean section, Am. J. Obst. & Gynec. 59:96, 1950.

Eastman, N. J.: The induction of labor, Am. J. Obst. & Gynec. 35:721, 1938.

Irving, F. C.: Ten years of cesarean section at the Boston Lying-In Hospital, Am. J. Obst. & Gynec. 50:660, 1945.

Manahan, C. P., Connally, H. F., Jr., and Eastman, N. J.: The experience of the Johns Hopkins Hospital with cesarean section, Am. J. Obst. & Gynec. 44:999, 1942.

Weinberg, Arthur: Midforceps operations, J.A.M.A. 146:1465, 1951.

CONFERENCE MATERIAL

1. How would you reassure a patient who was contemplating a hospital delivery concerning the identification methods for the newborn?

2. How would you help the patient who is having her first baby to "face" the experience of labor and delivery with less fear and apprehension?

3. If the patient goes into labor having made no arrangements for the care of her 2-year-old girl and her 12-year-old boy, what is the responsibility of the public health nurse or the hospital social service?

4. How can the public health organization in the community cooperate with the hospital in helping the patient to prepare for her delivery?

5. Why is prophylaxis for the eyes of the newborn required by law in most states? How would you go about finding out which states in the United States have passed this law?

6. How does the use of penicillin as prophylaxis compare with the use of silver nitrate?

7. What are the regulations established for working mothers and the length of time granted for convalescence after delivery? Where could this information be found?

8. How much information should be presented to lay groups (home nursing classes) to prepare them to care for emergency deliveries?

9. If the patient has planned to be delivered by the "natural childbirth" method, what is the responsibility of the nurse during labor and delivery? How best will the nurse be able to gain the patient's co-operation?

Situation Questions

Read through the entire question and place your answers in the parentheses.

1. Give the term or the phrase which best fits each of the following:
A. Enlargement of the external os to 10 cm. in diameter. (_____)
B. Maximum shortening of the cervical canal. (_____)
C. A type of drug used in obstetrics which blots out memory of whatever occurs under its influence. (_____)
D. A condition caused by failure of the uterine muscle to stay contracted after delivery. (_____)
E. A surgical incision of the perineum during second-stage labor. (_____)
F. Settling of the baby's head into the brim of the pelvis. (_____)

2. Many decisions are based upon the character, the frequency and the location of pain during labor.

A. In the case of a multipara, not in real labor but having false pains, check those items which most probably would serve to identify false labor pains.
   1. May begin as early as 3 or 4 weeks before the onset of true labor.
   2. Occur usually 3 or 4 days before the onset of true labor.
   3. Occur at regular intervals.
   4. Occur at irregular intervals.
   5. Are confined to the lower abdomen and the groin.
   6. Felt in high abdomen and back. (_____)

B. In the case of a primigravida in the beginning of the first stage of labor, check those items which most accurately would describe her labor pains.
   1. Occur at regular intervals.
   2. Occur at irregular intervals.
   3. Are confined to lower abdomen and groin.
   4. Located in small of back and abdomen.
   5. Occur at intervals of from 2 to 3 minutes.
   6. Occur at intervals of from 10 to 15 minutes. (_____)

C. In the case of a primigravida, in the final part of the first stage of labor, check those items which would most accurately describe her labor.
   1. Pains occur at regular intervals.
   2. Pains occur at irregular intervals.
   3. Less than a minute between pains.
   4. Pains occur at intervals of from 2 to 3 minutes.

    5. Duration of pains of from 45 to 60 seconds.

    6. Duration of pains from 50 to 100 seconds.

    7. First stage terminates after an average of 11 hours.

    8. First stage terminates after an average of 16 hours. (_____)

3. Labor is divided into the first, the second and the third stages.

  A. When is the first stage of labor considered to be terminated?

    1. When pains occur at 10- to 15-minute intervals.

    2. When the cervix is completely dilated.

    3. When the baby is delivered. (_____)

  B. When is the second stage of labor considered to be terminated?

    1. When the cervix is completely dilated.

    2. When pains occur at 2- to 3-minute intervals.

    3. When the baby is delivered. (_____)

  C. When is the third stage of labor considered to be terminated?

    1. When the baby is delivered.

    2. When the placenta is delivered.

    3. After the uterus has remained firm for 1 hour. (_____)

4. During the first stage of labor, unfavorable conditions which would cause the nurse to notify the physician would be:

  A. Elevation in temperature

  B. Plugs of blood-streaked mucus in vaginal discharge

  C. Bright blood in small amounts

  D. Pulse rate of 96

  E. Fatigue

  F. Continuous desire to urinate

  G. Sudden flow of water

  H. Passage of meconium

  I. Fetal heart rate of 140

  J. Chill (_____)

5. On admission of the patient to the obstetrical department, check those procedures which are usually carried out routinely:

  A. Check temperature, pulse, respiration and blood pressure.

  B. Direct patient to bathroom and have her void.

  C. Give patient tub bath.

  D. Cleanse, shave and disinfect vulvar and perineal area.

  E. Check fetal heart sounds.

  F. Prepare patient for vaginal examination. (_____)

6. Often it is the nurse's responsibility to decide when the patient shall be moved from the labor room to the delivery room. Which of the following signs signify that the second stage is very near?

  A. Patient has desire to urinate.

  B. Patient has desire to defecate.

  C. Patient begins to bear down with her pains.

  D. Pains occur at 5-minute intervals.

  E. Increase in amount of blood-stained mucus.

  F. Large amounts of bright-red blood.

G. Bulging of the perineum.

H. Pains last for 45 seconds.

I. Rupture of the membranes.

J. Emesis.   (_____)

7. A physician was busy draining mucus from the mouth of the baby immediately after its birth and asked the nurse to let him know as soon as the placenta seemed to be separated. Which of the following would indicate that it was separated?

A. Gradual rise of uterus into abdomen.

B. Gradual descent of uterus farther into pelvis.

C. Protrusion of several more inches of cord.

D. Softening of contracted pear-shaped uterus.

E. More firm, rounded uterus.

F. A sudden gush of blood.

G. Large clots of blood slipping out.   (_____)

8. A patient who was in a very poor condition hemorrhaged badly as soon as the baby was born. The physician immediately handed the baby over to the nurse to care for, as his every attention was needed to save the mother's life. In this emergency, the nurse should do some of the following. Indicate by numbering in order the sequence in which she should perform the necessary acts: (Assume sterility.)

A. Affix a clamp on the umbilical cord.

B. Affix two clamps on the umbilical cord close together.

C. Rub the baby's back carefully to stimulate crying.

D. Slap the baby's back sharply to stimulate crying.

E. Slap the baby's buttocks sharply to stimulate crying.

F. Wipe the nose and the external mouth to remove any fluid.

G. Hold baby up by his feet over a table.

H. Wait until pulsation in cord ceases.

I. Blow into baby's mouth if respirations do not start readily.

J. Wipe mucus out of the mouth with damp, sterile gauze.

K. Cut the cord between clamp and umbilicus.

L. Cut the cord so as to leave the clamp on the stump.

M. Wipe eyes with gauze moistened in boric-acid solution.

N. Adjust the infant so that he lies in a safe, warm bed.

O. Tie the stump within an inch of the navel.

P. Apply clamp to placental end of cord.

Q. Apply sterile dressing to stump.

R. Instill a drop of 1 per cent silver nitrate solution in each eye.

S. Wrap the infant in a blanket.

Additional steps:

T. Label baby for identification if in a hospital.

U. Watch heartbeat.

V. Watch cord.

W. Watch baby's color and breathing.

                                      (_____)

9. In addition to whatever the physician directs her to do during the first hour after the placenta has been expressed, if someone else cares for the baby, and the mother's condition is good, the nurse should do which of the following? (On the lines provided record any other duties not listed.)

A. Keep the patient warm and out of drafts.

B. Massage the fundus continuously.

C. Keep a hand on the abdomen over the uterus.

D. Administer one ampule of pituitary extract intramuscularly.

E. Cleanse the vulva and the perineum and the buttocks with antiseptic solution.

F. Apply sterile perineal pads.

G. Express clots that accumulate in the uterus.

H. _____

I. _____

J. _____   (_____)

10. Possibly the most dangerous stage of labor for the mother is the third stage because of the possibility of postpartum hemorrhage and shock.

A. Because there is a certain amount of blood loss, hemorrhage is said to take place when the loss reaches:

    1. 100 cc.

    2. 300 cc.

    3. 600 cc.   (_____)

B. The most common cause of postpartum hemorrhage is atony of the uterus. In a case of this type, the first thing to do is:

    1. Take a firm grasp on the uterus.

    2. Massage the uterus vigorously.

    3. Administer an oxytoxic drug.   (_____)

11. The doctor told the nurse to watch a patient during labor for evidence of a prolapsed cord which he feared might occur.

A. The nurse would consider that a prolapsed cord would be most likely to occur:

    1. During the second stage of labor.

    2. In breech presentation.

    3. If the presenting part was not engaged in the pelvic brim.

    4. If the amniotic sac were intact.

    5. If the mother were particularly fatigued.

    6. In a delivery by version.

    7. If the membranes had ruptured.

    8. In a multipara.   (_____)

B. If the nurse did discover the cord to be prolapsed, she should put the patient in:

    1. Knee-chest position

    2. Fowler's position

    3. The Trendelenburg position

    4. A prone position   (_____)

C. In addition, if the doctor is not present she may:
 1. Immediately wash the cord with warm antiseptic solution and re-place in vagina.
 2. Cover the cord with a wet sponge.
 3. Apply a clamp to the exposed cord and cover with a sterile towel.
 4. Keep the cord warm and moist by continuous applications of com-presses wrung from warm antiseptic solution.

D. The chief objectives of the emergency care given when prolapsed cord occurs are:
 1. To prevent cold air from prematurely stimulating respiration while the fetus is in the uterus. (_____)
 2. To prevent drying of the cord while it is still pulsating.
 3. To stimulate and restore circulation in the cord by vasodilation.
 4. To prevent or relieve pressure on the cord.
 5. To prevent the exposed cord from slipping back into the vagina.
 6. To prevent infection of the birth canal. (_____)

12. After the cervix is dilated the nurse should encourage the patient to:
A. Use the toilet facilities.
B. Remain in bed, and use the bedpan.
C. Use the bedpan on a chair close to the bed. (_____)

13. Frequently the patient is catheterized and given an enema during the progress of labor to:
A. Obtain a urine and a stool specimen.
B. Avoid straining as the patient bears down.
C. Prevent herniation of the underlying fascia. (_____)

Note: The key to the correct answers to these questions is given on page 644.

UNIT FOUR

NURSING DURING THE PUERPERIUM

ORIENTATION

The previous study of the generative organs should not only help the nurse to understand the progress of pregnancy and the development of the fetus but also should be a means of understanding how these organs and the various systems of the human body make the adjustment following this critical period of labor and delivery. The nurse must have the knowledge of the normal conditions, symptoms and changes of the puerperium in order to recognize the complications and the abnormalities that may follow. The patient will need surgical as well as obstetric care, and the nurse will have an opportunity to compare these two courses of study and to utilize her previous teaching. Her experience in medicine and surgery and in the operating room will be a very helpful background in carrying out the technics involved in the procedures necessary during the postpartum period. While pregnancy, delivery and the puerperium are all apparently normal physiologic processes, the nurse must be on the alert at all times for the ever-possible complications. This is especially important during the puerperium, because after the crisis of the delivery the attention of all concerned—the patient, the doctor and the nurse—is apt to be centered on the new baby. It must be remembered that the patient not only has to recover from the physical and mental strain and stress of pregnancy and delivery, but also has to make an emotional adjustment which includes the new baby. The nurse should seize this opportunity to emphasize to the parents that the mother, at the end of the in-bed period (be it home or hospital delivery), is then only entering her convalescent period. The mother now has a double responsibility, one to the new baby and one to herself. Too often convalescent care for the obstetric patient is neglected.

18

Normal Puerperium

DEFINITION

The puerperium (from *puer,* a child; and *parere,* to bring forth), also called the "lying-in state," is the period from the end of labor until the time when the genital organs and tract have returned to approximately their normal size and condition. This is about 6 to 12 weeks. Although this is a normal physiologic process, it is so near the borderline between health and disease that it must be watched carefully in order to avoid the development of any pathologic condition.

IMMEDIATE REACTION TO DELIVERY

Immediately after labor, the patient experiences a sense of exhaustion, normally followed by a feeling of relief. She usually passes from this state to sound and natural sleep.

Every effort should be made to encourage rest. The discomforts which may cause loss of sleep, such as after-pains, soreness of the vulva, hemorrhoids, etc., should be mitigated as much as possible.

A chill occurring immediately after labor is not uncommon. Such chills are due partly to nervous reaction and exhaustion, with a disturbance of equilibrium between external and internal temperature caused by the excessive perspiration in the stage of greatest muscular exertion, and partly to the sudden removal of the contents of the uterus from the abdominal cavity. A warm bed and hot-water bottles will do much to avoid this reaction.

The pulse shows a marked drop in frequency, due probably to greatly lessened arterial tension. The pulse count may be from 80 to 60 per minute. This is a favorable symptom; but a rapid pulse after labor may be an indication of shock or, possibly, of concealed hemorrhage.

The temperature of the patient ordinarily does not rise above 99° F., but occasionally a patient may have a somewhat higher temperature

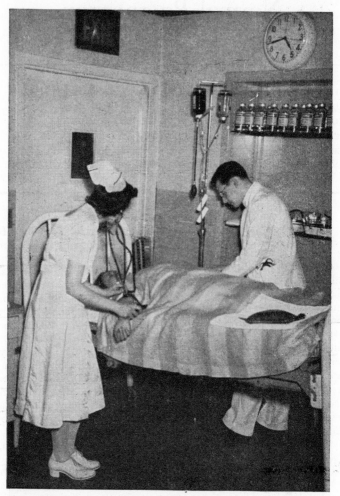

Fig. 246. Recovery room. (Millard Fillmore Hospital, Buffalo, N. Y.)

without ill effects. In judging the significance of the temperature, the pulse is the best guide; for in a puerperal patient with a slow pulse a slightly elevated temperature is not likely to signify a complication. Nevertheless, the nurse should report at once to the obstetrician a temperature of 100.4° F. or over or a pulse of over 100, and such a patient must be watched most carefully for the possible development of further unfavorable symptoms.

RECOVERY ROOM

In some hospitals a recovery room has been planned near the delivery room where there is access to any emergency treatment (Fig. 246). From the delivery room, the patient is transferred to the recovery room for several hours. Here she will be under the supervision of an experienced nurse who is responsible for reporting any departure from normal to the resident physician who is on call at all times. Reports from these hospitals state that their hemorrhage rate has definitely decreased due to this precautionary observation. In some hospitals the husband is permitted to stay with his wife during labor, to see the baby shortly after delivery and to see his wife as soon as possible.

PHYSICAL CHANGES

UTERUS

An understanding of the healing process by which the interior of the uterus becomes covered with a new lining membrane (endometrium) requires a description of the discharges, called "lochia," which are

eliminated from the uterus during this process. The separation of the placenta and the membranes from the uterine wall takes place through the outer portion of the spongy layer of the decidua, leaving the deepest or unaltered layer of the endometrium attached to the muscular wall, from which grows the new endometrial lining. The process is very like the healing of any surface, and there is oozing of blood from the small vessels on the surface—bleeding from the larger ones being controlled by compression of the retracted uterine muscle fibers and later by the formation of clots. As the oozing diminishes, the discharge becomes more watery or serous; as the new membrane (or endometrium in this case) grows over the whole surface, the discharge gradually ceases. With this discharge, or lochia, are cast off fragments of decidua and any small remnants of membranes that may have remained in the uterus. The lochia show these changes, and careful observation of the appearance and character is of the greatest importance as an index of the progress of the healing of the endometrial surface.

The Lochial Discharge. At first the lochia consist almost entirely of blood mixed with a small amount of mucus and particles of decidua which escape from the placental site. They should not contain large clots or membrane or be excessive in amount. This discharge lasts about 3 days, when it gradually changes to a pinkish color, due to the admixture of a considerable amount of serum from the healing surfaces. Toward the eighth or ninth day the lochia are thinner, less in amount, and of a brownish color with a characteristic stale odor; however, when the patient is out of bed for the first time there may be a definite increase in the discharge. By the end of the third week the discharge usually disappears, though a brown mucoid discharge may persist a little longer. The persistence of bright blood in the lochia, or the recurrence of fresh bleeding after the discharge has become dark and diminished in amount, should be reported to the obstetrician.

The lochia should never, at any time, have an offensive odor. The nurse should remember, however, that the discharge possesses a peculiar animal emanation which is quite characteristic. In quantity the lochia vary greatly with individuals, being more profuse in multiparae than in primiparae and with the mother who does not nurse her baby.

Suppression of the lochial discharge may be caused by cold or by fright, grief or other emotion. Such suppression usually is associated with a relaxed condition of the uterine muscle and should be reported at once to the obstetrician.

If the patient has any unusual discharge, it should be saved for the obstetrician to inspect.

Involution of the Uterus. The uterus begins to return to its normal condition with the beginning of labor. This process is called "involution" and consists partly in the contraction of the uterus and partly in the changes in the endometrium. A large part of the latter is eliminated, not only in the discharge of blood and serum but also by means of the general circulation. The normal process of involution requires several weeks; and at the end of that time the uterus should begin to regain (as nearly as it ever will) its normal state. The uterus never returns exactly to the virgin state; but it may approach it very closely if the patient has had a normal pregnancy, labor and delivery, and no lacerations of the cervix.

Progress of Involution. Immediately after labor, the uterus reaches to the level of the umbilicus and weighs about 2 pounds. By the time involution is complete, the uterus has shrunk so much that it lies entirely in the pelvis and should weigh only a few ounces. This involution may be watched by observing the height of the fundus, which may be felt through the abdominal wall. Immediately after the birth of the placenta, the fundus is felt at the level of the umbilicus or at 5 or 5½ inches above the pubes; and 12 hours later it probably will be found a little higher. Day by day careful measurements will show that it is diminishing in size, so that at the end of 10 days or so it cannot be detected by abdominal palpations. The approximate rate of decrease in the height of the fundus is a little over half an inch a day (1 cm.). Observation of this rate of involution is very important; any marked delay, especially if accompanied by suppression of the lochia or retention of clots, should be reported to the obstetrician. In measuring the height of the uterus, care should be taken that the observations are made after the bladder is emptied, as a full bladder will raise the height of the fundus.

Subinvolution of the Uterus. "Subinvolution" is the term used to describe the condition which exists

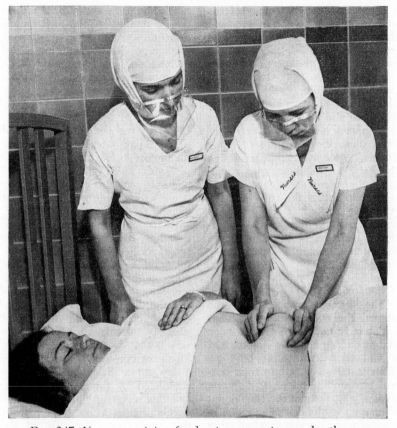

Fig. 247. Nurse examining fundus in puerperium under the supervision of a doctor. (Margaret Hague Maternity Hospital, Jersey City, N. J.)

when involution is not completed in the normal time. Poor muscle tone, general depletion, inadequate diet and lack of care may be contributing causes to this condition. Subinvolution is characterized by a large and flabby uterus, usually more or less chronically congested, which causes the patient much discomfort and disturbance of health until corrected.

After-pains. Normally, after delivery, the uterine muscle is in a state of contraction and retraction. This is an involuntary action of the muscle in an effort to expel the lochia and to return almost to its normal size. If there has been any marked distention or retention of blood clots, these contractions become active and are accompanied by pain. In multiparae a certain amount of tonicity of the uterine muscle has been lost, and these contractions and retractions cannot be sustained; therefore, the contraction and the relaxation of the muscle gives rise to the sensation of pain. These after-pains last from about 24 to 48 hours after delivery. They are also more noticeable after a pregnancy in which the uterus has been more distended than normal (twins or polyhydramnios). Putting the baby to the breast also stimulates the uterus to contract, and sometimes this is the only time the pains are noticed. When they are severe enough to disturb the patient's rest, the obstetrician should be notified, because a sedative may be necessary.

PELVIC CHANGES

The ligaments which support the uterus, the ovaries and the tubes which have undergone great tension and stretching are now relaxed, and it will take considerable time for them to return almost to their normal size and position. This is one reason why the patient should not remain up too long at one time. The vaginal walls, the vulva and all other tissues that have become hypertrophied during pregnancy also undergo a process of involution in their return to normal; and any abrasions and lacerations of the genital canal caused by the passage of the fetus should heal completely during the puerperium.

ABDOMINAL CHANGES

The abdominal walls recover partially from the overstretching during pregnancy. The striae usually remain. The abdominal muscles are often relaxed, and there may be a separation or diastasis of the recti muscle from the great distention during pregnancy. Rest, diet, prescribed exercise and good posture will do much to restore the tonicity of these muscles.

BREAST CHANGES

During the first, the second and the third days after the baby is born, the breasts secrete a small amount of yellowish fluid called "colostrum." Not until the third or the fourth day is the milk established. The amount of milk then increases rapidly; and, with the congestion that occurs at this time, the breasts often become tense, swollen, and sometimes painful. This congestion is caused not only by the pressure from the increased amount of milk in the lobes and the ducts but also from the increased circulation in the breast gland, producing a tension on the very sensitive surrounding tissues. This condition usually subsides after a day or two. Secretion is definitely stimulated by the baby's suckling, and this secretion will not continue for more than a few days without this stimulation. The care of the breasts at this time is very important.

ASSOCIATED CHANGES

DIGESTIVE

The digestive system shows some apparent reaction in that the appetite is diminished, probably due to the change in the digestive juices and the hydrochloric acid content of the stomach. As a result of the profuse perspiration and the loss of fluids during labor and delivery, the thirst is increased. In addition to the

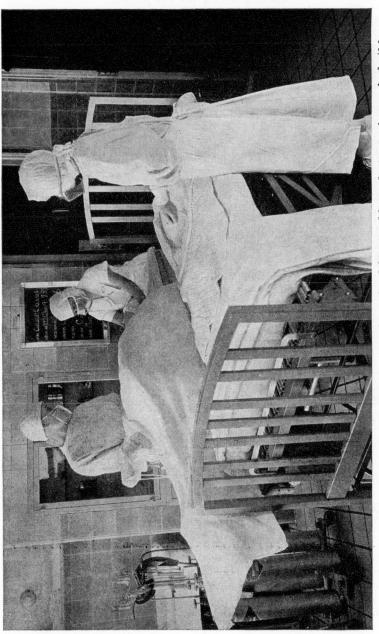

Fig. 248. Transferring the newly delivered patient from the delivery table to the patient's own bed. (Margaret Hague Maternity Hospital, Jersey City, N. J.)

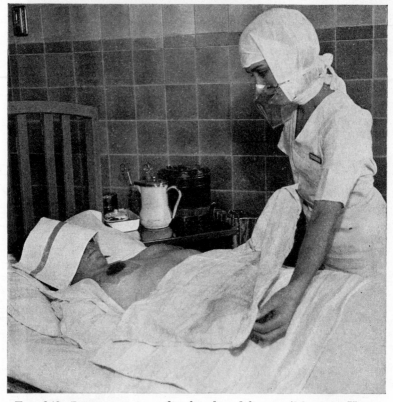

FIG. 249. Breast care immediately after delivery. (Margaret Hague Maternity Hospital, Jersey City, N. J.)

loss of weight at delivery, there is also the loss of weight during the puerperium due to the marked increase in excretions.

EXCRETORY

The excretory system is also affected by the result of labor and delivery. The release of the inter-abdominal pressure causes a relaxed condition of the intestinal and abdominal muscles and an inability to eliminate satisfactorily. It is also difficult for some patients to use the bedpan. The pressure on the rectum or tendency to hemorrhoids often causes discomfort during elimination. These conditions may be relieved by granting the patient bathroom privileges. Some obstetricians may order mild cathartics.

Pressure on the urinary meatus and the bladder during labor may produce an irritation and inflammation which inhibit any inclination to void. It is very important that the patient be urged to void shortly after delivery, for distention of the bladder interferes with uterine contractions and may cause postpartum hemorrhage. Early ambulation has minimized the need for catheterization.

Excessive perspiration during the puerperium is common, and night sweats may necessitate frequent changes of the patient's clothing and bed linen to prevent chilling and to add to her comfort.

POSTPARTUM EXAMINATION

The purpose of this examination is to determine with what normalcy the patient has completed her maternity experience. This examination, usually carried out about 6 weeks postpartum, should include a complete physical checkup, with special atten-

tion to the generative organs and the breasts, and should be checked with the initial prenatal examination, the results compared and the changes noted. This visit of the mother to her physician may have a definite relation to the patient's future health. If the nurse is conscious of the importance of this examination, it may be through her efforts that the patient will return to the obstetrician or the clinic. This return examination is an opportunity, too, for the patient to discuss with the obstetrician any symptoms or problems that she may have relating to her maternity experience. This 6 weeks' postpartum examination should be followed by another examination at the end of a year, at which time her system should have returned to normal. Many of the gynecologic ills may be entirely prevented or corrected when all patients realize the importance of this follow-up supervision.

SUGGESTED READING

Eastman, N. J.: Williams Obstetrics, New York, Appleton, 1950.

McLean, Lewis F., McDowell, H. C., and Sadugor, Marvin G.: The use of the recovery room in lowering maternal mortality, Am. J. Nursing 49:136, 1949.

19

Nursing Care During the Puerperium

INTRODUCTION

The observation and the nursing care of the patient during the puerperium is very important and is much the same as that which is given to a surgical patient. The difference, however, is that the nurse is responsible, not only for the comfort, the cleanliness and the nutrition of the mother but also for the procedures which are specifically obstetric, such as the breast care and the perineal care. In the hospital the nurse may not necessarily have the responsibility for both the mother and her new baby; nevertheless, the new baby must be considered in relation to this care. In the home the nurse will have the responsibility of both mother and baby. It should be remembered that the mother is not only adjusting physically from the experience of pregnancy, labor and delivery but is also making an emotional adjustment.

IMMEDIATE CARE

During the actual delivery of the baby and the third stage of labor, in all probability the nurse will be asked to observe the fundus by placing her hand on the patient's abdomen. This observation of the fundus is usually continued for an hour after the delivery of the placenta.

As a rule, the obstetrician prefers to be responsible for the fundus for the first 15 or 20 minutes. After this, the nurse will have the opportunity of making the patient comfortable. Some hospital routines include transferring the patient to her own bed while under the influence of the anesthetic or soon after delivery. However, before the patient is moved from the delivery room, there are certain nursing procedures to be followed. The patient should be bathed, made dry and comfortable; and special routines should be followed in the care of the breasts and the perineum. While giving this care, the nurse must always be on the alert for any changes in the patient's condition, such as her color, character of pulse, state of fundus and bleeding. After the temperature, the pulse and respiration have been taken, the patient is ready for the much-needed rest and sleep.

NURSING CARE

DAILY ROUTINE

The daily routine procedures for the postpartum patient vary in the different hospitals. However, certain details of the patient's care during this period should be noted every day, whether the patient is in the hospital or at home. These include the recording of the temperature, the pulse and respiration; observation of any changes in the breasts and the nipples; the character, the amount and the color of the lochial discharge; the height of the fundus; the condition of the perineal sutures, if any; and a record of the elimination, both intestinal and urinary. A report should also be made on how the patient sleeps and any emotional or nervous disturbances she may have. Attention should be paid to the patient's appetite and general

comfort. Many of these observations may be made during the daily bath. In addition, the nurse should note any deviations from the normal.

GENERAL CARE

Temperature, Pulse and Respiration. These routine records are usually made every 4 hours for the first few days; after that every night and morning, if the patient is progressing normally. If either the temperature or the pulse is above 100, the obstetrician should be notified.

Nutrition. The two factors which the nurse must bear in mind in arranging for the patient's diet are (1) the general nutrition of the patient and (2) providing enough nourishing food to stimulate the breast milk. If she has had nourishing food, the patient's convalescence will be more rapid, her strength will be recovered more quickly, the quality and the quantity of her milk will be better, and she will be better able to resist infections. The vitamin and mineral needs of the mother are even greater during lactation than they are during pregnancy (in pregnancy, 2,500 calories; in lactation, 3,000 calories). Foods which the patient knows from experience disagree with her should be avoided; but the old belief that foods, acid fruits particularly, will ensure colic in the infant is now much discredited. However, certain drugs may be excreted in the mother's milk. In addition to the regular food, the nursing mother should have at least 1½ quarts of liquid daily.

Rest and Sleep. After the exertions of labor, the patient should be encouraged to sleep and rest and she

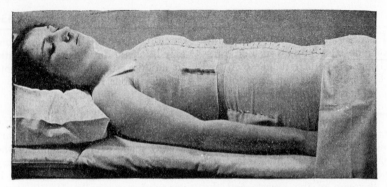

FIG. 250. Ace bandage. Breast binder, 8 inches wide, and an abdominal binder, 10 inches wide. (Becton-Dickinson Company)

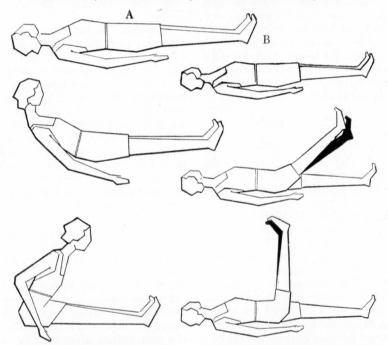

FIG. 251. Bed exercises. (A) Bed exercises for patients during the postpartum period; advised and regulated by the physician according to the individual patient's condition. These exercises are for the purpose of strengthening the abdominal muscles, preventing a pendulous abdomen, aiding involution and adding to the patient's general strength. (B) Both legs are slowly lifted to a position at right angles to the body, then slowly lowered. The legs are lifted alternately at first, and then both together. This series is repeated according to the physician's direction.

should be protected from worry. Making a patient comfortable and seeing that she is warm and has something hot to drink often bring the desired relaxation and sleep. Because of the routine peculiar to the nursing mother, emphasis should be placed on sleeping or relaxing whenever possible. Visitors, too, should be limited. A patient who is sleepless is always a source of anxiety. Septic conditions and mental disturbances are often preceded by sleeplessness, and marked or prolonged sleeplessness should be reported to the obstetrician. *only for hemorr* *of blood of bud*

Abdominal Supports. The abdominal binder is advised by some obstetricians and discouraged by others. A moderately firm binder, well applied, is a great comfort to some patients during the first day or so after delivery, for it permits turning without the disagreeable sagging sensation of the enlarged and heavy uterus. The reason for discontinuing the binder after the first day or so is that some obstetricians believe that it interferes with involution.

The binder, usually applied while the patient is in bed, is one made of unbleached muslin. The wide, 10-inch Ace bandage is also used with success. In an emergency a very good binder may be improvised from towels. Unless the binder is applied to give support, it is of little value. When the patient is first allowed out of bed, even for a short time, a snugly fitting abdominal support is not only a comfort but also prevents fatigue.

Exercise. Some physicians are now advising certain bed exercises during the puerperium to strengthen the abdominal muscles, to promote in-

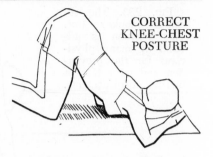

CORRECT
KNEE-CHEST
POSTURE

Chest on couch, bed, or floor. Knees apart. Thighs vertical. After taking posture external parts are drawn open to allow air to enter. (It escapes on return to upright posture.)

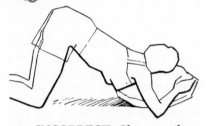

INCORRECT—Chest on pillow, thighs slant away from body.

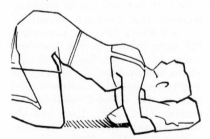

INCORRECT—Resting on elbows, thighs slant inward toward body.

Fig. 252. Knee-chest position may be advised if the uterus has not returned to its almost normal position.

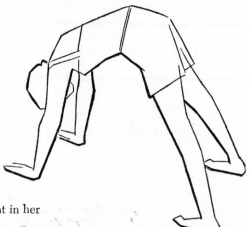

Fig. 253. The so-called monkey trot. This position is advised by many physicians for the prevention and correction of uterine displacements.

volution and to aid the patient in her convalescence.

Others are not emphasizing this routine but advise their patient during the early postpartum period to change her position often—lying on the side, taking the Sims' position (Fig. 128) and, later, lying on the abdomen and raising the head. Another exercise is to have the patient lie flat on her back with the top covers well tucked in at the foot and raise first one foot then the other, resisting the bedclothes. The next day she makes the effort to raise both legs at once in the same manner. The resistance offered by the bedclothes helps to accomplish the same results as the exercises. Later in the puerperium, if the uterus is retroverted, the obstetrician may recommend the knee-chest position for five minutes morning and evening (Fig. 252). Later the obstetrician may advise the "monkey trot" exercise (Fig. 253). If the patient has had an abnormal delivery or any extensive perineal repair, exercises may not be advisable. However, all exercises are advised by the doctor.

Bathing. The daily bath is refreshing, relaxing and stimulating, as well as a source of comfort to the patient. She may derive benefit from taking her own bath. This applies, of course, only if she has had a normal delivery and no repair has been necessary.

Elimination (Urinary). If the patient is allowed early bathroom privileges, urinary elimination may present no problem. However, the patient should be encouraged to urinate within the first 6 hours after delivery. This is of extreme importance, as a full bladder is considered one of the causes of postpartum hemorrhage. Every effort should be made to avoid the use of the catheter, because of the danger of infection, because there is a certain amount of soreness of the external genitals and also because catheterization tends to delay the time when natural urination can be accomplished. Within the first 6 hours efforts may be needed to excite normal urination. With some patients the presence of another person in the room interferes with concentrating and thus prevents urination. In such cases the nurse should leave the room after she has made the patient comfortable, telling her when she is to return or giving her a bell so that she will not be diverted by the sudden, unannounced return of the nurse. If these suggestions are not successful, the nurse may try the effect of the sound of running water, either letting water run from a faucet or pouring water from one pitcher to another. A partly filled hot-water bottle placed over the bladder while the patient is on a bedpan is another device often used with success. Using aromatic spirits of ammonia in the bedpan, or inhaling smelling salts, may sometimes provide the necessary stimulation. Sometimes just grasping a piece of ice in the hand helps. Irrigation of the external genitals is often stimulating.

Occasionally, a warm saline enema will relax the urethra, but the obstetrician should be consulted before giving an enema. Often the patient's inability to void is due to the fact that she is not accustomed to using the bedpan and would have this difficulty in using one at any time. This may be lessened by a sitting position, and the physician may allow the patient to be assisted to this position, if she has not a serious laceration.

As a distended bladder is fairly common during the puerperium, the nurse should make this one of her routine observations of the patient. She should offer the patient a bedpan at intervals and measure the urine at each voiding during the first few days. When a solution is used for cleansing the patient, it should be measured so that the amount of urine passed may be definitely ascertained.

CATHERIZATION. If the patient can once be made to void by voluntary effort, the subsequent use of the catheter should not be necessary; whereas, if the catheter has once been used, it may be necessary to continue its use for days. This increases the likelihood of infection of the birth canal, as well as of the urinary tract; this is because the urethral mucous membrane has been bruised by the enormous pressure to which it has been subjected, its resisting power is diminished, the vulvovaginal secretions abound in bacteria, and lochial decomposition soon begins.

Catheterization is a procedure demanding aseptic technic, because of the extreme danger of introducing bacteria into the bladder, and should not be done without an obstetrician's order. In preparing for catheterization, the patient should be warmly covered and draped as for a vaginal examination. If the patient's knees are supported at their outer sides by pillows, it adds greatly to her comfort. The light should be placed in an advantageous position. The tray should be conveniently located and should include the following items.

Sterile catheter dish (with cover) containing 1 thumb forceps, 2 rubber catheters (Fr. No. 16), 2 large cotton balls.
Sterile jar (with cover) 3⅛" x 2½" containing 5 small cotton balls.
2 curved basins 12" (1,000 cc.).
1 paper bag.
Towel.
Alcohol lamp and culture tube, if

specimen is to be taken for culture.

Technics vary in different hospitals, but in all cases extreme care must be taken to bring nothing unsterile in contact with the meatus. In general, the nurse prepares the patient as for a vaginal examination, except that the inner surface of the labia is carefully bathed with the cotton balls soaked with the green soap solution, using only downward strokes. Each cotton ball should be used only once. The meatus should receive special attention by sponging it carefully, using several pledgets. This is done just before the catheter is passed. The rounded end of the catheter always should be inspected before inserting to see that it is not broken or rough. It is dipped into sterile water or a lubricant and inserted very carefully 2 or 3 inches into the urethral opening, making sure that the other end of the catheter is draining into the sterile basin. Before withdrawing the catheter, palpate the fundus to see that the bladder is empty; then place one finger over the opening in the end of the catheter and remove it very slowly and gently (Fig. 171).

Intestinal Elimination. Because of pressure on the intestines during labor, the puerperal patient is almost always constipated. While obstetricians' orders vary, it is common to give an enema or a cathartic on the second morning after delivery. The physician may order a laxative that the patient ordinarily uses. If castor oil is ordered, it should be administered in the least objectionable way, e.g., in a glass with lemon in the

bottom and on top of the dose, or with soda and fruit juice. If cracked ice is given to the patient to hold in her mouth a few seconds, the medication is more easily taken. An oil enema followed by a soapsuds enema is sometimes ordered, especially where there has been a third-degree laceration and there has been no elimination for 3 or 4 days. A teaspoon of peroxide may be added to a pint of water in the soapsuds enema, as this breaks up the feces, making the material much softer and easier for the patient to expel. After the preliminary cathartic, there should be daily intestinal elimination.

EARLY AMBULATION

Out of necessity, there often develop routines and technics that change our former concepts. In such manner early ambulation came into being. During World War II, when there was a dearth of doctors and nurses and a shortage of hospital beds, patients were discharged from some hospitals after a stay of only 3 or 4 days or even less. To accomplish this state for release, patients were allowed out of bed 12 to 19 hours after delivery, with full bathroom privileges after 48 hours.

Although this abbreviation of hospital stay was an expedient introduced to meet special conditions, experience with this program has shown that it possesses certain intrinsic advantages for the mother. Patients seem to get their strength back more quickly and appear to be stronger on the sixth or the seventh day than they used to be on the twelfth or the fourteenth under the old regimen. It was found that with this increase in exercise for the newly delivered mother her circulation was stimulated, and there seemed to be practically no patients who needed catheterization. There were fewer complications of thrombophlebitis and morbidities of unknown etiology. Moreover, gastrointestinal function becomes more active with early ambulation, with the result that abdominal distention and constipation are less frequent.

The hospitals accepting early ambulation set up their individual routines and practices, such as the following:

1. The patient is "up and out" almost immediately.

2. Twelve hours, or the first day after delivery, the nurse assists the patient out of bed to stand and then circle the bed for 5 minutes, allowed to walk but not to sit. The following day the "time up" is increased to 20 minutes. Perineal care is given through the third morning, and then the patient is taught "self-perineal care." The patient is discharged after the fifth day.

3. After 48 hours the patient is allowed to stand for 1 minute but not permitted to dangle her feet from the side of the bed. Activity is increased each day, and the patient is discharged the seventh or the eighth day. Patients who have undergone cesarean sections usually are allowed up on the third or the fourth day and are discharged from the hospital about the tenth day.

4. About 19 hours after delivery the patient is assisted to stand and walk to a near-by chair to sit for 3 minutes. She is encouraged to be active in bed. Out-of-bed periods are increased gradually, and the patient is permitted to be up longer and do more walking. By the third day the patient is up at least 2 hours and is allowed bathroom privileges.

After labor the uterus is large and heavy, and the abdominal and pelvic muscles are stretched and relaxed; therefore, before the patient is allowed out of bed all day the fundus of the uterus should have disappeared behind the symphisis pubis (about 10 days); the lochia should be scant and not bright in color; the temperature and the pulse rate should be normal; and the patient should be sleeping and feeling well. It must be remembered, also, that pregnancy and labor are followed by the further responsibility of nursing and caring for the baby.

Nurses with public health experience will be concerned, no doubt, with what happens when the mother of the family returns home, not to convalesce as she should, but to assume at once the full responsibility of her family. The baby will need at least 7 hours a day of her time, and she may have to care for several young children. There will be household tasks, such as cooking, cleaning, washing and ironing, and all the other details that concern the upkeep of a home.

While many obstetricians are enthusiastic about early ambulation, this attitude is by no means unanimous, and the nurse will find various policies in vogue, both in regard to the time of getting up and the time of going home. Early ambulation under control seems to be reasonable and good, presupposing good pre-natal and delivery care. Mothers should be cautioned to proceed slowly in the postpartum period at home, resting a large part of the time. The mother will need house-hold help to take over the major responsibilities for 2 or 3 weeks. Teaching for this "getting back gradually" needs to begin early in the prenatal period, and plans for care should be made at that time. Fatigue and apprehension are the mother's main enemies, and much more help should be given to pre-pare her for this period. Here is where the public health nurses may make a great contribution in the fol-low-up supervision of these patients.

SPECIAL PROCEDURES

PERINEAL CARE

There is much discussion concern-ing the best way of caring for the perineum during the first days after delivery. Hospital technics differ greatly; a very good one from the Sloane Hospital for Women follows:

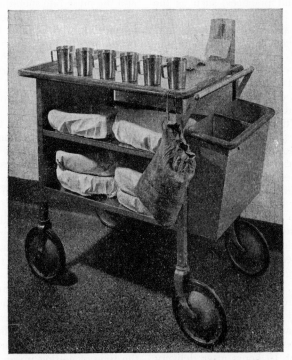

FIG. 254. Dressing carriage for perineal care. (Sloane Hospital for Women, New York)

PERINEAL CARE

Purpose:

1. To prevent infection of perineal wound
2. To promote healing of perineal wound
3. To cleanse perineum and external genitalia
4. To make patient comfortable
5. To prevent irritation of external genitalia from vaginal discharge

When Used:

Perineal care is given to both antepartum and postpartum patients.

1. Complete perineal care every morning; following voiding, defecation or enema
2. P.r.n. if perineum is inflamed or patient is uncomfortable from profuse discharge or complains of burning
3. Every 4 hours if patient is on third degree care (through 5th day), then p.r.n.
4. At other times during the day, following urination, the pitcher douche is omitted. The patient is dried with cotton balls, the bed pan is removed and a sterile pad is applied to the perineum.

Equipment:

1. Sterilized bedpan with clean cover
2. Sterile 500 cc. graduate with 400 cc. of warm tap water
3. Paper bag for waste
4. Package with dressing and three cotton balls
5. Clean fundus belt and two safety pins

Preparation:

1. Put on mask, roll up sleeves and remove watch
2. Wash and dry hands
3. Take all equipment to bedside. Place bedpan on chair protecting the chair with the cover. Other articles on over-the-bed table.

4. Screen patient and lower the bed
5. Turn covers back and inspect abdomen, measure height of fundus and notice position of uterus.
6. Unpin the pad in front, have patient turn on side; unpin pad in back. Remove pad from front to back noting the amount, odor and type of lochia, then discard in the bag.
7. Place patient on the bedpan, elevate the head of bed and make patient comfortable.
8. Open the dressing package before leaving bedside.
9. Lower bed when ready to give perineal care.
10. Record height of fundus before voiding and amount, color and odor of lochial discharge.
11. Fill sterile graduate with 400 cc. warm * tap water. Test on wrist.

Procedure:

1. Wash hands thoroughly, using brush on fingernails only. Do not dry hands. Pick up pitcher of water and put it on the over-the-bed table.
2. Drape patient using contaminated hand and pour entire contents of pitcher over perineum, using the other hand for the dressing.
3. Dry labia with cotton ball, using downward stroke on one side of perineum. Discard cotton in paper bag and repeat on other side of perineum.
4. Remove bedpan; place on chair and cover.
5. Have patient turn on her side. Separate gluteus maximus. Cleanse area, using sponge to remove drainage from perineum as well as anal region. Inspect perineum after cleansing.

* This applies to New York City's water supply. Sterile water may have to be substituted.

6. With patient on her back, adjust the fundus belt and pin the pad first in front, then in back.
7. While bed is still lowered, measure fundus after voiding.
8. Close paper bag and carry all articles used to dressing cart. Invert graduate. Place bedpans on lower shelf, paper bag in waste container and clean wrapper in clean container. If urine is to be measured, a slip of paper with patient's name on it is placed on top of bedpan cover.
9. If patient has defecation, discard contents immediately in bedpan washer.
10. Wash and dry hands.

Record:
1. Height of fundus before and after voiding
2. Character of lochia, amount, type, odor. Note presence of clots, pieces of membranes, excessive bleeding and a relaxed or boggy uterus.
3. Amount of urine
4. Condition of perineum. Tenderness of abdomen.

Care of Equipment:
1. Wash bedpans, place in sterilizer and boil for 10 minutes. Store in bedpan warmer. Wash pitchers and boil for 10 minutes in utensil sterilizer.
2. Place bags containing soiled materials in can and replace top. Save clean papers.

Procedure for Setting up Dressing Carriage:
It is more convenient to use a dressing cart when many dressings are to be done.

Preparation of Cart:
1. Put on mask, roll sleeves, remove watch, wash hands.
2. Place covered bedpans on lower shelves of cart.

3. On top shelf, place brown paper bags, clean fundus belts, packages of dressings and cotton balls, enema equipment, dressing list, and pencil.
4. When ready to do dressings, remove 500 cc. graduates from sterilizer. Place right side up on top of dressing carriage.

POINTS TO BE EMPHASIZED IN PERINEAL CARE

1. Both antepartum and postpartum patients receive same care.
2. Wash hands before beginning procedure and always between patients.
3. Assemble equipment to be used.
4. Never refuse patient a bedpan.
5. Patients should not be exposed unnecessarily. Instruct patient not to pin, unpin or adjust perineal pad while on q.4h. care.
6. Always leave patient comfortable.
7. Have patient flat in bed with arms at her sides when measuring fundus. Record findings immediately.
8. Have tap water at body temperature.
9. Cleanse area firmly but gently. Do not separate labia.
10. Separate gluteus maximus muscles to inspect perineum; cleanse area, using sponge from the perineum to anal region.
11. Apply pad from front to back. Pin ends of pad under the fundus belt.
12. Put all debris in paper bag supplied for this purpose.

SELF-PERINEAL CARE

Purpose:
1. To teach personal hygiene
2. To prevent infection

Articles Necessary:
1. Wicker basket or bag containing pads
2. Individual tissue

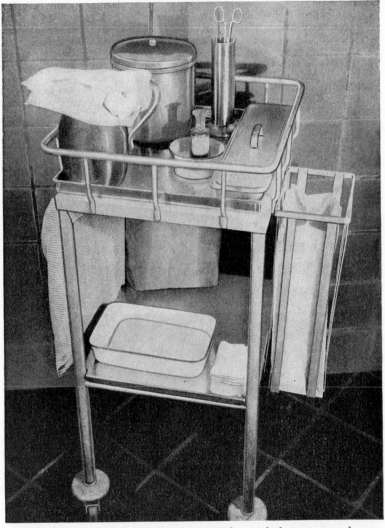

Fig. 255. Carrier for perineal care. This includes a covered tray with sterile forceps, tray for soiled forceps, covered can of cotton balls, receptacle for long dressing forceps (in sulfonaphthol solution 4%), covered pitcher ¾ filled with warm, sterile distilled water and enough sulfonaphthol solution to cloud the water (this solution to be in pitcher *only* at time of using) and a bag of sterile pads. (Boston Lying-In Hospital)

Procedure:

1. Take patient to bathroom. Show her where perineal pads are kept, and direct her to wash her hands.
2. Have patient unfasten pad, instructing her to remove it from front to back and place the pad in individual paper bag.
3. After voiding or defecation, pa-

tient cleanses herself from front to back with tissue, using a fresh piece for each stroke and discarding it in toilet. Flush toilet.
4. Demonstrate method for opening pad without contaminating the inner surface.
5. Instruct the patient to apply the perineal pad to the perineum,

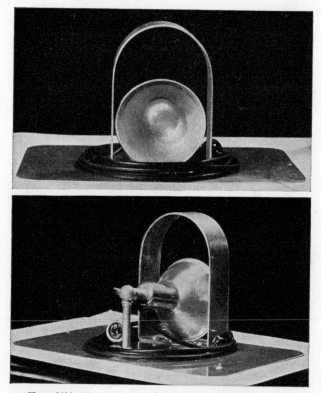

FIG. 256. Two views of a lamp designed for "light treatments" of the perineum. This lamp is equipped with a bracket which acts as a "cradle" over which the bedclothes may be supported. It is simple in design and inexpensive, especially practical for hospital or home use. The heat provided by such a lamp gives great relief in cases in which the perineal stitches are painful. The lamp was developed at the Western Reserve University Hospitals, Cleveland.

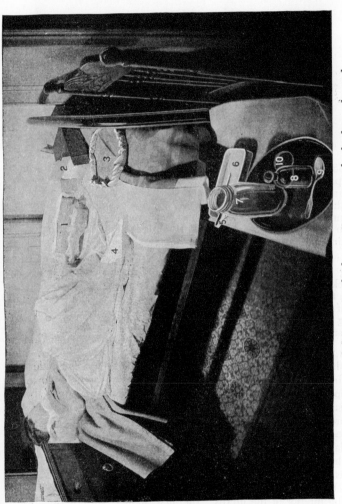

FIG. 257. Perineal dressing in the home. Patient on the bedpan draped.

1. Cotton in original package kept wrapped in a clean towel (towel open).
2. Perineal pads.
3. Paper pan for soiled pads and sponges.
4. Paper napkins on which to place clean pieces of cotton and perineal pad after the nurse has scrubbed her hands.
5. and 6. Sterile forceps in sterile basin.
7. Mason jar with prepared disinfectant. } on tray
8. Bottle containing disinfectant. } or plate
9. Spoon for measuring.
10. Tray or plate for jar, bottle, and spoon.

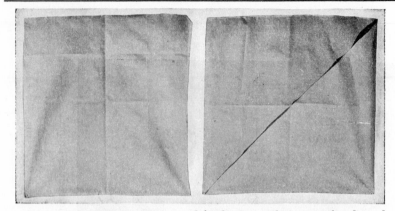

Fig. 258. Kneecaps. Front and back view. These may be draped over the patient's knees and used instead of sheet, thus saving time, laundry and rearranging of the sheet. A pair of kneecaps may be made of three 27-inch square diapers or 2¼ yards of unbleached muslin or flannelette 27 inches wide cut into squares. The third square is cut into two triangles and used for the insides of the two squares, thus making the "caps."

putting it on from the front to the back. Pin it in the front and then in the back. Place the gauze ends of the pad under the belt if using the fundus belt.

6. Wash and dry hands.

Physicians usually have special instructions which they wish carried out, and public-health organizations have developed routines which are used by nurses as guides in teaching the proper procedure to the patient's family. If the obstetric nurse realizes that, once labor is over, the chief danger to the puerperal patient is that of sepsis and that sepsis is due more to bacterial infection of raw surfaces in the interior of the uterus after the separation of the placenta and the membranes and to a lesser degree to lacerations of the cervix, the vagina and the perineum, she will understand why so much time has

been spent in evolving technics for the care of the perineum.

Steps in Perineal Care. The equipment should be prepared and arranged, and the patient should be screened. Place the patient in a dorsal position on the bedpan and drape. If a pillow is placed under her back she will be more comfortable. Remove the soiled dressings (always downward) and place them in the receptacle to be used for the soiled sponges. With sterile forceps take 5 pieces of sterile cotton and place them in a small sterile basin. Pour onto the cotton the antiseptic solution advised. Scrub the hands. Use the first sponge with a downward stroke over the vulva, then with the second and the third sponges cleanse between the labia majora and the labia minora, using one pledget on each side. Next, cleanse the center

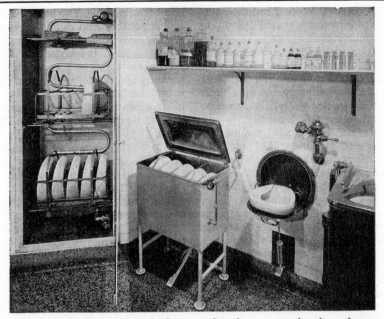

Fig. 259. After use, the bedpan is placed on a circular drop door—at the right. When the door is closed 7 gallons of cold water automatically flush the pan. It is then placed in a rack in the sterilizer. After sterilizing, the bedpan is kept warm in the closet where covers, etc., are also kept, as shown at extreme left. (Sloane Hospital for Women, New York)

of the vulva and the anus. The cleansing always is directed toward the rectum, each pledget being used for one stroke only. (If more sponges are needed, the cotton for them must be removed from the container with sterile forceps.) Apply the sterile pad and then remove the bedpan. Have the patient turn on her side; then dry the lower part of the back. Always leave the patient dry, tidy and comfortable. If she is soiled with profuse lochia on her thighs or back, she should be bathed with warm water and soap, for these parts do not have to be cleansed with the anti-septic solution. This procedure is used by many public health organizations for the care of the patient in the home.

BREAST CARE

The care of the breasts should be emphasized in the prenatal period (Chap. 8). Preventive measures consist in the preparation of the nipples during pregnancy, by cleansing and softening the nipples and supporting the breasts. In the very early postpartum period, this care includes the cleansing of the nipples before nursing, regulating not only the interval betwen feedings but the duration of the nursing period (from 3 to 5 minutes at first), and the proper position of the baby while nursing.

The breasts should be bathed daily with soap and water. The details of the technic used vary, but the objects of the care are always the same: to facilitate the baby's nursing, to add to the patient's comfort and to prevent sore nipples, which may lead to breast abscesses. According to some technics, the nipples should be cleansed with sterile water immediately before and after nursing. Clean pledgets should be used (hospitals use sterile pledgets); large swabs are very convenient for this purpose. Between nursings, each nipple may be protected by applying bismuth and castor oil paste and covered with a square of sterile glassine paper gently pressed against the nipple and held for a moment until the heat softens it enough to keep in place. These are discarded at nursing time, and generally the baby is allowed to nurse any remaining bismuth and castor oil from the nipple. The daily procedure at Sloane Hospital for Women and certain other hospitals is simply to wash the breasts at the time that the patient's daily bath is given. A breast towel is applied if there is any leakage. Short nursing periods are important in preventing sore nipples.

The Nursing Periods. The first nursing is usually after the mother has rested from the effects of labor and delivery. The mother should be made comfortable and the baby should be so placed that he is able to grasp the whole nipple rather than the end, for the nipple is delicate and easily injured by a baby's effort to catch hold. The baby should be comfortably held during nursing, making sure that his nose is not pressed against the breast, for this will make him drop the nipple repeatedly in order to breathe, and the extra manipulation necessary will often cause the nipples to become tender. Routines vary, but usually for the first 2 or 3 days the baby is not on the regular 3- or 4-hour schedule. This time element allows the nipples to become accustomed gradually to this manipulation.

When milk replaces the colostrum in the breasts (p. 426) they often become congested and tender. Breast feeding on a flexible schedule has become a part of the rooming-in method (p. 473).

Lactation. In endeavoring to increase lactation, the mother's health should be considered. Adequate rest, sleep, protection from worry, and diversion are essential. She should be shielded from grief, overwork or other causes of low vitality. Too much coffee should be avoided. Extra milk or cocoa should be taken between meals and at night before retiring. If too much milk disturbs the digestion, lime water or Vichy water may be added.

There is uncertainty regarding the value of galactagogues, which are foods or drugs used to stimulate breast milk. Certain patented foods are advised, but usually the well-balanced diet is more effective. Milk, cocoa, cereals (especially cornmeal) and a carbohydrate diet with large amounts of fluid may be suggested. Beets and all kinds of shellfish (especially crabs and oysters) are said to increase the quantity of milk to a marked degree. The tendency at present is to place emphasis upon stimulating the gland itself. The time to prepare for nursing the baby is during the prenatal period when the importance of diet, rest and general hygiene should be stressed. In the postpartal period, any emotional disturbance seems to have a very definite influence on the quantity and the quality of breast milk. Adequate nutrition during the lactating period conserves the health of the mother as well as providing the fundamentals for the health of the baby.

EFFECTS OF MENSTRUATION. Any change in the mother's milk during menstruation depends largely upon the amount of pain that the mother suffers at this time. Formerly, it was thought best to omit nursing entirely if the menstrual function returned during lactation, but today this is governed by the amount of pain that the patient suffers and by whether or not the baby is affected by the change in the breast milk during this time.

EFFECTS OF PREGNANCY. Should the mother become pregnant during this period, she should discontinue nursing her baby, for she cannot properly nourish herself, her baby, and the fetus in utero. This is too much of a strain for any individual, no matter how healthy she may seem to be.

Cracked Nipples. When a sore nipple is examined, it may be found to be fissured (cracked) or to have a small erosion (raw area). The primary treatment for either condition is rest, so as to avoid disturbing the nipple and to allow time for healing. In the majority of cases, a nipple shield (Fig. 261) may be used for

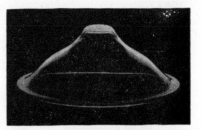

FIG. 260. Plastishields may be used in the routine postpartum breast care or for protection against external irritation, leakage or other factors. The shield is held in place by the patient's brassière or the usual hospital support. (Plastishields, Inc., Minneapolis)

FIG. 261. Anticolic nipple shield No. 773, frequently used in the treatment of cracked nipples. (Davol Rubber Co., Providence, R. I.)

protection and to allow the baby to continue nursing, but if there is any bleeding from the fissure or erosion, all nursing should be discontinued. Under such conditions, manual expression should be instituted to stimulate the breast and to relieve engorgement. The usual orders are to paint the fissure with a silver-nitrate stick after nursing; if there is a raw area, a paste of bismuth and castor oil, equal parts of each, may be applied. Other medications used are compound tincture of benzoin (applied with great care), balsam of

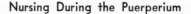

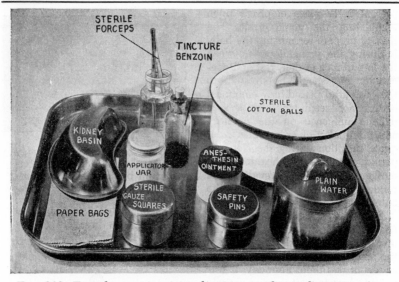

Fig. 262. Tray for use in giving breast care if complications arise.
(Sloane Hospital for Women, New York)

Peru, argyrol or alcohol. Many hospitals are now advocating the use of a thermalite (therapeutic) lamp for cracked or tender nipples; the afflicted breast is exposed for from 20 to 30 minutes morning and afternoon. Sore nipples should be watched very closely because very often they are the cause of breast abscesses.

Engorged Breasts. The lobules of the breast gland (Fig. 39) sometimes become distended, because the milk is not drawn off fast enough or else some of the milk ducts to the nipples are not clear or open. When the flow is interfered with, some part of the breast may become hard or "caked," while the rest of the breast is soft, or the whole breast may be engorged. This condition may be relieved and controlled by applying at intervals an ice cap over the affected area or by applying hot stupes to the breasts, especially before the nursing period. During this period of engorgement, a tight binder should be applied. These symptoms demand immediate treatment. After 2 or 3 days, the engorgement usually subsides. The regular emptying of the breasts by the baby's nursing and a comfortable support will then be all that is necessary. Nature usually makes the adjustment between the amount of milk secreted and the amount withdrawn. When the baby is not nursed for some reason, the whole breast may become engorged and painful, and a rise of temperature may accompany the condition.

Binders and brassières of various types may be used to support the breasts. The basic principle of them

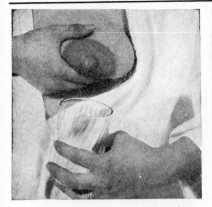

FIG. 263. First position in the expression of breast milk from a large, pendent breast, showing the thumb and fingers properly placed and pressing backward.

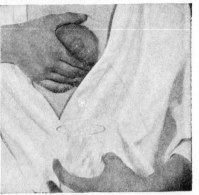

FIG. 264. Second position, showing the thumb and finger pressed deeply into the breast, at the same time compressing the breast well behind the nipple. This deeper pressure is necessary in a round, virginal-shaped breast.

all is the proper support of the whole breast in the natural position. When a breast is well supported, it not only is more comfortable but, if pendulous, the support aids in preventing congestion caused by the interference with the circulation (Fig. 250).

Preventive Measures. Too much emphasis cannot be placed upon the "preventive" measures in the care of the breasts. Abscess of the breast is very painful and often disastrous. Not only does it result in the suspension of nursing, with perhaps serious consequences to the baby, but it may destroy the functional activity of the breast and prevent the nursing of future babies. No one yet knows whether or not these breast conditions are a predisposing cause of carcinoma of the breast. The nurse should make every effort to recognize the early symptoms of breast compli-

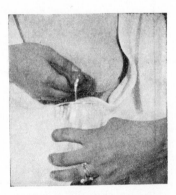

FIG. 265. Second position, showing compression of the breast between the thumb and fingers, well behind the nipple, and the milk coming in streams.

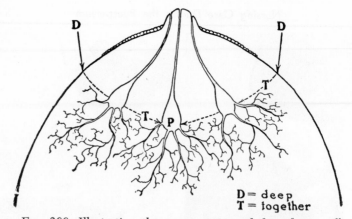

FIG. 266. Illustrating the movements needed to force milk out of the little pockets "P" in which it collects. Place a finger and a thumb on opposite sides of the nipple at "D" and "D." Press deeply into the breast in the direction of the black arrows. Then compress the breast together in direction of the dotted line toward point "P." This will force the milk out of the ducts in streams. "Deep" and "together" express in two words the motions required. (U. C. Moore, Nutrition of Mother and Child)

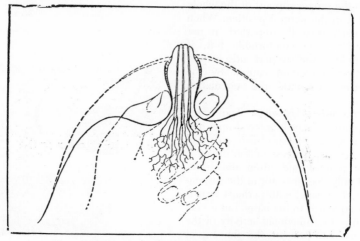

FIG. 267. Diagram showing the method of expressing the milk from the breast by compressing the milk pockets between the thumb and forefinger. The three unused fingers may be folded as indicated or used to support the breast. This represents the second or "together" motion. (U. C. Moore, Nutrition of Mother and Child)

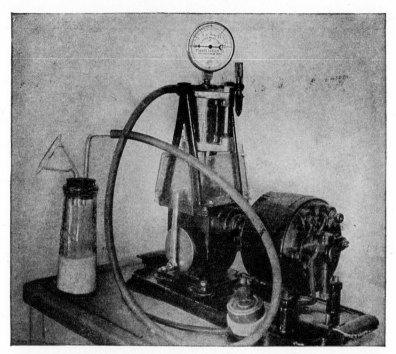

FIG. 268. Electric breast pump, using the principle of intermittent negative pressure. (Jeans, P. C., Rand, W., and Blake, F. G.: Essentials of Pediatrics, ed. 4, Philadelphia, Lippincott)

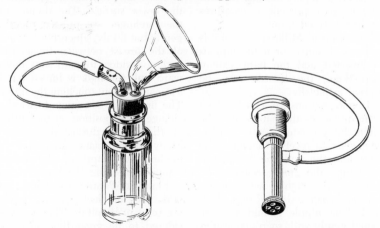

FIG. 269. Line drawing of a vacuum pump. This type of water pressure pump for the expression of breast milk may be used to great advantage in the home. (The Directory for Mother's Milk, Inc., Boston)

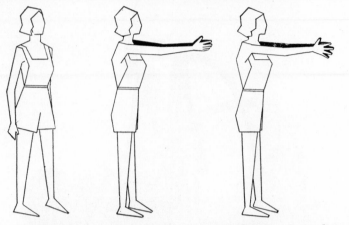

Fig. 270. Breast exercise. After breast feeding has been discontinued the breasts seem to be soft and flabby; these simple exercises may help to restore firmness of tissues. Stand with feet apart, toes turned in slightly, abdomen in and up, buttocks tucked under and head held high. Hold fingertips together, with arms at shoulder level. Press fingers together sharply and firmly. Relax and repeat ten times.

cations; the patient should also be instructed to report the first discomforts, so that preventive measures may be instituted at once.

Expression of Milk. If the baby is too weak to nurse, or if the nipples are inverted and the baby cannot grasp them, the breasts may be emptied artificially.

MANUAL EXPRESSION can be done by the nurse, or the patient may be taught this procedure. After sterilizing a glass to receive the milk, the hands and the nails of the person expressing the milk should be scrubbed thoroughly with warm water and soap and dried on a clean towel. The nipple should first be washed gently with soap and water, and then rinsed and dried. Then the breast is grasped gently just back of the areola, with the ball of the thumb in front and the forefinger beneath the lower surface. The thumb and the forefinger are pressed together gently but firmly, squeezing that part of the breast between them; then with a sudden forward and downward pull the milk is forced out in a stream without touching the nipple. The fingers do not move forward or change their position on the surface of the breast during the process. Many obstetricians advocate this method of emptying the breasts rather than using the breast pump.

ELECTRIC-PUMP EXPRESSION. Several types of electric breast pumps are used in hospitals. They are considered to be great time savers as well as useful in controlling the milk supply in the breasts. They are used

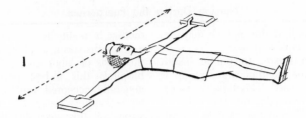

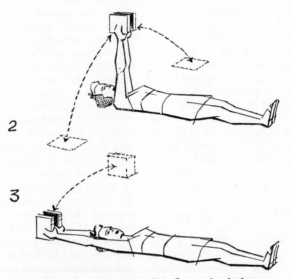

FIG. 271. Breast exercise. Lie flat on back, legs out straight in front, feet together, spine touching floor, keeping stomach flat. Breathe naturally. (1) Holding a book in each hand, stretch out arms level with shoulders. (2) Raise books slowly, keeping arms straight. Lower them just as slowly. (3) Raise books slowly again and carry them held together to floor over the head. Repeat. Stop all exercises before feeling tired.

mainly to increase the supply of milk, but in some cases they are advised for reducing engorgements, and with very gentle suction for fissured or sore nipples. Low suction will express the milk without discomfort or added injury to the nipple. For what-ever purpose the electric breast pump is used, the suction should be increased gradually to prevent irritation of the nipple and needless shock which might cause nervousness and retard the flow of milk. Some organizations lend electric breast pumps so that the mother may express her milk at home.

WATER PUMP. In public health nursing the vacuum water pump is sometimes used. This type of water-pressure pump for the expression of breast milk may be used to advantage in the home, especially where the mother has to express her milk and send it to the hospital.

BREAST EXERCISES. Patients are sometimes concerned about the temporary increase in the size of the breasts during lactation. When breast feeding has been discontinued the breasts soon approximate their previous size and firmness. However, there are exercises which, if done regularly, will help to hasten the return of the breasts to normal. These exercises should be limited at first and increased as the patient can tolerate them without fatigue.

CONVALESCING CARE

One of the most neglected phases of the present-day maternity care is the convalescing period. After the soul-stirring excitement of the delivery is over, if it has been more or less normal and the danger of complications is over or past, the major attention is more often than not directed to the baby. It is true that the normal obstetric patient appears to recover from her delivery with amazing rapidity, which may be accounted for by the fact that there is a great emotional reaction to the new baby which acts as a real stimulus. Besides, there is also born with the baby a responsibility for his protection and care which may add to this so-called stimulation. These facts help to obscure the fact that the mother in reality is recovering from a 9-months strain of pregnancy plus the crisis of labor and delivery. In hospitals this in-bed period is a generally accepted routine. In the home mothers today are more conscious of this necessity, but both groups neglect the following days of convalescence.

For the patient who has had a major surgical operation, there is a planned convalescent period, but for the obstetric patient little emphasis is placed on this convalescent care. Instead, the maternity patient arrives home, assuming more rather than less responsibility for her new baby, family and home. Convalescent care emphasizes the need for rest, nourishing food and protection from worry, which is almost imperative for the new mother. Parents seem to be under the impression that once the delivery is over, normalcy is restored almost immediately. However, it is agreed that it may be weeks before the generative organs have returned to their almost normal size and position, and months before the calcium loss has been restored. The emotional and endocrine adjustments may be even more delayed. Nurses may have the opportunity to emphasize this phase of care to the parents during the prenatal period so that better plans can be made to facilitate this very important phase of the maternity cycle.

Emphasis on care during the postpartum period should be made not only during the prenatal period but also during the hospital stay, at the time of dismissal from the hospital and at home. If the patient has been delivered in the hospital, ideally she should be discharged to a nursing agency for checkup care during her convalescence and before the post-partum examination. If nursing care is not available, the patient should be informed of what to expect at this time, with emphasis on the prevention of fatigue, apprehension about the baby, why she is physically below par and emotionally unstable, and anything that might cause nervous tension. The patient should be prepared for this formidable adjustment, especially the "slump" that occurs about 2 to 3 weeks or more after delivery. If, during the prenatal period, the parents have been taught how to handle and bathe the baby and some of the other important details of his care, they will have more assurance and self-confidence. If they have been given a source where they might telephone or write for answers to their questions, much of the apprehension and fear in connection with the new baby's care will have been bridged. Husbands who have accompanied their wives to parents' classes are so much more conscious of, and prepared for, this difficult period. Often they plan their time to be home to help assume some of the responsibilities. It is not so much the physical help that is needed as it is the cooperation gained by the partnership and the satisfaction of "sharing."

SUGGESTED READING

Adair, Fred L., Editor: Proceedings of the First American Congress of Obstetrics and Gynecology, Univ. Chicago Press, 1939.

——: Proceedings of the Second American Congress of Obstetrics and Gynecology, Univ. Chicago Press, 1942.

——: Proceedings of the Third American Congress of Obstetrics and Gynecology, Univ. Chicago Press, 1947.

Guerriero, William F.: Early Controlled Ambulation in Obstetrics, Proceedings of Third American Congress of Obstetrics, p. 81, 1947.

McCorkle, Mae: What is good postpartum care, Pub. Health Nursing (reprint), Dec., 1940.

Peck, Elizabeth: Perineal care after delivery, Am. J. Nursing 50:327, 1950.

Rosenblum, G., and Melinkoff, E.: Further studies in early puerperal rising, Am. J. Obst. & Gynec. 54: 325, 1947; also, J.A.M.A. 129:849, 1945.

20

Complications of the Puerperium

PUERPERAL INFECTION
HEMORRHAGE (See Chap. 16)
MASTITIS
BLADDER COMPLICATIONS

MENTAL DISTURBANCES (See Chap. 11)
EMBOLISM

PUERPERAL INFECTION

Following completion of the third stage of labor, the site of previous placental attachment is a raw, elevated area, deep red in color and about 4 cm. in diameter. Its surface is nodular, due to the presence of numerous gaping veins, many of which are occluded by clots. These form excellent culture media for bacteria. At this time, furthermore, the condition of the entire endometrium is peculiarly favorable to bacterial invasion, since it is less than 2 mm. thick, is infiltrated with blood and presents numerous small wounds. Since the cervix rarely escapes some degree of laceration in labor, it is another ready site for bacterial invasion. Vulvar, vaginal and perineal wounds offer still other possible portals of entry.

When inflammatory processes develop in the birth canal postpartum, as the result of bacterial invasion of these highly vulnerable areas, the condition is known as "puerperal infection." It is really a wound infection of the birth canal, usually of the endometrium. As is true of other wound infections, the condition often remains localized but may extend along various pathways to produce diverse clinical pictures. Febrile reactions of more or less severity are the rule, and the outcome varies according to the portal of entry, the type, the number and the virulence of the invading organisms, the reaction of the tissues, and the general resistance of the patient.

Puerperal infection is one of the most common causes of death in childbearing. Frequently used (but less satisfactory) synonyms are: puerperal fever, puerperal sepsis, puerperal septicemia and childbed fever.

Causative Factors. The vast majority of puerperal infections are caused by the streptococcus, but most of the well-known pathogenic bacteria—such as the staphylococcus, the colon bacillus and the Welch bacillus—may be responsible for the disease.

What are the sources of these bacteria? The late Dr. John Osborne Polak, of Brooklyn, N. Y., used to teach that there are "eleven causes" of puerperal infection—the ten fingers and the nasopharynx. He meant by this that the attendants themselves are most likely to carry infection to the parturient uterus. The physician may inadvertently do so in two ways. In the first place, gloved and sterile though his hands may be during the vaginal examinations or the operative manipulations, he may carry bacteria already in the vagina upward into the uterus. Secondly, his hands and the instruments he uses may become contaminated by virulent streptococci as the result of droplet infection, dispersed by himself or some of the attendants, and in this manner he may be responsible for introducing bacteria into the birth canal. Even in modern obstetrics, the latter is a very common mode of infection, and unless the utmost vigilance is used in masking all attendants in the delivery room (both nose and mouth) and in excluding therefrom all persons suffering or recovering from an upper respiratory infection, it is a constant source of danger.

Although a less common means of transfer today than a few decades ago, careless physicians and nurses have been known to carry bacteria to the parturient from countless extraneous contacts: from other cases of puerperal infection, from suppurative postoperative wounds, from cases of sloughing carcinoma, from patients with scarlet fever, from infants with impetigo neonatorum,

from umbilical infections of the newborn and, finally, from the autopsy table. The physician himself may have the infection on his own person, such as an infected hangnail or felon. Recently, a Baltimore midwife with an ulcer on her finger gave a patient a fatal case of puerperal infection.

Among certain groups, coitus late in pregnancy is more common than ordinarily believed and may introduce extraneous organisms to the birth canal or carry upward bacteria already present on the vulva or in the lower vagina. Tub baths, particularly in multiparae with gaping vulvae, may permit the bath water to gain access to the vagina and thus introduce surface bacteria from the whole body.

During the second stage of labor, the chances of fecal matter being transferred to the vagina are great, of course—another constant source of danger.

Puerperal infection is much more common if the patient has had a postpartum hemorrhage or a traumatic, operative delivery. Therefore, hemorrhage and trauma must be regarded as important predisposing conditions.

Types. There are four main types of puerperal infection: endometritis, thrombophlebitis, peritonitis and pelvic cellulitis (or parametritis).

1. ENDOMETRITIS is a localized infection of the lining membrane of the uterus. This is the common form and may be regarded as the parent type from which the other three forms develop as the result of extension.

2. THROMBOBOPHLEBITIS is an infection of the veins with clot formation in the blood contained therein.

It may be of two types: pelvic thrombophlebitis, an inflammatory process involving the ovarian and the uterine veins, or femoral thrombophlebitis, in which the femoral, the popliteal or the saphenous vein is involved. The latter type of thrombophlebitis is often spoken of as "phlegmasia alba dolens" (painful white swelling) and also very frequently as "milk leg"—a term once given to the condition by physicians in the belief that it was due to the collection of milk in the affected leg.

Femoral thrombophlebitis presents a special group of signs and symptoms. It is a disease of the puerperium characterized by pain, fever and swelling in the affected leg. These symptoms are due to the formation of a clot in the veins of the leg itself, which interferes with the return circulation of the blood. When "milk leg" develops it usually appears about two weeks after labor, the most common time being the eleventh or the twelfth day. As in all acute febrile diseases occurring after labor, the secretion of milk may cease when phlegmasia alba dolens develops.

The disease is ushered in with malaise, chilliness and fever, which are soon followed by stiffness and pain in the affected part. If it is in the leg, the pain may begin in the groin or the hip and extend downward or it may commence in the calf of the leg and extend upward. In about 24 hours, the leg begins to swell and, although the pain then lessens slightly, it is always present and may be severe enough to prevent sleep. The skin over the swollen area is shiny white in color.

The acute symptoms last from a few days to a week, after which the pain gradually subsides and the patient slowly improves.

The course of the disease covers a period of from 4 to 6 weeks. The affected leg seldom returns to its normal size but remains permanently enlarged and troublesome.

The prognosis is usually favorable. In some of the very severe cases, however, abscesses form, and the disease may become very critical or even be fatal. In very rare instances the clot may be dislodged and carried to the heart, causing instant death.

The treatment of femoral phlebitis consists in rest, elevation of the affected leg or arm, the use of ice bags along the course of the affected vessels, sedatives, as indicated, for the pain, and penicillin. A "cradle" should be used to keep the pressure of the bedclothes off the affected part. Some physicians apply warm wet dressings covered with cotton and oiled silk or rubber. The heat may be maintained by electric coils or hot-water bottles. These dressings are applied well inside the thigh. Under no circumstances should a nurse rub or massage the affected part; and it should be handled with the utmost care when changing dressings, applying a bandage, making the bed or giving a bath. As the acute stage subsides, general tonics, nourishing food and the most carefully regulated hygienic conditions are needed to build up the patient's strength. As recovery is usually tedious, skillful nursing care is required to preserve the tissues of the body.

These patients are usually mentally depressed and discouraged. If the nurse is conscious of this complication, she will make every effort to keep the patient contented and have her realize the value of immobilization, even though the convalescing period is prolonged. The nurse may also make helpful suggestions to the family. Early ambulation may help to prevent this complication.

3. PERITONITIS is an infection, either generalized or local, of the peritoneum. Here, as a rule, the infection reaches the peritoneum from the endometrium by traveling via the lymphatic vessels; but peritonitis may also result from the extension of an endometrial infection via the lining membrane of the fallopian tubes.

4. PELVIC CELLULITIS, OR PARAMETRITIS. This is an infection of the loose connective tissue which surrounds the uterus. It may result in the formation of a pelvic abscess.

In its typical form each of these four types of puerperal infection presents a very characteristic set of signs and symptoms; but it not infrequently happens that one form of the disease is combined with another. The distinctions between these different types are of interest and importance to the physician, for not only the treatment but also the prognosis depend upon the particular form of infection.

Symptoms and Signs. So far as the nurse is concerned, it is highly important that she recognize immediately the onset of the disease in order that the doctor may be notified at once and that proper treatment may be instituted without delay.

When puerperal infection develops, it usually manifests itself about the third or the fourth day after delivery. The patient may have no complaints in the milder forms of endometritis but simply a rise in temperature to 101° or 102° F., yet often she complains of malaise, headache, backache and general discomfort. The more virulent infections are often ushered in by a chill, or at least by a chilly sensation, followed by an abrupt rise of temperature to 104° or 105° F.; and they are often accompanied by a rapid pulse.

In mild cases of endometritis the temperature elevations persist for 3 or 4 days and then subside. On the other hand, when extension of the infection occurs, particularly in pelvic thrombophlebitis and cellulitis, the disease may persist for many weeks, often with a hectic temperature curve and repeated chills. If extension occurs to the peritoneum with development of generalized peritonitis, the course is likely to be rapid and fatal.

Treatment. The treatment of puerperal infection first of all is preventive. This consists in the most scrupulous care in carrying out the strictest rules of surgical cleanliness during labor and delivery and in guarding against infection with the same careful precautions during the puerperium. Similar care must be exercised in preventing the transfer of infection from one patient to another. Ideally, a nurse who is caring for a case of puerperal infection should not attend another obstetric patient. If it is impossible to arrange for such complete segregation, the nurse must consider every patient with puerperal infection as in isolation and follow a technic which will prevent transfer of infection. The hands need special attention. After caring for such a mother, they should be washed, scrubbed and soaked in antiseptic solution; and when in attendance on such a case, a special gown which is left in the patient's room should be worn. It never should be worn outside. Under no circumstances should a nurse go from a patient with puerperal infection to one in labor.

The curative treatment, of course, rests with the physician, but good nursing care is essential. The patient should be kept as comfortable and as quiet as possible, for sleep is important. Conserving the patient's strength in every way, giving her nourishing food, increased amounts of fluids, fresh air and sunshine will help to increase her powers of resistance. Her mouth will require careful attention—lemon and glycerine solution for the mouth and lips is excellent. The head of the bed usually is elevated to promote drainage, and sometimes ice-bags are applied to the head and the abdomen at intervals. Penicillin is lifesaving in many of these cases and is employed in most of them. One of the sulfa drugs may also be used. Blood transfusions are often given as auxiliary, supportive measures.

HEMORRHAGE

These complications are discussed in Chapter 16.

MASTITIS

Mastitis, or inflammation of the breast, may vary from a simple congestion to a suppurative process which results in the formation of multiple abscesses in the glandular tissue.

The cases of simple congestion may be due merely to oversecretion of milk and consequent distention and congestion of the mammary gland; but the inflammation accompanied by suppuration is always due to septic infection, which usually enters through a denuded or diseased nipple. The first symptoms of mastitis are a feeling of malaise and pain in the breast, followed by chilliness or a distinct chill and by a sharp rise of temperature—up to 105° or 106° F. Investigation shows that the gland is tense, hard, nodular, red and extremely painful.

About the third day after delivery, the congestion or distention of the breast is apt to cause intense pain. It is not altogether due to the amount of pressure caused by an increase in the milk supply but is caused chiefly by glandular swelling and by engorgement of the blood vessels and lymph spaces around the glands. The tenderness to touch is extreme, and nursing may be impossible.

For the heavy enlarged breasts, the usual treatment is a snug support. Obstetricians usually prescribe salines to lessen the venous and lymphatic engorgement and the application of ice bags or hot stupes intermittently to the breasts. The breast pump may or may not be used.

When Mastitis Appears. There are three periods when mastitis may appear, although it may occur at any time during lactation. The periods of greatest frequency are (1) during the first month, and especially in the third week; (2) whenever nursing is stopped suddenly, and the breast becomes engorged with milk; (3) at the end of lactation, either because of hypersecretion of milk due to careless management when the infant is weaned or because the baby, being dissatisfied with the quality or the quantity of the milk, irritates the nipple.

Nursing Care. If treatment is begun at once, it is often possible to check the condition at the onset. The obstetrician must be notified immediately. If the nurse is not able to do this, she may apply a snug breast binder and an ice cap over the affected part. These ice bags must be filled lightly with slush ice. They may be supported by small pillows at either side. The patient frequently complains of chill under this treatment, but she should be in bed and external heat should be applied. In some hospitals hot stupes are used instead of ice. A saline cathartic, such as magnesium sulfate (Epsom salts), ½ oz. in half a glass of water, or magnesium citrate, 6 to 12 ounces, may be given. Penicillin is specific in this condition and often works a cure overnight. Nursing is usually discontinued at the affected breast; and milk-making foods are restricted until all the symptoms have disappeared. Stilbestrol is often used to aid in the suppression of lactation.

If begun at once, this treatment is usually successful; but it must be instituted without a moment's delay if it is to be effective. Under the prescribed treatment—rest, tight bandaging and ice caps, with saline cathartics and penicillin—the inflammation usually subsides at the end of a day or two, at which time nursing may be resumed.

Abscess of the Breast. When infection occurs, there is pain and tenderness of the breast. The patient usually complains of general malaise and headache, and the breast may show an isolated, inflamed area. The patient may have a chill, followed by an elevation of temperature and an increased pulse rate. The obstetrician should be notified at once, and treatment should be instituted immediately. The treatment may be the same as the one suggested previously for engorged breasts: support, ice or heat applied directly, saline catharsis and penicillin. Most obstetricians advise removing the baby from the breast so as to decrease the functional activity of the glands; however, others hold that cessation of nursing causes engorgement. In some cases, the breasts are pumped or expressed manually, and the nursing is discontinued.

Surgical Care. If the treatment outlined above is unsuccessful and suppuration occurs, the treatment is necessarily surgical; then the nurse will follow the directions of the obstetrician. In operating, a radial incision is made, the pus is evacuated, and a small drain is inserted. The reason that breast abscesses occur more often late in the puerperium may be due to the fact that the patient does not always report the condition as promptly as does the nurse who is in attendance during the early part of the puerperium. Every patient should be instructed to report the first sign of breast discomfort.

BLADDER COMPLICATIONS

The two most common bladder complications in the puerperium are retention of urine (inability to void) and residual urine. In the former, the patient is unable to void at all; in the latter, she is able to void certain amounts of urine but is unable to empty the bladder. In the latter condition, large amounts of urine (from 60 to 1,500 cc., as shown by catheterization) may remain in the bladder even though the patient may think that she has voided completely.

Retention of urine, or the inability to void, is very common after operative delivery. It often lasts 5 or 6 days but may persist for 2 weeks or longer. Edema around the urethra is probably the main cause. As already stressed, the nurse should make every effort to have the patient void within 6 hours after delivery (see p. 434). If the patient has not done so within 8 hours, the physician usually will order catheterization. In some hospitals this is routine if voiding has not occurred within 8 hours postpartum. Repeated catheterization may be necessary for several days; or the doctor may request the insertion of an indwelling catheter which will provide constant drainage.

If 60 cc. or more of urine still remain in the bladder after the patient has voided, it is usually considered that the voiding has been incomplete. This is a frequent complication of the puerperium, and it is not uncommon in such cases for catheterization to yield 800 cc. or so of residual urine. The condition is very likely to occur when the patient first begins to void following several days of catheterization. It is due primarily to lack of tone in the bladder wall. A distended bladder may be a predisposing cause of postpartum hemorrhage.

In many cases of residual urine the patient is without symptoms, but in others there is suprapubic or perineal discomfort, frequent scanty urination and sometimes a low-grade fever. Some physicians treat this condition with catheterization after each voiding until the residual urine becomes less than 60 cc.; others employ constant drainage by means of the indwelling catheter for several days.

MENTAL DISTURBANCES

These are discussed in detail in Chapter 11.

EMBOLISM

Embolism, or "heart clot," may be formed originally in the right ventricle or may be due to a thrombus which is washed along in the blood current until it becomes lodged in the heart. The clot obstructs the passage of blood into the lungs, either wholly or in part, and the patient may die of asphyxia within a few minutes. The condition may follow severe hemorrhage, septic infection, shock or general exhaustion, and it may occur after exertion or at any time during the puerperium.

Symptoms. The symptoms are sudden, severe pain over the heart; great dyspnea; syncope; feeble, irregular or imperceptible pulse; pallor in some cases, and cyanosis in others. Death may occur at any time from within a few minutes to a few hours, according to the amount or degree of obstruction to the pulmonary circulation. Very few patients recover.

Treatment. The treatment consists, first, in preventing the accident by careful attention to all details of surgical asepsis and to the proper management of labor and delivery; and secondly, in the free administration of stimulants. It is essential that the patient be kept absolutely quiet and on her back, for the slightest movement may result fatally. If the patient survives the attack, she must be kept warm by the use of external heat; absolute rest is mandatory;

and a light, nourishing diet is given, in the hope that the clot may be absorbed. In some instances it is almost impossible to prevent embolism, because the patient may be recovering without elevation of temperature and without complications and yet, on the seventh or tenth day, suddenly cries out, passes into a coma and succumbs.

SUGGESTED READING

Duckman, Simon, and Hubbard, John F.: The role of fluids in relieving breast engorgement without the use of hormones, Am. J. Obst. & Gynec. 60:200, 1950.

Eastman, N. J.: "Puerperal Infection," Lewis' Practice of Surgery, Vol. 10, Hagerstown, Md., Prior, 1942.

Guibeau, Joseph A., et al.: Aureomycin in obstetrics, J.A.M.A. 143:520, 1950.

Hodgkinson, C. P., and Nelson, R. E.: Penicillin treatment of acute puerperal mastitis, J.A.M.A. 129:269-270, 1945.

Matthews, H. B.: "Puerperal infection," Nelson's New Loose-Leaf Surgery, vol. 7, New York, Nelson, 1944, p. 15.

Newton, Michael, and Newton, Niles R.: Postpartum engorement of the breast, Am. J. Obst. & Gynec. 61:664, 1951.

Wolfe, S. A., and Pedowitz, P.: Late postpartum hemorrhage, Am. J. Obst. & Gynec. 53:84-99, 1947.

CONFERENCE MATERIAL

1. What provision can be made by the hospital to keep the patient informed about conditions at home and the care of the children, if they are at home or in a shelter or boarding home?

2. If the patient develops a rash three days after delivery and a diagnosis of scarlet fever has been made, what would you consider to be the method of managing this problem?

3. What instruction should be given to the patient and her husband concerning her care following delivery and discharge from the hospital? How can the public health nurse emphasize this instruction to secure the husband's co-operation?

4. How do you account for the high maternal mortality rate due to postpartal complications? What contribution can the nurse make toward improving these conditions?

5. If you have a patient whose pregnancy was complicated by cardiac or kidney condition, tuberculosis, syphilis or diabetes, and who has been dismissed from the hospital in satisfactory condition, what would be the responsibility of the hospital and the public health organization in the community?

6. What arguments would you use to convince parents of the importance of breast feeding? What are the responsibilities of the doctors, nurses and parents?

7. Why is the postpartal examination important, and how long is the convalescent period following normal delivery?

8. How best can parents prepare for the convalescent period to avoid fatigue, emotional disturbances, etc.?

9. What are the pros and cons of "early ambulation" for the obstetric patient? How does the obstetric patient compare with the surgical patient in relation to "early ambulation"?

Situation Questions

UNIT FOUR: NURSING DURING THE PUERPERIUM

Read through the entire question and place your answers in the parentheses.

1. Soon after a patient was normally delivered the nurse observed that she had a chill. In addition to calling the doctor, the nurse should have:

A. Provided external warmth to the patient with blankets and hot-water bottles to the feet.

B. Given a heart stimulant.

C. Prepared to give oxygen.

D. Given a hot drink.

E. Put the patient in shock position.

F. Viewed the chill as an alarming symptom of impending danger.

G. Viewed the chill as a symptom of internal hemorrhage.

H. Viewed the chill as a symptom of infection.

I. Viewed the chill as a not uncommon occurrence immediately after delivery.   (_____)

2. If a patient making satisfactory progress has a pulse rate of 90 just before delivery, what rate or rates would be considered to be favorable soon after delivery?

A. 60

B. 70

C. 80

D. 90

E. 100

F. 110

G. 120   (_____)

3. In the space provided place the letter corresponding to the period of time when the lochial discharge described normally occurs:

A. First day.	1. Clotted blood with strings
B. From 1 to 2 days.	of membrane. (_____)
C. From 4 to 7 days.	2. Brownish color, thin,
D. From 8 to 14 days.	scanty. (_____)
E. Third week.	3. Blood mixed with small
F. Seventh week.	amounts of mucus. (_____)
G. Not at all.	4. Pinkish color; moderate
	amount. (_____)
	5. Yellow, creamish color. (_____)

    6. Dark-brown with occa-
      sional bright-red.   (_____)
    7. Characteristic stale odor.   (_____)
    8. Characteristic foul odor.   (_____)

4. A good understanding of the physiologic changes taking place in the mother during the puerperium is a basis for good nursing. Indicate which of the following are believed to be true. The involution of the uterus is accomplished by:

A. The contraction of stretched muscle fibers.

B. The sloughing off of external layers of muscles.

C. The squeezing off of external layers of muscles.

D. The absorption of endometrium into the blood.

E. The elimination of endometrium along with blood and serous discharge.

F. The formation of healing scar tissue on the lining of the uterus.

G. The peeling off of the outer portion of the spongy layer of the decidua.

H. The formation of new endometrium.   (_____)

5. The nurse should be able to recognize and report abnormal conditions which may occur during the puerperium. Which of the following would you consider to be indicative of normal progress of involution?

A. Immediately after birth at level of umbilicus.

B. Twelve hours after delivery—1 cm. above the umbilicus.

C. Second day after delivery—6 inches above pubis.

D. Fourth day after delivery—3 inches above pubis.

E. Eighth day after delivery—2 inches above pubis.

F. Tenth day after delivery—1 inch above pubis.

G. Fourteenth day after delivery—palpable at level of pubis.

                                                   (_____)

6. Although opinion is not unanimous concerning early ambulation, which of the following seem to be the advantages to be gained from this procedure?

A. Minimizes the need for catheterization.

B. Mothers seem to regain their strength more readily.

C. Minimizes the chances of hemorrhage.

D. Reduces the amount of lochia.

E. Hastens involution of the uterus.

F. Lessens incidence of thrombophlebitis.

G. Reduces occurrence of abdominal distention and constipation.

                                                   (_____)

7. Perineal-care routines for patients without sutures vary in some respects from hospital to hospital but they do not vary in respect to:

A. Method of draping patients.

B. Requiring the nurse to scrub her hands surgically clean.

C. Requiring the nurse to wear a mask.

D. Endeavoring to protect the patient against infection from external sources.

E. Endeavoring to combat infection due to ever-present skin bacteria.

F. Endeavoring to make the patient comfortable.

G. The nature of the solution used.

H. Using an antiseptic solution internally.

I. Requiring a surgical technic.

J. Requiring the disinfection of all raw surfaces.

K. Using forceps to sponge the vulva.

L. Requiring that all sponging should be directed downward toward the anus.

M. Requiring that sterile cotton pledgets be used for all sponging.

N. Requiring that each pledget be used for one stroke only.

O. Requiring that pads, if used, be sterile when applied.

P. Requiring that a perineal pad be applied.   (_____)

8. The chief danger from cracked, sore nipples is:

A. Infection of the infant from nursing.

B. Invasion of bacteria resulting in abscess of the nipple.

C. Invasion of bacteria through nipple deep into the breast tissue, resulting in abscessed breast.

D. Formation of scar tissue which will prevent normal nursing thereafter.

E. Formation of a permanent fissure in the nipple.   (_____)

9. In the spaces provided write the term or the phrase which best fits each of the statements below:

A. A suppurative process in the glandular tissues of the breast.   (_____)

B. A localized infection of the lining membrane of the uterus.   (_____)

C. An infection of the loose connective tissue which surrounds the uterus.   (_____)

D. Cessation of lochial discharge during the first week after delivery.   (_____)

E. Failure of the uterus to return to normal condition as rapidly as expected.   (_____)

Note: The key to the correct answers to these questions is given on page 644.

UNIT FIVE

THE NEONATAL PERIOD

ORIENTATION

One of the stimulating phases of the obstetric experience is the opportunity to observe and to care for the "brand" new baby. Before birth the baby is protected physically from jars and injury by the amniotic fluid and has been in an environment where the temperature was most suited to his growth and development. His birth may be anticipated by the mother with the greatest of joy or his arrival may be looked forward to with agony or an almost indifference. What effect this reception may have upon the baby is not known. The birth process is bound to be a painful one for the baby (as well as for the mother), and the readjustment which has to be made may be the most drastic and dramatic that he ever will be called upon to make. What fears or inhibitions may be carried over from this experience is a conjecture. At birth, the baby's brain is more than one-fourth its adult size, and his nervous system is in an impressionable state. The care of this new baby, which for the student nurse extends through the delivery and the baby's hospital stay, should be one of real consideration. It is very often during this time that much is determined in the way of habits for the new baby. It should be remembered that during these first days the nurse is introducing the baby to a new way of life and laying some of the foundations, thereby shaping his behavior. Beginning habits are very significant. The co-operation of the doctor, the nurse and the parents in instituting breast feeding may be only one of these milestones in the baby's future. Needless to say, the most careful and thoughtful attention on the part of the nurse should be given to aid this new baby to make these adjustments.

21

The Nursing Care of the New Baby

INTRODUCTION

The ten most important months of a baby's life are the nine months before he is born and the first month after birth. During pregnancy, the baby has been protected and nourished by the mother, but at birth the baby becomes an "independent" individual. Dr. Emerson Stone states: "Up to the moment of delivery, the fetus lives a parasitic existence, but with the assumption of an independent career at birth, it undergoes the most profound physiological changes that are encountered at any period of life. Certain of these alterations are immediate and others are delayed, but they are all permanent and therefore significant." It is necessary to use the utmost care in handling the baby, keeping him warm and protecting him from exposure and injury.

INITIAL CARE

In the delivery room, or before the baby has been removed to the nursery or to his own bed, the initial care has been given to the eyes, the mouth and the cord, and, if birth has taken place in a hospital, identification has been added. The baby should be watched to see that he is kept warm (a most important detail), that respirations are normal, that color is good, and that there is no bleeding from the cord.

471

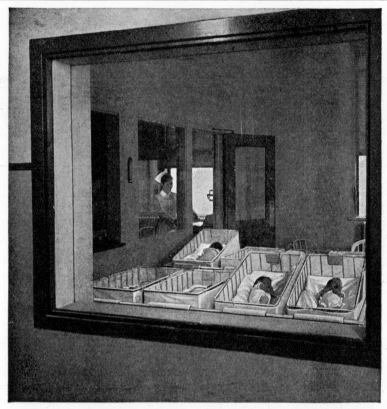

FIG. 272. The layout of the nursery from the hospital corridor. Note the use of glass, facilitating supervision and minimizing possible contagion from visitors. Babies are given care in their own individual beds. In the rear left is the doctor's treatment room. (Sloane Hospital for Women, New York)

PHYSICAL EXAMINATION

Immediately, or within the next few hours, the doctor will give the baby a complete physical examination. This usually includes the following: head (fontanels, overriding of skull bones); mouth (lingual frenum, precocious dentition, cleft palate and harelip); heart; lungs; abdomen; extremities; genitalia (imperforate meatus, phimosis, malformations); and anus (imperforate). The measurements of the baby are noted, such as the circumference and diameter of head and shoulders, and weight and length. The average boy baby weighs from 7 to 7½ pounds (about 3,300 Gm.) when he is born; girl babies weigh a little less. The

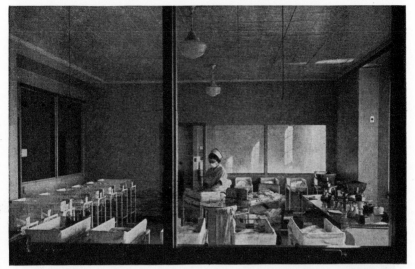

Fig. 273. Nursery in the Chicago Lying-In Hospital. Individual care is given to the baby in his bed. Nursery cart containing all supplies stands near by. One end of the cart has a container for waste, and the other a bag for soiled clothing.

average length of a baby at birth is about 20 inches (51 cm.).

The physician will examine the baby carefully for any deformity, injury or abnormality. If a deformity or injury is found, the obstetrician will advise concerning the baby's care. Usually, the father will be told at once, and the mother will be informed by him or the physician.

DAILY CARE

NURSERY CARE

In today's modern nurseries (Figs. 272, 273 and 274) some of the protections offered new babies are: the beds or units with individual equipment and greater space separation; air conditioning and humidifying ap-

paratus; sterilization of all articles used for the baby; heated bath tables and regulation by thermostatic control of any water used for babies; limiting the number of individuals who enter the nurseries; culturing the throats of nurses and doctors before assigning them to this service; and provision for isolation for any suspicious or questionable infections of eyes, mouth, skin, and intestinal conditions. Some hospitals have an observation nursery where babies are kept until any question of infection is eliminated.

ROOMING-IN

"Rooming-in" is the name given to the present plan of having the new baby share his mother's hospital unit. It is the present custom for any so-

Prep & water 1st da. (delivery day)

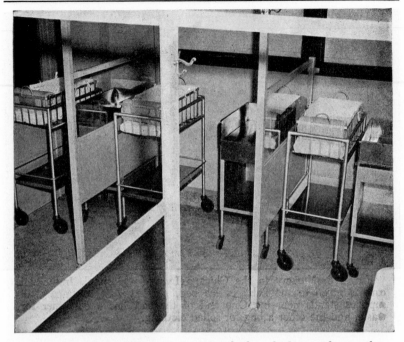

Fig. 274. Observation nursery with cubicles which provide complete isolation for each infant. Each unit is complete, containing all the equipment necessary for the care of the baby. (Margaret Hague Maternity Hospital, Jersey City, N. J.)

called new idea in medicine to be written up immediately in the popular magazines and newspapers, with and without factual basis. This leads the public to make demands of the profession often before hospitals are equipped to meet these requests. Rooming-in is not new. Years ago one of the differences between the private and the public pavilions of some hospitals was that the private patient was allowed to keep her baby in her room; whereas, the babies belonging to the mothers in the ward were segregated in a nursery. At that time some doctors thought that the mother very often was exhausted after the crisis of delivery and that she was not able to get sufficient rest with the new baby in her room. The obstetric patient was accustomed to having considerable nursing care for herself, and the baby was also cared for entirely by the nurse. The mother assumed no responsibility for herself or her baby. There were other patients who planned to have a nurse for the baby; therefore, they had no intention of assuming this care. Then, too, if the baby were not up to par physically, a real emotional complication arose. Visitors also created a

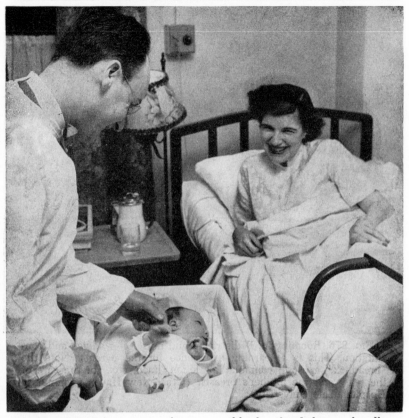

Fig. 275. Rooming-in makes it possible for the father to handle and become acquainted with the new baby. (French Hospital, New York; photo by Three Lions, Inc.)

problem. Then the hospitals provided nurseries where the babies could be placed and where it was thought that standards for better care might be set up.

To put rooming-in into practice calls for long preparation of the staff. Generally, it demands a different architectural arrangement and administrative planning. Different types of rooming-in projects are being developed, such as single-room arrangements, 4-bed units and the larger wings which accommodate a greater number of patients. Excellent experienced nurses, with understanding and interest, are needed to teach the new mother about the care and the handling of the new baby. Rooming-in requires 24-hour nursing service. Much of the practical care of the new baby must be learned by the

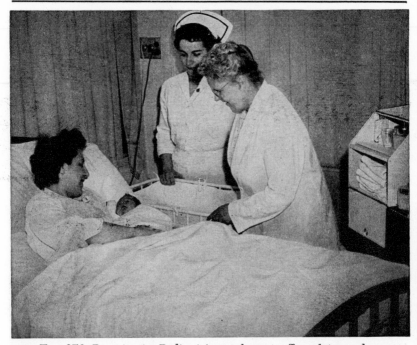

FIG. 276. Rooming-in. Pediatrician and nurse offer advice and consultation. This is a learning experience for the parents. Note the "breadbox," a useful container for lotion, linen, etc., for the care of the baby and the mother's breasts. (Grace-New Haven Community Hospital, Yale University)

new mother during her brief hospital stay to supplement the theoretical knowledge that she has gained during the prenatal period. At this time the new mother needs close supervision in order that she may learn the correct methods of care for the baby, and she should not be dependent on learning from the other patients in the unit.

Individual mothers, too, have to be taken into consideration. It is only natural that a mother will want her baby with her so that she may get to know him and learn to care for him under skilled guidance. The father, also, may experience and share the thrill of being with the new baby and, at the same time, learn a great deal about the baby's care. There may be some mothers who will not want to take over the care of the baby in the hospital because they appreciate this opportunity for rest and freedom from responsibility. Many mothers enjoy rooming-in but do not feel that they want the care or the responsibility of the baby. There may be others who are not sufficiently mature to assume this

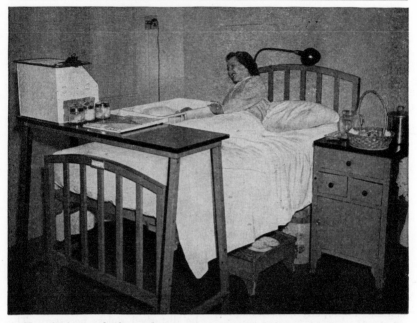

FIG. 277. A cubicle in the rooming-in unit of the Grace-New Haven Community Hospital. (Photos by John J. Curran)

charge immediately. To such a mother the baby may be considered a toy for her amusement. This group will need much more time and instruction. In the rooming-in plan, the baby also must be considered. It is important that the baby be handled properly and have sufficient undisturbed rest.

There are advantages to rooming-in, in that the mother and the baby are cared for by the same doctors and nurses, thereby eliminating the confusion which often results from the contacts with so many different people. With this experience, parents of first babies do not feel so helpless when they return home. There also seems to be an increased desire for mothers to nurse their babies. The mothers generally seem to be happier, and the babies are said to appear more contented. Up to the present time, hospitals report that there have been no skin infections or gastro-intestinal disturbances.

The parents who have planned their babies and shared their experiences during the prenatal period and have prepared together for the baby's arrival will appreciate rooming-in. These shared experiences certainly are a preparation for stable and secure family relationships.

CARE OF THE SKIN

At birth the baby is covered with a cheesy material called "vernix caseosa," which has been a protection to his skin while floating in amniotic fluid in utero. On the body, too, there may be a growth of fine downy hair called lanugo, which usually disappears within the first week or so. His skin may be of a bluish-pink, reddish or pale color, and often it is wrinkled and has a water-soaked appearance but becomes a normal color within 2 weeks. His skin is thin, delicate, extremely tender and very easily irritated. Since the skin is a protective covering, breaks in its surface may initiate troublesome infection, hence skin disturbances constitute an actual threat to the baby's well-being. The baby's skin may be irritated by rough clothing, improperly washed diapers, oil that is not pure or soap that is not mild.

The new baby does not perspire, usually, until after the first month, and he does not react to cold by having "goose flesh." In warm weather, or if the baby is dressed too warmly, he may develop prickly heat, a pimply rash on the face and the neck or other parts of the body. Fewer clothes and sodium bicarbonate or bran baths will help to relieve the discomfort. The nurse should observe very carefully the condition of the baby's skin and report to the physician any questionable appearance, such as pallor, cyanosis or jaundice.

BATHING

The baby's first bath is usually an oil bath to remove the vernix caseosa. This also prevents unnecessary evaporation from the skin and chilling of the body. The oil (sweet oil, mineral oil or some special preparation used by the hospital) for this purpose should be poured into a container, which is placed in hot water and allowed to stand until it is thoroughly warm. The nurse should apply the oil gently but rapidly all over the parts where the baby has much vernix. She should pay special attention to the scalp and all creases at the neck, behind the ears, under the arms, the palms of the hands and between the fingers and the toes, under the knees, the soles of the feet, and in the groins, the buttocks and the genitals. The excess oil should be removed with a soft towel. If there is a scaling of the superficial layer of skin, this may be helped by applying oil after the baby's bath and by giving him "drinks" of water regularly. The cord dressing should not be disturbed unless necessary. The baby should be handled as little as possible and must be kept warm. In some hospitals this initial oil bath is followed by a soap-and-water bath with only the daily oil bath thereafter. In others the initial oil bath is followed by the daily soap-and-water bath. In still others the bath is omitted altogether until the day of discharge, at which time a soap-and-water bath is given.

SLEEPING

After the profound experience of being born, the baby will need rest and sleep. If he is well and comfortable, he should sleep much of the time and wake regularly for his feedings. His clothes should be light in weight, warm but not too warm, and free from wrinkles and bunches. His position should be changed often,

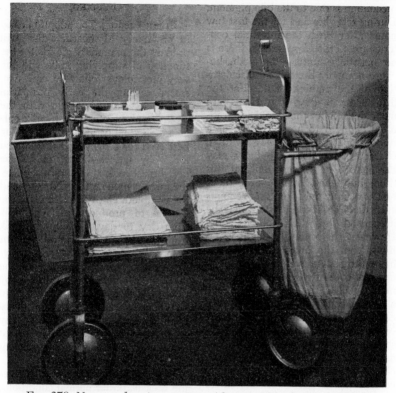

FIG. 278. Nursery dressing carriage (designed by Miss Lottie Morrison) for the care of babies in their individual beds. The carriage is equipped with a foot pedal to raise cover on laundry bag for soiled clothing (right). Bag for waste (left). The upper shelf contains: shirts, thermometers, oil, and diaper liners in place of washcloths for baby's buttocks. The lower shelf holds diapers, pads and bed linen. (Sloane Hospital for Women, New York)

from side to side and on his back, but never on his abdomen. A baby who is allowed to sleep on his abdomen may smother. This position may also interfere with the normal development of his rapidly growing jaws. These sleeping or resting periods are very important because during the early weeks these habit patterns are established.

ELIMINATION

Intestinal. During fetal life the content of the intestines is made up of brownish-green tarlike material called "meconium." It is composed of epithelial and epidermal cells and lanugo hair that probably were swallowed with the amniotic fluid. The dark greenish-brown color of the

Yellow stool, too much caries of elimination(?) [handwritten annotation]

meconium is due to the bile pigment. During fetal life and for the first few hours after birth the intestinal contents are sterile. Apparently, there is no peristalsis until after birth, because normally there is no discoloration of the amniotic fluid. For the first 2 or 3 days the stools are meconium. After this, the color gradually changes to a soft yellow of a smooth pasty consistency with a characteristic odor. The baby may eliminate 3 or 4 times daily at this time; but when he is a little older he has usually only 1 or 2 movements each day. The type of stool may be influenced by the mother's diet. However, there may be slight variations from the normal, which may have little significance if the baby appears comfortable and sleeps and nurses well. If the baby's stools have a watery consistency, are of a green color and contain mucus or gas, the condition may be an evidence of some digestive or intestinal irritation and should be reported to the physician. The number, the color and the consistency of the stools should be recorded daily on the baby's record.

Urinary. Urinary activity of the fetus is evidenced by the presence of urine in the amniotic fluid. The baby usually voids during delivery or immediately after birth, but the function may be suppressed for several hours. However, if the baby does not void within 24 hours, the condition should be reported to the physician, as suppression of the urine may be due to an imperforate meatus. After the first two or three days, the baby voids from 10 to 15 times a day. Any discoloration or change in the amount of urine eliminated should be noted on the record and reported to the physician.

FEEDING

Breast Feeding. The adoption early in pregnancy of measures that will prepare the mammary glands for the function of supplying milk, and the very meticulous follow-up care necessary during the early postpartal period, have much to do with the mother's ability to furnish milk sufficient in quality and quantity. The best food for a baby is that designed for it by nature—breast milk. The best breast milk is that furnished by the infant's own mother. Nursing and the complete emptying stimulate the breasts to produce sufficient milk from day to day. Usually the milk from one breast will be enough for a feeding for a very young baby; therefore, alternate breasts should be used for each nursing. As the baby grows older, it may be necessary to put him to both breasts at every feeding. This may be done at any time when the milk of one breast alone does not seem to be sufficient to satisfy the baby.

When the nursing period arrives the breasts, under normal conditions, should be firm and tense but never painful, and at this time a very slight pressure should be enough to cause the milk to flow. Many mothers need help with this new experience of nursing, and many babies must be taught to nurse. Therefore, the nurse has a definite responsibility in relation to breast feeding.

ADVANTAGES OF BREAST MILK. Breast milk is to be preferred to any modified milk, which at best is only a substitute. The advantages are:

Lower mortality and morbidity rates for breast-fed infants, as compared with the artificially fed infants

Exactly the correct composition for babies

Higher nutritional value of human milk

Free from bacteria

Convenient and economical

Constantly available, no preparation necessary

DEMAND FEEDING (self-demand, self-regulating), as it is popularly referred to, is being used more and more frequently as an increasing number of hospitals are adopting the rooming-in plan. Demand feeding is

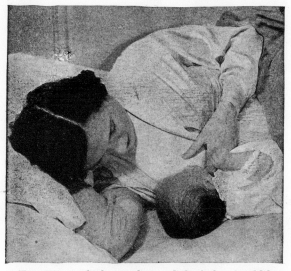

FIG. 279. Both the mother and the baby should be comfortable during the nursing period. The mother should hold the breast so that it does not interfere with the baby's breathing. When he cannot breathe freely, he becomes irritated and may refuse to nurse altogether.

Even temperature

Contains immune bodies (according to some authorities)

Lowered incidence of allergy

Earlier involutionary processes in the mother after the termination of pregnancy

Lowered incidence of carcinoma of the breast in women who have nursed their babies

Emotional satisfaction, which is very important in establishing parent-child relationships.

the idea of putting a baby on a nursing schedule that seems to fit his individual needs, instead of the previous concept of putting all babies on one rigid schedule of every 4 hours. No one set feeding program can suit all babies nor can it suit all mothers. Dr. Edith Jackson suggests that this demand feeding is "closely spaced rather than irregular." It must be remembered that all new babies are a bundle of demands and that food is only one of them,

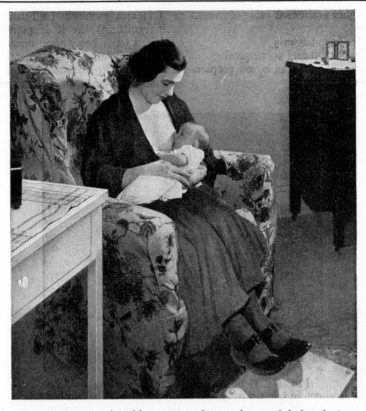

Fig. 280. A comfortable position for mother and baby during nursing. Note footstool for added comfort.

and also that it takes time for milk to digest and the stomach needs rest. All babies should have a well-adjusted start but they are immature and need guidance to attain a reasonable feeding pattern. The baby is usually put to the breast when the mother has had a sufficient rest from the effects of her delivery. At first, the breast secretes colostrum, which is characterized by a greenish-yellow color. It contains more proteid material and salts, and vitamin K, but less fat than normal milk, while its sugar content is about the same. It is important to the baby because of its cathartic properties. Some authorities state that babies who nurse this colostrum have less initial weight loss, and that it contains certain protective antibodies in which the newborn is deficient.

Position During Nursing. If the baby is to nurse satisfactorily, he must be held properly by the mother; while some mothers seem to know how to support a baby at the breast, many are awkward, and definite instructions are helpful. First of all, both the mother and the baby must be comfortable and in such a position that the baby can grasp the whole nipple without any effort—not just the end of it. If the mother is lying down, she should be on her side with her arm raised and her head comfortably supported. The baby should lie on his side, flat on the bed, or supported by pillows. When the mother is sitting up to nurse the baby, she should use a comfortable chair with a stool to support her feet, and, if necessary, a pillow may be used to support her arm or may be placed under the baby. The mother should guard against feeding the baby either too rapidly or too slowly, or allowing

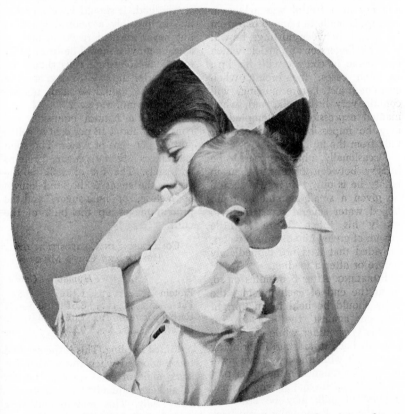

Fig. 281. "Bubbling" the baby. Holding the baby upright against the shoulder immediately after nursing and gently patting his back to bring up air.

his position to interfere with his breathing.

HUNGER. If the baby is not getting enough food, he will wake before his regular nursing time and be obviously hungry. He will cry and fret, refuse water with apparent disgust and, when nursing is permitted, seize the nipple ravenously and nurse with great vigor.

He may continue to nurse long after the breast is empty, in his effort to secure enough food; and he will cry in a fretful way when an attempt is made to remove him from the breast. Between nursings, he will suck his fingers or any article which may come in contact with his lips. In such cases, the breast, when examined just before nursing, will contain very little milk, and, when manual expression is attempted, it may be impossible to express any milk from the nipple.

Occasionally, a baby appears to be hungry between feedings when in reality he is only thirsty. He should be given a small amount of tepid boiled water several times daily to satisfy his thirst. There is little danger of giving him too much water, provided that it is not immediately before or after a feeding.

BUBBLING. After 5 minutes or so, or at the end of each nursing, the baby should be held in an upright position against the nurse's (or mother's) shoulder while she gently pats his back to aid him in bringing up any air which he may have swallowed. Gas remains in the lower part of the stomach; that it why a small amount of milk may be eructated with the gas. If the baby is put back in his crib before he is bubbled, he may regurgitate most of his feeding with the bubble.

REGURGITATION. Regurgitation, which is merely an overflow and occurs immediately after nursing, should not be confused with vomiting, which may occur at any time and is accompanied by other symptoms. This regurgitation is the means of relieving the distended stomach and indicates that the baby has either taken too much food or has taken it too rapidly.

COMPOSITION OF MILK. Mother's milk, as it leaves the breast, is a sterile fluid. It should have an alkaline or possibly a neutral reaction, but never an acid reaction, and its specific gravity should be from 1.027 to 1.032. Colostrum cells should be absent after the twelfth day, and the fat globules should be small, numerous and of uniform size.

Milk is a natural emulsion and consists of about 13 per cent of solids and 87 per cent of water. The solid substances are fat, sugar, proteins and salts. The fat of milk is the cream, the sugar is the kind known as "lactose," or "milk-sugar," and the protein makes up the bulk of the curd.

COMPARISON IN COMPOSITION OF HUMAN AND COW'S MILK

	Human	Cow's
Protein	1.15%	3.5%
Fat	3.5%	3.5–4.0%
Carbohydrate	7.0%	4.0–5.0%
Salts	0.2%	0.75%

Mixed Feeding. This is the method to be adopted when the mother has some milk, of good quality, but not in sufficient quantity to satisfy the baby fully. This may be either a complemental feeding (feedings of modified cow's milk given immediately after the breast feeding) or supplemental feeding (feeding which is

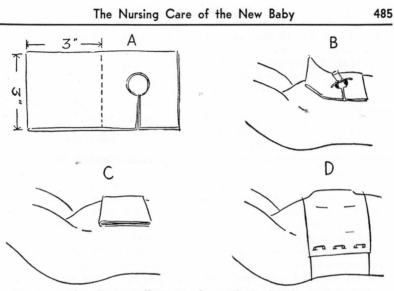

Fig. 282. This diagram illustrates the method of making and applying the cord dressing.

given in place of the breast feeding).

The hours for feeding, according to the age of the baby, are the same whether the baby is at the breast or on the bottle, and if the mother has not milk enough to satisfy her baby at every feeding, often she can omit one or two breast feedings and give instead a supplemental feeding.

MODIFIED MILK. The modified milk to be used in mixed feeding is prepared in the quantity and proportions suited to the age of the baby and given as complemental or supplemental feedings.

It is well to have a formula from the physician that may be used in an emergency. The following formula is used by several well-known pediatricians.

2 parts cow's milk (e.g., 14 oz. milk)

1 part water (e.g., 7 oz. water)

2 tablespoonfuls granulated sugar (when the quantity is for a full day's feedings, i.e., 21 oz.)

GENERAL OBSERVATIONS

EYES

In the daily care of the baby, no special treatment is given the baby's eyes unless there is a discharge. Any discharge should be reported and recorded on the chart. There may be some reaction from the prophylaxis, but the physician will prescribe the treatment.

CORD

Usually, babies do not receive a tub bath until the cord has separated and the umbilicus has healed. Usually the cord dressing is not changed unless it becomes soiled. It is well to ask the obstetrician's advice concerning changing the dressings. Most obstetricians advise the nurse to sponge the surrounding area with alcohol and to apply a dry sterile dressing. If the surrounding area is inflamed, apply a wet dressing of alcohol (50 per cent) and notify the obstetrician; but unless the dressing becomes soiled (e.g., with urine or meconium), it may be allowed to come off with the cord when it separates.

No attempt should ever be made to dislodge the cord before it separates completely. If it is necessary to remove the dressing, only such of the gauze as can be freed from the cord need be removed, and the fresh dressing is then applied. The cord usually becomes detached from the body between the fifth and the eighth day after birth, but its detachment may be delayed until the tenth, the twelfth, or even the fourteenth day without causing any concern, unless signs of inflammation appear. The nurse will usually find the cord in the umbilical dressing when she removes the binder to bathe the baby and there may also be a slight stain of blood. If the bleeding continues—as it may in very rare instances—the obstetrician should be notified. In most cases, the umbilicus is depressed somewhat and absolutely free from any evidence of inflammation. No further treatment is required except to keep the part clean and dry. When moisture is present, the umbilicus is cleansed with alcohol, and a dry sterile dressing is applied. For a moist umbilicus, some obstetricians advise cleansing with alcohol and then applying aristol powder (thymol iodide). On the day the cord separates, and daily thereafter, the condition of the umbilicus should be recorded. In some hospitals no cord dressing is used. However, the daily inspection of the condition of the cord and umbilicus should be noted.

GENITALS

Adherent Foreskin. In a male infant, adhesions between the prepuce and the glans penis are very common. The foreskin may be extended beyond the glans. Reduction to a very small opening is spoken of as a "phimosis." A curdy secretion, called "smegma," may form in considerable amount and collect under the prepuce behind the glans. Also small amounts of urine may be retained. Any of these conditions favor irritation and, if found, should be reported to the obstetrician. He may perform the delicate operations of separating the adhesions, stretching the prepuce or circumcising the baby.

If daily dressings are to be done following a circumcision, the obstetrician will leave the necessary orders. Boric dressings or sterile petrolatum are sometimes used. The manipulation following dilation and retraction is difficult, at first, and should be done gently. A gauze sponge lubricated with sterile petrolatum is used to retract and replace the foreskin. The foreskin must be replaced immediately; if not, edema may result, rendering the replacing difficult. Cold compresses are used in such an emergency.

Care of Girl Babies. Similar adhesions are sometimes found about the clitoris in female infants and, when observed, should be reported

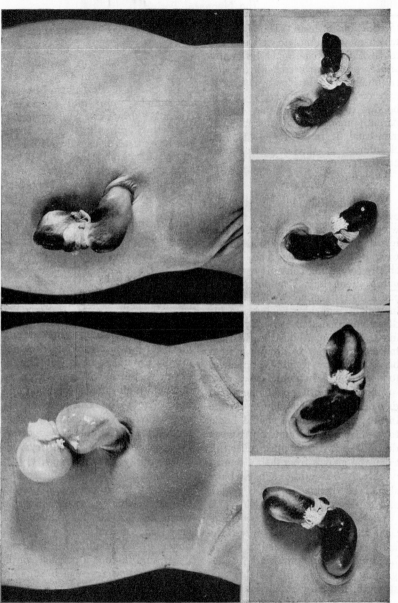

Fig. 283. The umbilical cord drying.

to the obstetrician. The smegma which may accumulate between the folds of the labia should be gently and carefully cleansed with oil. Occasionally, a slight bloody discharge may come from the vagina. It may be due to injury or it may be apparently menstrual in character. If menstrual, it rarely reappears, and cleanliness is the only treatment necessary.

WEIGHT

The baby should be weighed every day or every other day and his weight recorded accurately. The first few days after birth he usually loses weight because his food, being chiefly colostrum, contains very little nourishment but is important because of its laxative effect. This loss in weight may also be because his digestive apparatus is barely learning to function. About the time the meconium begins to disappear from his stools, the weight commences to increase and, in normal cases, does so regularly until about the tenth day of life, when it may equal the birth weight. Then he should begin to gain from 4 to 6 ounces per week during the first 5 months. After this time, the gain is from 2 to 4 ounces weekly. At 6 months of age, the baby should be double his birth weight, and triple it when a year old. This is one way to note the baby's condition and progress, and when the baby is not gaining, that fact should be reported to the physician. Besides gaining regularly in weight and strength, the baby should be happy and good-natured when awake but inclined to sleep a good part of the time between nursings.

PULSE AND TEMPERATURE

The clinical record of a normal baby should show a variation in pulse of from 110 to 150. Only experience can teach a nurse to count an infant's pulse rate accurately. Touching his wrist will generally startle him and noticeably accelerate the heart beat. It can always be felt at the temporal artery to best advantage, particularly during sleep. The rectal temperature may normally vary a whole degree, from 98° to 99° F. A premature baby may have a temperature below this, from 97° to 98° F.

CRIES

After the baby is born and has cried lustily, he becomes quiet and usually sleeps. After the eyes, the cord and the skin have received the necessary care, he is dressed and placed in a warm crib and does not usually cry unless he is wet, hungry or ill. A nurse will soon learn to distinguish an infant's condition and needs from the character of his cry, which may be described as follows. A loud, insistent cry with drawing up and kicking of the legs denotes colicky pain; a fretful cry, if due to indigestion, will be accompanied by green stools and passing of gas; a whining cry is noticeable when the baby is ill, premature or very frail; a fretful, hungry cry, with fingers in the mouth, is easily recognized; and there is a peculiar, shrill, sharp-sounding cry which suggests injury. A nurse should make every effort to recognize any deviation from the usual manner in which a baby announces his normal requirements.

SUGGESTED READING

Bartlett, F. H.: Infants and Children, New York, Rinehart, 1946.

Bauman, Elaine: The visiting nurse views rooming-in, Pub. Health Nursing 42:263, 1950.

Children's Bureau Publication Number 242: Appraisal of the Newborn Infant.

Cornell University Bulletin for Homemakers, Number 715, Living with Baby, May, 1947.

Hickcox, Verda F.: Changing maternity and newborn care in the hospital, Pub. Health Nursing 42:435, 1950.

Jeans, P. C., Rand, Winifred, and Blake, Florence G.: Essentials of Pediatrics, ed. 4, Philadelphia, Lippincott, 1946.

Kenyon and Russell: Healthy Babies, Boston, Little, 1952.

McBryde, Angus: Compulsory rooming-in in the ward and private newborn service at Duke Hospital, J.A.M.A. 145:625, 1951.

Macy, I. G., et al.: Human milk studies. Implications of breast feeding and their investigations, Am. J. Dis. Child. 70:135-141, 1945.

Moloney, J. C., Montgomery, J. C., and Trainham, G.: The newborn, his family and the modern hospital, Mod. Hosp. 67:43-46, 1946.

Richardson, Frank Howard: Breast feeding, J.A.M.A. 142:863, 1950.

Rooming In, Today's Health 28:24, 1950.

Slobody, Lawrence B., and Wallace, Helen M.; Principles and facilities for the care of newborn infants in the hospital, J.A.M.A. 146:1462, 1951.

Stone, E. L.: The Newborn Infant, Philadelphia, Lea & Febiger, 1945.

Taylor, Stewart E., and Lubchenco, Lula O.: Joint responsibilities of obstetrician and pediatrician, Am. J. Nursing 50:275, 1950.

Weymuller, C. A., Beck, A. C., and Ittner, E. J.: Measures for the protection of newborn infants, J.A.M.A. 133:78-84, 1947.

Zabriskie, Louise: Mother and Baby Care in Pictures, ed. 3, Philadelphia, Lippincott, 1946.

22

Nursing Care of the Premature Baby

DEFINITION

A premature infant is arbitrarily defined as any infant, of single or multiple birth, born prematurely, at term or even past term, with a birth weight of 2,500 grams (5½ pounds) or less. Such an infant is usually less than 48 centimeters (19 inches) in length and usually has been born prior to the thirty-sixth week of gestation. The suggestion has been made that the dividing line for Negro infants should be lower than for white, since Negro infants are reported to weigh proportionally less at birth than white infants. Infants over this empirical weight, even though apparently born at full term, occasionally may be diagnosed by a physician as "premature" on the basis of other

considerations, such as faulty maintenance of body temperature, particular feeding difficulties or certain physical characteristics. This may apply particularly to infants born to diabetic or prediabetic mothers. Although the upper limit of weight has been established, the lower never has been accepted by any authoritative group, and the level at which a dividing line is drawn between abortions and premature infants remains a matter of personal or local preference. The lower limit will depend on the definition of abortion, but the 1,000 gram figure is the one most frequently used. If the baby is from 6 to 8 weeks or more premature, the diagnosis is comparatively easy because of his weight, length and physical characteristics. It is the baby who is from 2 to 4 weeks premature who is usually neglected; yet he, too, will suffer from the lack of intra-uterine protection of the last weeks which he so much needs. The closer to full term, the greater the life chances.

CAUSES OF PREMATURITY

Since more than half of the neonatal deaths in the United States are due to prematurity and since these rates have remained constant for many years, the emphasis on preventive care must be stressed. If the money expended on premature care were applied to preventive care, it would be interesting to prognosticate the results. However, the causes of prematurity present a challenging problem. Some of the causes are of maternal origin: i.e., exhaustion, emotional crises, faulty nutrition and injury. Multiple pregnancy is the most common single cause of prematurity. Other causes are chronic nephritis, toxemia, infectious diseases (such as syphilis and tuberculosis), acute abdominal conditions resulting in surgical interference, cardiac and diabetic diseases and thyroid disturbances.

Pregnancy itself also has its contributing causes. Malformation in the embryologic development, erythroblastosis fetalis dependent upon the Rh factor and faulty nutrition of the fetus. Abnormalities of placental structure resulting in the rupture of the membranes, placenta previa, abruptio placenta and hydramnios, may cause prematurity. Then, too, there is a fairly large group of premature births due to undiagnosed causes.

Prematurity from analysis of the causes is very definitely an obstetric problem, because it occurs during pregnancy and terminates in a premature delivery.

CAUSES OF PREMATURE DEATHS

The causes of the deaths of these infants may be due to immature development of the vital centers, exposure, or to faulty resuscitation methods. Other causes are pulmonary conditions, such as pneumonia, atelectasis with and without hyaline, malformations, cerebral hemorrhage, erythroblastosis, anoxia and trauma. At the time of delivery the use of outlet forceps and episiotomy are recognized as means of preventing cerebral hemorrhage. These methods alleviate the pressure of the baby's head against the massive pelvic structures. The blood vessels of the premature baby lack the supporting wall structure and, therefore, are very easily damaged.

PREVENTION OF PREMATURITY

Edith L. Potter, M.D., of Chicago, says: "The ideal solution to the problem of prematurity is through the mother; more important than salvaging the life of a premature infant is the prevention of a premature birth. In many instances there is no recognizable cause of premature labor, although in a study of mortality made at the Chicago Lying-In Hospital, the common causes were toxemia, placenta previa and premature separation of the placenta. Prevention of these conditions would aid materially in decreasing the number of premature births." * Other authorities state that poor or inadequate diet and lack of rest are predisposing causes of prematurity.

DESCRIPTION AT BIRTH

As there are many degrees of prematurity, so also are there various stages of anatomic and physiologic development. Many of the symptoms described below may vary in infants of approximately the same fetal age, depending on the cause of prematurity and the physical condition of the mother and the infant. At birth the premature baby lacks the subcutaneous fat which is deposited during the last two months of intrauterine development. This gives the skin a transparent appearance with the blood vessels easily seen through the skin, which is often of a deep red color, sometimes with a cyanotic hue. These premature babies are prone to develop icteric skin changes, also. Because of the wrinkled appearance of the skin, these babies are often referred to as "old-looking." Lanugo is usually abundant all over the skin surface but disappears within a few weeks. The skin, especially around the nose, is peppered with small white nodules, which are due to the inactivity of the excretory glands of the skin. These nodules are called "comedones."

The external ears and the nose are very soft, due to the underdeveloped cartilage. The ears lie very close to the head. The skull is round in contrast with the long anteroposterior skull diameter of the full-term infant. The fontanels are large, and the sutures prominent. The finger- and

* Engle, Pregnancy Wastage, Springfield, Ill., Thomas, in preparation.

toenails may be immature, often not reaching the ends of the fingers and the toes.

The infant may be puny and small or he may approximate full-term weight, yet the internal organs may be imperfectly developed, and these babies appear reluctant to assume the responsibility to live. The respirations are shallow and irregular, due to the lack of expansion and proper interchange. There are often periods of apnea. Due to the irregular respirations and the poorly developed function of swallowing, there is danger of aspiration of milk or vomitus, causing cyanosis and predisposing to pulmonary infections. The premature baby regurgitates his food readily because the stomach is tubular in form, and the sphincters are poorly developed. The urine is usually scanty.

The walls of the blood vessels are weak, and the tendency to hemorrhage is great. Since the central nervous system is not fully developed, the premature infant is sluggish, must be wakened to be fed, and the muscular movements are feeble. The temperature is usually subnormal and fluctuating, due to the underdeveloped heat-regulating center. The cry is monotonous, whining, "kittenlike" and effortless, showing a lack of energy. All these symptoms are evidenced in varying degrees, according to the stage of prematurity.

IMMEDIATE CARE

The care given the premature baby at birth may differ from that given to the full-term baby, depending upon his condition. For the very small and feeble premature baby, the urgency of providing immediate warmth may precede the care of the eyes and completion of the care of the cord. Whenever possible, it is advisable to wait until the cord pulsation weakens before clamping it, so that the baby will benefit from the placental blood. The cord should be tied with special care because of the softness of the tissues, leaving space for a second ligature close to the body. The cord should be inspected at frequent intervals for bleeding, because prematurity is a predisposing cause of secondary hemorrhage. Since premature babies are also more susceptible to infections, asepsis is imperative.

As soon as the head emerges, the eyes should be wiped with moist sterile gauze. The instillation of prophylactic drops may have to be deferred until the condition of the baby warrants this treatment.

Because of the baby's underdeveloped and delicate structures, the resuscitation of the premature infant must be managed with extreme care and gentleness. Perhaps the method of resuscitation will determine the baby's chances to live. The mucus should be removed from the nose and the throat with great care. Any injury to the delicate tissues is an avenue to trauma and infection which may lead to pneumonia.

Since the maintenance of body heat is so essential, the baby should be wrapped in a warmed blanket, and a heated bed or incubator should be ready to receive him. When the baby's condition permits, his temperature and weight should be recorded, and his body oiled with warm oil. Oil on the skin is preferable to water because it prevents irritation and loss of heat. At all times, he should be handled as little and as gently as possible.

NURSING CARE

MANAGEMENT

Because of the nationwide interest in reducing deaths among premature infants, there have developed special premature nurseries and special premature referral centers in municipalities and other major health jurisdictions. Space is usually allotted in the hospital separate from the nursery for the full-term babies. Some centers concentrate on the care of the smaller babies. Generally, provision is made for the safe transport to and from the hospital. At the time of discharge plans are made for the follow-up care in the home. In these programs all premature infants spend the initial period in an incubator. These plans include: providing skilled medical and nursing care with the least possible amount of handling, maintaining adequate oxygenation, stabilizing the body temperature, safeguarding the baby against infection, supplying proper nutrition and feeding, maintaining a fluid and electrolyte balance and recognizing early abnormalities and infections.

Most hospitals have special premature nurseries which are air-conditioned in respect to temperature (85° to 90° F.), ventilation and humidity (50 to 65 per cent) control. Both electric incubators and specially prepared beds are used with good results. The principle of all incubators is the same, the only difference being in the construction details of various kinds. An incubator

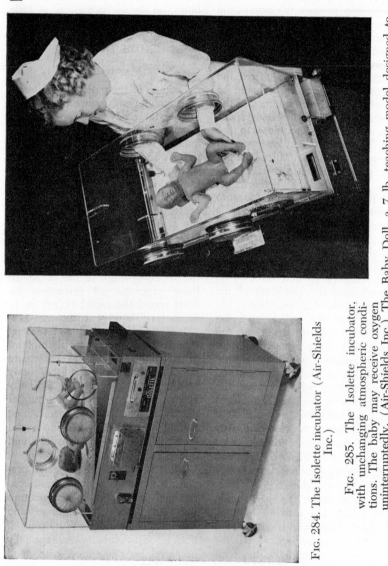

Fig. 284. The Isolette incubator (Air-Shields Inc.)

Fig. 285. The Isolette incubator with unchanging atmospheric conditions. The baby may receive oxygen uninterruptedly. (Air-Shields Inc.) The Baby Doll, a 7 lb. teaching model designed to resemble a new baby, including fontanels and "wobbly" head. (Sculptor Abram Belskie)

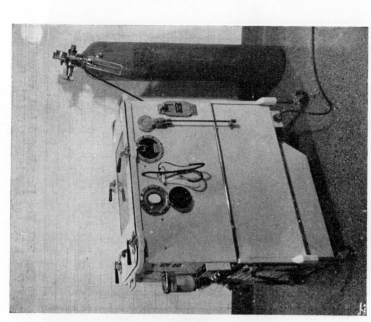

Fig. 287. Davidson incubator. (Sloane Hospital for Women, New York)

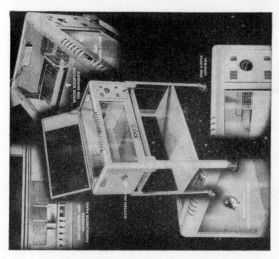

Fig. 286. Armstrong portable baby incubator, automatically controlled. (Gordon Armstrong Co.)

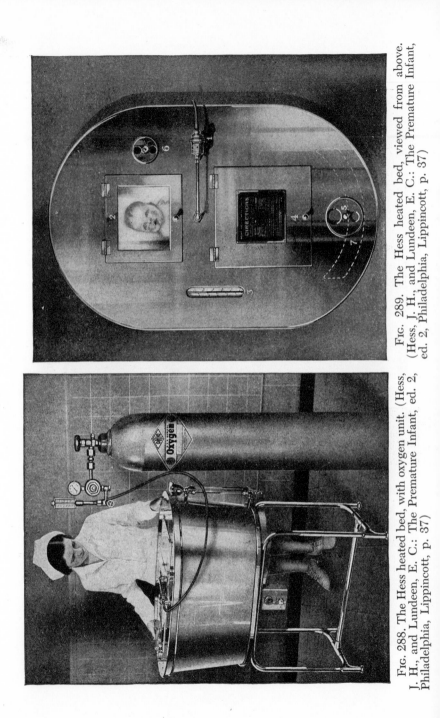

FIG. 288. The Hess heated bed, with oxygen unit. (Hess, J. H., and Lundeen, E. C.: The Premature Infant, ed. 2, Philadelphia, Lippincott, p. 37)

FIG. 289. The Hess heated bed, viewed from above. (Hess, J. H., and Lundeen, E. C.: The Premature Infant, ed. 2, Philadelphia, Lippincott, p. 37)

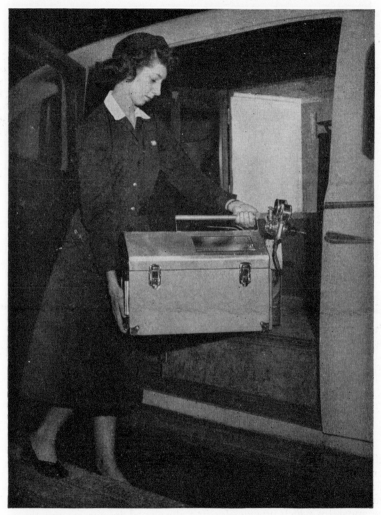

Fig. 290. Nurse of the New York City Department of Health placing the portable premature incubator into the Department's Premature Transport Service Ambulance. (City of New York, Department of Health; photo by George Doherty)

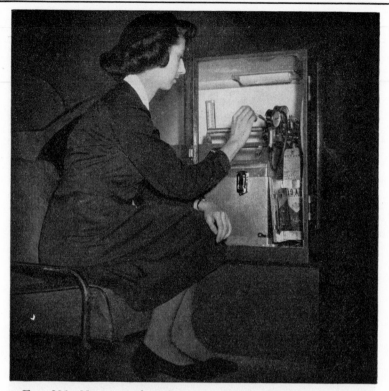

Fig. 291. Nurse regulating oxygen in portable incubator in the heated compartment of the Premature Transport Service Ambulance of the New York City Department of Health. (City of New York, Department of Health; photo by George Doherty)

is a miniature room in which the infant can lie, and the interior always can be inspected through the transparent windows. Another essential feature of a satisfactory incubator is the apparatus which provides for its thorough ventilation and the administration of oxygen, often so life-saving at this time. The incubators are so constructed that the temperature can be regulated to any desired degree.

Many persons have the impression that, once the baby is placed in a good incubator, no further special precautions need be taken. This is a mistaken idea. Premature or under-developed infants require the most solicitous care in every way; merely to keep them at a proper temperature will avail nothing unless the other details of their care are executed carefully. The maintenance of asepsis in every detail is essential for these inadequately fortified babies. It is also urgent that doctors, nurses or anyone caring for a delicate premature baby should avoid contact with any possible source of infection which might be transferred to the baby.

Rest is a most important factor, and the baby must be shielded from excitement and disturbing influences. Light should be curtailed, and loud or sudden noises should be avoided. All routine care is given in the premature bed whenever possible to limit the amount of handling, such as changing his clothing, administering nourishment, altering his position, or bathing him. The skin is extremely delicate and tender; and if diapers are used they should be changed as soon as they become wet or soiled. Sometimes only a small pad is placed under the baby. If the baby's condition warrants, a daily warm oil bath is usually given. If an incubator is not available he is dressed in a jacket of cotton and gauze or flannel. The weight and the temperature of the baby are both matters of importance and are carried out according to the hospital routine.

FEEDING

When planning the feeding schedule for the premature infant it is important to establish a food tolerance

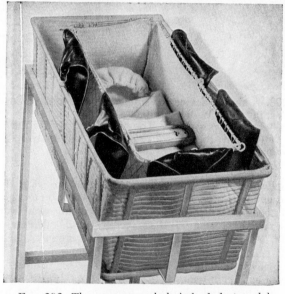

FIG. 292. The premature baby's bed designed by Lila J. Napier. The hot-water bottles regulate the temperature of the bed. The vapor-meter registers the temperature and moisture in the room, so that they may be regulated. This bed may be improvised from boxes, baskets, etc., and used in the home.

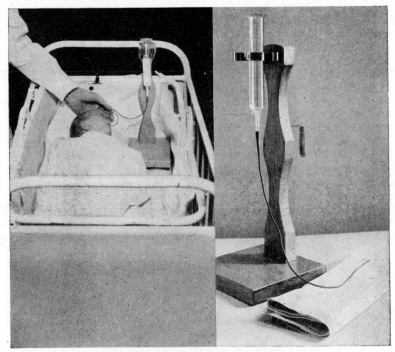

Fig. 293. A simple device for supporting the tube while giving a gavage feeding. This stand is attached to the top of the crib and thus facilitates the procedure. The nurse has both hands free to manage the baby and introduce the tube. (Lying-In Hospital of the Pennsylvania Hospital, Philadelphia)

since the intestinal tract (as well as other organs) is underdeveloped. The caloric needs of the premature baby are estimated according to the body weight. At first, the feeding should be in small amounts and increased gradually to the amount that will produce a consistent gain, since vomiting, distention and diarrhea may be due to overfeeding.

According to some authorities the general plan involves an initial period of rest, followed by small amounts of water at frequent intervals; gradual replacement of water feedings by milk feedings; gradual increase in amounts of milk and water at each feeding until caloric and fluid requirements are met. Some physicians advise adding a 5 per cent glucose solution to the drinking water. Undiluted raw breast milk has been found to be the best food for the premature baby. Boiling the milk destroys the enzymes so needed by the baby. Carbohydrates may be added to provide a more concentrated food in smaller amounts at a feeding. The mother's diet should be selected carefully, since diarrhea in the baby may result from her diet. While this may not affect the full-term baby, it may be serious for the premature baby. If the mother's breast milk is not available, every effort should be made to obtain it from another source. In many communities, frozen breast milk is available (p. 539). As a last resource, the physician may order a formula as a substitute. In addition to the feeding, some premature diets include vitamins A, B, C, D and K and some iron preparation. These will be added to the diet very gradually and not until the baby is able to tolerate them. The premature baby is usually fed every 2 or 3 hours. The stomach of the premature baby needs rest between feedings as much as that of the full-term baby; therefore, the interval should be regulated accordingly. The schedule should be as near that of a normal infant as is compatible with his progress.

The method of feeding depends on the baby's general condition and his ability to suck and swallow. When the swallowing reflex is not yet developed or if the baby becomes cyanotic when being fed or if the feeding takes too long and the baby becomes fatigued, gavage feeding may be necessary.

In gavage feeding, a sterile soft rubber French catheter (No. 10-12) is used. The distance between the bridge of the baby's nose and the estimated area of the stomach should be measured and marked on the catheter. The catheter is lubricated and introduced very cautiously, making sure that it has not been passed into the trachea. The catheter should be so controlled that no air will precede the milk. It is always a wise precaution to wait to make sure of the baby's reaction. The food should be introduced very slowly, and at the correct temperature. When removing the tube, it should be pinched to prevent the milk from escaping and entering the trachea. After the feeding, the baby's head should be elevated slightly and the body turned to the right side to aid the passage of the food into the intestines.

If a medicine dropper is used, the glass tip should be protected by rubber tubing which extends one-quarter of an inch beyond the tip. Before each sterilization, the tubing should be removed for cleansing and testing the glass tip. If gentle pressure is made on the back of the tongue with

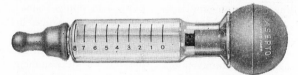

Fig. 294. The Breck Asepto infant feeder with midget or petite size nipple. Capacity one ounce, and graduated in eighths. While it greatly facilitates the feeding of infants too weak to nurse, it must be used with great caution. (Becton-Dickinson Company)

the rubber tubing on the end of the dropper, it may stimulate the baby to swallow.

The Breck Asepto infant feeder is a graduated glass tube with a small rubber nipple at the smaller end and a bulb at the larger. The bulb serves as an air reservoir, and, when the nipple is placed in the infant's mouth, slight intermittent pressure on the bulb will enable the baby to get the milk without any effort whatever, except that of swallowing. The nipple and the bulb are removed for cleaning and sterilization each time it is used. The Breck feeder should be used with great care and only by an experienced person. Whatever method of feeding is used, the baby's head should be raised.

PRECAUTIONS

Since the life of the premature baby may depend on his nursing care, the nurse should realize the seriousness of this responsibility during this period of her nursing experience and make every effort to increase her knowledge and develop her skill.

Often the first hours of the premature baby's life determine the outcome. He needs warmth, meticulous care, gentle handling, precise and careful feeding, and protection from infection. It must always be remembered that the word "premature" means that this baby has arrived before he had the opportunity to develop completely and, if he is to live, this intricate development has to be completed against odds almost unsurmountable—under conditions difficult even for the normal full-term

baby. It is important that home conditions be investigated by the visiting nurse or social worker before the baby is discharged from the hospital.

GROWTH AND DEVELOPMENT

Growth and development of the premature baby is dependent upon the prenatal causes, trauma at birth and the conditions arising in the postnatal period. Much will depend on the ability of the infant to meet the conditions attendant at birth and to adjust to the changes in his new environment. Those infants who react well to prompt treatment and care make their adjustment by the end of the first year, but there are others who may require 5 or more years to meet the normal child at that age.

The nurse is often asked if a premature baby will ever develop as well and become as strong and sturdy as one born at term. While the premature baby is slower in regaining his birth weight, by the end of the first year his weight should approximate that of the normal baby. Evidences of progress in his development are temperature stability, the increased vigor of his cry, stronger muscular activity, evidence of appetite and hunger, more normal periods of sleep, changes in the appearance and the character of his skin due to the addition of the subcutaneous fat, the development of reflexes and general signs of health. Authorities differ in opinion that it may take from 2 to 7 years for the premature to attain the physical and mental status of a full term baby's growth and development at a comparable age. There is no reason why the premature baby should not ultimately be as healthy as any other baby. There are today several noted people who were premature babies.

SUGGESTED READING

Bakwin, Harry: The home care of the premature infant, J. Pediat. 34:654, 1949.

Baumgartner, Leona: Nation-wide plan for reduction of premature mortality, J.A.M.A. 146:893, 1951.

Dunham, E. C.: Premature Infants, A Manual for Physicians, U. S. Federal Security Agency, Washington, D. C., Publication No. 325, 1948.

Dunham, E. C., and Bierman, J. M.: The care of the premature infant, J.A.M.A. 115:658, 1940.

Eastman, N. J.: Prematurity from the viewpoint of the obstetrician, Am. Pract. 1:343, 1947.

Gesell, A.: Behavior aspects of the care of the premature infant, J. Pediat. 29:210-212, 1946.

Greene, Doris M.: Caring for the premature baby, Am. J. Nursing 50:458, 1950.

Herbolsheimer, Henrietta: Mortality and cost experience with premature infants in 1948, J.A.M.A. 144:542, 1950.

Hess, J. H., and Lundeen, E. C.: The Premature Infant, Its Medical and Nursing Care, ed. 2, Philadelphia, Lippincott, 1949. (An excellent and practical book designed especially for nurses.)

Losty, Margaret A., Orlofsky, Irene, and Wallace, Helen M.: A trans-port service for premature babies, Am. J. Nursing 50:10, 1950.

McKellar, B.: A simple and inexpensive carrier for premature babies, Am. J. Obst. & Gynec. 37:343, 1939.

Parke, Priscilla C.: Naso-gastric tube feeding for premature infants, Am. J. Nursing 51:517, 1951.

Potter, Edith L.: The Relation of Premature Delivery to Death in the Neonatal Period, Committee on Human Reproduction of the National Research Council, Jan. 19, 1951.

——: Pathology of prematurity, J. Am. M. Women's A. 5:391, 1950.

Smith, Clement A.: Nutrition of premature infants, Nutrition Rev. 8: 353, 1950.

Stone, E. L.: The Newborn Infant, Philadelphia, Lea & Febiger, 1945.

Taylor, E. Stewart: The prevention of deaths from prematurity, Pub. Health Nursing 42:280, 1950.

Wallace, Helen M., Losty, Margaret A., and Wishik, Samuel M.: Prematurity as a public health problem, Am. J. Pub. Health 40:41, 1950.

Wallace, Helen M., Rascoff, Henry, and Knobloch, Hilda: Pilot study of maternal and neonatal factors in premature infant mortality, J.A.M.A. 146:886, 1951.

23

Disorders of the Newborn

ASPHYXIA NEONATORUM
INJURIES
INFECTIONS
MALFORMATIONS

ERYTHROBLASTOSIS AND THE RH
FACTOR
MISCELLANEOUS DISORDERS

ASPHYXIA NEONATORUM

Normally, the baby cries immediately after delivery—often when the shoulders are being born. If respiration has not begun within 30 seconds or so after birth, the condition usually is referred to as *asphyxia neonatorum*. This complication may show various gradations from brief, transitory apnea (absence of respiration) to fatal respiratory failure. In the milder cases the baby's face and often the entire body are of a livid hue, and the vessels of the umbilical cord are distended with blood; the tone of the muscles is good, so that any attempt to move the extremities or open the mouth will meet with some resistance. This stage of the process is known as *asphyxia livida*. In severe cases the baby's face and body are of a deathlike pallor, the vessels of the cord empty and the muscles relaxed so that the infant

is entirely limp. This stage is known as *asphyxia pallida*.

Failure of the baby to breathe at birth usually is due to one of three main causes, or to a combination of them:

1. Anoxia (deprivation of oxygen)
2. Cerebral injury
3. Narcosis

Anoxia. Since the baby in utero is entirely dependent upon the placenta for its oxygen supply, any interference with the function of that organ or with that of the umbilical cord will put the baby in grave danger because of anoxia. If the oxygen supply is entirely cut off for more than a very few minutes, fetal death in utero results; if only partially curtailed, the baby is born in an asphyxiated state and (like all asphyxiated persons) does not breathe.

Intra-uterine asphyxia may be produced in a number of ways. The umbilical cord may prolapse and become pinched between the pelvic brim and the fetal head, with the result that the umbilical vein becomes compressed and unable to carry oxygen to the baby. Premature separation of the placenta often disrupts placental function entirely so that the baby suffers complete deprivation of oxygen. Extremely severe uterine contractions may so squeeze the placental site as to jeopardize the infant's oxygen supply.

Cerebral Injury. This is a very common cause of apnea at birth, particularly after difficult operative deliveries. Not only may the associated brain hemorrhage damage the respiratory center itself, but other vital centers may be injured. As already indicated, the most frequent cause of cerebral injury at birth is difficult operative delivery, such as midforceps operations, version and extraction and breech extraction. Likewise, disproportion between the size of the head and that of the pelvis may bring about such compression of the fetal skull as to damage the brain. Cerebral injury may also result from long, difficult labor when no instruments are used.

Narcosis. The narcosis produced in the fetus by analgesic and anesthetic drugs given to the mother is a frequent cause of sluggish respiration at birth. As a rule, however, this is quite transitory, and statistics indicate that these babies do as well subsequently as infants whose mothers received no such drugs. This explains why nurses with adequate experience should closely supervise these patients.

Prevention of Asphyxia Neonatorum. Preventive treatment is very important but is largely the responsibility of the obstetrician. It begins with the first prenatal visit when he measures the pelvis and makes sure that it is large enough to allow passage of the baby's head without compression. Good diet and hygiene contribute greatly to the health of the infant at birth. During labor, the physician can do much to prevent asphyxia of the baby by avoiding as much as possible the more difficult types of operative delivery and by care in the use of analgesic and amnesic drugs. Moreover, by listening regularly to the fetal heart tones, he may detect early signs of impending fetal distress (slow rate) and, with this warning, it may be possible for him to deliver the infant before serious trouble develops. The passage of meconium-stained amniotic fluid is another sign of fetal distress but is of no value in breech presentations, since the passage of meconium —ordinarily pure meconium—is the rule in breech cases.

Many physicians believe that the administration of vitamin K to the mother late in pregnancy and during labor tends to prevent cerebral hemorrhage in the newborn by improving the clotting power of the fetus' blood. This antihemorrhagic vitamin passes readily through the placenta and raises the prothrombin concentration of the fetal plasma which is ordinarily low. Since prothrombin is known to be essential to proper blood coagulation, this measure is theoretically a sound one, and the practical experience of a number of obstetricians suggests that it may prove to be a valuable procedure.

Treatment of Asphyxia Neonatorum. In treating a baby which does not breathe at birth, there are five main principles to be kept in mind.

1. GENTLENESS. These infants are often in a state of shock, and rough attempts to resuscitate them—as by vigorous spanking, plunging in ice water and shaking—may do more harm than good. Methods of physical stimulation should be limited to gentle rubbing of the back, to snapping the feet with one's finger and, at the most, to light patting of the buttocks.

2. WARMTH. Hot-water bottles,

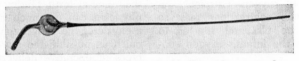

FIG. 295. Catheter and glass bulb with a trap, for aspirating mucus in the treatment of asphyxia. (Chicago Lying-In Hospital)

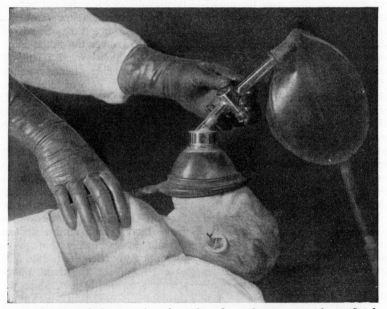

FIG. 296. Inhalation of carbon dioxide and oxygen with artificial respiration in partial asphyxia. Suction is applied through a soft rubber catheter introduced into the pharynx. An infant's size breathing bag is then filled with carbon dioxide and oxygen, the inhaler is placed on the face and gentle pressure, at intervals, applied to the chest. The color changes to pink, respiration becomes established and the infant attempts to cry. (Eastman, N. J.: Williams Obstetrics, New York, Appleton)

Fig. 297. The E. & J. Resuscitator and Inhalator, used at the Lying-In Hospital, Pennsylvania Hospital, Philadelphia.

The apparatus is a combination of automatic breathing machine and simple inhalation device. As a resuscitator, it reproduces respiration by setting up in the lungs a continuing sequence of alternating fixed positive and negative pressures. The rhythm is controlled by the intrapulmonary pressures of the baby and, therefore, automatically adjust itself to the lung capacity. As an inhalator, it supplies to the baby a constant flow of oxygen or oxygen-carbon-dioxide mixture. By means of a control lever, it is possible to switch instantly from insufflation-suction to straight inhalation and vice versa.

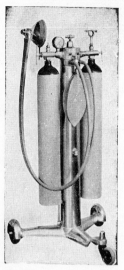

warm blankets and other means of maintaining body warmth must be in readiness. This is particularly important to remember because the measures employed to resuscitate infants, unless care be taken, tend to expose their completely naked bodies (accustomed to a temperature of 98.6° F.) to room temperature; and this may aggravate the state of shock. The body of the baby should be kept covered as much as possible.

3. POSTURE. Most obstetricians hold the baby up by the feet momentarily after birth in order to expedite drainage of mucus from the trachea, the larynx and the posterior pharynx. The baby is then placed on its back in a slight Trendelenburg position (head turned aside, lower than buttocks), also to favor gravity drainage of mucus.

4. REMOVAL OF MUCUS. Cleansing the air passages of mucus and fluid is essential. Since posture alone is often not adequate for this purpose, suction of one type or another is frequently necessary. An ordinary catheter is used, size 14 or 15 French; in premature infants a smaller size (10 or 11) is advisable. A glass trap (Fry) is inserted into the catheter to arrest mucus which otherwise might be drawn into the operator's mouth. Milking the trachea upward will help bring mucus and fluid into the posterior pharynx, where it may be aspirated by the catheter. Gentleness is essential, since the mucous membrane of the baby's mouth is delicate. Although the physician occasionally does so, the nurse should not introduce the catheter farther than the posterior pharynx. Mechanical suction devices are provided with most of the modern machines for infant resuscitation and are very convenient.

5. ARTIFICIAL RESPIRATION. This may be carried out in a number of

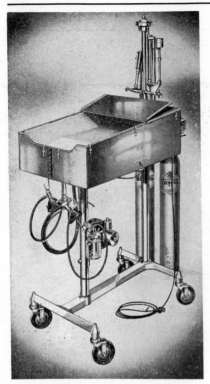

Fig. 298. Kreiselman infant resuscitator (Ohio Chemical and Surgical Equipment Co.)

ways. Gentle compression of the chest with the hand followed by sudden release may be tried a few times, but unless this produces spontaneous breathing immediately, more efficient methods should be employed. Slow, repeated flexing of the infant's thighs against the abdomen coupled with bending the head forward so that the chin impinges against the sternum is a more satisfactory way of compressing the chest. When the compression is released in either of these methods, negative pressure is established in the lungs, and air is drawn in.

Probably the oldest and most widely used method of resuscitation is mouth-to-mouth insufflation, but this is disapproved by some physicians. Although this procedure is ordinarily performed by the doctor, the nurse may be asked to carry it out if the available physicians are busy attending the mother. The operator stands or sits back of the infant's head. After placing two or three layers of gauze on the baby's face, the operator bends over the infant and puts his opened mouth over the infant's mouth and nose, the gauze intervening. He now exhales gently into the baby's respiratory tract. It is advantageous to follow this with light compression of the chest, insufflation and compression being alternated. One does not "blow" into the baby's mouth but simply exhales more or less naturally. Blowing into the baby's mouth with any degree of force is highly dangerous and may rupture a pulmonary alveolus.

Many hospitals are now using mechanical devices for the resuscitation of the newborn. Such apparatus permits the administration of pure oxygen to the baby's lungs at pressures which are controlled mechanically within safe limits. Instead of oxygen, some obstetricians prefer oxygen containing a small admixture of carbon dioxide, but others disapprove of the carbon dioxide.

Atelectasis. Prior to birth, the lungs contain no air and are in a state of collapse. With the first breath, expansion of the lung tissue begins and continues progressively for several

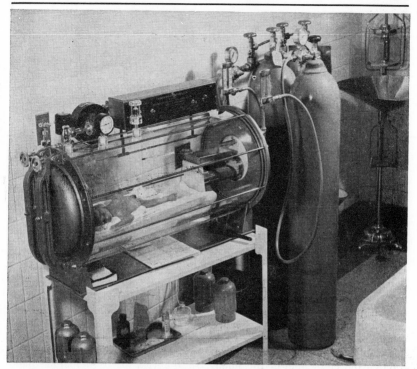

FIG. 299. Bloxsom air lock. (Allen Bloxsom, M.D., St. Joseph's Maternity Hospital, Houston, Texas)

days until all parts of the lung are expanded. Feeble respiratory action after birth may expand the lungs only partially, leaving large areas in a collapsed state. This condition is known as "atelectasis." It is particularly common in premature infants. Cyanosis is usually present because the small areas of expanded lung are inadequate to oxygenate the blood properly. Atelectasis is treated best by continuous administration of oxygen, frequent change of position and occasional attempts to stimulate deeper respiration. However, the

outlook in most of these cases is poor.

Bloxsom Air Lock. The Bloxsom air lock (Fig. 299) consists of an airtight, transparent cylinder, the interior of which is controlled automatically in regard to temperature and humidity. The special feature of the apparatus is that oxygen and air in about equal proportions can be introduced under "cycled pressures." By this is meant that the pressure of oxygen within the cylinder is allowed to build up until it reaches about 3 pounds, when an automatic valve allows the oxygen mixture to

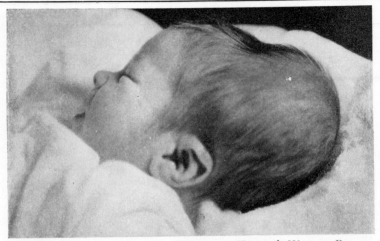

Fig. 300. Caput succedaneum. (Maternity Hospital, Western Reserve University Hospitals, Cleveland)

escape so that the pressure falls back to 1 pound. This building up of oxygen pressure and its release is carried out in cycles of about 1 minute each. The principle is that oxygenation thus produced will diffuse through the epithelium of the small bronchioles and other epithelial surfaces to reach the capillary blood of the infant's lungs. In addition, favorable diffusion gradients are set up for the outward diffusion of carbon dioxide from the infant's blood as well as inward diffusion of oxygen. In the case of a premature baby whose sternum is retracting because

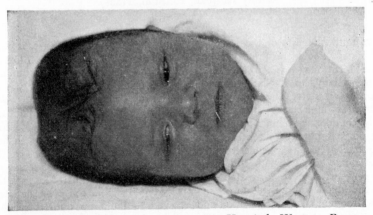

Fig. 301. Cephalhematoma. (Maternity Hospital, Western Reserve University Hospitals, Cleveland)

of atelectasis, the objective of the diffusion mechanism is to supplement the faulty alveolar oxygenation and so take a certain load off the overworked respiratory process until the alveoli become distended.

INJURIES

Caput Succedaneum. Prolonged pressure on the head during a protracted first stage, where the membranes rupture before the os is fully dilated, causes a swelling of the scalp over the area where it is encircled by the cervix. This is called "caput succedaneum," and in its milder forms is very common—so common that it may be regarded as normal.

It is due to an extravasation of serum into the tissues of the scalp at the portion surrounded by the os uteri during labor and free from pressure. The term is not confined to vertex cases; the corresponding swelling which forms on any presenting part is also, for the sake of uniformity, known as caput succedaneum. The condition always disappears within a few days without treatment.

Cephalhematoma. Another swelling of the scalp which resembles caput succedaneum in certain respects is caused by an effusion of blood between the bone and the periosteum. This explains why the swelling appears directly over the bone. It is most common over the parietal bones. It is seldom present when the baby is born and may not be noticed for 2 or 3 days; it increases gradually in size until about the seventh day after labor, when it remains stationary for a time and then begins to disappear. This condition is termed "cephalhematoma," and the baby usually recovers without treatment. It may be due to pressure in normal labor, or by forceps; but also it is seen occasionally in breech cases in which no instruments were used or prolonged pressure exerted on the aftercoming head. Such cases, however, are not common.

Intracranial Hemorrhage. (Synonyms: cerebral hemorrhage; brain hemorrhage.) In contradistinction to the two conditions just described, intracranial hemorrhage is one of the gravest complications encountered in the newborn. Indeed, it is the commonest immediate cause of stillbirth and neonatal death. It may occur any place in the cranial vault but is particularly likely to take place as the result of tears in the tentorium cerebelli with bleeding into the cerebellum, the pons and the medulla oblongata. Since these structures contain many important centers (respiratory center, etc.), hemorrhage in these areas is very often fatal.

Intracranial hemorrhage occurs most often after prolonged labor, especially in primiparae, and is particularly likely to take place in difficult forceps deliveries and in version and extractions. It is also seen more commonly in precipitate deliveries as the result of the rapid propulsion of the baby's head through the birth canal. It is due primarily to excessive or unduly prolonged pressure on the fetal skull. This causes excessive molding of the head and such overriding of the cranial bones that the delicate supporting structures of the brain (tentorium cerebelli, falx cerebri, etc.) are torn, with consequent rupture of blood vessels.

The development of symptoms in cerebral hemorrhage may be sudden or gradual. If the hemorrhage is severe, the infant is usually stillborn; if less marked, apnea neonatorum may result, often with fatal outcome. Many infants which are resuscitated with difficulty at birth succumb later from brain hemorrhage. On the other hand, the baby may appear normal after delivery and develop the first signs of intracranial hemorrhage several hours or several days later.

The nurse should be familiar with the common signs of cerebral hemorrhage, which are described as follows.

1. _Convulsions._ These may vary from mild, localized twitchings to severe spasms of the whole body. Twitching of the lower jaw is characteristic, particularly when associated with salivation.

2. _Cyanosis._ This may be persistent but is more likely to occur in repeated attacks.

3. _Abnormal Respiration._ Grunting respiration is characteristic; or it may be irregular, of Cheyne-Stokes type, or very rapid and shallow, or very slow. Very slow breathing usually is associated with cyanosis, suggests respiratory paralysis due to pressure on the medulla oblongata, and is a grave sign.

4. _A Sharp, Shrill, Weak Cry._ This is similar to that seen in meningitis.

5. _Flaccidity._ If persistent, this usually portends a fatal outcome.

TREATMENT. Prevention is most important but is largely the responsibility of the physician. It consists in protecting the infant from trauma, particularly in difficult operative delivery. As stated previously, many obstetricians believe that the administration of vitamin K to the mother before delivery decreases the likelihood of cerebral bleeding. Moreover, following operative delivery, often it is given to the infant hypodermically as a prophylactic measure.

Curative treatment is rarely effective, since considerable damage, as a rule, already has been done to the brain tissue when the signs of the condition first develop. Complete rest, with the very minimum amount of handling, is imperative. Infants suspected of having a cerebral hemorrhage should not nurse the breast and should not be weighed or bathed. Since shock is often present, external heat is frequently indicated. Feeding should be carried out in such a manner as to impose on the infant the least possible effort; some of these babies have to be gavaged. Usually the physician will order some form of sedative for convulsions and will prescribe the administration of oxygen for cyanosis. The head of the baby should be kept a few inches above the level of the hips, because this position is believed to lower intracranial pressure. It would be interesting if some research could ascertain the number of children who survive accidents of this type and become anything like normal individuals when they grow up.

Facial Paralysis. Pressure by forceps on the facial nerve may cause temporary paralysis of the muscles of one side of the face so that the mouth is drawn to the other side. This will be particularly noticeable when the baby cries. The condition is usually transitory and disappears in a few days, often in a few hours.

Arm Paralysis. Injury to the brachial plexus, inflicted in the course of breech extraction, may cause paralysis of one arm. In the majority of cases, this disappears within a few weeks but may be permanent. It is called "Erb's paralysis" (or "Erb-Duchenne's paralysis"). In order to reduce tension on the brachial plexus, the doctor usually will place the arm in a splint or cast in an elevated, neutral position.

Fractures and Dislocations. Fracture of a long bone or dislocation of an extremity may be the result of a version; or it may occur following a breech delivery in which the arms were extended above the head and are brought down into the vagina. Fractures of the clavicle ("collar bone") or of the jaw, or dislocation of either of these bones, may follow forcible efforts to extract the after-coming head in cases of breech presentation. These cases, of course, occur when the physician is present, and their treatment is his responsibility.

Fractures in the newborn baby usually heal rapidly, but it is often difficult to keep the parts in good position during repair. Dislocation should be reduced at once, or there will be great danger of permanent deformity in the joint. Follow-up supervision is necessary in order to prevent permanent deformity. Physiotherapy under orthopedic direction is important.

INFECTIONS

Ophthalmia neonatorum is a serious condition which may result in total blindness, but if suitable treatment is adopted at the very outset of the disease and intelligently carried out, usually the sight can be saved. The entire treatment is, of course, under the direct supervision of the physician.

Ophthalmia neonatorum is usually of gonorrheal origin and is characterized by a profuse, purulent discharge due to infection, generally from the genital canal at the time of birth. This is not always the case, however, and the lack of proper hygiene by the doctor or the nurse or the mother may carry the infection to the eyes of the baby. Until the use of silver nitrate prophylaxis was established, from 25 to 30 per cent of all children in schools for the blind suffered impaired sight as the result of a gonorrheal infection.

If the infection occurs at the time of birth, the disease appears within 2 or 3 days; but as the septic discharge may be introduced into the eye at a later period by neglect of the proper care of the baby, the onset may be later. Both eyes are usually affected; and at first they are suffused with a watery discharge and considerable inflammation of the eyelids. Within 24 hours the lids become very much swollen, and a thick, creamy, greenish pus is discharged. Later, unless treatment has been instituted early, the swelling becomes so marked that the eyes cannot be opened, opacities of the cornea occur, the conjunctiva is ulcerated and then perforated, and the eye collapses and finally atrophies.

The preventive treatment consists in the use of 1 per cent silver nitrate, which is instilled into the eyes immediately after birth, or penicillin is administered in the form of aqueous drops or ointment. Penicillin is widely reported as effective as silver nitrate for use at birth. Favorable reports are given for aureomycin also. Penicillin may also be given as intramuscular injections. If the infection persists, intensive penicillin administration should be carried out. Thanks to this drug, gonorrheal ophthalmia, which used to be one of the most stubborn and grave of afflictions and demanded the utmost in elaborate and prolonged nursing and medical care, is now cured within from 12 to 24 hours. The swelling and the pus usually disappear in even less time than this.

Ophthalmia neonatorum is a distinctly infectious disease, and there is extreme danger of conveying it to others. This applies not only to other babies' eyes but to the genital tract of other mothers. Even the eyes of

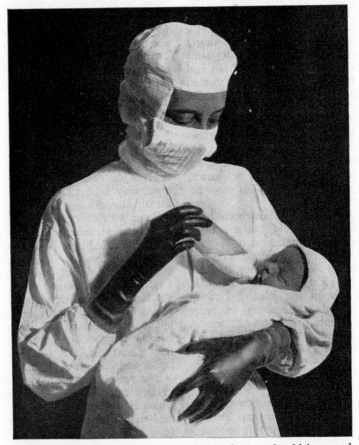

Fig. 302. A baby with any infectious disease should be cared for with isolation technic. When the baby is feeding, its hands are protected by a wrap-around sleeveless gown or blanket.

the nurse herself may become infected, unless she is most conscientious in her methods. The baby should be isolated, and all articles used should be sterilized. Gloves, cap and gown should be worn by the nurse, and she should handle all dressings with forceps. Staphylococcus of resistant types occasionally cause purulent discharge; all such cases should be under the care of a physician until recovery.

Impetigo. Impetigo is a skin disease of infectious origin and not infrequently occurs in epidemic form in the nursery. For this reason, it is often called "impetigo contagiosa." The condition manifests itself by the eruption of small, semiglobular vesicles or pustules. While these may appear on any part of the body, they are most frequently encountered on moist opposing surfaces, such as the folds of the neck, the axilla and the groin. Thence they may spread rapidly by auto-inoculation to any part of the body. The lesion is small and varies from the size of a pinhead to a diameter of half an inch. It contains yellow pus. The bacterium involved is usually the staphylococcus or the streptococcus.

The treatment is essentially preventive, and cases rarely occur if the nursery technic has been meticulous. The nurse and the doctor must wash their hands carefully before handling any baby, and every possible source of skin infection must be eliminated. Constant vigilance is necessary if these cases are to be prevented. In some hospitals, the following technic is employed to prevent impetigo: immediately after birth and following a soap and water bath, the infant receives an inunction of ammoniated

mercury ointment (2 to 5 per cent). In others, no bath or inunction whatsoever is given, and the vernix caseosa is allowed to remain in place. This substance protects the skin from infection; indeed, it is apparently Nature's way of providing protection for the delicate skin.

As soon as a lesion develops which resembles impetigo even slightly, strict isolation of the infant is imperative. The doctor should be notified at once. He probably will open the blebs or lesions and apply either gentian violet or sulfathiazole ointment. Light treatment often halts the infection quickly. Local applications of penicillin dressings or pads are also used successfully. If properly treated, the superficial lesions heal quickly with little scarring. Special penicillin preparations given by mouth have been effective in 2 days. A high nutritional level must be maintained and scratching should be controlled. It is important for the nurse to remember that it is the fluid within the bleb which spreads the infection. When impetigo develops in a nursery it may be stubborn to eradicate, and occasionally it may even become necessary to close the nursery for a few weeks.

Thrush or Sprue. The mouth or the tongue may be affected with small white patches due to a fungus growth. This condition, known as "thrush," is favored by lack of cleanliness in feeding, in the care of the mother's nipples, or in the care of the bottles and the nipples. It is most likely to occur in weak, undernourished babies. The baby's mouth must be kept clean, but great gentleness is required to avoid further injury to the delicate epithelium. Some physicians advise painting the spots with boric solution, soda solution, tincture of myrrh, a weak argyrol solution or gentian violet (aqueous solution 2 per cent). This is done by barely touching the spots with a sterile swab saturated with the selected solution. The doctor will direct details of such care.

Epidemic Diarrhea of the Newborn. During recent years, a number of highly fatal epidemics of diarrhea have occurred in nurseries for the newborn throughout the country. Among babies so affected, almost half have died. The mortality rate in premature infants is twice the rate in full-term infants. The onset is sudden, with profuse, watery yellow stools which increase in frequency. Associated with the diarrhea, a precipitous weight loss occurs—often a pound within 24 hours. The appearance of the baby changes rapidly from that of a healthy baby to one of a markedly dehydrated and emaciated infant. In a severe case, death may occur in a day, but more often the baby lingers on in a semicomatose condition for 4 or 5 days. The spread of the disease is very rapid, and half the infants in a nursery may succumb within a fortnight. Many of the epidemics accordingly are described as "explosive" in character.

The disease seems to be a special type of diarrhea which affects newborn infants and is quite different from the diarrhea from which older babies sometimes suffer. It is now certain that this disease is due to a virus. The symptoms and the mortality rate differ from bacterial types of dysentery or diarrhea. One of the most important predisposing factors is overcrowding in the nurseries. Faulty nursery technic is another—that is, failure to wash the hands before touching a baby, failure to sterilize rubber nipples properly, etc. The guiding principle involved is that everything coming in contact with the baby's mouth and nose should be in a surgically aseptic condition. All obstetric and nursing technics must be planned accordingly. Various health departments have set up rigid regulations along these lines in the hope of preventing epidemics. No visitors should be allowed while newborn infants are being fed or nursed by their mothers, and no visitors under 14 years should be allowed at any time. Small units for infant and maternity patients are desirable. Mask technic should be rigid.

When a case is discovered, immediate and absolute isolation is necessary, and the doctor is notified at once. Before the discovery of the curative action of sulfathiazole, which can cure a case in 24 hours and help prevent the spread through the nursery, emphasis was placed on starvation diets. Recently (1951) feeding rather than starvation has been recommended by some physicians. Dehydration must be overcome, water being given by increasing 5 cc. amounts until the full water requirement is met. The infant is also given 10 per cent glucose in water; and protein milk or skim milk is added. If the illness does not subside, food may be withheld for 12 hours, water supplied by clysis and the sulfathiazole medication renewed.

If an outbreak occurs there should be a follow-up of all infants discharged in the preceding 2 weeks and any infants needing treatment should be readmitted. All infants exposed at the time of an outbreak should be given sulfathiazole. Complete control of this disease which formally led to closing of the nursery can be gained by prompt reporting, rigid technics and sulfathiazole treatment.

Syphilis. Syphilis of newly born infants shows lesions only if the child has early prenatal syphilis. They may be present at birth or may appear from a few days up to 4 months of age, predominantly on the face, the buttocks, the palms and the soles. Mucous patches occur in the mouth, and condylomata about the anus. These lesions are highly infectious. The eruption is usually maculopapular and not quite so generalized as in acquired syphilis. Bullae may appear on the palms and the soles, a type of lesion never found in acquired syphilis. The palms and the soles may desquamate as a result of the lesions. Less frequently seen are papular lesions or purely macular or, very rarely, vesicular or somewhat pustular ones. The nails may be deformed, and alopecia may be present. In such cases the blood test for syphilis is usually strongly positive. In addition to the cutaneous manifestations of syphilis, other signs and symptoms may arouse suspicion of the presence of the disease. The infant becomes restless, develops rhinitis (snuffles) and a hoarse voice. The baby does not gain weight as it should. The lymph nodes are enlarged, especially the epitrochlear nodes. The liver and the spleen are enlarged, as are also the ends of the long bones.

In the treatment of syphilis of the newborn, the doctor will rely chiefly on penicillin, which has largely replaced the arsenic and bismuth formerly used.

Babies born to mothers who have been treated early in the prenatal period for syphilis are seldom born with the disease.

MALFORMATIONS

In one case in 200, approximately, an infant is born with some kind of malformation. Congenital deformities may range from minor abnormalities such as supernumerary digits to grave malformations, incompatible with life, such as anencephalus (absence of brain), hydrocephalus (excessive amount of fluid in the cerebral ventricles with tremendous enlargement of head) and various heart abnormalities. In the case of hydrocephalus, grave dystocia may occur because of the inability of the huge head to pass the pelvic inlet. Congenital malformations of the heart are a common cause of cyanosis in the newborn. Clubfoot, imperforate anus and meatus, harelip and cleft palate are other fairly frequent congenital deformities.

Harelip and Cleft Palate. Before the baby with harelip or cleft palate or both is referred for surgical treatment, he will need special care during feeding. Nursing (sucking) is difficult and may be impossible, depending on the degree of malformation. For some babies the Breck feeder, a medicine dropper or special nipples (cleft palate) fitted with a rubber flap may be used. Others may need gavage feeding. Because of difficulty in swallowing, great care must be exercised to prevent choking and nasal vomiting, but food is especially important in preparation for surgery. Therefore, definite time must be allowed to give adequate care to these babies. Some authorities think that these deformities are due to a lack of vitamin A in the prenatal diet.

Frenum Linguae. The frenum linguae is a vertical fold of mucous membrane under the tongue. If this membrane is short the activity of the tongue is limited, and this interferes with nursing. This condition should be observed at the time of the complete physical examination or during the nursing period. The doctor will "snip" the membrane with sterile blunt scissors.

Spina Bifida. Spina bifida is a rather common malformation and is due to the congenital absence of one or more vertebral arches, usually at the lower part of the spine. This allows the membranes covering the spinal cord to bulge, forming a soft, fluctuating tumor filled with cerebrospinal fluid. The tumor is diminished by pressure and enlarges when the baby cries. The disease is usually fatal, although a few recoveries have been recorded. When the tumor is very small and shows no signs of increasing in size, it may merely be protected from injury and infection by carefully applied dressings; but the more severe cases must be treated surgically.

Umbilical Hernia. Umbilical hernia, or rupture at the umbilicus, may appear during the first few weeks of life. The associated protrusion of intestinal contents may be made to disappear entirely on pressure, but it reappears when the pressure is removed or when the baby cries. This is due to a weakness in the abdominal wall caused by nonunion of the recti muscles. The condition usually disappears spontaneously, but should the protrusion of omentum persist, the abdomen may be strapped, using a 2-inch strip of adhesive plaster or a suitable cord bandage.

The graver congenital malformations are always a cause of keen disappointment to the family and sometimes produce serious psychologic disturbances in the mother. Such cases demand the utmost in sympathy and understanding on the part of the nurse, who will do well, as a rule, to endeavor tactfully to direct the mother's thoughts to other interests.

Obstructions of the Alimentary Tract

PYLORIC STENOSIS. This is a congenital anomaly and usually manifests its symptoms from the first few days to the second or the third week by the onset of vomiting which becomes projectile in character and occurs within 30 minutes after every feeding. The baby loses weight, the bowel elimination lessens, highly colored urine becomes scanty, and the symptoms of dehydration appear. Upon examination, gastric peristalsis is present and the pyloric "acornlike" tumor can be palpated. Usually, thick cereal feedings are prescribed. If no improvement is noted it is necessary to resort to surgery. Since it is not usually an emergency operation, there is sufficient time for supportive treatment to prepare the baby for surgery by vein and hypoclysis. The preoperative preparation includes intravenous blood and plasma. If the hemoglobin is below 70 per cent transfusion is indicated. Gastric lavage, from 1 to 2 hours before operation, should be done until returns are clear. Maintaining body heat before and after the operation is essential. After the operation the baby should be in the Trendelenburg position to avert aspiration. Transfusion should be given if indicated. The doctor usually orders from 5 to 10 cc. of water to be given within a few hours, then alternated with 10 cc. of breast milk or formula. As soon as the baby is gaining and consuming from 3 to 4 ounces at each feeding, he is ready for discharge.

OBSTRUCTION OF THE DUODENUM AND THE SMALL INTESTINE. These conditions are relatively easy to diagnose. Vomiting occurs with the first feeding, and no meconium is eliminated. The vomitus may or may not be bile-stained, depending upon whether the obstruction is high or low in the intestinal tract. If the obstruction is low, usually there is marked distention. An x-ray picture is used to confirm the diagnosis, and immediate surgery is indicated. However, the newborn infant should be allowed at least 12 hours for the respiration and kidney function to become established. The operation is usually accompanied by continuous venous drip and plasma, and blood should be available if needed. Postoperative care includes maintaining body temperature, intravenous fluids until peristalsis is established (about a week), followed by mouth feedings as given in pyloric stenosis. If distention occurs, nasoduodenal suction may be necessary. If the distention is severe, the baby should be in an oxygen tent.

INTUSSUSCEPTION. Acute intussusception is the most frequent type of intestinal obstruction and often may be unrecognized. There is usually intermittent abdominal pain, mild or severe, accompanied by blood and mucous intestinal elimination; and the baby may vomit. Upon abdominal examination a mass can be palpated. Immediate surgery is usually indicated. In preparation for surgery a gastric lavage is done, and an indwelling gastric catheter is inserted. Shock, if present, should be treated. An intravenous gastric drip may be ordered, and plasma and blood should be available for transfusion. After the operation the baby is placed in the Trendelenburg position, and the arms and the legs should be restrained. Hypoclysis may be given for 24 hours, followed by water by mouth. Feedings may be started on the third day if retained. Antibiotics may be ordered for the first 3 to 5 days and vitamin C to stimulate healing. The baby should be kept on his back for 10 days.

German Measles as a Cause of Malformations. As the result of observations made in an Australian epidemic of German measles in 1941, it seems clear that when German measles occurs during the first 3 months of pregnancy, a substantial proportion of the fetuses will show malformation, principally cataracts, heart disease, deaf-mutism and microcephaly. It should be noted that the disease which produces these harmful effects is German measles or rubella, and not rubeola measles, which has no such action. It should also be observed that German measles exerts these effects mainly when it occurs very early, usually before the twelfth week of pregnancy; and even then not all babies are affected. Just what proportion of babies are injured cannot be stated in the present stage of our knowledge. All that can be said is that when an expectant mother suffers from German measles during the first 12 weeks of pregnancy, there is a good—but by no means certain—chance that the infant will suffer from one of the malformations mentioned.

ERYTHROBLASTOSIS AND THE RH FACTOR

Erythroblastosis Fetalis. Erythroblastosis fetalis is a disease affecting the blood-forming organs of the newborn. The name is derived from *erythros,* "red," and *blastos,* "a formative cell." It occurs approximately once in every 400 deliveries and is responsible for about 3 per cent of all fetal deaths. The disease may manifest itself in three different forms.

1. *Hydrops fetalis.* The baby is tremendously edematous and invariably succumbs.

2. *Icterus gravis.* The infant is born with jaundice which deepens progressively; an anemia is also present. With repeated blood transfusions, many of these babies may be saved.

3. *Congenital anemia.* A marked anemia with consequent pallor is the characteristic feature of this type. Here, also, blood transfusion may save a certain number of infants.

Erythroblastosis fetalis is very likely to repeat itself in subsequent pregnancies, and some unfortunate mothers give birth to a series of such infants. Its cause, which has been discovered only recently, is immunologic in character and is based on the fact that the mother in these cases develops in her blood certain antibodies which attack a substance in the baby's red blood corpuscles known as the "Rh factor" (Fig. 149).

The Rh Factor. The Rh factor is a certain substance which most people have in their blood. It derives its name from the first two letters of the scientific term for the common monkey, the rhesus monkey, in the blood of which the factor is always present. The proportion of the white race which have the Rh factor is about 85 per cent; these people are called Rh positive. The remaining 15 per cent, who are without the factor, are called Rh negative.° The Rh factor is a hereditary characteristic, being transmitted as a Mendelian dormant.

When the blood of an Rh-positive person is introduced, through blood transfusion or otherwise, into the blood stream of an Rh-negative individual, the latter develops antibodies against the Rh factor present in the blood administered. Antibodies are substances which the body manufactures as a protective mechanism to counteract the effect of various kinds of new materials which may be introduced into the blood and the tissues. For instance, when bacteria gain access to the blood stream, antibodies against that particular kind of bacteria are usually developed and, sooner or later, destroy the bacteria. Antibodies may be regarded, accordingly, as a sort

° Only 7 per cent of Negroes are Rh negative, and about 1 per cent of Chinese.

of defensive army which the blood and the tissues muster against foreign, invading forces. It is these antibodies which cure most infectious diseases from the common cold to typhoid fever. Moreover, they often remain present in the blood and the tissues long after the disease has been combated successfully, making the person immune to that particular type of infection; in other words, should the same bacterium or material which incited the original manufacture of the antibodies be again introduced into the body, these defensive substances now stand ready to attack and destroy it.

As stated above, when an Rh-negative person is given a blood transfusion from an Rh-positive donor, antibodies are developed by the recipient against the Rh substance present in the administered blood. But, as is true when bacteria invade the body, these antibodies against the Rh factor do not form instantaneously but only after a period of time. Consequently, with the first transfusion, nothing out of the ordinary occurs. However, should this Rh negative recipient receive at some later date another transfusion from an Rh-positive donor, antibodies probably will have been developed and these will immediately attack the Rh factor. Since the Rh substance is an integral part of the red blood cells, this "battle" causes a violent commotion in the blood stream with the destruction of many red cells. As the broken-down products of these fragmented red cells are disseminated throughout the body, they exert a poisonous effect, and, as a result, the recipient of the blood transfusion suffers a reaction usually

manifested by a chill and fever but sometimes by more grave symptoms. In World War II, when many Rh-negative soldiers had to be given repeated blood transfusions, this Rh problem was a serious one. It was met by using Rh-negative donors for transfusions of Rh-negative persons— in other words, by administering blood without any Rh factor in it to cause the trouble described above. Nowadays physicians and surgeons everywhere are careful to determine the Rh status of any prospective recipient of a blood transfusion; if it is negative, blood from an Rh-negative donor is employed.

But what has all this to do with pregnancy? Once in every several hundred pregnancies, as the result of an extraordinary combination of chance factors, the Rh substance may be responsible for a chain of events which exerts a harmful effect on the fetus. A number of circumstances must be present before this singular action on the fetus can be exerted. In the first place, the woman must be Rh negative. As indicated above, there is only one chance in seven that any member of the white race belongs to this minority group. In the second place, her husband must be Rh positive; the chances are good— 6 out of 7—that he does belong to the positive group, but he may not. In the third place, the fetus must be Rh positive; because the husband is Rh positive it does not necessarily follow that the baby is positive, because if any large group of Rh positive men are studied it will be found that the spermatozoa of about one half are partly Rh negative and will produce an Rh-negative infant. In the fourth place—and this is the most unlikely circumstance in the lot—the Rh substance from the Rh positive fetus must find its way through the placenta and into the blood stream of the mother and build up antibodies therein, as occurs with an Rh-positive blood transfusion. Once these antibodies are developed in the mother they pass through the placenta into the fetal blood stream where they cause varying degrees of damage to the infant's red blood cells. Finally, the woman must have had a previous pregnancy or a previous blood transfusion because, as we have seen, it takes some time for the antibodies to develop.

From the above facts the following rather comforting conclusions can be drawn. Six out of seven women are Rh positive, and for them there is no possibility whatsoever of complications occurring from this source. Likewise in first pregnancies, even if the expectant mother is Rh negative, the possibility of trouble developing is quite remote unless she has had a previous blood transfusion with Rh-positive blood. But if a woman is Rh negative and has had previous pregnancies or previous transfusions, what is her outlook in subsequent pregnancies? So many factors enter into this question that it is impossible to answer it with great precision, but all authorities agree that the vast majority even of this group—from 90 to 95 per cent— go through pregnancy after pregnancy without any suggestion of a complication.

If the patient is Rh negative and has had a previous blood transfusion with Rh positive blood (or blood of unknown Rh character which was probably Rh positive), great caution must be exercised in prophesying the outcome of future pregnancies, since sometimes these patients carry Rh antibodies for many years after the blood transfusion.

In the great majority of cases, accordingly, the nurse can allay any fears that the patient may have in regard to the Rh factor. However, she is not justified in so doing under one circumstance, namely, if the woman has had a previous erythroblastotic baby, because the probability is good that this condition will repeat itself. The outcome will depend on whether the husband is homozygous (spermatozoa all Rh positive) or whether he is heterozygous (spermatozoa half Rh positive and half Rh negative). If he is homozygous, the outcome is almost certain to be another erythroblastotic infant. If he is heterozygous and an Rh-negative spermatozoan happens to be the one to fertilize the ovum— a 50 per cent chance—the fetus will be Rh negative and, having no Rh substance for the Rh antibodies of the mother to act upon, suffers no harm and develops normally.

Since knowledge of the Rh factor has developed, the following changes have taken place in obstetric practice. (1) It is customary to determine the Rh of every prenatal patient. (2) If she is Rh negative, the Rh of the husband is ascertained, and it is possible in some cases, but not always, to determine if he is homozygous or heterozygous. (3) In the latter half of pregnancy the blood of the mother is sometimes studied for the presence or the absence of antibodies by way of forecasting the outlook for the baby. (4) A patient who is Rh negative never is transfused

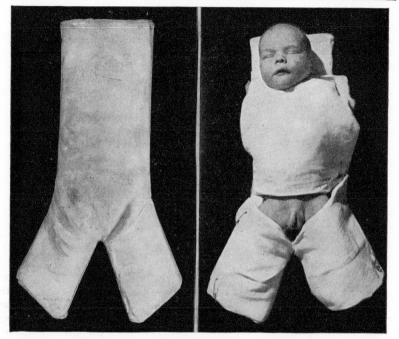

Fig. 303. Preparation of the baby for circumcision. (*Left*) Board, padded and covered with oilcloth, as used in many hospitals for circumcision. (*Right*) The baby, bound on the board with towels, ready for circumcision.

except with Rh-negative blood; this holds good not only in obstetric work but in the case of any Rh-negative person who is transfused, especially a female between birth and 45. (5) If the circumstances are such as to indicate that the fetus is or may become erythroblastotic, elaborate preparations are made to salvage the baby, especially by means of blood transfusion.

Treatment in Erythroblastosis. In live births, that is, except in *Hydrops fetalis*, the life of the child may be saved by mass or exchange transfusion with Rh blood. About 500 cc.

of blood, which is twice the normal blood amount of a newborn infant, will give a 90 per cent or higher exchange of blood. In some cases additional transfusions are needed. Transfusions should be given promptly. The new blood is sometimes given through a vein in the ankle while the infant's blood is withdrawn from the radial artery.

Donors in well-regulated areas are licensed, provided with a record book containing a photograph, types of blood, physical condition (weight, hemoglobin or iron content) and freedom from diseases transferable by the blood, such as malaria; the record also includes the dates of blood donation to prevent too great a depletion of red cells when the donor is engaged. It is agreed that mothers giving birth to erythroblastic infants should not nurse their babies.

MISCELLANEOUS DISORDERS

Icterus Neonatorum. Icterus neonatorum is an exceedingly common

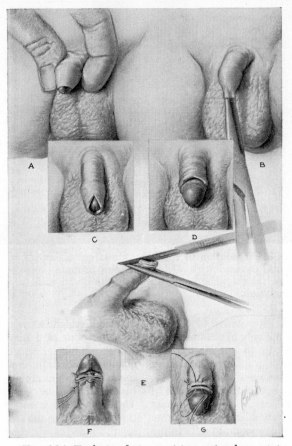

Fig. 304. Technic of circumcision, using hemostat, scalpel and sutures. After cleansing penis and surrounding area, the prepuce is stripped back with the help of a partial dorsal slit (A to D). The prepuce is now clamped and excessive prepuce cut off (E). The suture material used is plain 00 or 000 catgut in a very small needle (F and G), but some physicians prefer silk.

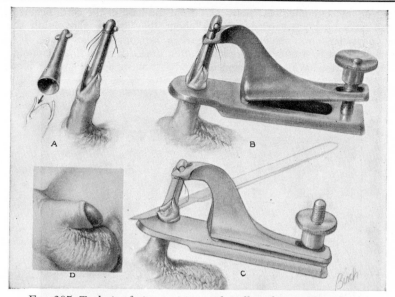

FIG. 305. Technic of circumcision with Yellen clamp. After cleansing area and stripping back prepuce as shown in Figure 304, the cone of the Yellen clamp is placed over the glans and the prepuce put on a stretch with sutures (A). The prepuce is now drawn through the beveled hole of platform (B). Screwing down clamp crushes prepuce, producing hemostasis. Three to 5 minutes of such pressure is necessary to prevent subsequent bleeding. The excess of the prepuce is then cut away (C) and the clamp removed (D). (Yellen, H. S.: Am. J. Obst. & Gynec. 30:146)

condition during the first ten days of life and, as the name implies, is characterized by jaundice. It makes its appearance, as a rule, on the third or the fourth day of life and disappears without treatment about the seventh or the eighth day. Almost one baby in three shows icterus, which is often called "physiologic jaundice." The cause is not known clearly, but some authorities attribute it to inadequate liver function, others to a certain destruction of red cells which takes place during the first week of life. The mother always may be assured that the condition is of no significance and will clear up within a few days.

Phimosis. In many male infants, the orifice in the foreskin of the penis is so small that the foreskin cannot be pushed back over the glans. This condition is known as "phimosis." While it is rarely of sufficient degree to obstruct the outflow of urine or cause any immediate symptoms, it is undesirable because it prevents proper cleanliness. Phimosis may be corrected either by stretching the orifice of the foreskin with a hemo-

stat, or by circumcision. Both of
these procedures are carried out by
the physician, but sometimes the
nurse is asked to stretch the foreskin
every day after having first received

from the base of the cord, occurs at
about the fifth to the eighth day
when separation takes place. It is
often preceded by a slight jaundice;
and is not an actual flow of blood

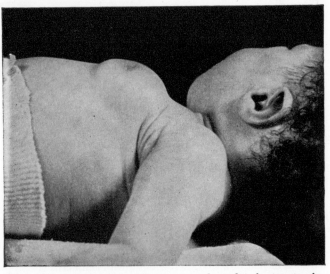

Fig. 306. Hypertrophy of breast in infant developing in the
neonatal period.

detailed instructions from the doctor.
Preparation of an infant for circumcision as well as two common methods of performing the operation are
here depicted.

Hemorrhage from Cord. Hemorrhage from the cord may be of two
types: (1) primary, due to the slipping or loosening of the ligature, and
(2) secondary, coming from the base
of the cord when it separates from
the body of the baby. In the first
instance, the bleeding is from the
end of the cord and not from its
base and can be controlled by the
proper application of a fresh ligature. The secondary hemorrhage,

but a persistent oozing which frequently resists treatment. This variety of hemorrhage, which is of rare
occurrence, is usually due to one of
two causes: (A) the baby may be
syphilitic, or (B) the peculiar condition known as the "hemorrhagic
diathesis" may be present. In this
condition, the baby's blood shows no
disposition to coagulate, and bleeding from any denuded surface is persistent and often profuse.

The nurse's responsibility in the
treatment of secondary hemorrhage
from the cord consists in applying to
the bleeding surface a piece of cotton saturated with a styptic—prob-

ably liquor ferri subsulfatis or solution of the subsulfate of iron, which may be secured from any druggist. The physician should be notified promptly; and if, by the time he arrives, the use of the styptic has not effectually controlled the oozing, he will doubtless ligate the base of the umbilicus and apply an antiseptic dressing. When this form of bleeding is at all severe and persistent, recovery is doubtful; and even if the umbilical hemorrhage is controlled, bleeding may appear in the nose, the mouth, the stomach, the intestines or the abdominal cavity; or purpuric spots may develop on various parts of the body. The prompt administration of vitamin K has greatly improved the prognosis in these cases.

Breast Engorgement. Engorgement of the breasts is common during the neonatal period, in both male and female infants. It is due to the same causes which bring about mammary engorgement in the mother—that is, endocrine influence. In the case of the infant, its breasts have been acted upon throughout pregnancy by the estrogenic hormone which passes to it through the placenta from the mother. This is the same hormone which prepares the mother's breasts for lactation. When it is withdrawn after birth, changes in the infant's breasts take place similar to those in the mother.

Mammary engorgement in the newborn subsides without treatment, but sometimes persists for 2 or 3 weeks.

Menstruation occasionally occurs in newborn girls and is due to estrogenic hormone, as described above. It usually amounts only to slight spotting and need cause no special concern.

SUGGESTED READING

Book, J. A., and Reed, S. C.: Empiric risk figures in Mongolism, J.A.M.A. 143:730, 1950.

Davidson, H. H., Hill, Justin A. H., and Eastman, N. J.: Penicillin in the prophylaxis of ophthalmia neonatorum, J.A.M.A. 145:1052, 1951.

Goodwin, Mary S., and Moore, J. E.: Penicillin in prevention of prenatal syphilis, J.A.M.A. 130:688, 1946.

Hellman, L. M., Shettles, L. B., and Eastman, N. J.: Vitamin K in obstetrics, Am. J. Obst. & Gynec. 43:921, 1942.

Ingraham, N. R., et al.: Penicillin treatment of the syphilitic pregnant woman, J.A.M.A. 130:683, 1946.

Kohn, Jerome, and Olson, Elsie: Whooping cough, Am. J. Nursing 50:723, 1950.

Lancaster, Walter B.: Crossed eyes in children, Am. J. Nursing 50:535, 1950.

Poncher, H. G.: Treatment of anemias in infancy and childhood, J.A.M.A. 134:1003-1007, 1947.

Potter, Edith: Rh: Its Relation to Congenital Hemolytic Disease, Chicago, Yr. Bk. Pub., 1947.

Ryan, Elizabeth K.: Nursing care of the patient with spina bifida, Am. J. Nursing 51:28, 1951.

Schneider, Charles L., et al.: Rh antibody stimulation with an Rh-negative fetus and its significance to the newborn, Am. J. Obst. & Gynec. 59:543, 1950.

Stevenson, Jessie L.: Orthopedic conditions at birth (Handbook), Joint Orthopedic Nursing Advisory Service, 1943.

Watts, Samuel G., and Gleich, Morris M.: Prophylaxis against gonorrheal ophthalmia, J.A.M.A. 143:635, 1950.

Wyatt, Oswald S.: Intestinal obstruction in the newborn and infant, J.A.M.A. 146:236, 1951.

Zettelman, H. J.: Initial fetal atelectasis, Am. J. Obst. & Gynec. 51:241-245, 1946.

*10 m. imp. mos. of baby's life —
9 mos of preg. & 1st month of birth*

24

After-Care of the Baby

IMPORTANCE OF AFTER-CARE

The after-care of the baby usually means the care given when the baby comes home from the hospital or when the mother assumes the responsibility if the baby is born at home. In either event, certain adjustments must be made. The mother has the physical care of the baby as well as her own emotional adjustment to make. This period may present different reactions. Overattention may be given the baby by the father and the mother may be disturbed by the lack of consideration; or the father may feel neglected for the same reason. On the other hand, the children in the family may resent the baby who requires so much of the parents' time and attention. Then there is the completely welcome baby whose mirac-ulous presence brings not only joy but great anxiety. At this time, too, the mother is convalescing from the crisis of the maternity cycle. All of these experiences occur at a time when the greatest responsibility of all must be met: that of caring for, protecting and training this new little individual. The co-operation and the understanding of the father in sharing these responsibilities will do much to make this period less difficult for the mother.

The baby's immediate or neonatal care has been described already, but from now on a plan for his daily care should be arranged and followed carefully. Everything that is done for him, to him, and about him affects his development, both physically and psychologically. His behavior patterns are in the making, and this is only another of the responsibilities that the parents assume when the baby becomes a part of the family. Babies are unable to make known their discomforts and wants; therefore, it is important for the parents or the person caring for the baby to anticipate and be conscious of this fact as well as to give the needed routine care.

DAILY SCHEDULE

This scheme should include feeding, sleep and rest, bathing, dressing, fresh air and sun, exercise and play. The following schedule is suggested to show the activities for the normal baby in a 24-hour period. The timing for the various activities should be so planned that they may be accommodated to the routine of the parents' plan for their day. It must be remembered that if the baby is to become a part of the family, this is the time to start with the idea by instituting changes or routines which will be simplifying rather than complicating. As the baby grows, there will of necessity be many changes in his schedule. The following is merely a suggested plan. There will be variations and adjustments to suit individual families.

6:00 A.M.   First feeding (or when the parents' day begins).

9:00 A.M.   Cod-liver oil—orange juice (when awake). Bath usually precedes next feeding.

10:00 A.M. Second feeding—followed by nap (in a well-ventilated room or outdoors)

2:00 P.M.   Third feeding — followed by nap. Exercise and play— holding the baby or putting him on a bed where he can kick and roll (carefully watched). Followed by sponge bath.

6:00 P.M.   Fourth feeding—bed.

10:00 P.M. Fifth feeding (this feeding may be given at the parents' bedtime).

2:00 A.M.   Sixth feeding (may or may not be necessary to give this feeding. When the baby wakes he should be fed so as not to disturb the sleep of the rest of the family).

Formerly, a very strict schedule was adhered to by many parents. Today the prevalent idea is to adopt a more lenient routine. A schedule that makes the baby a part of the family and allows the mother time to carry out her responsibilities will be more satisfactory.

FEEDING

ROUTINE

The baby's feeding schedule will be directed by the pediatrician. He may prescribe a flexible demand schedule to determine the approximate interval which suits the individual baby best. Since the baby's stomach needs rest, it is important that there be a reasonable period between feedings. There are other reasons than hunger why a baby cries. As the baby grows older, the amount of food needed depends upon his weight, size, age, vigor and general progress. If the baby is breast-fed, the mother may be assured that the mammary glands are so constructed by nature that the supply meets the demand. The amount of milk apparently is in-

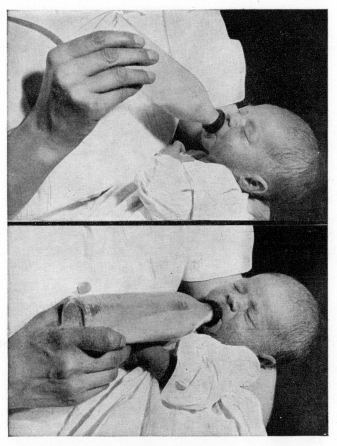

Fig. 307. (*Top*) The right way to hold a bottle. The baby's head should be turned slightly to one side, and the bottle held so that the baby will grasp the nipple squarely. To prevent the baby from swallowing air, the neck of the bottle should be filled with milk at all times.

(*Bottom*) The wrong way to hold a bottle. If the bottle is held flat, air enters the nipple, and the baby may suffer as a result of swallowing air.

creased, as well as its strength and quality. The same principle must apply if the baby is on artificial feedings. Not only is an increased quantity of formula given, but it is also

and, for such babies, artificial feeding must be prepared, either for part breast and part bottle or for bottle feeding altogether. In such cases, the type of feeding is prescribed by the

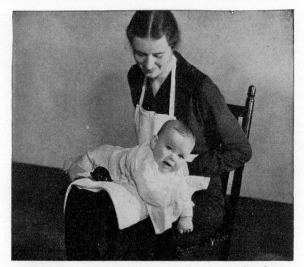

Fig. 308. Application of the hot-water bottle to the baby's abdomen. The bottle should always be covered. If the baby is placed in this position he will rest on the hot-water bottle rather than have the weight of the bottle on his abdomen.

increased in food value. As the baby grows older, also, the interval between his feedings will be lengthened. The first feeding to be discontinued will be the night feeding (2 A.M. or thereabout), then the evening feeding (10 P.M. or bedtime). Thereafter, the baby usually has 4 or 3 feedings per day. If, during these first few months, the mother's breast milk proves to be inadequate, a formula may be complemented or supplemented for one or two feedings. A few mothers cannot nurse their babies satisfactorily,

obstetrician or the pediatrician.

Only the proper amount of modified milk for one feeding should be put in a bottle; then it should be warmed to body temperature by placing the bottle in a bottle warmer or a pan of hot water. In cold weather a warm flannel cover may be used around the bottle to keep the milk from getting cold toward the end of the feeding, or it may be rewarmed. Under ordinary circumstances a normal baby should take the entire quantity of food prepared for one feeding in about 20 minutes.

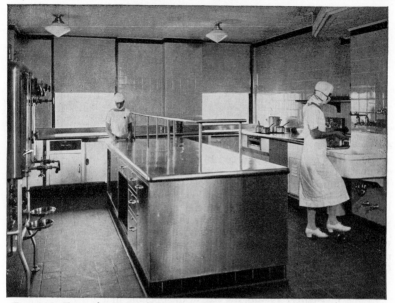

Fig. 309. Formula room. (Margaret Hague Maternity Hospital, Jersey City)

Any leftover food should not be used again.

If the infant refuses to take his food, there is usually some reason, such as new or different type of nipple, temperature of food, or strange surroundings. However, if he persists in refusing his food, the doctor should be consulted.

Indigestion. Gastric indigestion is very uncommon if the baby is breast fed. However, it may follow ill-advised supplementary foods, an emotional upset, swallowing air or too much excitement. The baby appears to be uncomfortable and regurgitates his food. All feedings should be interrupted for from 12 to 24 hours, giving fluids freely at intervals. If other symptoms are present, this attack may be the forerunner of a more

serious illness and should be reported.

Hiccoughs are due to swallowing air, taking food too rapidly, taking food that is too hot or too cold or irritation by food that collects in the esophagus. The gas formed in the stomach makes pressure which stimulates the spasmodic contractions of the diaphragm. Simple remedies are bubbling the baby, giving tastes of tepid water from a spoon and applying a hot-water bottle to the abdomen. This is usually a temporary discomfort and it is seldom that the physician needs to be consulted.

ARTIFICIAL FEEDING

In artificial feeding, it is necessary to modify the milk to approximate as nearly as possible the chemical and

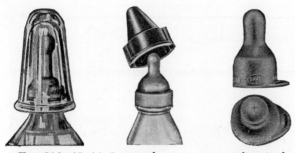

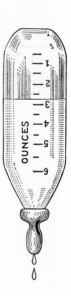

Fig. 310. (*Left*) Steri-seal cap to protect the nipple, eliminating the need for corks, cotton or rubber caps. This cap must be applied when wet. (Steri-seal Corporation) (*Center*) Baby-All shielded nurser, with holes or with the nonclogging crucial cut. Complete unit—bottle, screw-on nipple and new shield—seals nipple and formula against contamination until used. (Sanit-All Corporation) (*Right*) Davol "Anti-Colic" nipple with crucial cut, prevents clogging sometimes caused by terminal sterilization. (Davol Rubber Co.)

Fig. 311 (*Right*). Testing the size of the opening in a nipple. Milk should drop, as indicated, and not flow in a stream.

physical characteristics of human milk. Any milk except breast milk is a substitute. Certain patented baby foods may be prescribed by the physician, who will give specific directions for their use. Many large cities have laboratories which fill prescriptions for modified milk. They are known to be reliable, and the physician feels assured that there will be no error in the product. For this reason, where available, the feedings are purchased as ordered. Some hospitals maintain a formula service for the benefit of physicians requiring such a convenience. All public health nurses give instructions in milk modification. If mothers receive the proper instructions, they can prepare these formulas at home.

DIRECTIONS FOR MAKING FORMULA

The hands should be washed before assembling the equipment. All equipment used for the preparation of the formula should be kept separate. If bottled milk is used, the outside of the bottle should be washed with soap and cool water as soon as received, and the bottle should be placed in the refrigerator. If canned milk is used, the top of the can should be washed with soap and water, using friction, and then thoroughly rinsed. Hot water should be poured over the top just before it is opened. All equipment should be washed thoroughly in warm soapy water and rinsed well so that no milk film remains to hold bacteria.

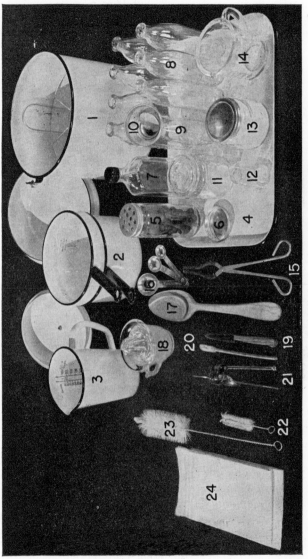

Fig. 312. Formula equipment. Sterilizer with bottle rack, double boiler, graduate, tray, nipple jar with perforated and plain covers, bottle for drinking water, seven 8-ounce bottles, one 4-ounce bottle (for water or orange juice), funnel with removable strainer (or tea strainer), covered jar for used nipples, 8 nipple protectors, jar of sugar for formula, small graduate or jar (to hold sterilized forceps, spoons, etc.), forceps, measuring spoons, wooden spoon or stirring rod (to stir formula while cooking and cooling), can opener (if canned milk is used), nipple brush, bottle brush and clean tea towel.

Bottles and Nipples. The 8-ounce bottle is a good size to use and should be graduated in ounces and half ounces, so that it will be possible at all times to know exactly how

The holes in the nipple are usually small, but they may be made the required size by heating a fine sewing needle with its eye fixed in a cork used as a handle. The point is

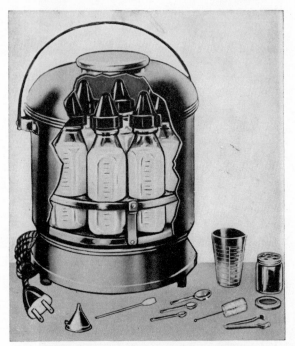

FIG. 313. Electric model of "Baby-All" formula and sterilizer outfit which may be used for regular or terminal sterilization. A nonelectric model is also obtainable. (Sanit-All Products Corporation)

much food the baby has taken. A sufficient number of bottles and nipples should be sterilized to supply the feedings for the 24-hour period. It is always safer to have one or two extra bottles and nipples in reserve in case of breakage.

The shape of the bottle should be such that every part of the inner surface can be reached with a brush to facilitate cleaning.

held in the flame until red hot, then accurately plunged into one of the three holes and withdrawn quickly. It needs practice before holes of proper size can be made. Some nipples have crucial incisions instead of punctured holes to prevent them from clogging.

The test of proper hole size is made by holding the bottle, filled with milk and with the nipple attached, upside down. The milk should escape drop by drop, and if it runs in a stream, the hole is too large. The objection to the large hole is that the baby nurses too rapidly, which causes indigestion, colic and other disorders. If the stream is very rapid, the baby may have difficulty in swallowing.

Preparation of Equipment. The equipment may vary with the type of formula prescribed. Wash in hot soapy water and rinse thoroughly in clear hot water and place the following articles in the sterilizer half-full of cool water: enamel graduate, measuring cup (or glass jar), measuring spoon, wooden spoon, two 4-ounce bottles (water and orange juice), water bottle, funnel, nipple protector, can opener (if canned milk is used) and forceps (place in sterilizer last to be removed first). Bring water to a boil, and boil vigorously for ten minutes.

In one method the bottles, the nipples and the equipment used in making the formula are sterilized before the formula is prepared. The formula is then made according to directions and is cooled. A specific amount of the formula is put into each bottle. The bottles are then nippled, capped and refrigerated.

Terminal Sterilization. In this method the formula is prepared under a clean but not aseptic technic. The bottles, the nipples and the nipple protectors are washed thoroughly but are not sterilized. The formula is prepared and poured into the bottles, and the nipples and the protectors are applied loosely. They are then placed in the sterilizer and heated to a temperature of 212° F. for 15 minutes. In this method the formula, the bottles, the nipples and

the protectors are all sterilized in one operation. Before the formula is refrigerated the nipple protectors should be made secure. However, some hospitals prefer to use the pressure autoclaving method, but in the home the above procedure is used. In both methods the formula must remain sterile and the nipple untouched and sterile until it reaches the baby's mouth.

There is a variety of bottles and nipples on the market, many of them sold as "units" (bottle, nipple and nipple protector).

MILK

In the various states, milk is usually graded by letter or special names to show differences in butter fat and bacteria allowed, and it is supplied in bottles or other sealed containers. Many cities recognize two grades of milk for general use: Grade A and Grade B. Others, e.g., New York City, recognize only one grade, Approved Milk, for the general milk supply.

Mixed milk or milk from a herd of cows is now considered better than from one cow, because it is more uniform in quality.

Loose Raw Milk. Loose raw milk or dipped milk usually comes from uninspected dairies. If raw milk is purchased for the baby it should be bottled certified milk; if not certified and not pasteurized, it should be pasteurized at home.

Certified Milk. Certified milk is produced under the supervision of medical commissions, which operate throughout the United States. As an added safety factor, certified milk may be pasteurized. The cows have been tested for tuberculosis and undulant fever, and the milkers and the dairies are inspected regularly. The bacterial count may not exceed 10,000 per cc. at the time of delivery to the consumer. It is the best bottled milk to be had in any community and can be relied upon at all times. In New York City a law was passed making it illegal to sell unpasteurized certified milk without a physician's written prescription for raw milk.

Vitamin D Milk. Vitamin D milk is produced by feeding the cows irradiated yeast or by exposing certified or Grade A (or Approved) milk to the direct rays of an ultraviolet lamp. In each quart of this milk, there is supposed to be the equivalent of 1¼ teaspoons of cod-liver oil. Some dairies now add to the milk a cod-liver oil concentrate, so thoroughly agitated that all of the milk is treated equally.

Skimmed Milk. Skimmed milk is milk from which all of the cream (fat) has been removed. Sometimes it is ordered for babies who have simple diarrhea but it should be used only when prescribed by the physician.

Pasteurized Milk. Pasteurized milk is milk of any grade which has been heated to a temperature of from 142° to 145° F. and kept at that heat for half an hour and cooled promptly. This is sometimes done at home in a double boiler. Pasteurized milk is not boiled, since it is heated to a temperature from 142° to 145° F. only. Pasteurized milk offers excellent protection, for it destroys the common disease organisms as well as most of the spoilage organisms which cause souring, bad flavors, etc. Where there is any question of milk quality, pasteurization is a safe measure.

Sterilized Milk. Sterilized milk means milk that is boiled for at least 10 minutes, during which few, if any, bacteria survive. It should be stirred constantly while boiling, so that there will be no loss of the proteins which otherwise may stick to the sides of the pan. The nutritive value is reduced somewhat, especially through the effect of heat on vitamin C, and orange or tomato juice and cod-liver oil always should be added to the diet, replacing this loss.

Three-Minute Boiled Milk. This shorter time of boiling produces less change in the milk than the boiling for 10 minutes, but it is still considered wise to add orange or tomato juice and cod-liver oil to the baby's diet. Boiling does not change the fats or the solids of milk. The protein goes through certain changes, but not enough to prevent the milk from providing the nourishment which its protein should furnish.

Frozen Milk. Some physicians think that milk which has been frozen should be boiled before using, because they find that babies may get severe diarrhea from drinking frozen milk, and boiling seems to correct this. If, during the cold weather, the milk is often frozen, it may be safer to use powdered or evaporated milk. Frozen milk should be thawed in cold water.

Buttermilk. There are two kinds of buttermilk. The ordinary buttermilk is the milk left after butter has been made. Artificially prepared buttermilk is whole or skimmed pasteurized milk to which acids or sour milk bacteria have been added. Although babies in certain eastern countries are fed sour milk, in this country it is used only if ordered by the physician. Buttermilk should also be supplemented by orange juice or tomato juice.

Lactic-Acid Milk. This is an artificial preparation of buttermilk. It can be made by adding a small amount of lactic acid to whole milk, usually a few drops to a quart (on physician's order).

Evaporated Milk. Evaporated milk is cow's milk which has been evaporated in a vacuum at high heat and is completely sterilized milk. It may be bought in cans and is about two times as concentrated as fresh milk and very convenient when traveling. Orange juice or tomato juice always should be given if evaporated milk is used. The change from fresh milk to evaporated milk may be made immediately, but the change from evaporated milk to fresh milk should be made gradually.

Homogenized Milk. Homogenized milk is merely regular milk which, just before pasteurization, has been forced through a tiny opening under tremendous pressure. This breaks up the butter fat globules into much smaller ones and distributes them permanently throughout the milk. As a result, cream will not rise on homogenized milk, and so the last drop of it is as rich and nourishing as the first.

Powdered Milk. Powdered milk is milk from which all the fluids have been removed. It consists of the 12 to 13 per cent solids that are found in milk, for the 87 per cent of water is eliminated by the drying process. Powdered milk is obtainable in various forms: powdered whole milk, partially skimmed milk, modified milk, protein milk, lactic-acid milk

and other special preparations. These are very simple to use when traveling, for all that is necessary is to add the specified amount of boiled water. The physician should be consulted before powdered milk is given to the baby.

Protein Milk. Protein milk is powdered whole milk treated with liquid rennet or junket tablets and dried to a powder. It is diluted and given according to the doctor's directions.

Mothers' Milk

FROZEN MOTHERS' MILK. When the need comes it is frequently not a question of money but of organization, without which the need might well not be met at any price.

Healthy nursing mothers who have more milk than their own babies require, can help less fortunate premature and sick babies, who for various reasons are deprived of this food, by selling their surplus milk.

There are at present 18 stations in the United States for this purpose; all are charitable organizations controlled by a board of directors and a group of consulting physicians.

MOTHERS' MILK BANK. The preservation of Mothers' Milk was the outgrowth of a great demand for such milk and involved the problem of finding a method whereby a surplus, when available, could be preserved. The roller process and the spraying process were tried first; the freezing process seemed to be superior to the drying as applied to human milk. The present widespread use of frozen-food lockers, "deep freezes" and other forms of equipment for preserving foods of all sorts in a frozen state, and the availability of "dry ice" make storage and transfer problems minimal. Frozen milk can be transported to the ends of the earth in dry-ice containers.

Technic. The nurse must wear a headgear and mask, then follow a sterile technic for both preparing the milk for freezing and also after the milk has been brought back into liquid.

Procedure. Any amount up to 14 ounces of pooled mothers' milk may be put in a sterile jar; the rubber ring and the cover are put in position, not clamped, and they are placed in an autoclave and sterilized by nonpressure steam at from 180° to 210° F. for 15 minutes. Before removing it from the autoclave, put one clamp in position to hold the cover; now place the jar in hot water, gradually reducing the temperature until the jar can stand absolutely cold water; when well chilled, remove and label "Mothers' Milk" with the date of freezing. Place in holding cabinet or locker that maintains a temperature of from 10° to 15° F.; the freezing time is from 30 to 90 minutes. After the milk is solidified, the jar can be sealed securely by the second clamp put in position. (This prevents breakage due to expansion of the milk during the freezing.)

This frozen milk can be kept indefinitely, provided that the cabinet or the locker has maintained the required temperature.

THAWING THE FROZEN MOTHERS' MILK. Place the jar in *cold* water and gradually increase the temperature to tepid. This will take from 30 to 45 minutes. Wipe the jars after taking from the bath. Flame the cover of the jar before removing.

Remove the cover and the rubber ring, flame the edge and the side of the jar, pour the contents into sterile nursing bottles and cap the bottles. Place in the refrigerator at 40° F. If the frozen supply looks as if all the cream had separated it will emulsify when heated before feeding.

It is advisable to take baceterial recounts to make sure that the milk has not been contaminated. This and other technical procedures of human milk collection and preservation are more fully discussed by Clement A. Smith, M.D., of Boston, in his article, "Human Milk Technology" (see Suggested Reading, p. 588).

ADDITIONAL FOODS

As the baby progresses, mothers are advised to give him other foods which supply vitamins and minerals in addition to those in the milk. These foods include cod-liver oil or its concentrates, fruit juices, cereals, vegetables, soups, beef juice and liver. Any new food should be introduced into the baby's diet in very small amounts, hardly enough to call a taste.

Cod-liver Oil. Cod-liver oil, which has been called "bottled sunshine" because it is thought to have much of the same value as direct sunshine, aids in the baby's growth, helps to prevent infection and prevents and cures rickets. Physicians usually advise cod-liver oil when babies are about a month old. The amount should be increased gradually, beginning with 3 to 5 drops, so that, when the baby is 4 to 6 months old, he is getting 2 teaspoonfuls twice a day. If a cod-liver oil concentrate is ordered the dosage is considerably smaller. If a dropper is used to give the oil, it may be dropped inside his

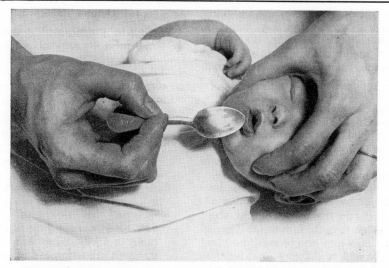

FIG. 314. How to give the very young baby cod-liver oil. Open the baby's mouth by pressing the cheeks firmly but gently between the fingers and thumb of the left hand. Pour the oil into a teaspoon held in the right hand, and give it to the baby little by little. If given just before the bath, when completely undressed, the stain and odor of cod-liver oil will be avoided.

cheek with little danger of spilling. Babies often spit out oil, but seldom really vomit. If disposable tissues are used, stains on the towels and the clothing will be prevented.

Fruit Juices. One of the first fruits to be given the baby is orange juice. Others, such as tomato, prune, apricot, pineapple, and other cooked fruits, may be prescribed for variety and to relieve constipation. Some juices are more effectual than others with individual babies. However, by comparison, they may contain less vitamin C and, therefore, a larger amount would be necessary to give the same vitamin content. For babies who are unable to take juices, concentrates are sometimes prescribed, such as ascorbic acid.

Orange juice is a very important supply of the antiscorbutic vitamin C. When the baby is about two weeks old, the doctor probably will order one teaspoonful of freshly extracted strained orange juice to which an equal amount of boiled water may be added to prevent the baby from "choking." Sweet oranges, to which no sugar has been added, should be used. The amount of juice is increased by one teaspoonful each week until the third month, when the amount is 2 or 3 ounces daily. A small glass or spoon may be used to give the baby the experience of drinking as well as sucking. If strained canned tomato juice is used, twice the amount is necessary.

Cereals. The next food to be added

is cereals. When they are first introduced into the diet they should be strained. There are on the market prepared precooked cereals (dry and canned) to which only water or milk need be added. Cereals should be soft when served to the baby, but thick enough to encourage the baby to chew. Usually, cereals are offered at breakfast time and for supper. Dark cereals are used to counteract constipation; they also contain more vitamin B.

Soups. Soups made from beef stocks and vegetables are other additions to the baby's diet at about the fourth or the fifth month. Canned varieties may also be used. Soup not only adds a different fluid but also acts as a vehicle for vegetable content, vitamins and minerals.

Beef Juice. Beef juice for the baby may be made by cutting round steak into small pieces, broiling it slightly, then squeezing it slightly in a potato ricer, a few pieces at a time. Salt to taste and heat by putting it in a cup and standing it in hot water.

Vegetables. Strained vegetables are given babies at about the third or the fourth month. Spinach, peas, wax or green beans and carrots are added to the diet, depending upon the baby's progress. Chopped foods are given when the child is a little older. These vegetables have been prepared by several reputable firms and are sold in glass jars or cans. A little seasoning may be added before they are served. If vegetables are prepared at home, they may be cooked in patapar paper or a pressure cooker, as these methods help retain the vitamins and prevent their loss into the boiling water. They are then puréed and seasoned.

DIET DURING ILLNESS

When a baby appears ill, it is always advisable to suspend regular feedings and substitute barley water until the advice of the physician can be obtained. Barley water may be made as follows:

Whole barley: add 2 teaspoonfuls of washed whole barley grain or pearl barley to a pint of water; boil slowly to two thirds of a pint, and then strain.

Barley flour: add 2 tablespoonfuls to 1½ pints of water in a quart saucepan; boil slowly to one pint. Strain and allow the liquid to set to a jelly. When warmed for use it will return to a liquid.

WEANING

The increased variety and quantity of foods introduced into the baby's diet makes weaning a very gradual and simple process. Weaning is best accomplished gradually by eliminating one breast feeding or one bottle feeding at a time in favor of a substitute. If this process is begun about the fourth month, by the time the baby is completely weaned, he is on three meals a day. If the baby has been accustomed to drinking from a glass, the weaning process is much simpler.

When, for any reason, it is necessary to wean the baby while the breasts are still secreting milk, it will be necessary to "dry up" the breasts. In general, the breasts should be emptied as completely as possible, a snug breast binder applied, and milk-making fluids restricted. To aid the process, the physician may order Epsom salts or citrate of magnesium. The milk should disappear in a few

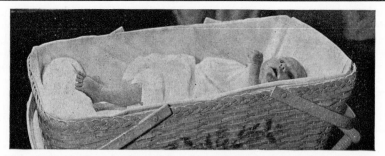

FIG. 315. A roll at the foot of the crib protects the baby's feet from the pressure of the covers.

days, but if the breasts become engorged, the doctor should be consulted immediately. He may order ice caps to be applied to the breasts or he may give stilbestrol or both.

SLEEP AND REST

The "brand-new" baby has the reputation of sleeping most of the time; that is, from 19 to 21 hours a day. But, like adults, babies vary in the amount of sleep needed; some need more than others. A baby should be put to sleep at stated intervals and left undisturbed to sleep or rest quietly. Before putting the baby to bed, either for his night's sleep or for his daytime sleep or rest, he should be made comfortable. Bathing his face and hands, rubbing his back, smoothing wrinkles, removing his outer clothing, seeing that he is dry, making sure that he has not too many covers, changing his position and leaving him in a well-ventilated room are all sleep-producing aids. A baby usually sleeps well if he is comfortable, warm and regularly fed.

The baby's position should be changed from side to side and on his back every time he is diapered or put to bed. This encourages symmetric muscular activity and growth. If this habit is instituted before he is able to turn over by himself, he will develop the habit of sleeping in different positions. When he is awake and being watched, or during his playtime, he may be placed on his abdomen for a change. Authorities state that, for the young baby, the habit of sleeping on his abdomen and face may interfere with the normal development of his fast-growing jaws. There is always a chance, too, of the baby's smothering when sleeping on his abdomen. This position also interferes with the normal position of the feet and may cause them to turn inward or outward. As soon as he is able to choose his favorite position in which to sleep, it is difficult to change his habit of lying in his preferred position.

It cannot be emphasized too strongly that the baby's intricate nervous system needs protection during these early months of development and this is accomplished chiefly by planned periods of sleep and rest. Babies become fatigued very easily. Too much handling, stimulation and excitement are very exhausting and often interfere with the normal rest and sleep. While the baby should be conditioned to the ordinary noises of the household, his environment should provide an opportunity for relaxation, rest and sleep.

BATHING

INTRODUCTION

The baby's bath should be one of the most interesting procedures that the nurse has to learn and to teach. It is both a task and a pleasure to give the baby his bath. This experience must first be acquired by the nurse before she can impart to the mother or the parents the necessary information concerning the important details. The nurse should perfect the procedure before attempting to demonstrate skillfully and explain the details. In her teaching, the nurse must keep in mind that the mother is convalescing, that she is learning a new procedure and, at the same time, making a great emotional adjustment to the new member of the family.

The bath may be anticipated as a difficult procedure, but actually learning to handle the baby, gently and carefully, with the head and the neck supported, is more difficult. The utter helplessness of the new baby makes it paramount that he be handled protectingly and correctly. No nurse or mother can expect to be proficient without practice; and this is particularly true of the baby bath procedure. The fear and dread of handling the new baby subsides with this practice. Proper bath equipment

not only simplifies the learning process but also makes it safer for the baby. The manner of bathing the baby should be the one most satisfactory for the mother and the baby; but since this procedure must be learned, the method which conserves the mother's energy and is safer for the baby seems to be most logical.

If the mother (or parents) has had the opportunity of attending classes and actually learning how to bathe the baby, the nurse's teaching (in the hospital or in the home) will be more effectual. The bath should be given at the same time every day. It should be given at the mother's convenience, at a time when she will be uninterrupted, and always before a feeding. It always should be given in the same order; not only because it may be given more quickly, but because the baby, too, learns this order and responds, before long, by putting up a hand or foot to be bathed at the proper time.

For the baby this daily bath should be refreshing and an aid to his development. A bath not only helps to keep his skin in good condition but also stimulates his circulation and affords an excellent form of exercise. The daily bath also sets a standard for cleanliness.

TYPES OF BATH

Sponge Bath. The sponge bath is usually given before the cord has separated and the umbilicus has healed. It may be given also when the mother may not feel well or the baby appears not well. If a water bath is given to a premature baby (2 to 4 weeks premature), it is usually a sponge bath rather than the tub bath. In certain types of skin ir-

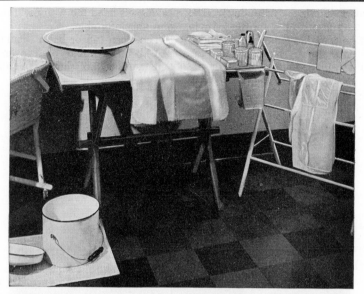

Fig. 316. Setup for a table bath. If the table is backed to the wall and the articles are arranged as shown at the ends of the table, so that the baby lies between them, there is less chance of his rolling off the table. (Maternity Consultation Service, New York)

ritations the sponge bath may also be suggested. The bath procedure is much the same except that the baby is not rinsed in the tub.

Table Bath. If this type of bath is given, it is important that the setup be so arranged that the three sides of the table are protected, and the baby never, for any reason, is left unguarded on the table. The table should be against the wall; the tub on one end, the tray and the clothes on the other; and between these two there should be a comfortable pad on which to place the baby. The chief objections to this method of bathing the baby are that the individual expends more energy while standing and that it is less safe for the baby.

Also, if the mother learns to handle the baby by this method, she will stand while dressing and diapering him, which means that she will be standing many hours when she should be conserving her energy during this convalescent period.

Lap Bath. The lap bath has many advantages. For the mother, who is really convalescing, it is less tiring. If she learns to bathe the baby while sitting, she will also dress and change him on her lap or a low table. The mother can learn to relax while giving the bath and she needs to economize in energy expended. She also needs to learn to handle her baby. It is one more way of getting acquainted with him, and all babies need mothering (parenting). The lap bath also is safer for the baby in that he is on the mother's lap, and if an emergency should arise the mother will have to put him in a safe

having his head too warm will make him uncomfortable.

The clean tub or basin should be placed on a table of convenient height. The tub should be about

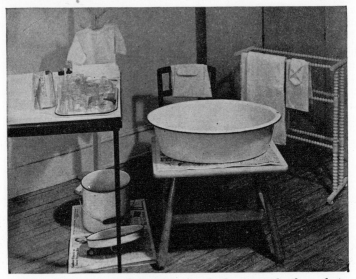

Fig. 317. Setup for giving a lap bath. Note the low chair without arms, the bathtub at a convenient height and equipment accessibly arranged. (Maternity Consultation Service, New York)

place before leaving him. The warmth from the mother's body, too, adds to the baby's comfort.

EQUIPMENT. Before bathtime, all the articles to be used during the bath should be in readiness. The room should be warm (75° to 85° F.). If the room is drafty, a screen may be used to protect the baby, or a couple of chairs draped with a sheet or a blanket may serve this purpose. On cold days the baby should be bathed before a heater or open heated oven and held so that his feet are nearest the heat, because

three quarters full, or perhaps less, of warm water from about 105° to 100° F. The safest method is to test the temperature of the water with an accurate thermometer. However, this is not always possible; in such a situation, water may be used that feels comfortably warm to the elbow.

A coffee table, a toddler's table (table-and-chair combination), a stool, a low hamper, or an ordinary box are all possibilities as a tub table. The chair selected should be the correct height and comfortable for the mother, and her lap should slant toward her. Placed conveniently at the right should be the diaper pail, so that the soiled cotton clothing may be put to soak immediately in plain cold water. A newspaper will protect the floor. Also, within easy reach, on a table, low chest, or substitute, should be the baby's toilet tray (Fig. 124). The outfit of clean clothing should be arranged in the order to be used on the baby. The bath towel, the receiving blanket, the face towel and the washcloth may be arranged on the table, the clothes rack or the costumer. A waterproof or water-repellent apron is a great convenience for the mother.

BATH PROCEDURE

This detailed series of bath pictures is presented to help the nurse to teach and to demonstrate the method of bathing and handling the baby. The following pictures (with the exception of Figs. 320 and 321) were taken at Sloane Hospital for Women, Medical Center, New York, in the mothers' classroom, which is beautifully equipped and attractively decorated in pastel colors. It is important that during either the prenatal period or her hospital stay the patient be taught the details of this procedure.

In teaching this procedure the nurse should emphasize the importance of washing the hands before handling the baby or any of his equipment and clothing. The reason should be explained; the baby needs to be protected while gradually building up his own resistance to his new surroundings; and he should also be protected from colds and infections. In many hospitals the nurse is masked while giving care to the baby. In the home this precaution is used where there is a question or possibility of a cold or a sore throat. Cleanliness is one of the basic fundamentals in the baby's care.

Before beginning the bath, the bath set-up should be checked to be sure that it is complete, and the water should be tested to check the temperature. When the baby is picked up, the bath towel inside the receiving blanket should be wrapped about him after the dress, the pettiskirt or the nightgown (if these are worn) have been removed.

If the baby seems to be restless, he may be offered some water to drink just before beginning the bath.

The baby's nose should be cleansed before the bath and at bedtime and when otherwise indicated. Dryness and irritation in his nose may make him very uncomfortable, and sneezing is very often his only means of relieving this annoyance.

With one hand, the baby's head is steadied to prevent wriggling while the nose is being cleansed. The cotton applicator * or "q-tip" is tested to see that the point is well covered and it is slightly moistened with oil and introduced barely inside the nostril and turned gently. This moistens the mucous membrane and aids

* Although the cotton applicator affords the most efficient means of cleansing the baby's nose and ears, some authorities disapprove of this method on the grounds that a sudden movement of the baby may result in injury. The Children's Bureau, United States Department of Labor, Publication No. 8, "Infant Care," suggests using a piece of moistened twisted cotton and inserting it in the baby's nostril with a twisting motion of the fingers, keeping hold on one end of the cotton so that it does not get out of reach.

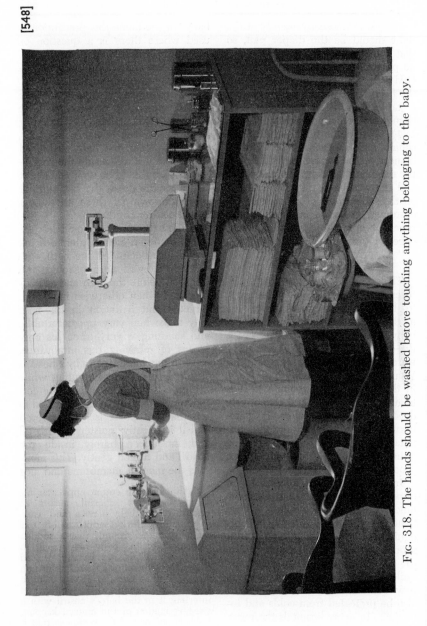

Fig. 318. The hands should be washed before touching anything belonging to the baby.

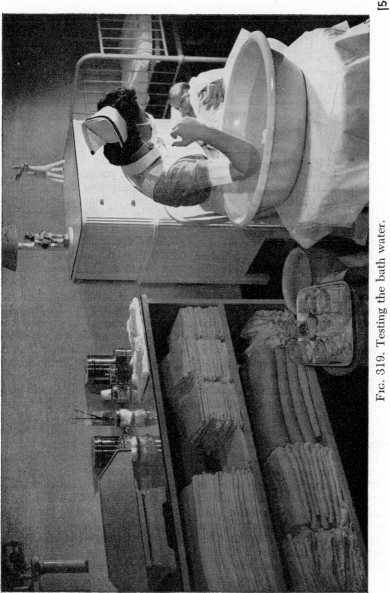

Fig. 319. Testing the bath water.

[549]

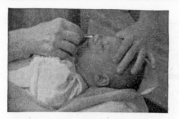

Fig. 320. Cleansing the baby's nose.

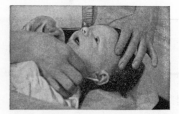

Fig. 321. Cleansing the baby's outer ear.

in loosening any dry particles. Water used on the applicator is drying, while the oil is lubricating. If mucus has collected, the baby may sneeeze and then, with a clean applicator, the mucus may be removed. A clean applicator is used each time and for each nostril, to prevent the possibility of transferring from one nostril to the other any material which might cause an infection. This procedure not only makes the baby more comfortable but, if always a part of the daily routine, he will not resent this treatment should he contract a cold. It may be also a preventive of the "nose-picking" habit.

The baby's ears should be cleansed daily with an applicator moistened with oil, using the oil in the creases of the outer ear and behind the ear where the skin surfaces touch. The reason for using oil instead of water to cleanse the external ear is to prevent the danger of getting water in the ear canal. Water in the baby's ears is not only uncomfortable (and he cannot tell you about it) but it may be the cause of later ear complications. His head is supported in the same manner as when caring for the nose. (These two daily procedures are omitted in the routines of many hospitals.)

Before washing the baby's face, the face towel is placed under the baby's chin. No soap need be used. If the washcloth is square, the corners should be gathered into the palm of the hand. A small round washcloth is easier to use and prevents the possibility of cold wet corners dangling over his face. The nurse should instruct the mother that no special treatment is given the baby's eyes unless there is a discharge, which should be reported to the doctor for his advice. However, it is a good precaution to cleanse the eyes from the nose outward with the clean washcloth, using a clean part for each eye. The baby's mouth should be inspected, but no cleansing treatment given. Mothers should be told that most babies have a whitish coating on the back of the tongue but that if there are any isolated white cheesy spots, any redness or irritation, the doctor should be consulted. The soft, absorbent face towel is used to pat the skin dry. Before the hair and the scalp are bathed, the bath towel should be wrapped carefully about the baby's neck.

The baby's hair and scalp should be washed daily with soap and rinsed carefully. During this procedure his head and neck should be well sup-

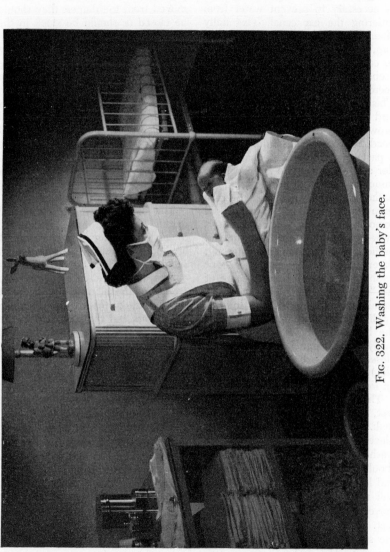

Fig. 322. Washing the baby's face.

ported over the tub. Special vigilance is necessary to prevent water from entering the ear canal. This daily shampoo is a preventive of "crib cap," which is easier to prevent than to correct. This condition, known as "seborrhea capitis," is due to an over-secretion of the sebaceous glands. This oily secretion mixes with dust and lint and forms a yellowish-brown waxy-looking crust on the head. However, if it should be found, a paste of sodium bicarbonate powder and water may be applied for 5 minutes; then the scalp should be bathed thoroughly and carefully with soap and water. Another method of removing this crust is to apply warm sweet oil to the scalp at night and bathe it carefully the next morning. Parents may be apprehensive about washing the baby's head because of the "soft spot" (fontanel). The nurse should explain that if the soap is applied with the palm of the hand the baby cannot be injured. (Normally, the fontanel is not entirely closed until the baby is 18 months old.) Thorough drying of the hair is an important detail.

The diaper is removed, and, if wet, is put into the diaper pail to soak. If it is soiled, it should be placed on the newspaper to be washed before soaking. The buttocks should be cleansed with the cotton and lotion (or oil), so that the band will not become soiled as it is removed over the buttocks and the feet. This is done before removing the shirt and the band, to prevent exposure. The pad and the waterproof protector should be left under the baby until he is put into the tub.

The nurse should stress the safety pin technic. Whenever pins are removed from the diaper, they should be closed or should be stuck in the soap pincushion which not only protects the points but also lubricates as well. No extra safety pins should be on the tray or lying about. Only those used in the diaper will then have to be accounted for. The shirt and the band should be removed and placed on the newspaper, and the baby should be wrapped in the bath towel and the receiving blanket. In applying the soap to the baby's body very little is needed, only enough to lubricate the hand.

The baby's body can be soaped readily with the hand under the towel, uncovering only one part of his body at a time. Special attention should be paid to the little creases of the neck, under the arms, the creases of the elbows, the palms of the hands, in the regions between the fingers and the toes, and in the groins. If the fingers and the toes are well soaped during the bath, it is very easy to clean the fingernails and the toenails with a blunt end of a toothpick or a blunt orangewood stick. This is the beginning care of the hands and the feet.

After the baby has been soaped, he is ready to be placed in the tub carefully, buttocks and feet first, so as not to frighten him.

The nurse should emphasize the position in which the baby is held while he is being put into the tub, during the rinsing, and until he is brought back on the lap. The left wrist supports his neck and head, and his left arm is held securely with the thumb and the fingers of the left hand. This position of the left hand

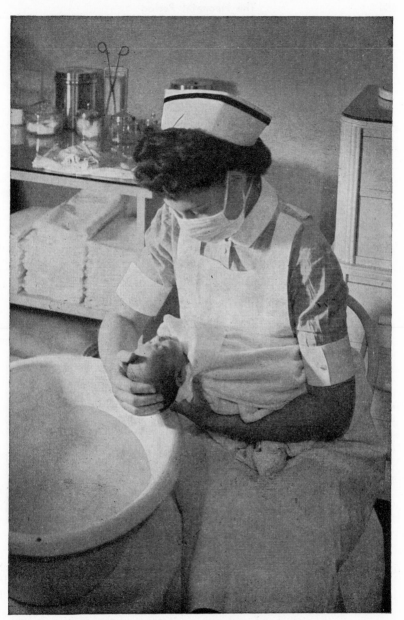

Fig. 323. Washing the baby's hair and scalp.

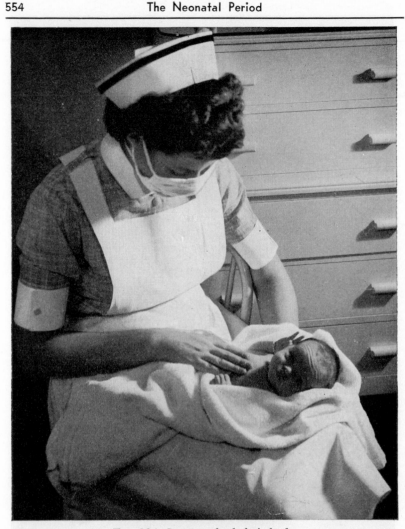

Fig. 324. Soaping the baby's body.

is not changed from the time the baby is put into the tub until he is brought back on the lap. His head and shoulders are thus well supported, and the right hand is placed under the buttocks as he is lifted in and out of the tub. This method of holding a slippery, soapy baby is comfortable for both the baby and the mother.

Because of the position in which he is held it is not necessary to turn

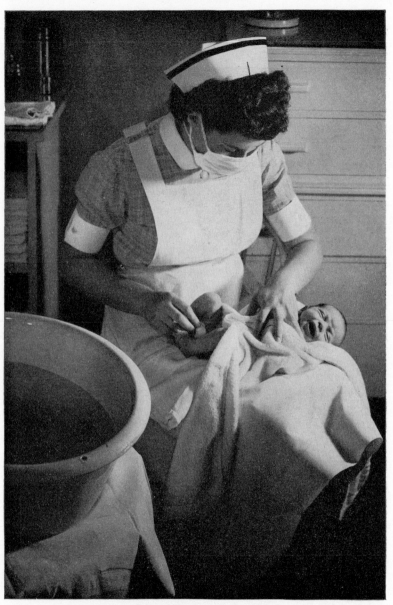

FIG. 325. Cleansing the buttocks.

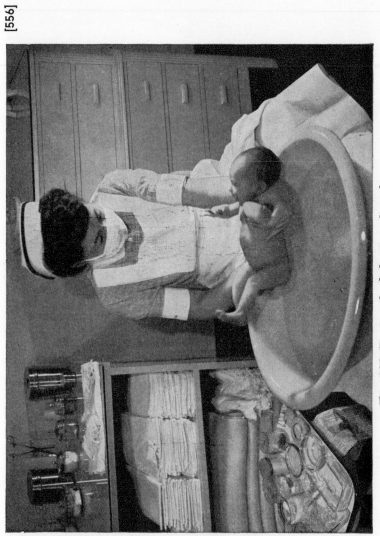

Fig. 326. Putting the baby into the tub.

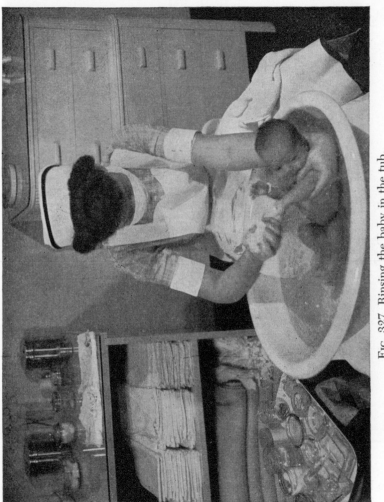

Fig. 327. Rinsing the baby in the tub.

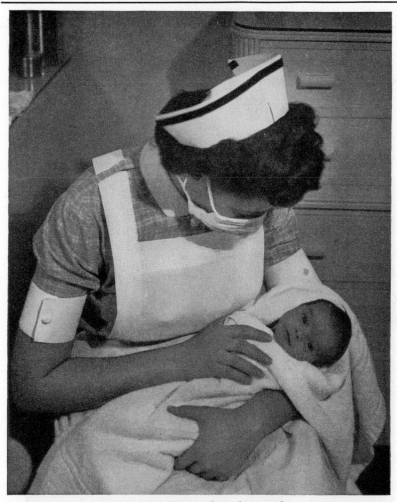

Fig. 328. Wrapped in the towel.

the baby over to rinse his back. It is also easy to steady his entire body and to keep his head and ears out of the water. The baby needs to be in the tub only long enough to rinse him thoroughly; special attention should be given to the creases and between the fingers and the toes. Since the baby is easily frightened, splashing water on the chest may startle him, therefore rinsing his chest should be done very gently. Just before taking the baby from the tub, the pad and the protector should

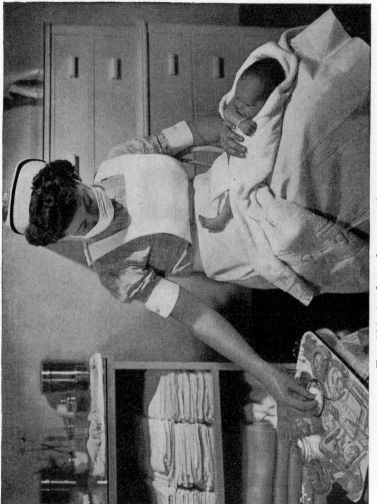

Fig. 329. Applying lotion to the creases.

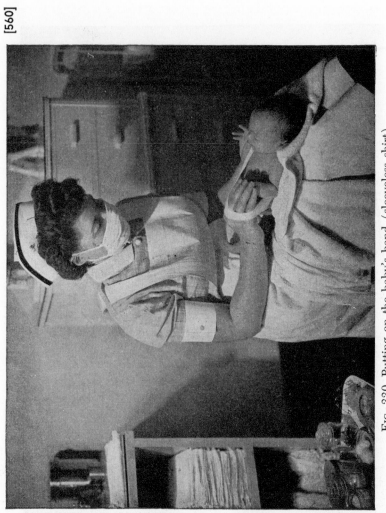

Fig. 330. Putting on the baby's band (sleeveless shirt).

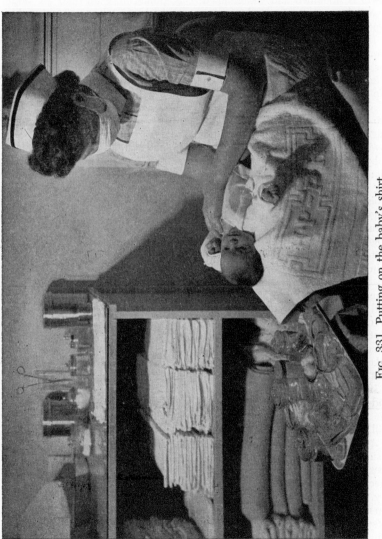

Fig. 331. Putting on the baby's shirt.

[561]

be placed in the diaper pail. If the towel is smoothed and straightened, it will be easier to wrap him more quickly when he is lifted to the lap.

If the towel is wrapped snugly around the baby and if he is held for a few minutes, the towel will absorb much of the moisture from the surface of the body. The soft absorbent face towel is used to dry the creases and in between the fingers and the toes. The damp bath towel should be removed and the baby wrapped in the receiving blanket. The neatest way of applying lotion is to use a cotton pledget moistened with lotion, and with the fingers apply the lotion to the creases and massage it around the fingernails and the toenails. When cotton is used, particles stick to the skin surface. Any excess lotion may be removed with the small towel. The skin area around the genitals and the buttocks needs more lotion in order to shed the urine and to protect the skin. Powder, unless applied sparingly, has a tendency to cake and to retain the urine in contact with the skin.

If the baby is dressed in his band and shirt before the care is given to the umbilicus and the genitals, he will be more comfortable.

After the umbilicus is healed, the resulting scar is usually in a depressed area. It is important to inspect this daily and to keep this area dry. This is another detail that the nurse must bring to the mother's attention. If it is not kept dry, the skin becomes soft, and the area may become irritated.

Daily care of the genitals is also necessary. In the case of a boy baby, the foreskin should be retracted gently each day, taking care that it is pulled forward into its original position after the mucous membrane on the end of the penis has been cleansed with lotion. If the foreskin is tight, the doctor should be consulted. Many parents wish to have their baby circumcised. These arrangements should be made during the mother's hospital stay. In the case of a girl baby, the labia should be separated and the mucous membrane carefully cleansed with lotion, always directing the sponge toward the anus. This is an important detail for the nurse to emphasize in teaching the mother this care. If there is any discharge, it should be reported to the doctor.

After the bath the baby is dressed in a band, a shirt and a diaper (sometimes he also wears a dress, a kimono, a sacque or a nightgown) and is wrapped in a cotton receiving blanket.

Before completing the dressing, the baby should be turned over and his clothing smoothed; the pad and the protector should be placed next to the diaper to protect the clothing. Babies are wrapped in a cotton receiving blanket, which aids in keeping the feet and the abdomen warm. Fewer clothes mean less handling for the baby and less work for the mother. After the bath, most babies are usually fed and then are ready for a nap.

Care of the Baby's Nails. Because parents find it difficult to cut and keep the baby's nails clean, the nurse should emphasize this as a part of the baby's daily care. The nails function to protect the ends of the fingers and the toes. Keeping the nails cut straight across even with the ends

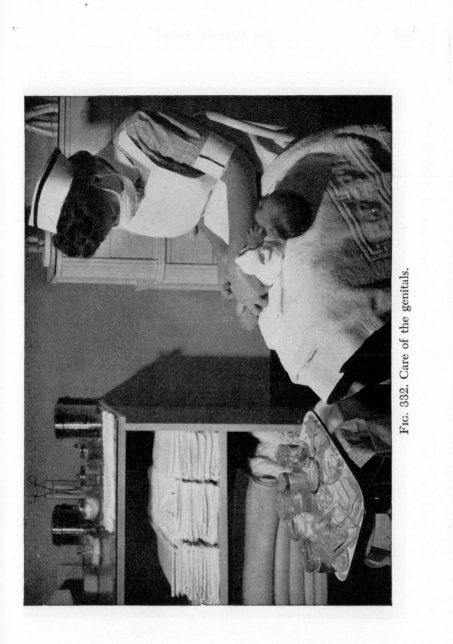

FIG. 332. Care of the genitals.

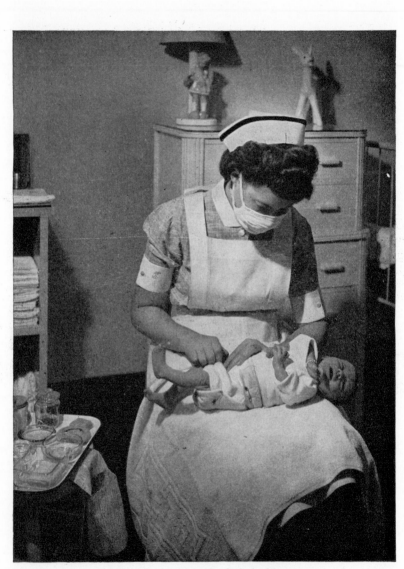

Fig. 333. Pinning the baby's diaper.

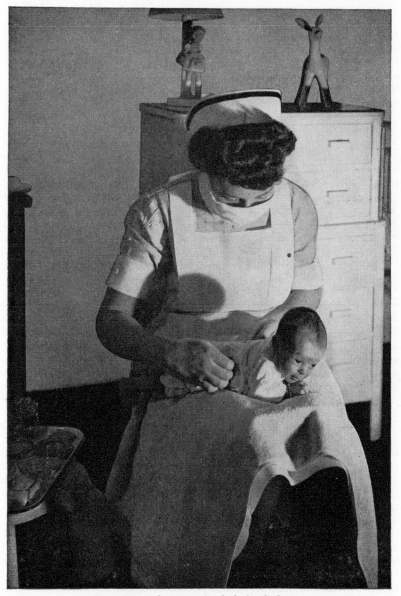

FIG. 334. Adjusting the baby's clothing.

of the fingers and the toes and keeping the cuticle soft and smooth will help to prevent hangnails and ingrowing nails. To cut the nails, the baby's whole hand should be enclosed in the mother's hand, exposing one finger at a time. This is best accomplished when the baby is asleep or when he is most rested. The nails should be kept smooth with a fine emery board, to prevent scratching. A blunt smooth toothpick or blunt orangewood stick may be used to clean the nails. If this care is given daily, it is accepted by the baby as a part of his routine and it is the beginning care to develop well-shaped fingernails and toenails.

CLOTHING AND DRESSING

Effect and Purpose of Clothing

The purpose of clothing is to protect the body from cold, heat, sunlight, rain, mechanical injuries, dirt and insects. Clothes, too, may serve as ornamentation, and babies are often overdressed for this reason. The baby should be so dressed that he is comfortable, warm (but not too warm), his activities not interfered with and his postural development not inhibited. He should also be dressed according to the external temperature. The function of clothing, therefore, is to assist the skin in the maintenance of normal body temperature with the maximum of comfort. Food, muscular activity and emotional outbreaks, such as crying and fretting, increase the body heat, whereas rest and diminished muscular action result in less heat production. Environmental factors, such as temperature and humidity, also affect body heat. Perspiration is a continual physical phenomenon of the skin, and its nonabsorption or nonevaporation may cause too rapid a chilling of the body. Wool absorbs moisture most satisfactorily; cotton less so. When woolen material becomes moist, the layer of air between the garment and the skin is still maintained, thereby diminishing body chilliness or heat loss. On the other hand, cotton sticks to a moist skin and allows for a rapid escape of body heat, or chilling, at low temperatures. For this reason, a cotton and wool or silk and wool mixture sometimes is advised for the baby's bands and shirts.

The young infant, especially during the first 10 or 12 weeks, and before the heat-regulating center is completely developed, requires relatively more clothing than does the older infant. During this period the baby's voluntary muscular movements are comparatively few, and he lies in a crib which is usually well-padded, thereby furnishing additional warmth. If he does not lie in a crib he is usually held, and this contact also furnishes warmth. The older infant usually develops a certain amount of subcutaneous fat which serves to conserve body heat; therefore, less clothing may be required.

If the baby is underdressed, his skin feels dry, his extremities are cold and gray in color, and his temperature is subnormal. On the other hand, if he is overdressed, he is uncomfortable, irritable, restless and cross. His face may be flushed, body extremities hot and sometimes moist, and temperature elevated. Often there is a loss of appetite. Prickly heat and colds may follow in the

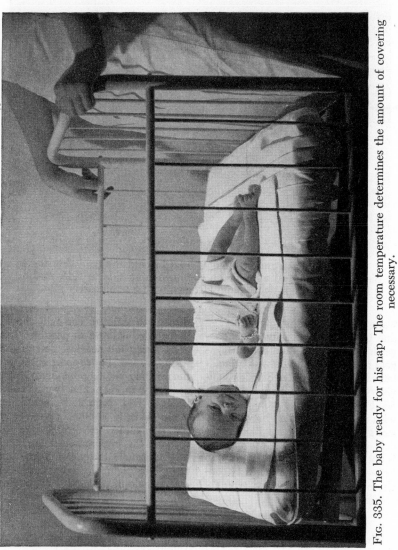

Fig. 335. The baby ready for his nap. The room temperature determines the amount of covering necessary.

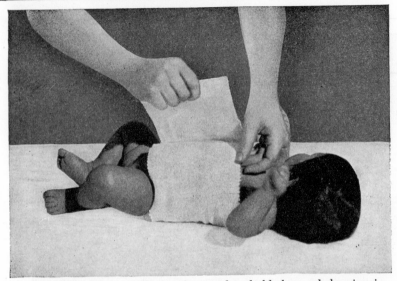

Fig. 336A. The straight band is used to hold the cord dressing in place. It is wrapped around the abdomen from side to side, making it fit snugly but not tightly, and fastened with 3 small safety pins.

wake of overdressing. Overheating due to overdressing may cause congestion of the nose and the pharyngeal mucous membrane which facilitates bacterial invasion. Scientists advise that when the temperature is 86° F. or above, the skin is cooler with a layer of clothing between the sun and the skin.

If the baby's feet are warm, if he is not perspiring and if he appears to be comfortable, the mother may conclude that he is dressed warmly enough.

Technic of Dressing

The skill in dressing the baby, like the art of bathing him, is acquired through experience. The baby should be handled as little as possible. The head, being the heaviest part of the body, should be supported at all times. Only the amount of clothing necessary to keep him warm, comfortable and protected should be worn. This is another opportunity for the nurse to demonstrate to mothers the importance of learning how to handle the young baby and also to explain the advantages of each article of his clothing. To provide clearer detail for the nurse, this series of pictures (Fig. 336 A-K) was taken dressing the baby on the table instead of on the lap. (See p. 198, for complete layette.)

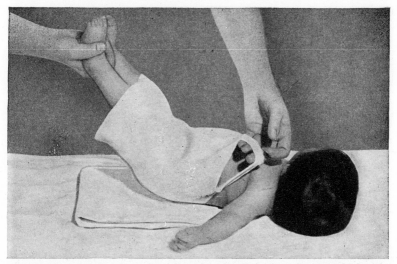

FIG. 336B. This band or sleeveless shirt is used after the straight band is discarded and is put on over the feet. The neck of the band should be so constructed that the "pull" on the shoulder will be close to the neck—an aid to good postural development. It is a waist to pin the baby's diaper to, and keeps the baby's abdomen warm.

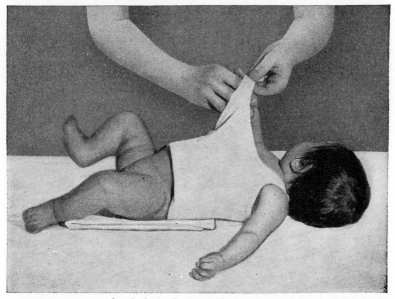

FIG. 336C. Protect the baby's fingers when slipping them through the armhole.

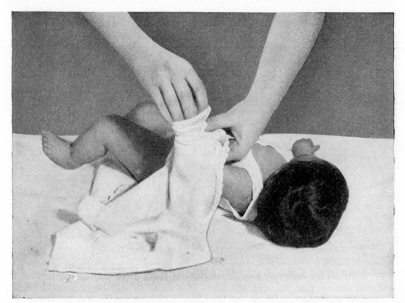

Fɪɢ. 336D. In putting on the shirt, the baby's whole hand should be grasped and pulled through the sleeve to prevent injury to the baby's fingers. The open shirt means less handling for the new baby. Slip-over shirts should be put on over the feet.

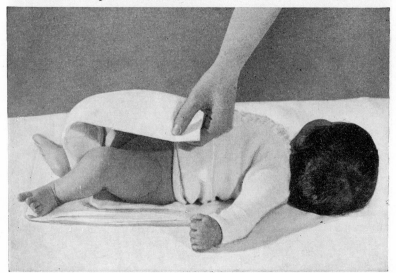

Fɪɢ. 336E. Fold the diaper oblong and place it under the baby, drawing up the lower half between the thighs.

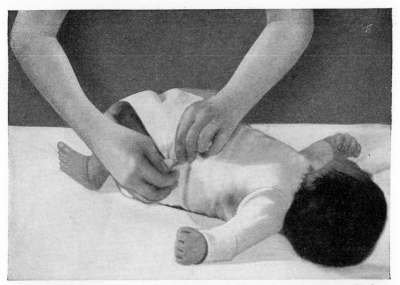

FIG. 336F. In pinning the diaper, protect the baby from pinpricks by guarding the point of the pin with the finger.

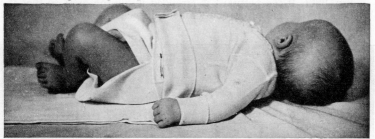

FIG. 336G. The back is pinned over the front, and the band is pinned on the outside of the diaper to prevent it from becoming soiled.

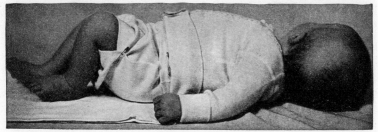

FIG. 336H. The diaper should be adjusted with safety pins at the waist and knee. There will be no pressure on the genitals if the diaper is not fastened too high or too tightly.

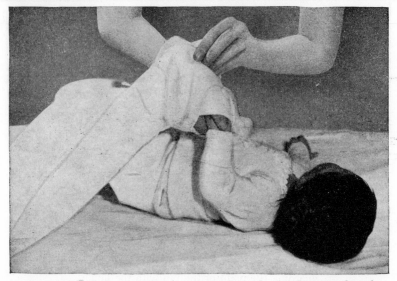

Fig. 336I. If the pettiskirt is arranged inside the dress so that the sleeves may be put on as one garment, it means less handling of the baby.

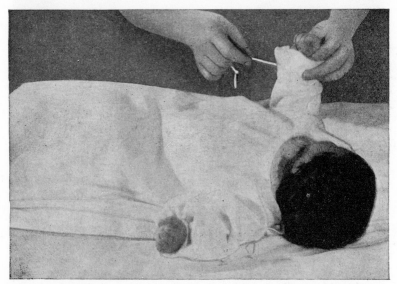

Fig. 336J. Sleeves may be tied at the wrist, so that the hands will not slip through.

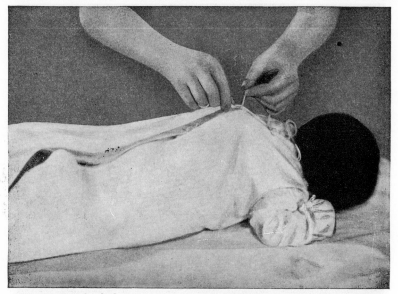

FIG. 336K. The baby is turned on his abdomen to adjust his clothing and smooth out the wrinkles.

FRESH AIR AND SUN

Fresh Air. Fresh air is one of the baby's greatest requirements, because oxygen is needed to aid in the utilization of food. In fact, fresh air has the same beneficial effects on babies that it has on adults. In the baby's room the air should be kept fresh and moving, but the baby should be protected from drafts. When he is taken out, he should be dressed to suit the weather. Warm hands and feet and a tendency to sleep while out are good indications that the baby is clothed properly. During the cold weather, windproof material under the mattress and over the covers offers added protection.

Sun. Today much is being said about putting the baby in the sun.

This routine is usually started about the third or the fourth week, depending, of course, on the climate; and should be given before 10 A.M. and after 3 P.M. In warm weather the sunbaths may be given out of doors, but in cool weather the baby may be dressed appropriately and placed before a screened window. A great part of the beneficial or ultra-violet rays of the sun do not penetrate plain glass. The exposure of the skin surface of the baby to the sun's rays should be progressive, or until he has acquired an even tan all over his body. He should be so placed that the sun or glare is never permitted to shine directly in his eyes; and he always should be protected from the wind. During the winter in cold latitudes, when the ultraviolet

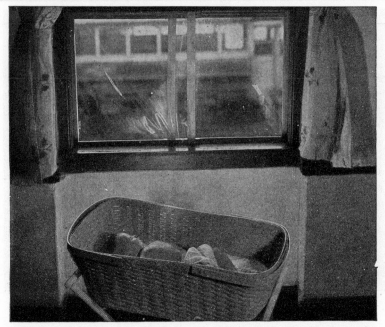

FIG. 337. Screen for the baby's sun baths during cooler weather. The basket has two handles and may be used with or without the stand.

rays of the sun are negligible, cod-liver oil or its equivalent ("bottled sunshine") should be given to supply the needed vitamin D which aids in the utilization of calcium and phosphorus.

EXERCISE AND PLAY

Value. The baby's crying is a necessary physiologic form of exercise. The apparent aimless waving of the arms and the vigorous kicking of feet and the legs are exercises which are developing the muscles that the baby will use later for sitting, creeping and walking. New babies, also, get much of their exercise merely by being held for a little while each day, perhaps before bedtime when the father is home and he can become better acquainted. A baby should not be tossed about, played with, or handled unnecessarily. An intelligent way of holding and carrying the baby constitutes good exercise for him. If babies are well and normal and not forced into activities before they are ready for them, usually they will develop their muscles through their own exercise. A healthy baby left to his own resources will take all the exercise he needs.

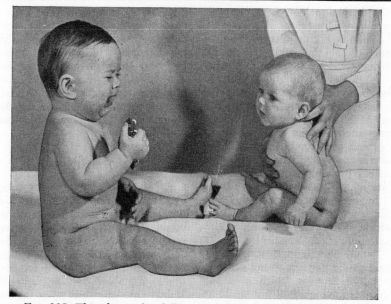

Fig. 338. This shows the difference between the posture of a baby (8 months old) whose muscles have developed and who is able to sit up alone and that of one (4 months old) who is too young to sit alone.

If tne baby is held in the sitting position before he is ready, his back is rounded, making pressure on the internal organs, the head extends forward, and his neck is thickened. He will sit up by himself as soon as his muscles have developed to the point where he can use them for such purposes. The stumbling, falling, poorly balanced toddler is usually the child who has been helped to sit up and aided in walking before he is ready. The leg muscles are strong enough to walk long before the baby tries to walk. The leg muscles will support the baby's weight at 9 months; but the baby cannot learn to walk until the nerve centers in his spinal cord mature sufficiently to co-ordinate the movements of his legs. The co-ordinating nerve centers which help to hold up the head mature first, then those for sitting up, then those for standing. The walking reflexes are the last of the series to mature. Walking requires complicated co-ordination of many groups of muscles. When the foot is moved forward the toes are automatically lifted slightly. Nothing is gained by trying to make a baby walk before these nerve centers are ready. Like so much of the child's development, he should not be pushed ahead of nature's schedule. Few parents realize that when the baby begins to stand, he is making one of the greatest physical achievements he will ever have to make.

While it is true that nature does much to help the child adjust to this change, it is equally true that many children develop injurious habits at this period. Mothers frequently fail to detect these habits before damage has been done. Every mother recognizes such obvious faults as bowed legs and can correct them with the help of the doctor, who, watching for rickets, probably will prescribe cod-liver oil. But other defects are likely to have their inception at this time which are less easily recognized but which, as the child grows older, may have serious consequences.

It may be true that, while his leg muscles are perhaps strong and normal, the muscles which help him hold his back straight are weak. So he may lose his balance because of muscular inadequacy in his back rather than in his legs. If this is true, and if he continues to use his legs while the rest of his body is not quite ready for its new erect position, he may fall into posture habits which tend to develop round shoulders, flat chest and a prominent or sagging abdomen. Normal babies are born structurally perfect. Their normal development is dependent upon many factors, such as proper feeding, correct sleeping position, unrestricting clothing and type of handling.

PLAY

The habit of play begins early. Even during the first weeks a playtime should be planned when the baby can rest or learn to amuse himself. Perhaps putting him on his abdomen on a hard mattress and letting him do the perfectly normal lifting of his head and looking around that his curiosity prompts will be a good beginning. As he grows older, suitable toys for his different stages of development will not only amuse him and stimulate his interest but also will aid co-ordination and teach him resourcefulness and independence. It promotes companionship for parents to have a regular playtime with their baby.

HABITS

A habit is doing the same thing over and over again; and, to aim toward the ideal, habits must be established early and must be correct to have real value. Since babies and children are great imitators, parents and adults should set adequate examples to be imitated. Habits are dependent upon the environment and the experiences to which the individual has to adjust. The newborn baby begins to acquire habitual reactions very early in life—some say even before birth. Early habits are thought of in terms of eating, sleeping, bathing and elimination.

Eating Habits. Eating habits begin with the first nursing. The baby should be comfortable, but not allowed to dawdle, sleep or remain at the breast too long. If the baby's feedings are regular, he will develop the habit of waking when mealtime arrives. Good eating habits established early will carry over to the time when he is eating three meals a day. If the baby is held properly and fed regularly, and if his food is sufficient, he is not so apt to start the habits of crying and thumbsucking.

THUMBSUCKING is probably the most common of the undesirable

habits which babies form. He may begin to suck his thumb almost as soon as he is born or the first time he accidentally gets his thumb into his mouth. If it is prevented at the very beginning, the habit seldom develops. The thumb should be removed gently but persistently from the baby's mouth, but without making it an issue. If the baby's diet is adequate, if he is fed regularly, if he is not allowed to get too tired, and if he has a definite time for diversion or play and has a toy to hold, the thumbsucking habit may be prevented or overcome. Closing the ends of the sleeves may help to correct the habit.

Thumbsucking is a menace to the baby's health not only because the chief mode of infection is through the mouth (and babies' hands are not always clean) but also because the pressure of the thumb contributes toward deforming the developing jaw. At teething time the baby should be given a teething ring to guard against this habit.

WOOL SUCKING is a habit which develops as a result of having wool near or about the face. Wrapping the baby in cotton receiving blankets is a preventive.

PACIFIERS are another menace to the baby's health because they cannot be kept clean. Continuous sucking increases the saliva, which may interfere with the appetite, or he may swallow air. Pacifiers also have a tendency to spoil the shape of the mouth.

CRYING is both an exercise and a medium of expression. A baby may cry for attention or because he is hungry, thirsty, uncomfortable, nervous, ill, too hot or too cold, wet, needs his position changed or his clothes straightened. It is not always easy to determine the cause of crying. While a certain amount of crying is normal, a habit of crying may develop which is fatiguing. Added attention often only encourages the baby to cry, and "spoiling" is the fundamental reason for the habit of crying.

Toilet Standards. The subject of toilet standards for the baby has provoked so much discussion that it has caused great confusion and fear in the minds of some parents in anticipation of its achievement. This is regrettable, because toilet training is only another detail in the baby's education. Timing and habit are the key words of this accomplishment.

Some mothers prefer to begin this training as soon as they themselves feel able, and before the baby sits by himself. In that event, the mother simply holds the baby in her arms, so that his back is well supported and he is comfortable, with the pan from the toidey base in her lap. Other mothers wait until the baby sits by himself, when he can use the toidey seat attached to the bathroom seat. At this time, the mother stays with the baby, of course, until he has learned to think of being left alone as another of his accomplishments.

In either case, whenever training is begun, it is preceded by several days of careful checking on the exact time when the baby usually has his bowel movement; then he is taken up and simply held for ten minutes or so over the receptacle, which has been previously warmed. When he is successful, he is praised. When a failure occurs, it is ignored. It is es-

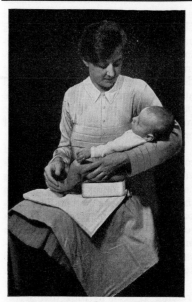

FIG. 339. The position for the younger baby who has attained regularity in his intestinal elimination.

sential that the baby be taken up at the same hour or at the same point in his daily routine, if the training is to be successful.

After the bowel training seems to be more or less established, the bladder training may be started similarly, by begining when the baby wakes from his naps. Babies usually void immediately upon awakening, and, if taken up at that moment, they will urinate. They soon learn to wait to be taken up (not long, of course). After this begining, it is timing and habit; before and after naps, first thing in the morning and last thing at night, before and after going out. No baby can be expected to indicate his needs; however, babies are individuals and react differently to this routine as to every other phase of their training. A few make their wants known at an early age; others allow their parents or those responsible for their care to think for them. They apparently find life too interesting to be bothered with this trifle.

There will be lapses, many of

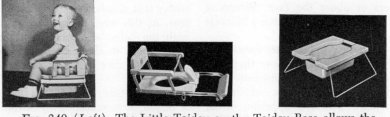

FIG. 340 (*Left*). The Little Toidey on the Toidey Base allows the toddler to help himself, thereby developing independence in toilet habits. (The Toidey Company, Fort Wayne, Ind.)

FIG. 341. (*Center*) The Little Toidey seat with the footrest (vital in bringing about proper squat position for easy functioning) may be used on base or toilet. (*Right*) The Toidey Base for the Little Toidey includes a removable pan and is a great convenience where there is only one bathroom or if the bathroom is on another floor. It folds for traveling. (The Toidey Company, Fort Wayne, Ind.)

them. Fatigue, undue excitement, breaks in the usual routine, cutting teeth, illnesses, new foods, sudden cold spells, confusion in the home and parents' carelessness all have an

DEVELOPMENT OF THE NEWBORN BABY

Psychologic Influences. Dr. Forsyth called attention to the fact that

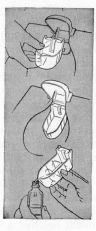

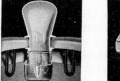

FIG. 342. Toidey specimen collector. (*Left*) A 2-ounce cup, made of transparent plastic, locks to Toideyette, the plastic deflector for the front of the Little Toidey. The collector is long enough to procure urine specimen's from both girl babies and boy babies; however, it is short enough to avoid contamination of the urine from feces. (*Top*) Collector attached: rear and side views. (The Toidey Company, Fort Wayne, Ind.)

effect. As with all training, it takes time, patience, perseverance and a relaxed attitude. To be clean, dry, comfortable and form a lifetime habit is a real achievement. Individual standards play an important role in this training. Later, when the baby is busy learning so many new things and his mind is so occupied with new interests, this "timing and habit" come to be accepted as a matter-of-fact routine.

Rest and Sleep. Rest and sleep are important to the baby's health and development and a protection to his nervous system. Rest and sleep are habits as are bathing, feeding, etc., but because parents do not recognize them as habits, they are often a neglected detail of the baby's routine.

a baby has a psychologic as well as a physical side; he stated that recently much new knowledge had been brought before us as a result of psychoanalytic investigation of adults. Many adult neurotic conditions have been traced to happenings in the first 5 years of life; and within the last few years it has been established that some of the severer mental affections were the product of psychologic mishandling in the first year. During that year, the baby is most impressionable, mentally as well as physically; and memories of the earliest years in adults have thrown a great deal of light on processes going on in the child's mind, the adult experiences being confirmed by watching the behavior of young children and comparing it with the statements of adults. It seems quite clear that impressions received in the first year were practically indelible and that the incidents of earliest infancy influenced more than anything else a child's development into a normal being.

Dr. Forsyth began by picturing the psychologic condition of an infant shortly before birth. Then, for the only time in his existence, the child lives under ideal conditions—asleep, warm, protected from danger, and with no need to fend for himself to get his food and oxygen. Then the baby was completely contented, and every need was supplied almost before it arose. Then came the process of being born. It is commonly supposed that the mother is the person most in need of sympathy at this time, and people are apt to overlook what it means to the baby.

Freud stated that from his analyses he had evoked memories of some terrifying experience which a child had already gone through at a very early age. Probably the birth process is the most terrifying experience that ever could happen, and it comes at the outset, when the baby is most impressionable. Not only is he liable to be crushed or hurt, but he is probably born half or three quarters suffocated, which is as terrifying to an infant as it would be to an adult. The child's first experience of this world, therefore, is not a happy one and is such as to make him wish to return whence he came.

Then he encounters difficulties; he has to do many things for himself, which hitherto his mother has done for him. The baby has to learn to breathe, and to become acquainted with the functions of hunger and

feeding, and of excretion from the bowel and the bladder. Those being the first two things a baby experiences, they must be expected to make a deep impression. At this stage, knowledge of the outside world is practically nil; a true description of an infant's intelligence would be to say that he has no idea that his body is his own and still less of an idea of the world outside himself. One of the first matters to occupy his intelligence is learning that certain things in his immediate surroundings are, and others are not, parts of his own body; and this knowledge takes many months to acquire. Babies in the first year of life have been known to bite their own forearms and to be surprised when it hurt. At first, the baby has no idea of his bodily attributes and spends months in eager experiment. Broadly, one might say that a newborn infant's intelligence is nil, but that emotionally he is as lavishly endowed as he is in adult life. His feelings are very strong and more impressionable than any later stage. Impressions received at this time are enduring and determine character in later childhood and adult life.

The Newborn Baby. The growth and the development of the baby from birth are very definitely associated with the kind of care that his mother has had during the prenatal period. Therefore, it would seem to be of prime importance to place emphasis on this period of maternity care.

The growth and the development of even a normal baby are extremely complex, and it should be remembered that there is a difference in the time in which perfectly normal babies develop their activities. One of the indications of his normal progress is the closure of the fontanels. The posterior fontanel usually closes when the baby is from 6 to 8 weeks old. The anterior fontanel closes when the baby is about 18 months old. If the baby is malnourished, the fontanels close earlier; or, if the baby has rickets, they remain open longer. If the baby is being examined regularly by a doctor, he will note any unusual condition and advise accordingly.

At birth, a normal baby can cry, nurse, sleep, lift his head slightly, and move his arms and legs. He probably can distinguish between light and darkness, but he is not able to focus his attention on an object. Many young babies have a squint in the eye, or, when trying to see an object, their eyes become crossed. This is because of the inability to control the eye muscles and the undeveloped muscular co-ordination.

His taste is not developed, but he is able to distinguish sweet, sour and bitter substances. His sensibility to touch and painful impressions is present but not as acute as in later childhood. The hearing is more acute, and loud noises startle him. In a short time, noises and voices can be recognized, but he cannot localize sounds for 2 or 3 months. The sense of smell is thought not to be developed. A new baby does not evidence cold by gooseflesh; therefore, the right amount of clothing and covering is regulated for comfortable warmth to avoid chilling as well as overheating.

The First Year. At 1 month the baby looks at his mother's face, his eyes follow a moving light, he lifts his head and will hold a finger or a large ring. At this age 1 baby out of 375 is said to smile.

At 2 months he smiles and coos, sheds tears, yawns, stretches and kicks. He turns his eyes toward a bright light and learns to blink. This again emphasizes the fact that his eyes always should be protected from the sun or glaring light. He turns his head in response to a speaking voice and reacts to changes in the tone.

At 3 months some babies laugh out loud. They can roll and wiggle so that it is unsafe to leave them unprotected. At this age the baby tries to make a variety of grunts, gurgles and other sounds. He can grasp a rattle when it is offered to him.

At 4 months he begins to see details, looks at his hands and feet with interest, holds his head quite steady (nevertheless, it should be supported), grasps objects and wants to play at feeding time.

At 5 months he differentiates between strangers and people he knows. He rolls from side to side and can pick up a rattle when he drops it. He can also hold a cup. At this time he begins to resent interference with his activities.

At 6 months he can sit for a moment without support for his back, sit in a padded chair, pick up a cup by the handle or grasp objects deftly. He reaches for things and bangs away on the table, pans, etc., and he enjoys playing with his toes and fingers.

At 7 months he expresses satisfaction vocally and is interested in sounds, such as banging or ringing bells.

At 8 months he may stand, play

peek-a-boo or pat-a-cake and is interested in throwing things.

At 9 months he sits alone and crawls on his hands and knees, or he may hitch along. When he hears music, it calls forth rhythmic movements. He can use his thumb and forefinger to pick up objects and can wave a bye-bye. He can make scold-ing sounds and noises that resemble words, using the inflection and the intonation of adult speech.

At 10 months he recognizes his own name. He can push himself backward.

At 11 months he may walk and repeat certain sounds; when laughed at, he "repeats his act."

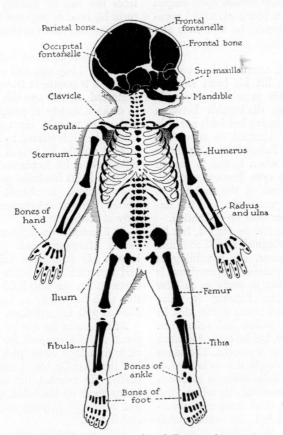

Fig. 343. Drawing of a full-term fetus which shows the amount of ossification yet to be completed. This demonstrates the importance of adequate diet and the necessity of developing good posture habits for the baby and young child.

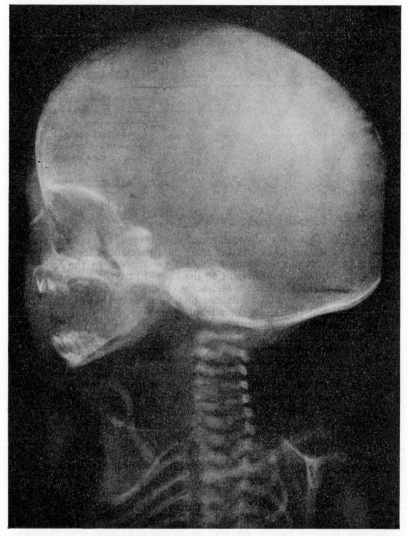

FIG. 344. This remarkable roentgenogram, taken of a developing fetus when his mother was 5½ months pregnant, should help to demonstrate the importance of adequate prenatal care. His teeth, which began to form at 7 weeks of pregnancy, show a definite degree of calcification. (T. Wingate Todd, Western Reserve University.)

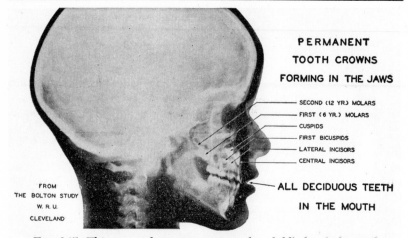

PERMANENT
TOOTH CROWNS
FORMING IN THE JAWS

SECOND (12 YR.) MOLARS
FIRST (6 YR.) MOLARS
CUSPIDS
FIRST BICUSPIDS
LATERAL INCISORS
CENTRAL INCISORS

FROM
THE BOLTON STUDY
W. R. U.
CLEVELAND

ALL DECIDUOUS TEETH
IN THE MOUTH

FIG. 345. This unusual roentgenogram of a child's head shows the erupted deciduous teeth and the unerupted permanent teeth in their stages of development. Since the teeth are present in the jaws at birth, their quality is dependent on the kind of care the baby receives during his prenatal existence and early childhood. This picture illustrates the importance of a balanced diet, early dental supervision and good hygiene. (B. Holly Broadbent, Director, The Bolton Fund, Western Reserve University)

At 1 year he may walk and, when standing, he can lower himself to the sitting position. He invents words, holds a cup and drinks from it and takes off his shoes and stockings.

Personality and Physical Development. During all the months that the developments just described have been noted, there has been another side of the baby that has also been developing—his personality, character and intellect. His good mental habits will depend largely on his surroundings, and for that reason parents should make every effort to surround the baby with the best possible influence.

A few odd notes on the baby's development may be of interest and may emphasize further the care that should be given to a baby. The baby is practically formed in its bodily structure by the end of the eighth or the ninth week of pregnancy. It is very tiny, not more than 1½ inches in length, but perfect in every external detail of fingers, toes, eyes and ears. At 7 weeks the baby's first teeth begin to form, and by 3 months calcification has begun to take place. When the baby is born, he is equipped physically with the foundation growth of all of his intricate systems, including more than 200 bones and about 50 teeth, and with enough iron, copper and iodine (and probably many other materials) stored in his body to last until he is able to eat foods which contain these elements. The nervous system and the sense organs have accomplished so much of their growth before birth that they increase only 4 times in all postnatal life. The heart, the liver and the spleen have also done much of their growing before birth and they increase only from 10 to 15 times from birth to maturity. The brain, at birth, is about a fourth of its adult size; at 18 months it is about a half of its full size or more; and at 6 years it is about $\frac{9}{10}$ of its adult size. The lungs, the blood and the skeleton grow at about the same rate as the body as a whole. The development of the eyeball is very rapid, and by the time the baby is 2 years old, the eyeballs are very nearly as large as they ever will be. The growth of the genital system is delayed and makes no rapid advances before an age of from 9 to 12 years. During this whole developing period (birth to about 18 years), the body multiplies its birth weight about 20 times.

Teething. The development of the baby's teeth begins when the mother is about 7 weeks pregnant. By the time the baby is born, each tiny toothbud of both his first and second sets lies imbedded in his jaws. As the baby grows, his teeth grow also, and they begin to erupt about the sixth or the seventh month. If they do not appear at this time, there is no need for concern, for the time for cutting teeth varies according to hereditary tendencies and the physical condition of the body. Teething is a normal process and usually is not accompanied by any disturbance. Giving the baby a hard rubber teething ring to chew on helps the teeth-

ing process. An object that permits the baby to suck instead of to chew is detrimental rather than helpful.

The most important things to remember about the baby's teeth are that they continue to develop from early pregnancy until the permanent teeth are erupted and that the mother's diet during pregnancy and the baby's diet throughout babyhood and childhood are all-important, as is his general physical condition. Most of the materials of which the baby's body is built and the means of providing energy and strength enter the body through the mouth, and the chewing process is a part of the utilization of these foods.

The care of the baby's teeth should begin as soon as the first tooth appears. A small toothbrush with soft bristles may be used and thus start a good habit. No toothpaste or powder is necessary in these very early days. Dental supervision should be instituted early.

PROPHYLACTIC MEASURES

The follow-up supervision includes such prophylactic measures as vaccination and immunization for the baby during the first year. Because such diseases as smallpox and diphtheria are a general public health problem, the nurse should be interested and should take advantage of the opportunity to discuss with the mother the advisability of these preventive measures.

IMMUNIZATION AND VACCINATION

The three most important immunizing measures for young infants are for smallpox, diphtheria and whooping cough. From 1 to 3 injec-

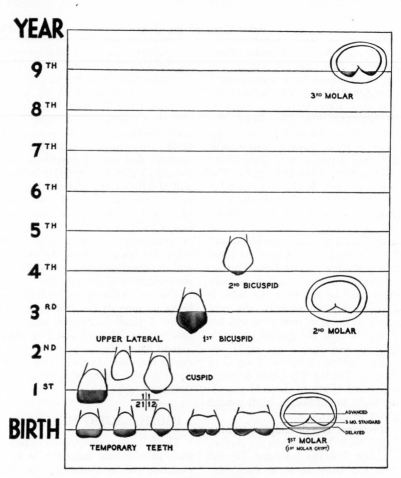

BOLTON STANDARD

Fig. 346. The Bolton Standard chart shows the time of the beginning of calcification of both the deciduous and permanent teeth; the shaded area indicates the amount of calcification at the several annual intervals.

This time table is based on x-ray interpretations and consequently lags behind the time tables based on histologic and anatomic dissections. The information has been accumulated by the Bolton Study in their serial examinations of nearly 5,000 healthy Cleveland children in contrast to the tables of calcification based on anatomic dissections of the skulls of dead children that are usually retarded through handicaps suffered during their lifetime.

With the exception of the upper and lower permanent lateral incisors, all the various kinds of permanent teeth commence to calcify at the same time; i.e., the upper and lower *(Continued on next page)*

586

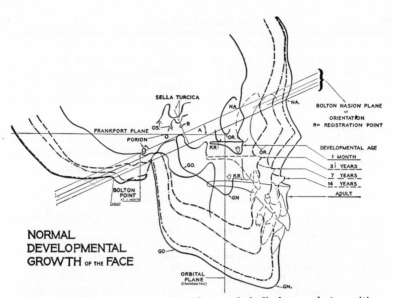

NORMAL
DEVELOPMENTAL
GROWTH OF THE FACE

FIG. 347. How the bones of the face and skull change their position in the process of growth and development. This illustrates how poor habits, such as sucking the thumb, or pacifiers and inadequate mastication, might influence this development. (B. Holly Broadbent, Director, The Bolton Fund, Western Reserve University)

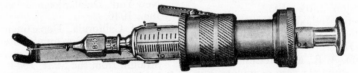

FIG. 348. Busher automatic injector which is especially good for giving hypodermics to children. The depth to which the needle can penetrate the muscle is controlled by a bracket, and the automatic release facilities the injection. (Becton-Dickinson Company)

FIG. 346 (*Continued*) central incisors commence to calcify at six months and form concurrently, the upper and lower cuspids at about the first year, while the upper lateral incisors do not begin to calcify until shortly after the first year. Also, the lower permanent lateral incisors begin their calcification at the same time as the permanent central incisors. Likewise, with the bicuspids and molar series, four teeth are added at the same time. They fall in the period shown on the chart, the first bicuspids next at about 2½ years, the second permanent molars shortly before the third year, the second bicuspids between the third and fourth year, while the third permanent teeth, or "wisdom teeth," usually begin to calcify during the eighth year. (B. Holly Broadbent, Director, The Bolton Fund, Western Reserve University)

tions are given at the time when any antibodies carried over from the mother are decreasing and will interfere least with the infant's response. Generally accepted ages are 6 months for smallpox and from 6 to 9 months for diphtheria and whooping cough, which may be given separately or combined. Some authorities advise injections for whooping cough at from 5 to 7 months or even earlier. Tetanus vaccination is sometimes given also in infancy. Later (1 or 2 years later for whooping cough) booster doses are usually given; e.g., on beginning school for diphtheria or when an outbreak for smallpox occurs.

The doctor should be consulted on one of the early visits.

SUGGESTED READING

Bartlett, Frederic: Infants and Children. Their Feeding and Growth, New York, Rinehart, 1946.

Connecticut State Board of Health: Child Development Chart.

Development of the Human Dentition, Distributed by American Dental Assoc., 222 East Superior St., Chicago 11, Ill.

Iowa State Department of Health, Des Moines: Teen Age Tooth Topics.

Kenyon and Russell: Healthy Babies, Boston, Little, 1952.

Modern Methods of Formula Preparation, Nursing World 125:283, 1951.

Nelson, A. R., and McCullagh, Ruth M.: Summer care of infants, Pub. Health Nursing 42:407, 1950.

Peto, Marjorie: Preventing nipple clogging, Am. J. Nursing 50:487, 1950.

Portune, Alicia: Children and animals go together, Am. J. Nursing 51:502, 1951.

Senn, Milton J. E., and Newill, Phyllis K.: All about Feeding Children, New York, Doubleday, 1944.

Smith, Clement A.: Human milk technology, J. Pediat. 20:616-626, 1942. (Also in reprint form.)

Spock, Benjamin: Common Sense Book of Baby and Child Care, New York, Duell, Sloane & Pearce, Inc., 1946.

State of California, Department of Public Health, Bureau of Maternal and Child Health, San Francisco: Straight from the Start, 1944.

Zabriskie, Louise: Mother and Baby Care in Pictures, ed. 3, Philadelphia, Lippincott, 1946.

CONFERENCE MATERIAL

1. How do you account for the high infant mortality during the first month of life?

2. What is the responsibility of the hospital and the nurse for the baby after he leaves the hospital in relation to the further supervision of his care and development?

3. What publications, pamphlets and books are available for the help of the mother in planning a routine for the care of her baby?

4. What advice would you give a mother who is leaving the hospital with a new baby and has an older child at home who has been exposed to whooping cough?

5. What advice and help could you give the mother to help her to adjust the new baby in the home and

to prevent a 2-year-old brother or sister from becoming jealous or suppressed?

6. What are the arguments for and against the mother returning to work following delivery and placing the baby in a day nursery?

7. What are some of the indices of normal development of the baby during the first year?

8. In discussing with men and women the question of birth injuries (as a result of poor obstetric care), how may men be convinced that the problem of better maternity care is a general one involving men as well as women and demanding their interest and co-operation?

9. What are the advantages and the disadvantages of "rooming-in," in relation to the mother, the baby, the hospital and the nursing service.

Situation Questions

UNIT FIVE: THE NEONATAL PERIOD

Read through the entire question and place your answers in the parentheses.

1. The most important months of the baby's life are:
A. 3 months after birth.
B. 6 months after birth.
C. 9 months before and 1 month after birth.
D. 12 months after birth. (_____)

2. Since "rooming-in" is so widely advertised in all magazines, the hospitals should adopt this plan of maternity care because:
A. All mothers need the experience gained thereby.
B. All babies need this added attention.
C. All mothers want this type of service.
D. Selected mothers and babies may profit where the plan could be adopted. (_____)

3. A. What type of initial bath is usually given the newborn baby?
1. Tub bath
2. Spray bath
3. Oil bath
4. Soap-and-water sponge bath (_____)
B. The reason for selecting this method is that:
1. Baby's skin is easily irritated.
2. It provides nourishment to the tissues.
3. It stimulates the circulation.
4. It is the best means of applying external heat. (_____)

4. A. If the physician feels that the baby is not in need of circumcision, the daily care of the genitals of the male infant should be to:
1. Wash externally with soap and water, otherwise let alone.
2. Retract and cleanse with oil under the foreskin.
3. Retract and cleanse with boric-acid solution under the foreskin.
4. Retract and cleanse with alcohol under the foreskin.
5. Apply petrolatum under the foreskin after the bath.
6. Stretch the prepuce, lubricate with boric ointment. (_____)
B. Reasons for the above:
1. To remove any accumulated urine.
2. To remove any accumulated smegma.
3. To increase the size of the prepuce.
4. To reduce swelling in the prepuce.
5. To break up the formation of adhesions. (_____)

591

5. The nurse caring for a baby during the first month or 4 weeks frequently interprets the baby's needs by means of his cry. Place at the right the letter corresponding to the need that you would be most likely to associate with the cry described:

NEED	CRY	
A. Wet diaper	1. A loud insistent cry—knees drawn	
B. Injury	up and kicking.	(_____)
C. Hunger	2. A whining cry—persistent.	(_____)
D. Colicky pain	3. A fretful cry with passing of gas	
E. Indigestion	and green stools.	(_____)
F. Illness	4. A sharp-sounding cry.	(_____)
	5. A fretful cry—fingers in mouth.	(_____)
	6. A shrill cry on inhalation—holding	
	breath.	(_____)
	7. Demanding cry—persistent.	(_____)

6. The principle underlying the concept of demand feedings for the newborn is:

A. Maintaining a rigid 4-hour schedule to establish eating habits.
B. Feeding every 2 hours to stimulate digestion.
C. Fitting individual feedings to individual needs.
D. Assuring an adequate nutritional intake.   (_____)

7. The young mother asks the nurse how she will know when her baby is hungry, to which the nurse could reply correctly:

A. "All crying indicates hunger."
B. "Feed the baby whenever he is awake."
C. "He will cry, fret, and refuse water and suck anything in contact with his lips."
D. "Try him first on water, and if he refuses the water, feed him."
          (_____)

8. The greatest period of weight gain for the baby during the first year is during the period of:

A. The first 1 to 5 days
B. First 5 months
C. Sixth to ninth months
D. Ninth to twelfth months   (_____)

9. The nurse would watch the baby's stools for indication of faulty digestion and abnormality. By numbering at the right, indicate the sequence of appearance of those of the following that you believe would be observed in a *normal baby* during the first 4 weeks or month:

A. Curdy, yellow . . . . (1. _____)
B. Smooth, yellow . . . . (2. _____)
C. Dark tarlike . . . . (3. _____)
D. Green, smooth, oily . . . . (4. _____)
E. Streaked with red . . . . (5. _____)

F. Yellow, watery ....(6. _____)
G. Mottled brown, soft ....(7. _____)
H. Green, curdy ....(8. _____)
I. Scrambled-egg color and consistency ....(9. _____)
J. Frothy green ....(10. _____)
K. Brown, formed ....(11. _____)
L. Clay-colored, soft ....(12. _____)
M. Milky white ....(13. _____)

10. Which one of the above (Question 9) would lead the nurse to believe that there was too much carbohydrate in the formula of the bottle-fed baby?   (_____)

11. Regardless of whether or not the baby is born prematurely, he is considered to need special premature care if at birth he does not weigh more than:

A. 3 lbs.   F. 5½ lbs.
B. 3½ lbs.   G. 6 lbs.
C. 4 lbs.   H. 6½ lbs.
D. 4½ lbs.   I. 7 lbs.   (_____)
E. 5 lbs.

12. The nurse is frequently asked about the probability of a premature baby surviving and being normal. Her answers would be based upon her understanding that, other things being equal:

A. A 7-month baby is more likely to live than an 8-month baby.

B. A baby born prematurely will not have as high an intellectual capacity as if he had been born at full term.

C. A premature baby is as well developed but considerably smaller than a term baby.

D. The earliest time at which an infant can be born with any prospect of living is after 7 lunar months.

E. With each successive week after the baby is viable the chances for life become progressively greater.

F. At full term the infant is completely formed and ready to perform the functions of respiration, digestion and excretion.

G. A baby born before term is able to perform some vital functions better than others.

H. A baby born before term is able to perform all vital functions but less effectively than at term.   (_____)

13. One of the methods of preventing cerebral hemorrhage in the new-born infant used currently with effective results is:

A. Use of vitamin B added to the mother's diet.

B. Use of vitamin A added to the mother's diet.

C. Use of vitamin K added to the mother's diet.

D. Use of vitamin C added to the mother's diet.   (_____)

14. The nurse would observe symptoms indicating cerebral hemorrhage in an infant through looking for:

A. Convulsions

B. Twitching of extremities

C. Bulging of fontanels

D. Rapid respirations

E. Rapid, thready pulse   (_____)

15. One of the communicable diseases in the mother's first trimester period which most often produces malformations in the newborn is:

A. Scarlet fever

B. Diphtheria

C. Measles

D. German measles   (_____)

Note: The key to the correct answers to these questions is given on pages 644 and 645.

UNIT SIX

ADDITIONAL MATERNITY INFORMATION

25

History of Obstetrics*

In the course of one chapter it is impossible to give a detailed history of obstetrics. This does not purport to be a complete account of the progress of obstetrics through the ages but merely a skeletal outline upon which the interested may place significant facts by additional reading reading. Sufficient references will be given where more complete information can be obtained.

For greater simplicity and more ready understanding, the ages of obstetrics have been divided arbitrarily as set forth at the beginning of this chapter.

OBSTETRICS AMONG PRIMITIVE PEOPLES

We know little about obstetrics among the primitive races but are

able from careful study of the customs of the aboriginal American Indians and the African Negroes to learn some of the customs which were part of the obstetric practice of the ancients. Childbirth in primitive times was a relatively simple process. The mother retired to a place apart from the tribe and there gave birth to her child without great difficulty. It is known that intertribal marriages were relatively rare; therefore, there was not the conglomeration of mingled races which exists today. A realization of this fact alone makes possible an understanding of the relative simplicity of childbirth under these circumstances. The fetal head and body were accommodated satisfactorily within the anatomic range of the maternal pelvis. The lack of mixed marriages prevented the resultant disproportion between passenger and pelvic passages. It became customary for women who

* By Douglas E. Cannell, M.B., B.Sc. (Med.), F.R.C.S. (C), Toronto, Canada.

had attended other women in labor to be asked to assist or accompany more of them, and they became the primitive counterpart of our latter-day midwife. The only real danger a primitive mother faced was that of abnormal presentation which usually terminated fatally for both mother and child. Toxemias and other complications are largely the products of more advanced civilization and were rarely if ever met among primitive peoples.

EGYPTIAN OBSTETRICS

In Egypt, a highly organized state of society existed and with it there arose a more complicated, if not more advanced, type of obstetrics. The priesthood in Egypt was interested in all the activities of society, and obstetrics was not neglected. They had a supervisory interest in it and took an active part in the care of abnormal or operative cases. They are known to have had obstetric forceps, performed cesarean sections on dead mothers, and podalic version was a part of their art.

ORIENTAL OBSTETRICS

Hindu medicine was probably the first authentic system of medicine to be given to the world. One of their most prolific writers and earliest men of whom we have written record is Susrata. The exact date of his existence is still a matter of dispute, but he is variously stated to have worked and written between 600 B.C. and A.D. 500, more probably about the latter date. His knowledge of menstruation and gestation was quite modern. He knew and described intelligently the

management of normal and abnormal labor. He described the use of forceps and cesarean section upon dead mothers to remove living children, and gave excellent prenatal and postpartum advice. He advised cleanliness on the part of the obstetrician; cutting the beard, the hair and the nails closely; the wearing of clean gowns; and thorough disinfection of the operating rooms prior to operation or delivery. His surgical antiseptic technic seems remarkable to modern students.

Chinese obstetrics was largely of a legendary nature until the publication of a Chinese household manual of obstetrics, *Ta Sheng P'Ien,* which, according to the author's own statement, "is correct and needs no change or addition of prescription." There were monographs on obstetrics prior to this, but none so complete. Many of his statements are unfounded; in fact the knowledge is scanty or incorrect, but the author had the saving grace of objecting to unnecessary interference and counseled patience in the treatment of labor. He had a poor opinion of midwives in general, stating that "the majority of them are fools." The reviews of Chinese obstetrics and obstetric drugs by Maxwell are excellent and give a detailed account of an interesting phase of obstetrics, which for lack of space we are forced to dispense with in this account.

GRECIAN OBSTETRICS

Prior to Hippocrates, the Asclepieads, or followers of Aesculapius, the Father of Medicine, had a slight and largely supervisory interest in obstetrics. Abortions were not illegal.

There is little definite knowledge concerning this period, but it seems probable that obstetric treatment was of a primitive nature.

The Hippocratic Period. During this age, normal obstetric cases were handled by midwives under the supervision of the physicians. Abnormal labor was entirely in the hands of the medical profession. To Hippocrates is accredited the Hippocratic oath which is still a part of the exercises for all students graduating from medical school. Treatises upon obstetrics attributed to Hippocrates are the oldest records available of the Western World's obstetric methods.

Greco-Roman Obstetrics. This period was one of progress which was due largely to the work of Celsus, Aëtius and Soranus (second century). The last re-introduced podalic version and is responsible for the first authentic records of its use in the delivery of living children. He gave an excellent technical description of the procedure and the indications for its use.

BYZANTINE, MOHAMMEDAN, JEWISH AND MEDIEVAL PERIODS

These may be said to have been characterized by a complete absence of progress, and as a corollary, a retrogression and loss of previously known practice resulted. This was due in large part to the general failure of science in the medieval period, but the interference of the Roman Church in secular matters, particularly those of a scientific nature, must be held responsible for a large share of it. The paucity of operative treatment in difficult labor may be judged from the recommendations contained in the only textbook of the day on obstetrics and gynecology, which read as follows: "Place the patient in a sheet held at the corners by four strong men, with her head somewhat elevated. Have them shake the sheet vigorously by pulling on the opposite corners, and with God's aid she will give birth." However, hospitals and nursing services were organized in this age.

While the ancient Jews gave very little assistance to the woman during labor and delivery, they were interested in the hygiene of pregnancy and cleanliness at the time of childbirth. Hygiene and sanitation were apparently a part of their religion. At the time of difficult deliveries, the women "were comforted until they died." The stool or obstetric chair was used at this time and continued to be used until about the nineteenth century A.D. Reference is made to this chair in the Bible, in the first chapter of Exodus, "when you do the office of the midwife to the Hebrew women, and see them upon the stools . . ."

THE RENAISSANCE PERIOD

The Renaissance was characterized by advances in medicine and obstetrics commensurate with those in other fields. During this time we have the first English text on obstetrics, the *Byrthe of Mankynde,* published by Raynalde. Both it and its German counterpart by Roesslin are copies of Soranus, and with their publication podalic version was re-introduced to obstetric practice.

Many famous men were responsible for the progress in obstetrics—among them Leonardo da Vinci (who made the first accurate sketches of the fetus in utero) and Vesalius (who accurately described the pelvis for the first time).

To Ambroise Paré, the dean of French surgeons and obstetricians, must go the chief credit for making podalic version a useful and practicable procedure. Due to his skill, he preferred its use to cesarean section in difficult labor. By his careful studies of its indications and technic, he made possible the removal of obstetrics from the hands of the midwives, where it had rested since the fall of the Roman Empire, and its establishment as an independent branch of medicine. Regulations were enacted for the practice of midwives, and schools were established during this period for their training. Paré's work on version and his discouragement of cesarean section were opportune.

Sections had been practiced since antiquity upon dead mothers, but the first authentic section performed upon a living mother is credited to Trautman, of Wittenberg, in 1610. This was done upon a woman with a large ventral hernia which contained the uterus. Prior to this, Nufer, a sow gelder, is reputed to have performed the operation on his wife, after obstetricians and midwives had failed to deliver her. It has been stated that Jane Seymour was delivered by a section done by Frère, a noted surgeon of the time, at the request of Henry VIII. That she died a few days after the birth of Edward VI adds credence to the story, but no absolute confirmation is available.

Due to the frightful mortality from hemorrhage, sepsis, etc., it did not become popular in spite of the advocacy of the Church. Through the following centuries it was done occasionally, but not until the advent of uterine sutures and aseptic technic did it become a practical procedure.

The origin of its name has been ascribed to Julius Caesar, but, as his mother lived many years after his birth, this seems improbable—considering the high mortality of all abdominal operations before the time of Lister. A more accurate explanation is that Numa Pompilius, one of the earlier Roman kings, passed a law making it compulsory to perform the operation upon all mothers who died while pregnant in order that the mother and the child might be buried separately. This was known as the "Lex Regis" and with the advent of the Caesars as the "Lex Casearis"—and subsequently "cesarean section." The name has been attributed to "cedere," the Latin verb meaning "to cut," but the former explanation seems to be more reasonable.

THE SEVENTEENTH CENTURY

This century was notable for many famous obstetricians. Mauriceau, of Paris, was the first to correct the view that the pelvic bones separated in normal labor. He was also the first man to refer to epidemic puerperal fever. His description of an obstetrician or rather of the qualities an obstetrician should possess is both interesting and amusing. He states:

He must be healthful, strong and robust; because this is the most laborious of all the Operations of Chirurgery; for it will make one sometimes sweat, so he shall not have a dry Thread, tho' it were the coldest Day in Winter. . . . He ought to be well shaped, at least to outward appearance, but above all, to have small hands for the easier Introduction of them into the Womb when necessary; yet strong, with the Fingers long, especially the Fore-finger, the better to reach and touch the inner orifice. He must have no Rings on his Fingers, and his Nails well pared, when he goeth about the Work, for fear of hurting the Womb. He ought to have a pleasant Countenance, and to be as neat in his Clothes as in his person, that the poor women who have need of him, be not affrighted at him. Some are of the opinion, that a Practitioner of this Art ought on the contrary to be slovenly, at least very careless, wearing a great Beard, to prevent the Occasion of the Husband's Jealousy that sends for him. Truly some believe this Policy augments their Practice but 'tis fit they should be disabused; for such a Posture and Dress resembles more a Butcher than a Chirurgeon, whom the woman apprehends already too much, that he needs not such a Disguise. Above all he must be sober, no Tipler, that he may at all times have his Wits about him. . . ."

Van Deventer, of Holland, has been called the Father of Modern Obstetrics and is credited with the first accurate description of the pelvis, its deformities, and their effect upon parturition. He also shares with Ould, of Dublin, the first description of the mechanism of labor. As time passed, customs changed and the term "accoucheur" replaced the objectionable "midman" and "man-midwife." Obstetric forceps were invented, probably about 1580, by Peter Chamberlen but were kept as a family secret until 1813 in an effort

of the Chamberlens to monopolize the field. In 1699 Hugh Chamberlen sold one-half of the instrument to Amsterdam but added fraud to infamy by selling the vector or worthless half. Prior to that, in 1670, he had demanded the equivalent of $7,500 for the secret and, in an attempt to show their worth, had killed a woman and baby before Mauriceau, who craftily chose for the demonstration a woman with a distorted pelvis, upon whom he previously had planned to do a cesarean section. After some hours of fruitless effort, Chamberlen failed in his attempts at delivery, with the resultant double fatality. When the Chamberlen forceps were finally revealed to the profession in 1813, their need had been met by other men, and the Chamberlens were thus justly punished for the discredit they had brought upon their calling.

THE EIGHTEENTH CENTURY

The eighteenth century was marked by a succession of famous men such as Palfyne, the Hunters, Smellie, White and others. The first named is credited with the invention of obstetric forceps, as he presented a copy in 1770 to the Academy of Medicine of Paris.

Smellie taught obstetrics with a manikin and made improvements on the obstetric forceps in use at that time, adding a steel lock and curved blades. He also laid down the first principles for their use and differentiated by measurement between contracted and normal pelves.

William Hunter, though a pupil of Smellie, was opposed to the use of forceps, and frequently exhibited his rusted blades as evidence of their uselessness. In conjunction with his brother, he laid the foundation of our modern knowledge of placental anatomy.

Charles White published an obstetric thesis advocating the scrubbing of the hands and general cleanliness on the part of the accoucheur; he was the pioneer in aseptic midwifery. John Harvie, 90 years before Credé, advocated external manual expression of the placenta, and it is known that a similar procedure was in use in Dublin at that time. One of the most active and famous English obstetricians of the time, John Clarke, had his fame commemorated in this epitaph:

Beneath this stone, shut up in the dark
Lies a learned man-midwife y'clep'd Dr.
    Clarke.
On earth while he lived by attending
    men's wives,
He increased population some thousands
    of lives;
Thus a gain to the nation was gain to
    himself
An enlarged population, enlargement of
    pelf.
So he toiled late and early, from morn-
    ing to night,
The squalling of children his greatest
    delight;
Then worn out with labours, he died
    skin and bone
And his ladies he left all to Mansfield
    and Stone.

There were many famous obstetricians on the Continent in this period, chief among them being Baudelocque, who invented the pelvimeter and named and described positions and presentations. In America, prejudices against men in midwifery were carried over from Europe; as late as

1857 a demonstration before the graduating class at Buffalo roused such a storm of criticism that the American Medical Association had to intervene. Their judgment was that any physician who could not conduct labor by touch alone should not undertake midwifery.

This eighteenth century produced such men as Moultrie, Lloyd and Shippen. The last was a pupil of Smellie and Hunter; in 1762 he opened a school for midwifery in Philadelphia, and, since he provided convenient lodgings for the accommodation of poor women during confinement, he may be said to have established the first lying-in hospital in America. With Morgan, he founded the School of Medicine of the University of Pennsylvania, becoming its first Professor of Anatomy, Surgery and Midwifery.

THE NINETEENTH AND TWENTIETH CENTURIES

The increased knowledge, interest and ability which physicians brought to obstetrics were largely offset by the increased mortality due to puerperal fever. During the seventeenth, the eighteenth and the nineteenth centuries it became a pestilence, at times wiping out whole communities of puerperal women. The mortality rates varied in the best European clinics at Paris and Vienna from 10 to 20 per cent. The origin and the spread of the disease were little understood or studied. Obstetricians wasted futile hours on a study of minor alterations in instruments or technic and ignored the vast loss of life from puerperal fever. Oliver Wendell Holmes, of Harvard, first presented his views on the contagiousness of puerperal fever in 1843, and in 1855 he reiterated them in a monograph on *Puerperal Fever as a Private Pestilence.* This was, and still remains, a medical classic on the subject. His statements aroused great controversy in America, and he received a great deal of abuse and criticism from Meigs and Hodge, two of the foremost American obstetricians of the day. One of them stated that it was ridiculous to conceive of any gentleman carrying contamination on his hands from patient to patient.

The following is Holmes' summary of his observations on the prevention of puerperal sepsis. Written in 1843, before the discovery of any human pathologic organism, and before the adoption of disinfection in surgical procedures, it is a truly remarkable summary.*

1. A physician holding himself in readiness to attend cases of midwifery, should never take any active part in the postmortem examination of cases of puerperal fever.

2. If a physician is present at such autopsies, he should use thorough ablution, change every article of dress, and allow twenty-four hours or more to elapse before attending to any case of midwifery. It may be well to extend the same caution to cases of simple peritonitis.

3. Similar precautions should be taken after the autopsy or surgical treatment of cases of erysipelas, if the physician is obliged to unite such offices with his obstetrical duties, which is in the highest degree inexpedient.

4. On the occurrence of a single case of puerperal fever in his practice, the

* From Abraham Levinson, Pioneers of Pediatrics.

physician is bound to consider the next female he attends in labor, unless some weeks, at least, have elapsed, as in danger of being infected by him, and it is his duty to take every precaution to diminish her risk of disease and death.

5. If within a short period two cases of puerperal fever happen close to each other, in the practice of the same physician, the disease not existing or prevailing in the neighborhood, he would do wisely to relinquish his obstetrical practice for at least one month, and endeavor to free himself by every available means from any noxious influence he may carry about with him.

6. The occurrence of three or more closely connected cases, in the practice of one individual, no others existing in the neighborhood, and no other sufficient causes being alleged for the coincidence, is prima facie evidence that he is the vehicle of contagion.

7. It is the duty of the physician to take every precaution that the disease shall not be introduced by nurses or other assistants, by making proper inquiries concerning them, and giving timely warning of every suspected source of danger.

8. Whatever indulgence may be granted to those who have heretofore been the ignorant causes of so much misery, the time has come when the existence of a *private pestilence* in the sphere of a single physician should be looked upon not as a misfortune but as a crime; and in the knowledge of such occurrences, the duties of the practitioner to his profession should give way to his paramount obligations to society.

While Holmes first conceived the correct idea of the nature of the disease, it is to Ignaz Philipp Semmelweiss that the glory must go of finally proving without question the nature of its source and transmission. He was an assistant in the Viennese clinic for women, and while his associates fussed with unimportant details of technic, he was studying and mourning the tremendous death rate among puerperal women in the clinic. He observed that the death rate in Clinic I where women were delivered by medical students or physicians was always higher than that of Clinic II where midwives officiated or received instruction. After fruitless study and manifold changes in technic in order to follow more closely that of Clinic II, the cause of the disease was brought home to him in a desperate and startling fashion. His friend, Kalletschka, an assistant in pathology, died after performing an autopsy upon a victim of puerperal fever, during which Kalletschka had sustained a slight cut on his finger.

At postmortem the findings were identical with those of puerperal sepsis, and Semmelweiss concluded that the disease was transmitted from the dead, by contact from the physicians and the students, who often went directly from the postmortem room to deliveries. Accordingly, he immediately instituted and enforced a ruling which made it obligatory that all physicians and students wash their hands in a solution of chloride of lime after attending autopsies and before examining or delivering mothers. In seven months he had reduced the mortality in Clinic I from 12 to 3 per cent, and in the subsequent year had a mortality lower than Clinic II, a hitherto unheard-of feat. Subsequently, he observed that puerperal sepsis could be transmitted from patient to patient by contact of contaminated material, or attendants, as well as from the postmortem room, and in 1861 he published his immortal work on *The Cause, Concept and Prophylaxis of Puerperal Fever.*

Medicine provides pitiful figures in profusion, but none, it seems, met such a cruel reception and ultimate fate as Semmelweiss. His colleagues (for the most part, but with a few notable and loyal exceptions) distorted and criticized his teachings. Had they stopped there it might have been bad enough, but they carried their distaste for his views to the stage of persecution. He was forced to leave Vienna and go to Budapest, where a similar attitude— if possible a more malignant one— awaited him. A disappointed man, he died in 1865 from a brain abscess which may have originated in an infection similar to that of his friend Kalletschka. To the tragedy of his life, his death added satire. His work, however, has lived on; Pasteur and Lister added to it; and with a more modern and tolerant age his worth has been recognized.

The organisms causing puerperal fever probably were seen by several early workers beginning with Mayrhofer, who, in 1863, described "cylindrical vibrios" or "strings of pearls" in the lochia of puerperal sepsis. In 1864, 310 deaths occurred in the 1,350 confinement cases in the Maternité hospital in Paris, and that "Vestibule of Death" had to be closed in 1865.

Pasteur, in 1879, saw "cocci in chain" in cases of puerperal sepsis and contributed definitely to our knowledge of the causal streptococci, demonstrating to doctors the "presence of the invisible foe" in a drop of blood obtained by a "simple pinprick on the finger tip of the unhappy woman doomed to die the next day" and recommending methods of aseptic technic for their control.

The nineteenth and the twentieth centuries were largely notable for their utilization of drugs to alleviate the pains of childbirth. The use of ether as an anesthetic was first discovered in America, but it was first utilized for childbirth by Simpson in Great Britain. He brought back the lost art of version by making it a safer procedure and eventually substituted chloroform for ether. As with almost every advance in medicine, it was opposed bitterly. The opposition was loudest and most vehement from the clergy, but in 1853 Queen Victoria accepted it for delivery and by her action silenced most of the criticism. Nitrous oxide had been used in 1880 and has continued to be popular ever since that time. More recently, ethylene and cyclopropane have been used in various clinics with great success. The latter has attained wide popularity because of the low concentration of anesthetic compared with the high oxygen content of the mixture. The dangers of explosive combinations cannot be discounted completely, but with proper precautions these may be avoided. Spinal anesthesia is of value in cesarean section, but few clinics use it in vaginal delivery. Local anesthesia is becoming more popular and has distinct advantages in toxemic and cardiac patients.

Obstetric analgesia has made great strides during the twentieth century. Morphine and scopolamine were used in 1902 and repopularized about 1920. This combination supplemented by inhalation or colonic anesthesia is probably the best method available at the moment. Barbiturates, particularly Amytal Sodium and pentobarbital sodium, have been widely used on this continent. The combination of barbiturates with scopolamine hypodermically, or paraldehyde rectally, has met with greater success in many centers. All forms of analgesia require closer attention to the progress of labor on the part of the obstetric and nursing staffs, if they are to be uniformly satisfactory.

The present century will be remembered largely for the development of antepartal clinics and the more concentrated care of the expectant mothers that came with them. The application of advances in general medicine, metabolism and public health to obstetrics has led to a marked decrease in mortality and morbidity from cardiac, pulmonic, metabolic, venereal and associated medical conditions complicating pregnancy. The consideration of adequate vitamin, mineral and caloric contents in connection with the diet of pregnant and puerperal women has not only decreased the morbidity but has enhanced the health of all mothers and children who receive adequate obstetric care.

Many other contributions have been made and are being added constantly to the science of obstetrics, not the least of which is more intensive training and study in this specialty demanded by the public as well as the medical profession. The advent of routine external expression of the placenta, silver nitrate prophylaxis in the eyes of the newborn, purified ergot and pituitary preparations in hemorrhage control and prevention are but a few of the methods and medications which have marked the early twentieth century.

The morphologic and anthropologic studies of Naegele, Roberts, Williams, Goodwin, Caldwell, Moloy and others has done much to improve our understanding of the various types of pelves and some of their importance in labor. Roentgenologic pelvimetry and cephalometry have greatly advanced our knowledge of the probable course of labor and delivery; Thoms, Caldwell and Moloy, Hanson, Jarcho and countless others have contributed to our advances in this field. This type of pelvimetry is the most accurate method available at the moment; but in its present state cannot, and probably never will, completely supersede clinical skill and judgment in the management of borderline cases of bony dystocia.

In a necessarily brief and incomplete fashion, an endeavor has been made to touch upon some of the more interesting phases of the history of obstetrics—a delightful and fascinating subject.

SUGGESTED READING

Findley, Palmer: Priests of Lucina, Boston, Little, 1939.

Finney, R. P.: Story of Motherhood, New York, Liveright, 1937.

Guttmacher, Allan: Story of Human Birth, Garden City, Blue Ribbon Books, 1937.

Heaton, C. E.: Obstetrics and gynecology in America, North Carolina M. J. **8**:35-37, 1947.

Heaton, Claude: Fifty years of progress in obstetrics and gynecology, New York State J. Med. **51**:83-85, 1951.

Williams, Whitridge: Sketch of the History of Obstetrics in America, New York, 1903. (Reprinted from American Gynecology 5:1903.)

26

Teaching Aids

INTRODUCTION

In this edition an effort has been made to present to the student nurse the subject of obstetrics and maternity care. With a thorough foundation of theoretical instruction and adequate practical experience in this branch of nursing, the nurse should be equipped to contribute one of the most interesting services life has to offer.

The foundation for all future developments, physical and mental, lies within the human body at birth; and, because maternity care involves the individual "in the making," there is this extraordinary opportunity for the nurse to share or have a part in helping to produce better human beings. This responsibility involves not only care and prevention of those diseases, accidents and abnormalities associated with pregnancy but also preventive work in the fields of eugenics, pediatrics, communicable diseases and mental nursing. Babies wanted and babies well cared for will be born into an environment which could be only an asset to their inheritance. With the present trend for premarital examinations and physical examinations required for marriage licenses (in some states) there should be the possibilities or potential qualities in both parents which would provide better physical health and increased mental stability.

The knowledge of the maternity situation as a whole may help the nurse to appreciate the fact that the care of the individual is the foundation for improving maternity care generally. In general, many people think that if women bore children and delivered themselves as do wild animals or savages, there would be no danger and no deaths from pregnancy. Of course, superficially, this sounds reasonable. There are no figures—nor could such figures be obtained—which show how many wild

607

animals die in giving birth, but it is known what happens under similar conditions. A study was made by Holland some years ago. Stratz, a Dutch physician, was sent to Solo, one of the East Indies, where everything was most primitive and as wild as can be imagined. Stratz found that there were ten times as many mothers who died during pregnancy and childbirth in Solo as in the mother country, Holland. Since doctors and nurses play such an important part in this maternity care, should they not assume some responsibility in obtaining better conditions for both mothers and babies during this whole period of pregnancy and the months following?

To provide adequate maternity care for the mothers of this country is a tremendous problem, no program for which has yet been developed.

At any given time there are more than 2,000,000 pregnant mothers distributed throughout the United States. These women are of all races, many of them living in a new climate and under conditions that are new and strange. The mechanical handicaps alone are difficult to meet. For example, in this country, there are 3,026,789 square miles of territory, including many whole communities, in which there is not one made road, and many homes are well-nigh inaccessible. As might be expected, health service facilities are often deplorably inadequate. There never has been sufficient trained professional care available to meet the needs of the American people, and with the present increasing demand for doctors and nurses, the conditions are even more serious. The distribution of doctors and nurses is uneven among geographic areas and economic strata of the people. While many large cities are well supplied, many rural areas are most inadequately provided with doctors, dentists and nurses; some are practically without access to these services.

A great deal is expected of the public health nurse who undertakes maternity and infant hygiene work. She is expected to organize a complete service, which includes finding mothers early in pregnancy and getting them under medical supervision, prenatal nursing supervision, teaching the fundamentals of general hygiene and preparations for the baby, helping the patient with delivery preparation (and in many cases attending the delivery) as well as follow-up care and supervision of the mother and the baby after delivery. While there is a growing consciousness of need for this care on the part of parents, many pregnant mothers and their families do not recognize the need for care much before the baby is expected. Therefore, the nurse's first responsibility is to teach the mothers and their families why care is necessary during the prenatal period and what the details of this care should be. The mother must be convinced of the value of this care to her baby and to herself before she is willing to spend her time and money. The father must be convinced also, in order that he may assume his share of the responsibility. Before the nurse can render this difficult service, she herself must know obstetrics and its many problems; and, because of her knowledge, believe in the necessity for obstetric

TABLE 2. BIR

Year	Fi
1920	31
1921	32
1922	28
1923	27
1924	28
1925	28
1926	27
1927	27
1928	2
1929	2
1930	2
1931	24
1932	22
1933	22
1934	2
1935	2
1936	2
1937	26
1938	2
1939	26
1940	2
1941	30
1942	31
1943	32
1944	28
1945	20
1946	34
1947	46
1948	39

* The rates
sands). Rates
number of Sta
1920 to date
tion area.

1935	1936	1937	1938	1939	1940	1941	1942	1943	1944	1945	1946	1947	1948	1949
16.9	16.7	17.0	17.6	17.3	17.9	18.9	20.9	21.5	20.2	19.6	20.3	25.8	24.2	24.0
22.0	21.0	21.3	21.4	21.7	22.2	22.7	24.7	28.2	27.5	25.5	30.9	32.0	31.8	32.0
22.5	23.5	25.5	26.4	22.2	23.5	24.1	24.7	25.5	24.8	26.2	25.5	27.9	27.0	27.9
17.9	16.6	17.2	18.2	18.2	19.7	20.7	22.0	23.7	24.2	23.9	25.8	27.0	26.5	24.9
13.4	13.9	15.3	16.5	15.3	16.2	18.1	21.3	23.0	22.5	22.9	22.5	24.1	23.0	23.4
17.7	17.1	18.3	19.2	18.6	18.8	19.1	21.7	22.9	22.6	21.8	25.6	27.4	27.5	26.3
13.0	12.8	13.1	13.7	13.9	14.7	16.7	21.0	22.3	19.6	21.5	21.9	23.5	21.3	20.4
15.8	15.1	16.7	17.0	16.7	17.2	19.2	20.5	23.0	21.9	20.2	22.8	24.9	22.9	23.1
18.2	18.9	19.7	20.6	21.3	23.1	24.7	18.4	19.5	19.0	22.4	20.9	23.6	23.7	23.6
17.4	17.1	17.7	18.6	17.6	17.8	19.8	20.7	23.8	24.0	21.3	22.7	23.5	22.9	23.0
20.8	20.1	20.8	21.0	20.7	20.8	21.8	23.7	26.4	25.8	22.2	26.7	28.8	28.3	27.8
19.8	21.1	20.0	22.9	21.5	22.3	22.3	24.0	26.5	26.3	26.0	27.2	31.2	29.2	27.9
14.3	14.3	14.6	15.6	15.0	15.6	17.0	19.7	20.7	18.9	22.3	21.7	23.7	21.8	21.9
15.4	15.6	16.1	17.3	17.1	18.1	19.3	21.2	22.4	21.2	24.1	23.5	25.8	24.2	24.2
16.2	16.8	16.5	16.9	17.4	17.9	18.4	20.0	20.8	20.8	23.5	23.6	26.3	24.4	24.3
16.3	15.9	15.7	15.9	16.0	15.9	16.7	19.7	21.3	21.1	23.9	23.0	25.5	23.8	23.5
20.3	19.3	19.2	21.2	21.5	22.3	22.3	24.3	25.3	25.6	25.2	27.1	28.6	27.3	26.6
19.9	20.7	21.6	22.9	20.8	21.5	23.1	24.0	26.7	26.4	25.3	27.3	28.8	28.2	28.7
18.6	17.9	17.8	17.8	17.8	17.8	18.7	21.1	23.8	22.9	26.1	22.0	24.3	21.7	20.9
16.3	15.9	16.5	17.3	15.8	16.6	18.8	23.1	23.9	22.1	22.6	22.2	24.5	23.3	22.9
14.4	13.9	13.9	13.8	14.5	15.3	16.3	19.5	20.9	19.3	21.5	21.3	23.4	20.6	20.0
18.5	18.5	19.0	20.1	18.3	18.9	20.5	22.5	23.5	21.3	21.8	23.8	26.6	25.1	25.1
17.5	18.1	18.1	18.9	18.2	19.0	19.5	22.1	22.9	22.5	22.6	24.8	27.1	25.5	25.4
24.1	24.6	25.8	26.5	23.8	24.1	24.9	26.8	30.2	28.9	24.7	30.9	32.0	31.8	32.0
14.6	14.1	14.3	14.7	15.6	16.4	17.5	19.0	20.1	19.5	23.4	21.8	23.7	22.2	21.8
18.9	19.6	19.0	19.8	19.7	20.5	20.4	22.8	24.0	23.8	23.1	26.0	29.3	28.1	27.3
17.1	17.4	16.3	16.4	17.0	16.8	16.9	19.1	21.1	21.2	21.8	23.0	26.0	25.1	24.6
14.4	14.2	17.2	18.7	18.0	18.7	19.8	21.4	23.7	22.8	25.8	23.0	26.4	23.2	23.1
15.5	15.1	15.0	15.4	16.2	17.3	17.8	19.3	20.7	19.1	22.5	22.7	26.7	24.5	22.8
12.7	12.4	12.6	12.9	13.6	14.1	15.8	19.4	20.2	18.8	21.4	22.0	23.6	21.0	20.8
31.3	30.6	32.8	33.9	27.2	27.7	27.8	27.3	31.1	32.1	21.8	33.1	35.4	34.7	34.2
14.3	14.1	14.3	14.6	13.9	14.6	15.7	19.0	19.7	18.6	22.3	21.2	23.0	21.0	20.4
23.0	22.0	22.6	22.9	22.4	22.6	23.7	26.0	28.1	27.3	23.6	28.0	30.1	28.5	27.4
19.5	19.3	17.9	18.5	20.5	20.8	21.0	22.8	24.9	25.7	22.8	28.2	30.9	29.5	28.9
15.1	15.4	16.0	16.7	15.8	16.6	18.3	20.8	21.1	19.7	20.8	22.7	25.4	23.4	23.7
17.4	16.5	16.3	17.3	18.6	19.1	19.5	21.3	23.9	24.0	27.6	23.7	25.0	23.8	23.4
13.1	13.7	15.1	15.8	15.5	16.4	17.6	20.7	21.9	20.5	20.0	21.6	24.6	23.8	23.7
16.0	15.7	15.8	16.3	16.4	16.7	17.6	20.3	21.3	19.5	22.6	22.4	24.8	22.2	21.6
15.0	15.0	15.0	15.5	14.9	15.1	16.2	19.7	21.1	19.9	20.9	22.7	24.2	21.5	20.8
22.1	21.1	21.7	21.9	22.6	23.4	24.8	25.8	30.1	29.0	24.0	28.9	30.3	29.3	29.2
18.6	18.6	17.2	17.1	18.0	18.1	18.1	21.3	23.4	23.8	22.4	26.4	29.0	27.8	27.8
18.9	17.7	18.0	18.5	18.6	19.1	20.8	22.3	24.9	24.4	24.8	25.3	27.2	25.4	25.4
18.9	18.2	18.8	19.6	19.1	19.7	21.2	22.5	26.3	26.5	24.8	25.9	27.1	26.1	26.4
24.7	24.3	24.5	25.5	24.0	24.6	25.0	28.2	29.6	27.7	23.1	28.6	33.3	31.2	31.3
17.5	17.0	16.5	16.5	17.8	18.6	18.8	21.1	22.9	22.0	20.7	24.5	27.4	26.2	25.3
19.5	19.2	19.2	16.9	19.6	20.6	21.9	22.3	26.2	25.0	23.0	24.7	26.8	25.2	25.2
13.7	14.2	15.1	16.1	15.6	16.2	17.6	22.0	24.0	23.2	20.1	23.1	25.7	24.0	23.8
23.0	22.3	22.6	22.8	22.0	22.1	23.0	23.9	24.8	24.2	25.5	26.6	29.0	27.4	27.1
18.1	18.1	18.3	18.8	17.4	17.5	18.2	20.5	21.8	21.0	20.2	23.9	26.1	25.0	24.9
18.8	20.4	19.3	21.0	19.8	20.1	20.7	23.9	25.2	24.1	22.7	24.2	28.4	27.6	27.1

State Area	8	1939	1940	1941	1942	1943	1944	1945	1946	1947	1948
Area	40	38	32	26	26	23	21	16	13	12	
Alabama	59	61	52	33	34	37	34	26	26	23	
Arizona	44	50	30	39	27	30	30	21	18	13	
Arkansas	57	49	40	37	39	28	29	21	18	21	
California	31	28	23	20	20	17	16	12	10	9	
Colorado	54	41	33	19	26	25	24	19	13	10	
Connecticut	26	28	20	18	16	15	12	9	7	6	
Delaware	41	54	23	16	24	15	32	13	8	11	
District of Colum	52	29	27	27	22	21	15	17	11	9	
Florida	65	65	63	41	37	33	30	30	22	19	
Georgia	56	57	48	41	39	36	32	26	25	21	
Idaho	22	36	27	26	23	25	20	16	10	8	
Illinois	31	30	25	21	21	18	17	14	10	8	
Indiana	36	29	25	24	20	20	17	13	11	10	
Iowa	30	35	27	19	17	18	18	11	9	8	
Kansas	37	37	28	26	21	18	19	15	10	8	
Kentucky	43	36	37	27	25	25	25	20	18	15	
Louisiana	62	53	43	35	32	34	25	20	19	17	
Maine	39	40	31	21	22	23	25	16	15	8	
Maryland	37	28	25	20	18	19	15	11	10	9	
Massachusetts	35	28	28	21	20	18	18	13	9	7	
Michigan	31	29	27	21	18	17	15	12	11	8	
Minnesota	29	22	20	16	14	14	14	9	6	7	
Mississippi	59	63	57	44	39	38	38	31	26	26	
Missouri	41	37	30	26	25	22	23	16	14	11	
Montana	32	30	16	22	18	15	16	14	11	9	
Nebraska	35	32	24	19	17	17	15	10	11	7	
Nevada	41	48	27	7	20	23	18	18	12	16	
New Hampshire	34	32	26	12	27	28	18	13	11	12	
New Jersey	32	30	27	20	19	16	16	13	10	8	
New Mexico	50	47	45	48	47	40	37	20	21	24	
New York	32	30	23	22	21	19	18	12	10	9	
North Carolina	47	52	40	34	32	30	28	20	17	19	
North Dakota	24	17	23	22	29	18	11	10	11	10	
Ohio	39	32	25	21	22	19	18	13	12	9	
Oklahoma	40	40	31	31	25	24	22	16	17	11	
Oregon	24	25	21	17	15	18	13	10	9	4	
Pennsylvania	38	32	31	27	25	25	22	15	13	10	
Rhode Island	34	25	22	18	22	18	14	14	9	13	
South Carolina	59	68	62	53	44	38	34	27	26	24	
South Dakota	29	34	26	20	16	18	13	10	10	10	
Tennessee	56	47	37	30	29	28	24	18	17	18	
Texas	49	46	36	30	26	25	23	16	15	15	
Utah	31	27	19	17	16	14	13	14	8	6	
Vermont	36	36	22	21	22	19	17	14	12	10	
Virginia	51	45	40	32	29	26	21	16	17	14	
Washington	36	31	18	17	16	16	17	12	11	5	
West Virginia	33	33	29	23	29	22	17	15	16	11	
Wisconsin	28	28	23	18	20	18	14	14	11	11	
Wyoming	35	42	21	23	15	9	9	16	8	11	

Source: Federa
* Dropped fron

Deaths assigned to pregnancy and childbirth per 10,000 live births

1935	1936	1937	1938	1939	1940	1941	1942	1943	1944	1945	1946	1947	1948
56	57	54	51	48	47	45	40	40	40	38	35	33	32
63	67	62	61	60	61	59	50	45	45	45	39	38	38
112	120	121	99	94	84	88	80	77	69	69	43	52	56
47	51	55	51	46	46	44	40	37	35	32	29	30	28
50	53	54	44	42	39	37	35	34	34	33	31	30	29
73	74	73	60	55	60	52	50	50	49	51	41	38	38
43	42	40	36	36	34	31	29	30	31	30	29	26	24
66	65	64	53	44	49	43	47	47	49	39	30	32	29
59	72	61	48	48	47	51	51	48	45	48	42	33	25
62	59	60	58	56	54	53	48	47	45	44	40	39	35
68	70	62	68	58	58	58	49	47	44	42	37	35	34
51	51	44	45	46	42	34	36	32	34	35	34	30	30
46	47	43	41	38	35	34	33	33	32	32	31	29	28
51	51	50	43	39	42	40	37	40	34	36	33	31	30
47	48	44	41	39	37	36	34	34	33	30	31	29	26
50	52	44	43	39	38	38	36	34	33	33	31	29	27
59	67	59	61	53	53	59	48	50	47	47	41	38	40
69	72	66	67	63	64	58	48	45	46	43	38	38	38
63	64	65	56	52	53	51	46	51	47	46	33	29	27
62	69	62	56	50	50	53	44	43	41	38	35	32	29
48	47	44	40	37	37	35	32	34	33	32	35	32	29
48	51	48	45	42	41	39	37	38	38	36	34	32	30
45	44	41	39	36	33	34	30	31	31	31	30	29	27
54	58	59	57	56	54	55	47	47	44	41	38	37	38
57	58	57	52	45	47	46	39	40	38	38	34	33	30
60	57	51	46	49	46	37	34	39	36	34	36	33	31
41	44	42	36	37	36	34	33	36	33	29	31	28	27
71	70	40	48	45	52	42	57	52	50	46	40	34	39
54	46	48	48	46	40	36	36	46	38	36	33	31	29
46	44	39	40	39	36	36	31	34	34	32	29	28	26
129	122	124	109	100	100	95	98	92	89	101	80	69	70
48	47	45	41	39	37	33	32	33	33	32	30	29	27
69	69	66	69	59	57	60	48	47	45	43	38	36	35
59	50	52	50	49	45	38	37	35	35	29	35	31	29
50	51	50	43	43	41	41	37	39	38	37	32	30	30
55	60	57	49	50	50	47	41	43	41	40	32	33	34
41	44	42	39	35	33	31	31	30	30	29	29	25	25
51	51	50	46	46	45	41	38	38	40	38	34	32	28
47	48	48	44	39	38	36	40	44	35	28	30	29	26
79	81	76	80	66	68	75	59	55	55	50	42	40	40
52	48	51	44	41	39	41	38	36	35	31	30	32	32
64	68	61	63	54	55	55	46	45	45	48	39	37	37
72	71	74	65	67	69	57	54	51	50	49	43	42	46
49	53	41	47	40	41	30	33	31	34	31	28	26	27
49	58	50	48	46	45	44	42	39	41	35	35	32	29
70	74	70	66	61	59	67	53	47	47	47	39	37	38
45	45	40	39	37	36	35	33	35	34	35	34	29	27
61	71	62	62	55	54	61	53	52	52	52	42	39	40
46	48	43	42	40	37	35	32	35	32	31	31	30	26
51	58	56	52	46	46	44	45	37	41	40	34	35	40

care, believe that she can teach the subjects she knows and be truly interested in each individual mother and her problems.

The part that the nurse will take in the actual supervision, care and instruction of the patients will differ in different communities. Exactly what it will be in any given community will depend on the medical and nursing facilities and the division of labor between the doctor and the nurse. The larger part of her duty lies in the definite demonstration and teaching of personal and general hygiene and in the care of the family. This is a large factor in the reduction of maternal and infant mortality and morbidity. In rural communities she usually will find quite different working conditions: scattered, small communities, doctors few in number, and transportation inadequate and difficult. In any of this work where the nurse often has to work alone, she will find use for the fundamentals of nursing she acquired in her hospital experience and for many improvisations to suit the various conditions she meets. The nurse is often asked by community boards, patients and others for advice on many questions. She may have had no definite previous training bearing on these special questions, but at least she should know where such information may be obtained. To aid the nurse, the following outlines, illustrations, visual aids * and suggestions have been included.

* The Cleveland Health Museum, Cleveland, Ohio, has many excellent teaching aids, such as the Dickinson-Belskie models.

SUGGESTIONS FOR CLASSES

PRELIMINARY PLANS

Nurses are often called upon to organize a series of classes for mothers, fathers or parents. In planning such a series, the resources of the community as well as certain other factors have to be considered. Some of these are listed below.

Consent of the organization or group or committee to sponsor the classes

Suitable location, such as:
Grange hall
Church
School
Library
Unoccupied store
Organization headquarters
Hospital clinic, etc.

Requirements for site selected:
No unnecessary steps
Adequate ventilation and heat
Bathroom facilities
Ample space for demonstrations
Storage closets for equipment (with locks)
Suitable chairs
Simple and attractive furnishings
Cordial atmosphere

Teaching equipment available:
Demonstration or illustrative material for each class
Resources of the community
Improvised equipment

Number and size of classes to be held, dependent on:
Group
Transportation facilities
Social and educational background of group
Time available

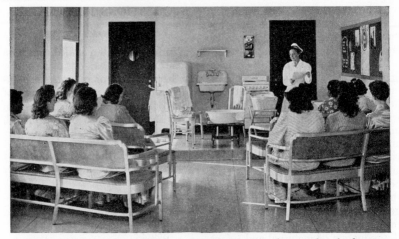

Fig. 349. This hospital has a special room for mothers' classes, equipped with all the essentials, kitchenette, stove, sink and refrigerator, as well as demonstration equipment for the care of the baby. This room is used for prenatal classes as well as for demonstrations to patients before discharge. Teaching of this kind is a routine part of the nurse's work in almost all hospitals. (Margaret Hague Maternity Hospital, Jersey City, N. J.)

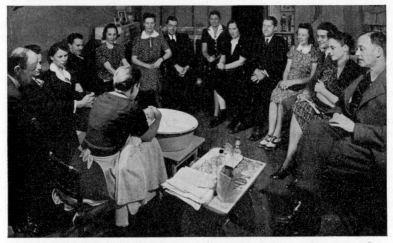

Fig. 350. When parents attend classes together and receive the same instruction, it strengthens their mutual interest and increases their understanding and co-operation. (Maternity Consultation Service, New York)

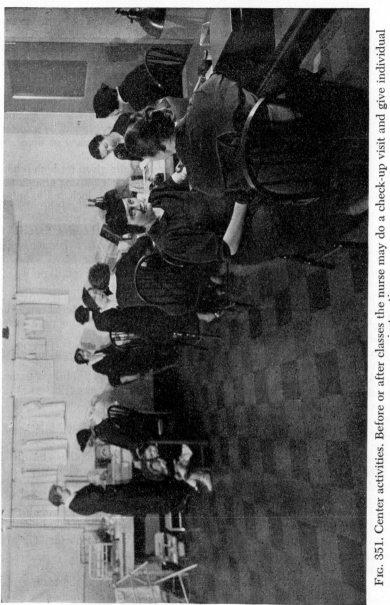

Fig. 351. Center activities. Before or after classes the nurse may do a check-up visit and give individual instruction.

Needs and interest of group
Number of applicants
Means of securing members:
Referred by doctors, nurses,
hospitals, clinics
Individual contacts and former
class members
Publicity, such as
Newspaper articles
Magazine articles
Posters and circulars
Announcements (churches,
public meetings, etc.)
Reading material:
Lending library
Public library
Scrapbooks
Pamphlets
Magazines
Federal and state literature

The content of subject matter to be covered in this series of classes should be divided according to the number of classes and the time allotted. To stimulate the interest of the various groups, the classes should be kept informal, and discussion should be encouraged. Interest in the individual patient creates a co-operative atmosphere. Some organizations have found that serving refreshments adds to the informal and social response of the group.

The nurse teaching the class should be familiar with the availability, locally or by mail, and the costs of articles exhibited and advised (such as layettes and equipment, mother's clothes, foods, etc.). In teaching, also, when technical terms are used, an explanation of these should be made in language which befits the patients' background and understanding.

When planning classes, the needs and the questions of the group should be considered. Sometimes a combination of classes or a change in the sequence is necessary. All illustrative material used for demonstration or exhibit should be chosen with thoughtful care. If commercial posters or pictures from magazines are utilized they should be selected from the point of view of accuracy and teaching value.

If classes are given for high school students or home-nursing groups, the following may be included as introductory classes:

Criteria for choosing friends
Opportunity for home-making
versus career
Preparation for marriage
Budgeting

The following material may be used as a basis in planning a series of classes.

PRENATAL CARE

Supervision *throughout* pregnancy
by a competent doctor:
Different individual reactions to
pregnancy
Difference in individual's health
status
Protection of mother's health
Prevention of complications
Advantages to the developing
baby
Complete physical examination
and what it includes
Routine visits to doctor and why
Dental care:
Daily care
Preservation of the teeth
Prevention of infection
Relation of nutrition to dental
health

YOUR PRENATAL CARE

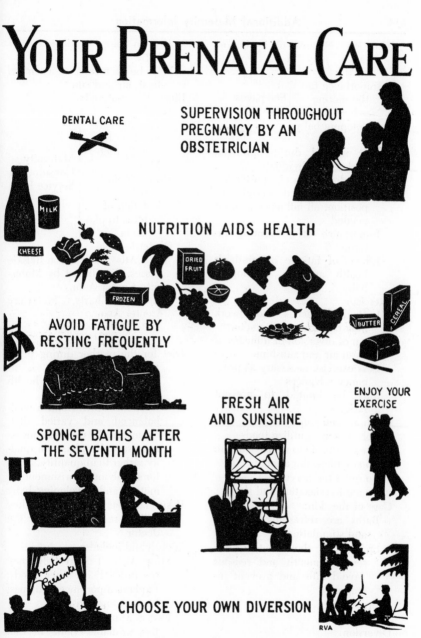

DENTAL CARE

SUPERVISION THROUGHOUT PREGNANCY BY AN OBSTETRICIAN

NUTRITION AIDS HEALTH

AVOID FATIGUE BY RESTING FREQUENTLY

SPONGE BATHS AFTER THE SEVENTH MONTH

FRESH AIR AND SUNSHINE

ENJOY YOUR EXERCISE

CHOOSE YOUR OWN DIVERSION

FIG. 352. Prenatal care outline.

Nutrition (because of its importance, may be a separate class):

Importance to the mother ⎤ See pages
Needs of the developing baby ⎦ 166-177

Rest:

Rest needed during prenatal period is individual

Dependent upon circumstances, habits, age, and nervous disposition; all influence amount needed

Importance of preventing fatigue

Effects of fatigue on mother's health and on developing baby

Exercise:

Individual needs — housework may constitute full amount

Form of diversion or a means of fresh air and sunshine

Less exercise necessary as pregnancy advances

May be limited to prevent fatigue

Fresh air and sun needed:

For oxygen to utilize foods

For vitamin D to utilize calcium

To stimulate the appetite

To quiet the nerves

To aid in relaxation and sleep

Care of the skin:

Baths are refreshing, relaxing and stimulating

Sponge or showerbaths after seventh month and reasons (avoid falls and prevent infections)

Breast care

Elimination

Diversion:

Helps to prevent worry and depression

Aids in happy anticipation of baby

May be a means of exercise, fresh air and sun

Illustrative material:

Posters ⎤
Prenatal care
Foods in the daily diet
Milk ⎬ Maternity Consultation Service Inc.
Developing baby
Relation of fetus to placenta ⎦

Obstetric table

"Birth Atlas," Dickinson-Belskie Series, distributed by Maternity Center Assn.

Anatomic Charts, Maternity Center Assn.

NUTRITION

Diet for the mother during pregnancy and lactation is of major importance for health of mother and baby

If mother has always had a well-balanced and varied diet, change in the diet will not be necessary. Emphasis on quality rather than quantity. Need for supplying nourishment for mother and developing baby

If special diets are necessary they will be recommended by the doctor

Diet should include:

MILK. About 1 quart daily—may be utilized in other foods. Explain importance to tissues, bones and teeth

FRUITS AND VEGETABLES. Varieties available—value in diet and elimination—importance of vitamins

TABLE 6. OBSTETRIC TABLE FOR DETERMINING THE DATE OF DELIVERY

Jan..	1	2	3	4	5	6	7	8	9	10	11	12	13	14	15	16	17	18	19	20	21	22	23	24	25	26	27	28	29	30	31	*Nov*
Oct..	8	9	10	11	12	13	14	15	16	17	18	19	20	21	22	23	24	25	26	27	28	29	30	31	1	2	3	4	5	6	7	
Feb..	1	2	3	4	5	6	7	8	9	10	11	12	13	14	15	16	17	18	19	20	21	22	23	24	25	26	27	28				*Dec.*
Nov..	8	9	10	11	12	13	14	15	16	17	18	19	20	21	22	23	24	25	26	27	28	29	30	1	2	3	4	5				
Mar..	1	2	3	4	5	6	7	8	9	10	11	12	13	14	15	16	17	18	19	20	21	22	23	24	25	26	27	28	29	30	31	*Jan.*
Dec..	6	7	8	9	10	11	12	13	14	15	16	17	18	19	20	21	22	23	24	25	26	27	28	29	30	31	1	2	3	4	5	
April..	1	2	3	4	5	6	7	8	9	10	11	12	13	14	15	16	17	18	19	20	21	22	23	24	25	26	27	28	29	30		*Feb.*
Jan..	6	7	8	9	10	11	12	13	14	15	16	17	18	19	20	21	22	23	24	25	26	27	28	29	30	31	1	2	3	4		
May..	1	2	3	4	5	6	7	8	9	10	11	12	13	14	15	16	17	18	19	20	21	22	23	24	25	26	27	28	29	30	31	*Mar.*
Feb..	5	6	7	8	9	10	11	12	13	14	15	16	17	18	19	20	21	22	23	24	25	26	27	28	1	2	3	4	5	6	7	
June..	1	2	3	4	5	6	7	8	9	10	11	12	13	14	15	16	17	18	19	20	21	22	23	24	25	26	27	28	29	30		*April*
Mar..	8	9	10	11	12	13	14	15	16	17	18	19	20	21	22	23	24	25	26	27	28	29	30	31	1	2	3	4	5	6		
July..	1	2	3	4	5	6	7	8	9	10	11	12	13	14	15	16	17	18	19	20	21	22	23	24	25	26	27	28	29	30	31	*May*
April.	7	8	9	10	11	12	13	14	15	16	17	18	19	20	21	22	23	24	25	26	27	28	29	30	1	2	3	4	5	6	7	
Aug..	1	2	3	4	5	6	7	8	9	10	11	12	13	14	15	16	17	18	19	20	21	22	23	24	25	26	27	28	29	30	31	*June*
May..	8	9	10	11	12	13	14	15	16	17	18	19	20	21	22	23	24	25	26	27	28	29	30	31	1	2	3	4	5	6	7	
Sept..	1	2	3	4	5	6	7	8	9	10	11	12	13	14	15	16	17	18	19	20	21	22	23	24	25	26	27	28	29	30		*July*
June..	8	9	10	11	12	13	14	15	16	17	18	19	20	21	22	23	24	25	26	27	28	29	30	1	2	3	4	5	6	7		
Oct..	1	2	3	4	5	6	7	8	9	10	11	12	13	14	15	16	17	18	19	20	21	22	23	24	25	26	27	28	29	30	31	*Aug.*
July..	8	9	10	11	12	13	14	15	16	17	18	19	20	21	22	23	24	25	26	27	28	29	30	31	1	2	3	4	5	6	7	
Nov..	1	2	3	4	5	6	7	8	9	10	11	12	13	14	15	16	17	18	19	20	21	22	23	24	25	26	27	28	29	30		*Sept*
Aug..	8	9	10	11	12	13	14	15	16	17	18	19	20	21	22	23	24	25	26	27	28	29	30	31	1	2	3	4	5	6		
Dec..	1	2	3	4	5	6	7	8	9	10	11	12	13	14	15	16	17	18	19	20	21	22	23	24	25	26	27	28	29	30	31	*Oct.*
Sept..	7	8	9	10	11	12	13	14	15	16	17	18	19	20	21	22	23	24	25	26	27	28	29	30	1	2	3	4	5	6	7	

Supposing the upper figure in each pair of horizontal lines to represent the first day of the last menstrual period, the figure beneath it, with the month designated in the margin, will show the probable day of confinement.

MEAT, FISH, EGGS, PROTEIN VEGETABLES. Building materials—value in mineral and vitamin content

CEREALS AND BREAD. Dark varieties more vitamin value

BUTTER FATS, CREAM, SALAD OILS. May need to be limited but rich in vitamin A

FLUIDS. Freely, unless restricted by doctor—function of fluids in relation to food absorption and elimination of waste

VITAMINS AND MINERALS. Why important?

Why food is so important for the pregnant mother:

1. To maintain daily strength and build resistance

2. To prepare for delivery (tone and condition of muscles—especially the uterus)

3. To hasten convalescence

4. To prepare to nurse the baby

5. To provide nourishment for the developing baby

Diet in relation to weight gain

Illustrative material:

Posters

Developing baby } Maternity
Foods in the daily diet } Consultation Service Inc.
Milk

National Nutrition Council and

Dairy, cereal and meat companies often offer usable material for visual aids

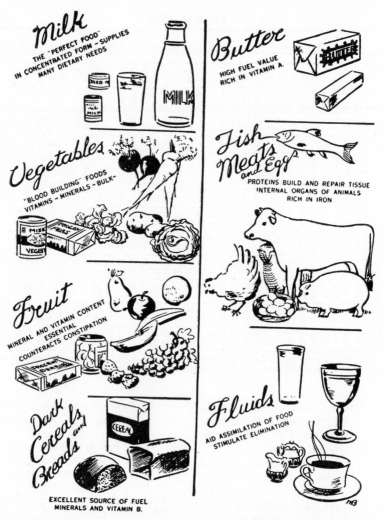

FIG. 353. Foods necessary in the daily diet during pregnancy: 1 pint to 1 quart of milk a day; taken as milk, used in gruel, cocoa, desserts, or added to soups. Vegetables—especially the green variety. Fruits—fresh, dried or canned. Dark cereals and dark breads—white bread may be used for variety. Butter. Fluids—water and other liquids. The pregnant mother should have an adequate diet: (1) to maintain her daily strength; (2) to prepare for labor (by building up the muscle tone of the body during the prenatal period to meet the crisis of labor and delivery); (3) to hasten convalescence after delivery; (4) to prepare to nurse her baby; and (5) to provide materials necessary for growth and development of the baby. The normal baby at birth has developed all the delicate and intricate foundations of the body—more than 200 bones, 50 teeth, as well as a brain which is about one quarter to one half the size it will be when he is an adult.

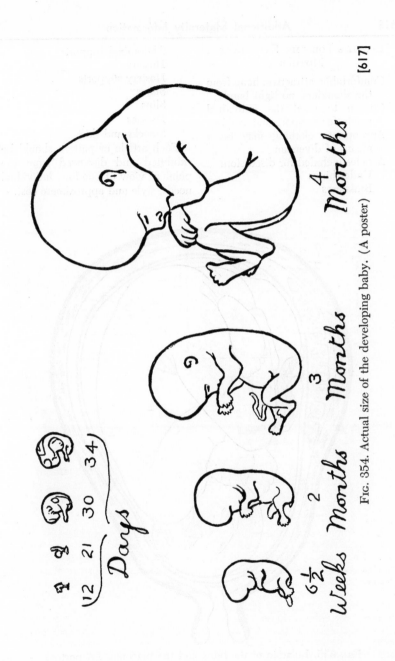

FIG. 354. Actual size of the developing baby. (A poster)

CLOTHES FOR THE EXPECTANT
MOTHER

Comfortable, attractive, hang from
the shoulders, no tight bands

Chosen to meet the individual
needs for support and comfort

Appropriate clothing may be a
means of diversion

Articles included for discussion:
Underthings
Brassières
Abdominal support
Hosiery
Hosiery supports
Shoes
Slips
Dresses
Smocks and skirt

Each article or pattern should be
exhibited and discussed from the
point of view of comfort, individual
needs, style and approximate cost.

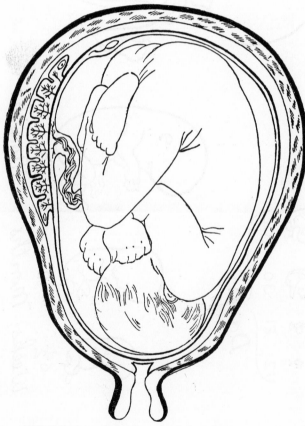

FIG. 355. Relation of the fetus and the placenta. (A poster)

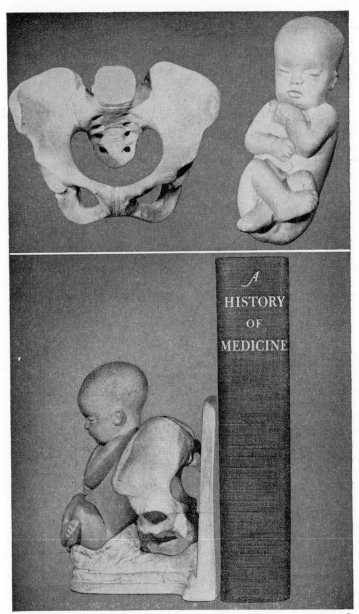

Fig. 356. Models designed by Dickinson-Belskie to be used in classes. Book ends when not being used for teaching purposes. (Cleveland Health Museum)

UNDERTHINGS. Should be light in weight, easy to launder, and nonrestricting. (Patient will probably need to make no change from what she is wearing)

BRASSIÈRES. Should fit the individual and support the breasts in the normal position. Choose the type which may be used before and after delivery

ABDOMINAL SUPPORT. Abdominal binder may be made of unbleached muslin or a support may be purchased—may be a girdle or a corset, depending on the amount of support needed

HOSIERY. Stockings and socks. Stockings should be supported by a shoulder garter or abdominal support (Figs. 111 and 115). Large enough to cause no restrictions. Socks more comfortable when the weather permits.

HOSIERY SUPPORTS. May be made or purchased

SHOES: Should be comfortable and have solid heels to prevent tripping

SLIPS. As pregnancy advances, the wrap-around slip will be more comfortable (Fig. 109)

DRESSES. One or two attractive maternity dresses may be a good investment. Advantages for comfort and diversion

SMOCKS, SKIRT AND SLACKS may have more appeal to some.

[This is an excellent time to include the information on the care of the nipples, showing the tray setup for that purpose. (Fig. 102.)]

Properly fitted brassières, supports and shoes all help to prevent fatigue when postural changes occur.

Illustrative material:

Posters
    May be made of attractive up-to-date pattern covers or advertisements of dresses, smocks, skirts
    Postural changes during pregnancy
    Exhibit material including brassières, supports, etc.
    Breast tray

THE BABY'S LAYETTE

Each article should be exhibited and discussed from the points of view of number needed (one on baby, one on line, one in reserve) (3-4 dozen diapers), style and materials.

Light in weight—complete outfit weighing not more than 16 ounces
Easy to put on and take off to prevent undue handling
Easy to wash, to dry and iron
Exclude all forms of the harness type
Articles included for discussion:
    Band
    Shirt
    Diaper
    Diaper pins
    Pads
    Waterproof protectors
    Dress
    Pettiskirt
    Receiving blanket
    Blanket
    Bunting
    Waterproof pants
(The list may include sweaters, sacques, nightgowns, etc.)

Because the baby's growth and development is so rapid, he does not need a vast amount of clothing, but he should have enough to make possible his being kept comfortable, warm, fresh, dry, and clean.

This is an excellent time to demonstrate correct handling and dressing of the baby.

Illustrative material:
Complete layette
Doll

NURSERY EQUIPMENT

Presented from the point of view of the baby's needs.

Each article should be exhibited and discussed from the viewpoint of comfort, safety, simplicity, postural development, convenience of the mother (easy to handle and keep clean), accommodation to the individual circumstances and purse.

Equipment may be purchased or many of the articles may be made or improvised.

Articles included for discussion:
Bed or basket
Mattress
Waterproof cover
Sheets or pillowcases
Bath set-up (tub, table, chair)
Diaper pail
Toilet tray
Clothes drier
Carriage
Netting
Bed: Basket, bassinet, kiddie-koop, crib
May be improvised by using box, carton, bureau drawer, etc.
If basket or box, etc., used on chair, emphasize precaution of tying chair legs
Mattress: Firm and flat (with no pillows) and why
Explain importance to baby's postural development
Folded bed pad or cotton

blanket may be substituted temporarily for basket or carriage mattress
Check kinds available in the community—Hair, hairflex, cotton, sponge rubber
Waterproof cover: Entire surface of mattress should be covered
Protects the mattress and prevents unnecessary odors
Sheets and pillowcases: Sheets for crib (may be made from adult sheets)
Pillowcases more convenient and economical for basket, bassinet, or carriage
Bath set-up: Enamel tub, easy to keep clean
Table may be coffee table, low hamper, sturdy bathroom stool, chest or wooden box
Child's table and chair combination, table may be used for tub, set used later for play and feeding table
Chair should be low enough to be comfortable and give the correct slant to the lap
Diaper pail: Makes washing easier because diapers may be put to soak as soon as removed
Prevents unnecessary odors
Clothes drier: or some planned place to dry baby's clothes
Toilet tray: Each article and its use should be explained as well as how to assemble it and its daily care (Figs. 124 A and B)
Discuss the many improvisations
Carriage: May be substituted for the basket or bassinet
Should be discussed from the point of view of need and the community resources

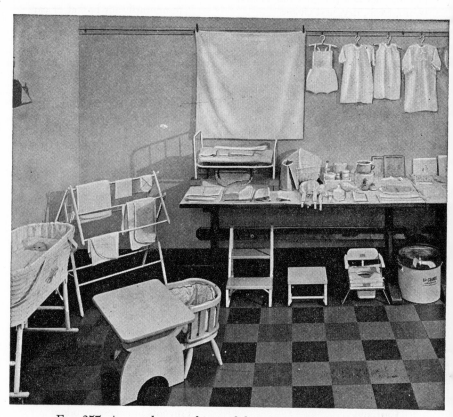

Fig. 357. A complete teaching exhibit. (It will be noted that several items are duplicated, due to photographic angles.) Arranged on the line are the necessary articles for the layette: Straight band (used only as a bandage to hold the umbilical dressing in place), diaper band (sleeveless shirt or V-band), shirt, diaper, hand-knitted soakers (used instead of waterproof pants), flannelette dress or nightgown, batiste gertrude, batiste dress (dress and gertrude made over the same pattern as the flannelette but using fine material), sun suit and flannelette square or receiving blanket.

On the table there is a variety of demonstration material. Baby's toilet trays (one improvised type), bunting, light-weight wool blankets, variety of approved diapers, disposable diapers, paper

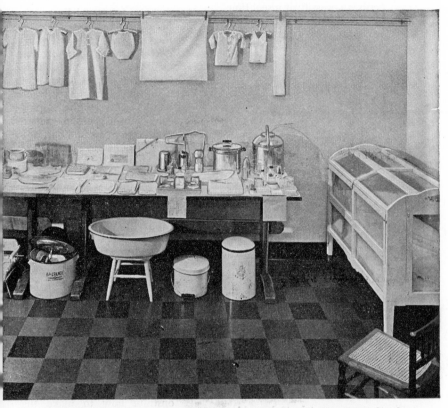

diaper linings, paper crib pads, huck toweling pads, shirt drier, bottle
warmers, sterilizers (electric and non-electric), bottle rack (used in
any large cooking kettle), training commode, baby shoes, bath towel,
washcloths, breast tray, brassières, abdominal supports, maternity
corset, shoulder garters, basket with miniature demonstration bed (to
show how to prepare for delivery), large cornucopia, paper pan, paper
pads (newspaper).

Other equipment and furniture includes: low chair to be used for
bath set-up (Fig. 317), kiddie-koop, 2 types of diaper pails, tub on
stool, electric washer, Toidey traveler, footstool, toddler steps, clothes
drier, basket on stand, and toddler's chair and table (instead of high
chair). (Maternity Consultation Service.)

Netting: for basket, carriage or crib, a necessity at insect time to protect the baby

(Much or little may be expended for these articles.)

Illustrative material:

All articles discussed if possible

Improvised material and equipment

Pictures

Posters

Toilet tray—if not possible to have toilet trays set up

Graphic illustration showing correct and incorrect posture of baby

THE BABY'S BATH

This should be demonstrated—using complete setup.

Emphasize the details, such as: preliminary preparations, advantages of type of baby bath to mother, advantages to baby, time for giving bath

Explain each step in the procedure

This is another opportunity to demonstrate the handling and the dressing of the baby. (For procedure, see page 566.)

Illustrative material: Tub, table, chair, toilet tray, diaper pail, complete set of clothes, extra receiving blanket, bath towel, face towel, washcloth, newspapers, bath apron, doll and bed

Pamphlet: "How to Bathe and Dress Baby," Maternity Consultation Service

NOTE: Because of the abdominal enlargement during pregnancy, it is often uncomfortable to practice this procedure before delivery.

DELIVERY PREPARATIONS

Hospital versus home delivery

For both groups a discussion of the symptoms of labor (which doctor probably already has explained) and preliminary "warnings"

When to call the doctor or when and how to go to the hospital

For the hospital group—certain preliminary preparations, hospital admission procedures and routines

For patients to be delivered at home—preparations to be prepared and articles which the patient can make

Each article should be exhibited and discussed from point of view of how improvised, prepared and used. (See illustrative material listed below.)

Other points for discussion would include: Selection of room, importance of good light, toilet facilities, necessity for additional help in the home at delivery and immediately following

This is an excellent time to demonstrate how to make the patient's bed for delivery

If talk is given to a group, some registered with hospital and others for home delivery, the interest of the hospital group may be stimulated by the fact that they are being prepared, perhaps, to help someone else in an emergency

Illustrative material (may be adjusted to fit the routine of the organization or the locality):

Doll-size bed with equipment

Newspapers for making paper

bags, Kelly pad, newspaper bed pads

Muslin covers for newspaper pads

Basins

Kettles and ladle

Perineal pads

Cotton in sterile package

Stockings for patient

Tray—pitcher or Mason jar, spoon, glass, saucer

Bedpan

Mother's tray—comb, soap dish, glass, toothbrush, toothpaste

Baby's outfit—basket or bed, set of clothes, receiving blanket with lining, provision for heating bed

Visual aid: "Birth Atlas," Dickinson-Belskie Series, distributed by Maternity Center Association, New York

NOTE: For some groups the nurse may wish to give the steps of the actual delivery, explaining the progress of labor.

POSTDELIVERY CARE

This class may be developed under two topics: (1) care of the mother and (2) care of the baby.

For the mother, emphasis should be placed on: the stay-in-bed period, adequate rest and sleep, nutrition, protection from worry and adequate household help

Reasons for special care of the breasts and perineum

Watchful care at the time of sitting out of bed should be explained

Special emphasis should be placed on the convalescing period as an aid to future well-being, ability to nurse the baby, and reassuming family responsibilities

The important role of the husband: sharing of responsibilities and interest (a most important detail in family development), assuming the responsibility of heavy work, protecting the mother from worry

Postpartum examination: What this includes and why necessary

For the baby, a plan for his daily care:

Feedings at regular hours during the day—wake if necessary

Cod-liver oil and orange juice given when awake

During night, feed baby when parents retire and when baby wakes (instead of 2 A.M. feeding)

Introduce all new foods in small quantities

Emphasis on not overfeeding baby

Sleep and rest—time set apart for sleep or rest

Change position often—side to side and on back

Make comfortable for sleep by bath or washing face and hands

Bathing is refreshing and relaxing and should be a daily routine at a specified time.

Special attention to nose, fingernails and toenails

Sun baths and fresh air—sun bath in summer before 10 A.M. and after 3 P.M.

Care to prevent sun and glare in baby's eyes

Sun baths and fresh air may be a part of his indoor routine

Exercise—all of the baby's natural movements of arms and legs are exercises preparing his muscles for sitting up, creeping and walking. Therefore, he should not be inhibited by clothing or harnesses.

Bathing, dressing and crying are forms of exercise for the baby

Play time—a time set aside which the baby may anticipate as "his own"

At first—this may be just "holding," later a time when toys are added

If at a time when the father is home—helps to develop family unity

Crying—discuss the different

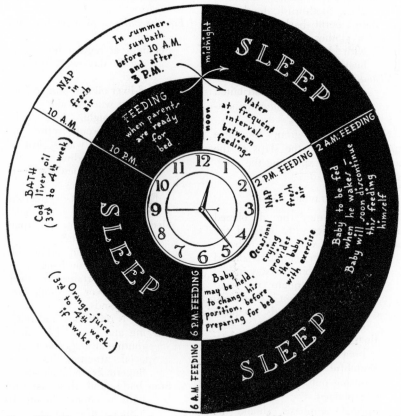

Fig. 358. Plan the baby's day (clockwise) to conform with your day. (A poster)

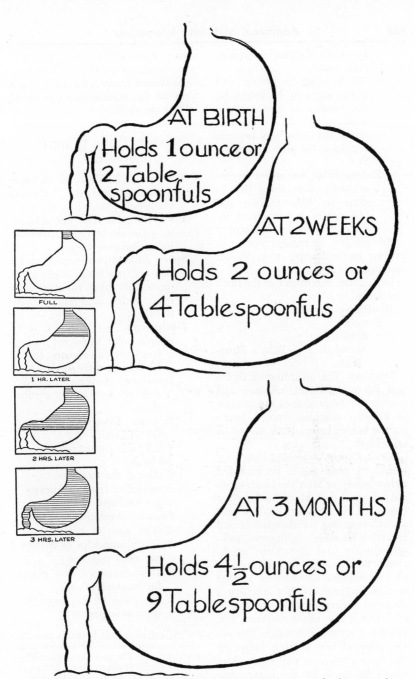

FIG. 359. A diagram of the actual size of the baby's stomach. (A poster)

types of crying and what they may mean

Toilet training is timing and habit—and may be begun by the mother as soon as she feels physically able and when the baby has become regular in his time of elimination

Habits—habit formation begins at birth. Everything that is done for him, to him and about him has a direct influence on his development

Advantages of regular and continuous medical supervision should be emphasized.

Discuss the importance of the birth certificate.

Illustrative material:

Posters

Baby's Day

Actual Size of Baby's Stomach

Diploma. The awarding of diplomas has a significant influence and may be the beginning of the interest in keeping complete record books for the babies before birth as well as after birth.

Craft Classes. A sewing class or a combined class might be included either before or after the class, or on some special day. Many mothers are interested in making binders and shoulder garters for themselves and receiving blankets, nightgowns, jackets, dresses and pettiskirts, washcloths, bath aprons, etc. Knitting may also be included for sweaters, knitted panties and afghans. Not only is it a financial saving to make these articles, but it also offers diversion and creates a greater interest in the anticipation of the coming baby. At this time a prenatal visit or checkup might be made by the nurse, thus saving time and energy. In some communities a combined class may be instituted where fathers may make some of the equipment. The possibilities are endless!

OBSTETRICS DURING EMERGENCY *

Temporary quarters for delivery should provide the following features:

Location: Near, but not actually in, a casualty station, convenient for ambulance service.

Space: At least two rooms—one for delivery, one for recovery (adequate light, heat, running water even under emergency conditions).

Equipment:

Simple solid table not over 3 feet wide (no stirrups, legs to be held by assistants)

Instrument sterilizer (to be approved by local medical chief)

2 cans (Sterno) emergency heating unit

Small table (instruments)

3 chairs

2 clinical thermometers

2 sponge or transfer forceps

2 jars for same

Germicidal solution for same

4 ¼-lb. cans of ether

6 10-cc. ampoules or bottles 1 per cent procaine

2 10-cc. syringes and needles for local anesthesia

Kelly pads to be improvised from newspapers

* Adaptations may be made from this emergency procedure for a home delivery service. (The American Committee on Maternal Welfare, Inc., Joseph H. Howard, M.D., Bridgeport, Conn.)

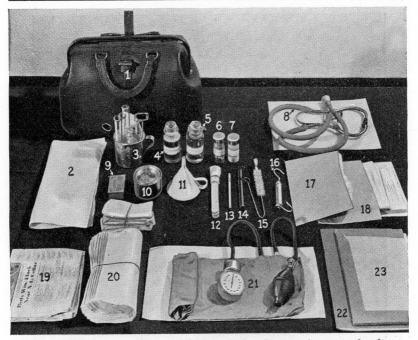

Fig. 360. A prenatal bag and contents for the nurse's use in the district or clinic nursing: (1) 14-inch leather bag; (2) apron in case; (3) tin cup * (urinalysis outfit containing: 2 test tubes, test tube holder, forceps, urinometer and glass, filter paper, litmus paper, acetic acid in dropper bottle); (4) bottle of green soap; (5) bottle of alcohol; (6) aristol powder; (7) toothpicks; (8) stethoscope; (9) matches; (10) Sterno; (11) funnel; (12) spatulae (one end protected with paper napkin); (13) mouth thermometer; (14) rectal thermometer; (15) test tube brush; (16) scale; (17) cotton in case; (18) literature in case; (19) newspaper cornucopias; (20) paper napkins (utility towels, etc.); (21) blood pressure outfit; (22) instruction book; (23) record case.

One bundle of tongue depressors

2 enema kits
2 bedpans
4 waste pails (at least 8-qt. capacity)
2 rolls of toilet paper
6 wash basins
12 cakes of white soap
1 simple strong box to store patient's valuables and birth records
12 sheets, single-bed size
12 woolen blankets, single-bed size
6 cotton blankets, single
24 hand towels
24 diapers

NOTE: An adequate supply of Kits Nos. 1, 2, 3 and infant layettes.

* Paper cups may be substituted.

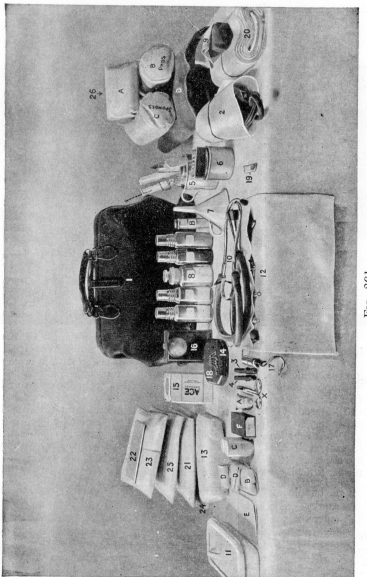

Fig. 361

Fig. 361. Combination delivery and prenatal bag used in the Tioga County, N. Y., Demonstration in Rural Maternity Work. (Directed by the Maternity Center Association, New York, and the N. Y. State Department of Health.)

1. Bag containing:
2. Blood pressure outfit
3. Mouth thermometer
4. Rectal thermometer
5. Urinalysis outfit
   cup
   urinometer and glass
   test tube holder
   test tube brush
   2 test tubes
   matches
   filter paper
   litmus paper
   acetic acid dropper bottle
6. Sterno
7. Funnel
8. Bottles containing:
   green soap ⎫
   lysol   ⎪
   alcohol   ⎬ in bottles
   boric solution ⎪
   salt tablets ⎭
9. Hand scrub in rubber cap
10. Stethoscope
11. Sterilizing basin
    (a) tube petrolatum
    (b) aristol powder
    (c) silver nitrate
    (d) extra cord dressing ties
    (e) cord dressing ties and binder (sterile)
    (f) hypodermic and needles
12. Instrument case containing:
    rectal tube

catheter
extra scissors
2 douche nozzles
1 connecting tip
extra forceps
1 medicine dropper
13. Sterile set
    2 clamps
    1 scissors
    1 forceps
    1 medicine dropper
    1 sterile cord dressing ties and binder
14. Safety razor
15. Bandage
16. Boy Scout spot light
17. Baby scale
18. Doz. medium and small safety pins
19. Tape measure
20. Paper napkins
21. Absorbent cotton in envelope
22. Toothpicks
23. Apron
24. Patterns for baby clothes
25. Abdominal binder in envelope
26. ⎧ (a) 2 sterile towels (done up singly)
    ⎪ (b) sterile case (6 pads)
    ⎨ (c) sterile case (12 cotton pledgets)
    ⎪ (d) (package of sterile supplies may be done up extra and carried in back of car)
    ⎩

KIT NO. 1

Sterile obstetric package:
   Package 1—2 masks, 1 brush.
Mother's supplies:
   Package 2—2 envelopes, each containing 2 dozen small balls of cotton.
   Package 3—2 towels.
   Package 4—2 towels.
   Package 5—3 vulvar pads.
Baby's supplies:
   Package 6—2 cord ties and dressings, 2 gauze bands, ½ dozen small balls cotton in envelope container (envelope can be made of muslin or paper), identification tag.

KIT NO. 2

Nonsterile equipment and supplies for physician's use at delivery:
Safety razors and blades
2 clamps (1 Kelly, 1 Kocher)
1 pair tissue forceps
1 pair scissors
1 bar soap
1 chromic catgut No. 0
2 No. 3 cutting needles
1 hypo syringe and needles
Ergot preparation
1 bag or container for supplies
Pituitrin
¼-lb. can of ether
1 can of Sterno
Silver nitrate
2—¼-lb. cotton rolls
2 pairs of No. 8 rubber gloves or finger cots for rectal examinations
Lubricant
Catheter
1 qt. size round basin
1 4-oz. bottle—thermometers in alcohol
Bedside birth record, List of Connecticut Obstetric Consultants,

Nurse's Routine for Delivery and Care of the Newborn.

KIT NO. 3

Additional supplies for operative deliveries (furnished by hospital staff obstetricians assigned to consultation service):
1 Simpson forceps or equivalent
1 needle holder
1 mouse tooth thumb forceps 5″
2 needles, No. 3, half round cutting
No gloves (10-min. scrub)
1 mask
6 towels (3 packages, 2 each)
1 catheter
1 hypo syringe, 2 needles
Ergot preparation
2 cans ether—¼-lb. cans
2 sponge forceps
2 Kelly clamps
1 scissors 5″ straight
2 needles, No. 2, half round
1 gown
1 cap
3 tubes of catgut—chromic No. 0
1 uterine pack, 5 yds. long, 4 in. wide, 4 thicknesses
1 ether mask
Pituitrin

NURSE'S ROUTINE FOR DELIVERY AND CARE OF THE NEWBORN UNDER EMERGENCY CONDITIONS

Procedure:
1. Cover table with newspaper for use of nurse and doctor.
2. Place coat on chair covered with newspaper.
3. Get history of labor from patient.
   a. When pains began, and how often they occur

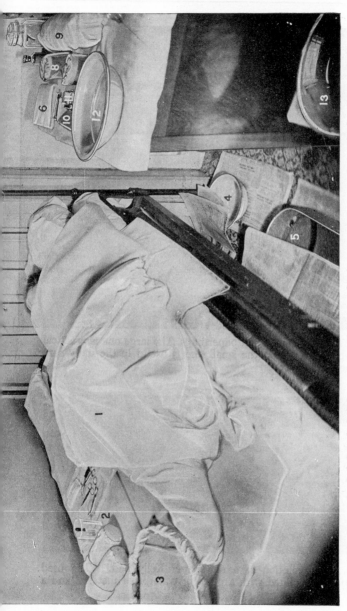

Fig. 362. Setup for left-handed delivery of patient in the home. (Reverse for right-handed delivery.)

1. Patient draped ready for delivery (fold of sheet may be lifted).
2. Tray with sterile pad, sponges, instruments for clamping and cutting the cord—cord ties, dressing and binder, medicine dropper, medicine glass, silver nitrate.
3. Paper pan or cornucopia.
4. Placenta basin.
5. Bedpan (placed between newspapers).
6. Ether cone—petrolatum, paper napkins.
7. Tray, Mason jar, disinfectant, spoon (to be used during post-partum care).
8. Two packages sterile perineal pads wrapped.
9. Sterile cotton wrapped in towel.
10. Enamel basin with sterile hypodermic set (ready).
11. Flashlight.
12. Basin of antiseptic solution, for sponging patient's genitals.
13. On chair, basin of antiseptic solution for doctor's hands.

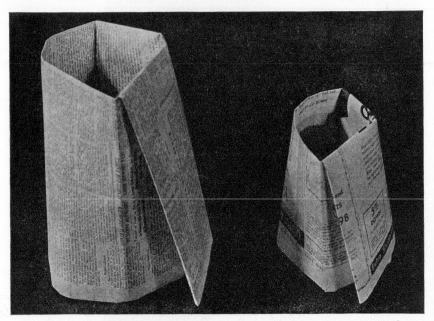

FIG. 363. The large and small paper bags. The large one is practical at the time of delivery and the small one is useful in the daily care of the mother and baby.

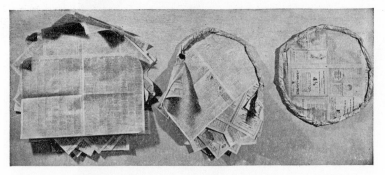

FIG. 364. The evolution of a newspaper Kelly pad. When used under a patient, it is lined with a piece of waterproof material and a towel.

b. Have membranes ruptured?

c. Time of last bowel movement

d. Time of last urinating

e. General condition of patient—cold, sore throat, etc.

f. Any evidence of bleeding

g. When foods or fluids were last taken

4. Setup for delivery

a. Put two large kettles of water to boil.

b. Cover sink board with newspapers and wash hands.

c. Take out bag of articles needed for delivery.

d. Boil hypo syringe and needles 5 minutes in a small covered pan and set aside in a sterile sponge.

e. Prepare rectal setup.

(1) Equipment

(a) One rubber glove or finger cot

(b) Lubricant

(c) Paper towels or newspapers

(2) Procedure

(a) Place glove or finger cot in paper towel or folded newspaper convenient for physician's use.

(b) After use, wash thoroughly with

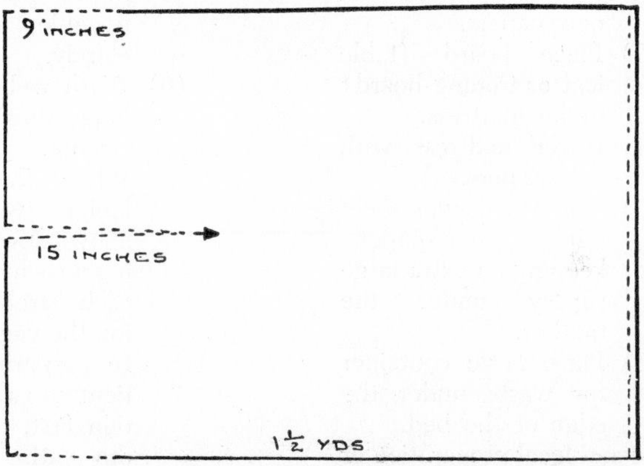

Fig. 365. Diagram showing how to make a clinic gown for patients. Three yards of outing flannel, 1 yard wide; fold in half crosswise, stitch sides, leaving 9 inches on each side at the top for armholes; put a one-inch hem at the bottom of the gown. Cut 15 inches in the center top, back and front for the neck, bind and reinforce with a triangular piece. A dressing-room may be improvised by arranging a three-panel screen for privacy. A coat hanger and chair may be included in the "enclosure" for convenience. This makes very inexpensive clinic equipment.

soap and water and dry glove or finger cot for use again.

f. Ask family to assemble the following:

(1) Tub or basin for waste receptacle
(2) Three basins or pans
(3) Board or ironing board
(4) Safety pins
(5) Baby's clothes
(6) Clean bed linen
(7) Cup, spoon and saucer
(8) Dinner plate or pie-tin cover

g. Arrangement of room

(1) Remove unnecessary furniture.
(2) Protect furniture with newspapers.
(3) Place board (table leaf or ironing board) under mattress.
(4) Cover mattress with newspapers.
(5) Cover bed over sheet with newspapers, keeping an extra large supply under the mother.
(6) Place large container for waste under the edge of the bed.

5. Shave and local preparation of patient

a. Equipment

(1) For shaving of patient
(a) Basin of warm, soapy water containing 4 cotton pledgets, and a razor
(2) For cleansing of patient

(a) One basin of warm soapy water containing 8 cotton pledgets
(b) One basin of warm water containing 8 cotton pledgets

b. Procedure

(1) Spread newspapers on the bed, with edges extending over the side.
(2) Place the patient crosswise on the bed, with feet on chairs.
(3) Place 3 basins for shaving and cleansing patient on chairs.
(4) Soap pubic area well.
(5) Shave pubic hair if possible; if not, clip closely.
(6) Wash well—abdomen, inner thighs and perineum.

When washing over labia, wash from above downward, using a clean pledget for each stroke, protecting the vaginal orifice. In preparing the patient, use a soapy solution first, then repeat the entire procedure with warm water.

(7) Turn the patient lengthwise in bed after completing the shaving and preparation.

6. Sterilization of equipment

a. Boil instruments 10 minutes in a covered kettle or saucepan.

2 clamps (1 Kelly, 1 Kocher)

1 pair of scissors

1 catheter

Rubber gloves

Drain and set aside for use at time of delivery.

b. Sterilization of basins to be used in local cleansing of patient.

(1) Place 3 or 4 cups of soapy water in the basin. Cover and boil 10 minutes. After it has boiled, set aside and keep sterile for use at time of delivery.

(2) Place 3 or 4 cups of clear water in a basin. Cover and boil 10 minutes. After it has boiled, set aside and keep sterile for use at time of delivery.

Alternate: If more convenient, the second basin may be inverted over the one containing the soapy water. After boiling, sterile water from reserve supply can be put in the second basin.

c. Boil cup, spoon and saucer and set aside for giving baby water by mouth. After boiling, place the spoon in the cup of sterile water and cover with a saucer. Keep sterile until needed.

7. Preparation for the baby

a. Prepare the baby's crib.

b. Assemble supplies for care of baby.

(1) Firm pillow or pad

(2) Soft gauze and cotton

(3) Sterile cottonseed oil and 2 per cent ammoniated mercury ointment. If oil and ointment are lacking, a single bath with castile soap and warm water may be given. It is safe to wipe a baby gently with sterile gauze and leave it without further cleansing. (See No. 12— Care of Baby, Item c.)

(4) Layette.

8. Final preparation for delivery to be carried out while doctor scrubs. If gloves are not supplied and are not available, physicans should scrub for 10 minutes.

a. Place sterile delivery package on bureau. Open outer cover and remove mask and scrub brush for physician's use.

b. Nurse puts on mask.

c. Nurse removes covers from 2 sterile solution basins and places basins on chair or table close to patient's bed, in a position convenient for physician's use. Place cotton pledgets from sterile obstetric package on chair, convenient for physician's use.

d. Place instrument basin at foot of bed. Basin should be inverted so instruments are lying on plate or pie-tin cover.

e. Place receiving blanket for baby at foot of bed.

f. Place Package V (vulva

pads) from sterile obstetric package on chair near basins.

g. Place Package VI (baby's supplies) at foot of bed if physician prefers to tie cord before delivery of placenta.

9. Assist physician during preparation of draping patient and while delivering baby.

a. Remove basin from instrument plate. Keep basin sterile to receive placenta.

b. After cord is clamped and cut, wrap baby in receiving blanket. See that he is breathing well and place him in a warm safe place.

10. Assist physician with third stage of labor.

11. Immediate postpartum care of mother

a. Watch fundus and pulse frequently.

b. Remove soiled newspapers from under mother and make her comfortable.

12. Care of baby

a. Assist physician with tying of cord and applying dressing and binder.

b. Assist with instilling silver nitrate in baby's eyes.

c. Wash off blood and cleanse gently in creases and folds with cottonseed oil and apply ammoniated mercury ointment.

d. Take rectal temperature.

e. Dress baby and wrap in blanket.

f. Give baby several teaspoons of sterile water.

g. Place baby in crib on right side with head lowered.

13. After-care of mother

a. Take temperature, pulse and respiration.

b. Give partial sponge bath.

c. Check fundus and watch for bleeding.

d. Give nourishment as ordered.

14. Clean up all equipment. Boil instruments and razor. Pack bag.

15. Instruct helper to watch:

a. Baby—for bleeding from cord.

b. Mother—for (1) excessive vaginal bleeding and for (2) inability to urinate.

FRONTIER NURSING SERVICE, INCORPORATED

Delivery Bag Equipment

Right Saddlebag

Bottles in pocket with medications as authorized
Four perineal pads in bag
One Higginson syringe in bag
Baby's bag
    Rectal thermometer
    6 ampoules silver nitrate
    2 pairs artery clamps
    1 pair scissors
    1 bottle cord ties
    Tape measure
    Scales
    4 sterile gauze dressings
    4 oz. olive oil
    Safety pins
    Catheter
Mother's bag
    Mouth thermometer
    1 2-inch bandage
    1 hypo syringe
    2 one-half-inch needles

1 pair rubber gloves
Medications as authorized
One delivery gown and cap
One bag of cotton and right-hand
glove
Paper napkins
Scrub-up rubber bag
Soap
Nail brush
Orangestick
2 oz. Lysol
1 rubber apron
2 towels
5 pus basins

Left Saddlebag

Supplies in pocket
Medical routines
Envelopes
Paper
Emergency Medical Aid Blanks
Copy of Delivery Bag Equipment
Pencil
One-pint measure—containing
1 urinalysis outfit
1 funnel
1 bag—containing
1 large catheter
Rubber tubing
Glass connecting tube
2 small catheters
1 douche nozzle
Sterile gauze packing
A Sterno outfit and safety matches
Emergency bag
1 sterile perineal suture
1 hypo syringe
2 2-inch needles
2 1-inch needles
Medications as authorized
2 tongue depressors
1 cotton apron
Rubber sheet
Newspapers

GENERAL NURSING BAG EQUIPMENT
FOR THE USE OF THE FRONTIER
NURSING SERVICE, INC.

Apron
Towel
Rubber cap—containing
Scrub brush
Soap in container
Orangestick
Lysol
Paper napkins
Bag of cotton
Set of instruments
Mouth thermometer
Rectal thermometer
Postpartum bag—containing
Scales
Tape measure
Boric acid powder
Benzoin
USP Alcohol
Gauze dressing
Urinalysis bag—containing
Tin cup
Sterno and matches
Dilute acetic acid
Test tube and holder
Dressing bag—containing
Gauze dressings
Bandages
Applicators
Tongue blades
Adhesive
Pus basin
Sphygmomanometer
Rectal bag—containing
Higginson syringe
Funnel and small rectal tube
Ointment bag—containing
Selection from authorized oint-
ments
Pill bag—containing
Selections from authorized pills
Bottles of medicines from authorized
list

Emergency bag—containing
  Cord ties
  Silver nitrate
  Rubber gloves
  Hypodermic syringe
  Hypo needles both ½″ and 2″

Catheters
Medicine as authorized
Antivenin serum (in summer)
Medical routine
Paper and pencil
Envelopes
Emergency Medical Aid Blanks

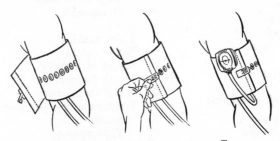

FIG. 366. New B-D security cuff.

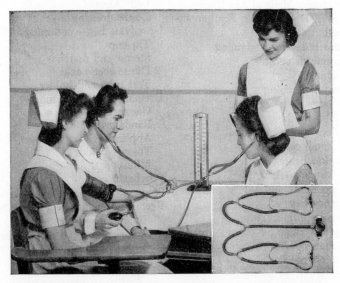

FIG. 367. Students using teacher's stethoscope. (Becton-Dickinson Company)

CARE OF HYPODERMIC NEEDLES

The care of hypodermic needles is, at best, a tedious and disagreeable task; and oftentimes after a hypodermic or other injection, the needle is laid aside to be cleaned and dried later. Usually when the deferred cleaning of the needle is undertaken, it is found to be clogged. Oxidation is the foe of all steel needles, but rust occurs only when needles are put away without being dried properly.

After using steel needles, they should be soaked in plain water, until they can be washed, boiled and then rinsed in alcohol. They may be dried either with compressed air or by the use of the Brunet needle drier. A wire dipped in oil or petrolatum should then be inserted. Steel needles treated in this way will last much longer and will not rust. Frequent honing of steel, erusto, platinum-iridium, gold and nickeloid needles on a fine oilstone will keep the points smooth and in good condition.

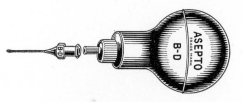

Fig. 368. Brunet needle drier.

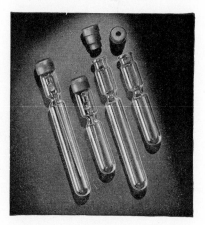

Fig. 369. Steri-tube for autoclaving needles. The needle is so held in the tube that the point is never dulled by contact with the tube. The syringe may be attached to the needle before it is removed from the tube, thus eliminating any chance of contamination. (American Hospital Supply Corporation)

Answer Key for Situation Questions

UNIT ONE

1: F
2: A
3: B
4: A. External conjugate
   B. Diagonal conjugate
   C. Intercristal
   D. Conjugate vera
   E. Intertuberous diameter
5: A: A; C; E
   B: B; D
   C: D
   D: D; E
   E: C
6: C
7: A: 4
   B: 3
   C: 1
   D: 2
8: C
9: A
10: A: 2
    B: 2
    C: 3
11: B
12: C
13: C
14: D
15: B; C; H
16: 1: A
     2: M
     3: O
     4: P
     5: C
     6: K
     7: I

16: 8: N
     9: B
    10: D
    11: G
    12: R
    13: E
    14: F
    15: S
    16: U
    17: L
    18: C
    19: P
    20: O
17: A
18: A: LOT
    B: LOA
    C: ROP
    D: LSP
    E: RMA
    F: RADP

UNIT TWO

1: Column I: A, C, D, F, I, M
   Column II: N, O
   Column III: E, J, L, M, P
   Column IV: H, J, K, Q
2: A: 2
   B: 3
3: B
4: B
5: F
6: C
7: C
8: A: 2
   B: 3
9: A: 1

9: B: 3
    C: 3
10: A: 3 and 4
    B: 1
11: B
12: D
13: A
14: B
15: A; B; D; H; L; N; O; P; Q; T
16: A: 1
    B: 1 and 2
17: A
18: A: 4
    B: 4
    C: 3
    D: 3
    E: 3
19: A

UNIT THREE

1: A: dilatation
    B: effacement
    C: amnesic
    D: atony
    E: episiotomy
    F: lightening
2: A: 1; 4; 5
    B: 1; 4; 6
    C: 1; 4; 6; 7
3: A: 2
    B: 3
    C: 2
4: A; C; G; H; J
5: A; D; E
6: B; C; E; G
7: A; C; E; F
8: F; J; G; C; H; B; L; O; Q; R; N
9: A; C; F
10: A: 3
    B: 2
11: A: 3; 7
    B: 1 or 3
    C: 1
    D: 4; 6

12: B
13: C

UNIT FOUR

1: A; D; I
2: A; B; C
3: 1: G
    2: D
    3: B
    4: C
    5: G
    6: G
    7: D
    8: G
4: A; D; E; G; H
5: A; B; D
6: A; B; F; G
7: B; D; E; F; J; L; M; N; O; P
8: B; C
9: A: mastitis
    B: endometritis
    C: pelvic cellulitis or parametritis
    D: suppression
    E: subinvolution

UNIT FIVE

1: C
2: D
3: A: 3
    B: 1
4: A: 2
    B: 1 and 2
5: 1: D
    2: F
    3: E
    4: B
    5: E
    6: F
    7: A
6: C
7: C
8: B

 9: 1: C   11: E
    2: G   12: D; E; G
    3: I   13: C
    4: B   14: A and B
10: D; H; J   15: D

Glossary

Note.—The definitions and pronunciations as indicated in the following paragraph in this Glossary follow Webster's International Dictionary.

āle, châotic, câre, ădd, *ă*ccount, ärm, ȧsk, sof*á;* ēve, hĕre, êvent, ĕnd, silĕnt, makēr; īce, ĭll, charĭty; ōld, ōbey, ôrb, ŏdd, sŏft, cŏnnect; fo͞od, fo͝ot; out; oil; cūbe, ŭnite, ûrn, ŭp, circ*ŭ*s, menü; chair; go; sing; then, thin; nat*ŭ*re; verd*ŭ*re; k = ch in German ich or ach; bon; yet; zh = z in azure

abdominal (ăb-dŏm′ĭ-năl). Belonging to or relating to the abdomen.
  a. delivery, delivery of the child by abdominal section. See *cesarean section.*
  a. gestation, ectopic pregnancy occurring in the cavity of the abdomen.
  a., intra, situated or occurring within the abdomen.
  a. pregnancy. See *gestation* above.
  a. section. See *cesarean section, celiotomy, laparotomy.*

ablatio (ăb-lā′shĭ-ō). Ablation. Removal of a part.
  a. placentae, premature detachment of a normal placenta.

abnormal (ăb-nôr′măl). Contrary to the usual or natural structure; contrary to the natural condition.

abortifacient (*á*-bôr″tĭ-fā′shĕnt). 1. Causing miscarriage. 2. A drug capable of causing a miscarriage.

abortion (*á*-bôr′shŭn). The expulsion of the fetus which is not viable; expulsion of the fetus during the first three months of pregnancy.
  a., criminal, an illegally induced abortion for the purpose of destroying the product of conception.
  a., habitual, an abortion which is repeated at about the same time in successive pregnancies.
  a., incomplete, an abortion which is followed by the retention of part or all of the placenta.
  a., inevitable, an abortion which cannot be prevented due to the progressive symptoms and expulsion of the fetus.
  a., missed, an abortion in which the embryo or fetus is dead, but is not expelled for two months or longer.
  a., spontaneous, an abortion which occurs naturally.
  a., therapeutic, an abortion performed by a physician because of some grave maternal disease endangering the life of the mother.
  a., threatened, an abortion in which the expulsion of the fetus is threatened, but the process is abated under suitable treatment.

abrasion (ăb-rā′zh*ŭ*n). 1. Attrition; a rubbing or scraping off. 2. A spot rubbed bare of skin or mucous membrane.

abruptio placentae (ăb-rŭp′shĭ-ō pl*á*-sen′-tē). Premature detachment of normally implanted placenta; accidental hemorrhage.

abscess (ăb′sĕs). A collection of pus contained in a cavity formed in any part of the body by the disintegration and stretching of the tissue.

accouchement (*ă*-ko͞osh′män). [French, *accoucher,* to put to bed, to deliver.] The act of being delivered; delivery.
  a. forcé (fōr-sā′), rapid delivery, artificially performed, requiring the forcible dilatation of the cervix of the uterus. The operation is rarely used today.

accoucheur (ăk″o͞o-shûr′). [French.] A male midwife; an obstetrician.

accoucheuse (ăk″ōō-shûz′). [French.] A midwife.

acetone (ăs′ĕ-tōn). Dimethyl ketone, a colorless liquid having a pleasant ethereal odor, found in small quantities in normal urine and occurs in larger amounts in diabetic urine.

acid (ăs′ĭd). 1. Sour, sharp to the taste. 2. Having the chemical properties of an acid. 3. In chemistry, a compound having the property of combining with an alkali or a base and thus forming a new compound.

    a. amino. Forms the chief structure of proteins; several of these acids are essential in .human nutrition.

    a. reaction, a reaction by which litmus paper or solution is turned red by the addition of an acid.

acidosis (ăs-ĭ-dō′sĭs). Clinical term commonly used to indicate a lowered blood bicarbonate with a tendency toward acidemia.

acinus (ăs′ĭ-nŭs; pl. acini—ăs′ĭ-nī). Any one of the smallest lobules of a compound gland, such as the mammary gland.

acme (ăk′mĕ). The highest degree or height of a disease; crisis.

acne (ăk′nĕ). Any inflammatory disease of the sebaceous glands. The inflamed glands form either small pink papules or pustules.

acrid (ăk′rĭd). Pungent; producing an irritation.

acromion (ă-krō′mĭ-ŏn). An outward extension of the spine of the scapula, used to explain presentation of the fetus.

acute (ă-kūt′). Sharp-pointed; ending at a point or in an angle less than a right angle; severe, as *acute* pain. In medicine the term is applied to diseases having violent symptoms attended with danger and terminating within a few days.

adhere (ăd-hēr′). To cling together; to become fastened; e.g., adherent placenta.

adnexa (ăd-nĕk′să). Appendages.

    a., uterine (ū′tĕr-ĭn), the fallopian tubes and ovaries.

after-birth (ăf′tĕr-bûrth″). The structures cast off after the expulsion of the fetus, including the membranes and the placenta with the attached umbilical cord; the secundines.

after-pains (ăf′tĕr-pāns″). Those pains, more or less severe, after expulsion of the after-birth, which result from the contractile efforts of the uterus to return to its normal condition.

agalactia (ăg′ă-lăk′shĭ-ă). Absence or failure of the secretion of milk.

albuminuria (ăl-bū″mĭ-nū′rĭ-ă). A condition in which albumin is present in the urine.

alkaline (ăl′kă-līn). Having the properties of an alkali.

    a. reaction, the reaction in which red litmus paper is turned blue by alkalies.

allantois (ă-lăn′tŏ-ĭs). A tubular diverticulum of the posterior part of the yolk sac of the embryo; passes into the body stalk through which it is accompanied by the allantoic (umbilical) blood vessels, thus taking part in the formation of the umbilical cord, and later, fusing with the chorion, it helps to form the placenta.

alopecia (al-o-pe′she-ah). Baldness; deficiency of hair, natural or abnormal.

alveolus (ăl-vē′ŏ-lŭs). An air sac of the lungs formed by terminal dilatations of the bronchioles. The acinus of a gland. A tooth socket.

alvine (ăl′vĭn; -vīn). Belonging to the belly, stomach or intestines.

    a. dejections, the feces.

amenorrhea (ă-měn″ŏ-rē′ă). Absence or suppression of the menstrual discharge.

amnesia (ăm-nē′zhĭ-ă). Loss of memory.

amnion (ăm′nĭ-ŏn). The most internal of the fetal membranes, containing the waters which surround the fetus in utero.

amniotic (ăm″nĭ-ŏt′ĭk). Pertaining to the amnion.

    a. sac, the "bag of membranes" containing the fetus before delivery.

analgesia (ăn″ăl-jē′zĭ-ă). Drug which relieves pain, used during labor.

anastomosis (*ă-năs″tŏ-mō′sĭs). A communication between two vessels.

anchylosis. See *ankylosis.*

androgen (ăn′drŏ-jĕn). Any substance which possesses masculinizing activities, such as the testis hormone.

android (ăn′droid). The term adopted for the male type of pelvis.

anemia (*ă-nē′mĭ-*ă). Deficiency of blood in quantity, either general or local; also, deficiency of the most important constituents of the blood, especially the red blood corpuscles.

anencephalus (ăn″ĕn-sĕf′*ă-lŭs). Form of monstrosity with absence of a brain.

anesthesia (ăn″ĕs-thē′zhĭ-*ă). 1. Loss of feeling or perception, especially loss of tactile sensibility. 2. The production of anesthesia.

anesthetic (ăn″ĕs-thĕt′ĭk). 1. Having no perception or sense of touch. 2. A medicine having the power of rendering the recipient insensible to pain.

angioma (ăn-jĭ-ō′m*ă). A tumor the cells of which tend to form blood or lymph vessels.

ankyloglossia (ăng′kĭ-lŏ-glŏs″ĭ-*ă). Tonguetied.

ankylosis (ăng″kĭ-lō′sĭs). The consolidation of the articulating surfaces of two or more bones that previously formed a natural joint; stiff joint.

annular (ăn′*ū-lēr). Shaped like a ring.

anomaly (*ă-nom′*ă-lĭ). Marked deviation from the normal standard.

anorexia (ăn′ŏ-rĕk″sĭ-*ă). Loss of appetite.

anovular (ăn-ōv′*ū-lēr). Not accompanied with the discharge of an ovum; said of cyclic uterine bleeding.

anoxia (an-ox′e-ah). Oxygen deficiency; any condition of insufficiency of tissue oxidation.

anteflexion (ăn″tĕ-flĕk′sh*ŭn). An abnormal curvature of an organ in which the upper part of the organ is bent forward, as of the uterus.

antenatal (ăn-tĕ-nā′t*ăl). Occurring or formed before birth.

antepartum (ăn″tĕ-pär′t*ŭm). Before delivery or childbirth; prenatal.

anterior (ăn-tēr′ĭ-ēr). Situated before or in front of.

anteversion (an″te-vûr′sh*ŭn). The forward tipping or tilting of an organ; displacement in which the organ is tipped forward but is not bent at an angle, as in anteflexion.

anthropoid (ăn-thrŏ′poid). Funnel-shaped; applied to a type of pelvis.

antibiotic (ăn′tĭ-bī-ŏt′ĭk). 1. Destructive of life. 2. A chemical compound which is produced by and obtained from certain living cells, especially lower plant cells, such as bacteria, yeast, molds, etc., and is antagonistic to some other form of life, such as pathogenic or noxious forms, being often biostatic or biocidal. Some of these substances are also produced synthetically.

antigen (ăn′tĭ-jĕn). Any substance which, when introduced into the blood or tissues, incites the formation of antibodies.

antihistamine (ăn-tĭ-hĭs′t*ă-mēn). Counteracting the effects of histamine, an amine (an organic compound containing nitrogen) which occurs in all animal and vegetable tissues.

antiluetic (ăn′tĭ-lū-ĕt′ĭk). Antisyphilitic.

antiscorbutic (ăn″tĭ-skôr-bū′tĭk). An agent used to prevent or cure scurvy.

antiseptic (ăn″tĭ-sĕp′tĭk). 1. Preventing sepsis or putrefaction. 2. A substance which prevents or retards putrefaction,—that is, the decomposition of animal or vegetable bodies with evolution of offensive odors. Among the principal antiseptics are: alcohol, creosote, carbolic acid, common salt, corrosive sublimate (bichloride of mercury), vinegar, sugar, charcoal, chlorine, boric acid and tannic acid.

a. dressing, a surgical dressing containing antiseptics.

a. surgery, surgery with proper antiseptic precautions.

anuria (*ă-nū′rĭ-*ă). Absolute suppression of urinary secretion.

aperient (*ă-pēr′ĭ-ĕnt). 1. Mildly cathartic. 2. A gentle purgative.

aphthae (ăf′thē). Thrush; more correctly,

the whitish spots in the mouth that characterize aphthous stomatitis.

A.P.L. 1. An abbreviation for anterior pituitarylike; applied to the gonadotropic principle of the urine of pregnant women or of the placenta. 2. A commercial chorionic gonadotropic preparation.

apnea (ăp-nē′ȧ). Cessation of respiration.

areola (ȧ-rē′ō-lȧ). The ring of pigment surrounding the nipple.

    secondary a., a circle of faint color sometimes seen just outside the original areola about the fifth month of pregnancy.

arterial (är-tēr′ĭ-ăl). Belonging to an artery.

    a. blood, the bright-red blood of the arteries which has been aerated (charged with oxygen) in the lungs.

    a. hemorrhage, hemorrhage directly from an artery.

articulation (är-tĭk″û-lā′shŭn). The fastening together of the various bones of the skeleton in their natural situation; a joint. The articulations of the bones of the body are divided into two principal groups,—*synarthroses*, immovable articulations, and *diarthroses*, movable articulations.

Aschheim-Zondek test (ăsh″hīm-tsŏn′-dĕk). A test for the diagnosis of pregnancy. Repeated injections of small quantities of urine voided during the first weeks of pregnancy produce in infantile mice, within 100 hours, (1) minute intrafollicular ovarian hemorrhage and (2) the development of lutein cells.

ascites (ȧ-sī′tēz). An accumulation of serous fluid in a cavity of the body; i.e., edema of the peritoneum; dropsy of the belly.

asepsis (ȧ-sĕp′sĭs). The absence of septic materials; exclusion of disease germs and other causes of septic poisoning.

aseptic (ȧ-sĕp′tĭk). Not septic; free from septic matter; not exposed to injurious effects of septic materials.

asphyxia (ăs-fĭk′sĭ-ȧ). Suspended animation; that state in which there is total suspension of the powers of body and mind, usually caused by interrupted respiration and deficiency of oxygen in the blood, as by hanging or drowning.

    a. livida (lĭv′ĭ-dä), the skin is livid (blue) from the presence of carbon dioxide in the blood, but the circulation continues.

    a. neonatorum (nē″ō-nȧ-tō′rŭm), "asphyxia of the newborn," deficient respiration in newborn babies.

    a. pallida (păl′ĭ-dä), the skin is pale, the pulse weak, and the reflexes are weak or absent.

assimilate (ă-sĭm′ĭ-lāt). To convert food into nutriment.

astringent (ăs-trĭn′jĕnt). 1. Binding; contracting. 2. A medicine having the power to check discharges, whether of blood, of mucus, or of any other secretion.

asynclitism (ȧ-sĭng′klĭ-tĭz′m). Oblique presentation of the head in parturition.

atelectasis (ăt″ē-lĕk′tȧ-sĭs). Imperfect expansion of the lungs at birth; also a partial collapse of the lung.

atony (ăt′ō-nĭ). The lack of tone or strength.

atresia (ȧ-trē′zhĭ-ȧ). Imperforation; absence or closure of a normal opening.

atrophic (ȧ-trŏf′ĭk). Relating to atrophy; characterized by atrophy or failure of nutrition.

atrophied (ăt′rō-fīd). Affected with atrophy; degenerated, wasted.

atrophy (ăt′rō-fĭ). Defect of nutrition; wasting or emaciation with loss of strength, unaccompanied by fever.

attitude (ăt′ĭ-tūd). A posture or position of the body. In obstetrics, the relation of the fetal members to each other in the uterus; the position of the fetus in the uterus.

auscultation (ôs″kŭl-tā′shŭn). The act of listening for sounds within the body.

avitaminosis (ā-vī′-tȧ-mĭn-ō′sĭs). Any condition due to a deficiency of vitamins in the diet, such as scurvy or beriberi.

axis (ăk′sĭs). 1. A line about which any

revolving body turns. 2. **Pelvic a.**, the curved line which passes through the centers of all the anteroposterior diameters of the pelvis.

bacteria (băk-tēr'ĭ-ā). The plural of *bacterium*. A form of microbes or plant micro-organisms.

bag of waters. The membranes which enclose the liquor amnii of the fetus.

ballottement (bă-lŏt'mĕnt). Literally means tossing. A term used in an examination when the fetus can be pushed about in the pregnant uterus.

Bandl's ring (Bän'dls). A groove on the uterus at the upper level of the fully developed lower uterine segment; visible on the abdomen after hard labor as a transverse or slightly slanting depression between the umbilicus and the pubis. Shows overstretching of lower uterine segment. Resembles a full bladder.

Bartholin's glands (Bär'tŏ-lĭn). Glands situated one on each side of the vaginal canal opening into the groove between the hymen and the labia minora.

basiotribe (bā'sĭ-ŏ-trīb″). An instrument for crushing the base of the fetal skull.

basiotripsy (bā'sĭ-ŏ-trĭp″sĭ). Crushing base of fetal skull with basiotribe.

Bednar's aphthae (bĕd'narz ăf'thē). Ulcerations or small yellow patches on the hard palate of the newborn and infants; showing a profound and marked state of constitutional disorder; general ill health and malnutrition.

bicornate uterus (bī-kôr'năt). Having two horns which, in the embryo, failed to attain complete fusion.

bimanual (bī-măn'û-ăl). Performed with or relating to both hands.

b. palpation, examination of the pelvic organs of a woman by placing one hand on the abdomen and the fingers of the other in the vagina.

biparietal (bī'păr-ī'ĕ-tăl). Pertaining to the two parietal bones.

birth (bûrth). 1. The act of coming into life; the delivery of a child. 2. That which is born. See *delivery*.

b. mark, a "maternal mark" or "mother's mark," a mark on the skin from birth—the effect, as some erroneously suppose, of the mother's longing for, or aversion to, particular objects, or of some accidental occurrence affecting her own person during pregnancy. See *nevus*.

blastoderm (blăs'tŏ-dûrm). Delicate germinal membrane of the ovum.

b. vesicle, hollow space within the morula formed by the rearrangement of cells, and by proliferation.

bleb (blĕb). Any bulla or skin vesicle filled with fluid.

blennorrhea (blĕn-ŏ-rē'ā). A discharge from mucous surfaces, especially gonorrheal discharge from the urethra or the vagina; also, gonorrhea.

blood plasma. The liquid portion of the blood in which the corpuscles are suspended. Plasma is obtained from whole blood by removing the corpuscles by centrifuging or by sedimentation. Plasma contains all the chemical constituents of whole blood except hemoglobin.

blood pressure. The pressure of the blood on the walls of the arteries, dependent on the energy of the heart action, the elasticity of the walls of the arteries, the resistance in the capillaries, the volume and the viscosity of the blood. The maximum pressure occurs at the time of the systole of the left ventricle of the heart, and is termed the maximum or the systolic pressure. The minimum pressure is felt at the diastole of the ventricle and is termed minimum or diastolic pressure.

bougie (boo″zhē'). A slender instrument resembling a catheter but solid instead of having a canal, primarily designed for introduction into the urethra. Now used for inducing labor.

Braxton-Hicks sign. Painless uterine contractions occurring periodically throughout pregnancy, thereby enlarging the uterus to accommodate the growing fetus.

B.-H. version, one of the types of

operation designed to turn the baby from an undesirable position to a desirable one.

breast, caked. See *mastitis.*

breech (brēch). Nates or buttocks.

   b. labor or **b. delivery,** labor or delivery marked by breech presentations.

bregma (brĕg′mȧ). The point on the surface of the skull at the junction of the coronal and sagittal sutures.

brim (brĭm). The edge of the superior strait or inlet of the pelvis.

bruit. A sound or murmur heard in auscultation.

   b. placentaire, a blowing sound heard in the pregnant uterus, caused by fetal circulation.

bulla (bŭl′ȧ). A large blister or cutaneous vesicle filled with serous fluid.

caked breast. See *mastitis.*

calorie (kăl′ō-rĭ). A unit of heat; the amount of heat required to raise 1 Gm. of water 1°C., i.e., from 15°C. to 16°C.

caput (kā′pŭt). 1. The head, consisting of the cranium, or skull, and the face. 2. Any prominent object, such as the head.

   c. distortum (dĭs-tôr′tŭm), torticollis.

   c. incuneatum (ĭn-cū-nĕ-ā′tŭm), impaction of the head of the fetus in labor.

   c. succedaneum (sŭk″sĕ-dā′nĕ-ŭm), a dropsical swelling which appears on the presenting head of the fetus during labor, caused by lack of pressure on that part.

caries (kā′rĭ-ēz). [Latin, "rottenness."] 1. Ulceration of bone. 2. Decay of the teeth, resulting in the formation of cavities.

caruncle (kăr′ŭng-k'l). Any fleshy eminence, whether normal or abnormal.

   lacrimal (lăk′rĭ-mȧl) **c.,** the red eminence at the inner angle of the eye.

   urethral (ū-rē′thrȧl) **c.,** a small red growth on the mucous membrane of the urinary meatus in women.

casein (kā′sē-ĭn). The most important of the proteins of milk; constituting the basis of cheese in a state of purity.

catamenia (kăt-ȧ-mē′nĭ-ȧ). See *menses.*

caudal (kô′dăl). The term applied to analgesia or anesthesia resulting from the introduction of the suitable analgesic or anesthetic solution into the caudal canal (nonclosure of the laminae of the last sacral vertebra).

caul (kôl). A portion of the amniotic sac which occasionally envelops the child's face at birth

celiotomy (sē″lĭ-ŏt′ō-mĭ). Abdominal section; surgical opening of the abdominal cavity.

cellulitis (sĕl″ū-lī′tĭs). Infection of the loose connective tissue.

cephalhematoma (sĕf″ăl-hē″mȧ-tō′-mȧ). A tumor or swelling between the bone and the periosteum caused by an effusion of blood.

cephalic (sĕ-făl′ĭk). Belonging to the head.

   c. pole, the cephalic extremity of a fetus.

   c. presentation, presentation of any part of the fetal head in labor.

cephalo- (sef′ȧ-lō). A combining form denoting relationship to the head.

cephalotomy (sĕf″ȧ-lŏt′ō-mĭ). Dissection of the head; also the cutting or breaking down of the fetal head.

cephalotribe (sĕf″ȧ-lō-trīb′). An instrument for crushing and extracting the fetal head in cases of difficult labor.

cephalotripsy (sĕf″ȧ-lō-trĭp′sĭ). The operation of crushing the fetal head with the cephalotribe.

cerebrospinal (sĕr″ĕ-brō-spī′nȧl). Relating to the cerebrum and the spinal cord.

   c. fluid, the clear, limpid fluid contained in the ventricles of the brain, the subarachnoid spaces and the central canal of the spinal cord.

cervix (sûr′vĭks). Necklike part; the lower and narrow end of the uterus, between the os and the body of the organ.

cesarean section (sĕ-zâ′rĕ-ăn). D livery

of the fetus by an incision through the abdominal or vaginal wall and the wall of the uterus.

Chadwick's sign (tshăd'wĭks). The violet color on the mucous membrane of the vagina just below the urethral orifice, seen after the fourth week of pregnancy.

chafe (chāf). To make sore or abrade by rubbing or friction.

chancre (shăng'kĕr). The primary lesion of syphilis, developing at the site of entrance of the syphilitic infection; appearing as a small papule which erodes into a reddish ulcer covered with a yellowish exudation.

chancroid (shăng'kroid). Soft chancre; an infection of the genitals caused by *Hemophilus ducreyi*. It begins as a pustule on the genitals, forming soon after inoculation, grows rapidly and finally breaks down into a virulent ulcer, discharging pus.

change of life. See *climacteric*.

chemotherapy (kĕm'ō-thĕr'ȧ-pĭ). The treatment of disease by administering chemicals which affect the causative organism unfavorably but do not injure the patient.

chloasma (klō-ăz'mȧ). Pl. *chloasmata*. A cutaneous affection exhibiting spots and patches of a yellowish-brown color. The term chloasma is a vague one and is applied to various kinds of pigmentary discoloration of the skin.

   c. gravidarum, c. uterinum, chloasma occurring during pregnancy.

chorea (kō-rē'ȧ). St. Vitus's dance; a convulsive disease characterized by irregular and involuntary movements of the limbs. It usually occurs in early life and affects girls more frequently than boys.

chorio-epithelioma (kō'rĭ-ō-ĕp-ĭ-thē-lĭ-ō'-mȧ). Chorionic carcinoma; a tumor formed by malignant proliferation of the epithelium of the chorionic villi.

chorion (kō'rĭ-ŏn). The outermost membrane of the growing zygote, or fertilized ovum, which serves as a protective and nutritive covering.

chromatin (krō'mȧ-tĭn). The more readily stainable portion of the cell nucleus.

chromosome (kro'mo-sōm). One of several small, dark-staining and more or less rod-shaped bodies which appear in the nucleus of the cell at the time of cell division and particularly in mitosis.

chronic (krŏn'ĭk). Long-continued; lasting a long time; opposed to acute.

cicatrix (sĭk'ȧ-trĭks). Pl. *cicatrices*. A scar; an elevation or seam consisting of a new tissue formation replacing tissue lost by a wound, sore or ulcer.

cilia (sĭl'ĭ-ȧ). Minute lashlike processes in the mucous membrane lining the fallopian tubes.

circumcision (sûr″kŭm-sĭzh'ŭn). The removal of all or part of the prepuce, or foreskin of the penis.

clamp (klămp). A surgical device for effecting compression.

   Willett's c. A special scalp clamp by which traction can be exerted on the presenting head during labor.

   Yellen c. A special clamp used in circumcision.

cleft palate (klĕft păl'ĭt). Congenital fissure of the palate and the roof of the mouth.

climacteric (klī-măk'tĕr-ĭk). A particular epoch of the ordinary term of life, marked by periods of seven years, at which the body is supposed to be peculiarly affected and to suffer considerable change; especially, the menopause or "change of life."

clitoris (klī'tō-rĭs). A small, elongated, erectile body, situated at the anterior part of the vulva. An organ of the female homologous with the penis of the male.

clonic (klŏn'ĭk). Applied to spasms in which the contractions and relaxations are alternate.

coaptation (kō″ăp-tă'shŭn). The fitting together of the ends of a fractured bone or the edges of a wound.

coccyx (kŏk'sĭks). The small bone situated caudal to the sacrum, the caudal and vestigial end of the spinal column.

coitus (kō'ĭt-ŭs). Sexual intercourse; copulation.

collapse (kŏ-lăps'). 1. A falling or caving in. 2. A state of extreme depression or complete prostration of the vital powers, such as occurs after severe injury or excessive bleeding.

colostrum (kŏ-lŏs'trŭm). A substance in the first milk after delivery, giving to it a greenish or yellowish color.

    c. corpuscles, large, granular cells found in colostrum.

colpeurynter (kŏl-pū-rĭn'tēr). A dilatable bag, used to stretch the vagina by introducing the bag in a flaccid condition and then distending it by the forcible injection of air or water.

colpeurysis (kŏl-pū'rĭ-sĭs). Dilatation of the vagina by means of a colpeurynter.

colporrhaphy (kŏl-pōr'a-fĭ). 1. The operation of suturing the vagina. 2. The operation of denuding and suturing the vaginal wall for the purpose of narrowing the vagina.

colpotomy (kŏl-pŏt'o-mĭ). Any surgical cutting operation upon the vagina.

coma (kō'ma). A state of lethargic drowsiness, produced by compression of the brain and other causes.

comatose (kŏm'a-tōs). 1. Having a constant propensity to sleep; full of sleep. 2. Relating to coma.

comedones (kŏm'ē-dō'nez). A plug of dried sebum in an excretory duct of the skin.

conception (kŏn-sĕp'shŭn). The impregnation of the female ovum by the spermatozoon of the male, whence results a new being.

condyloma (con-dil-o'mah). Pl. *condylomata*. A wartlike excrescence near the anus or the vulva; the flat, moist papule of secondary syphilis.

confinement (kŏn-fīn'mĕnt). Term applied to childbirth and the lying-in period.

congenital (kŏn-jĕn'ĭ-tĕl). Born with a person; existing from or from before birth, as, for example, congenital disease, a disease originating in the fetus before birth.

congestion (kŏn-jĕs'chŭn). An excessive accumulation of the contents of any of the blood vessels or ducts.

conjugate (kŏn'jōō-gāt). The antero-posterior diameter of the pelvic inlet.

conjunctiva (kŏn''jŭngk-tī'va). The delicate mucous membrane lining the eyelids and covering the external portion of the eyeball.

contraception (kŏn''tra-sĕp'shŭn). The prevention of conception or impregnation.

contraindication (kŏn''tra-ĭn''dĭ-kā'-shŭn). That which forbids the use of a remedy which otherwise it would be proper to exhibit. Any condition of disease which renders some special line of treatment or some particular remedy undesirable or improper.

convalescence (kŏn''va-lĕs'ĕns). The state or period between the removal of actual disease and the full recovery of the strength.

convulsion (kŏn-vŭl'shŭn). Violent agitation of the limbs or body generally marked by clonic spasms.

copulation (kŏp''ū-lā'shŭn). Sexual intercourse; coitus.

cornea (kôr'nē-a). The transparent structure forming the anterior part of the eyeball.

coronal (kŏr'ŏ-năl). Belonging to, or relating to, the crown of the head.

    c. suture, the suture formed by the union of the frontal bone with the two parietal bones.

corpus luteum (kôr'pŭs lū'tē-ŭm). The yellow mass found in the graafian follicle after the ovum has been expelled.

cortex (kôr'tĕks). The outer layer of an organ as distinguished from its inner substance.

cotyledon (kŏt''ĭ-lē'dŭn). Any one of the subdivisions of the uterine surface of the placenta.

couveuse (kōō''vûz'). An arrangement or apparatus designed for the preservation and development of infants prematurely born or otherwise feeble. An *incubator*, which term is in more common use in the United States.

cranioclasis, cranioclasm (krā'nĭ-ŏ-klă-sĭs, krā'nĭ-ŏ-klăsm). The crushing of the fetal skull.

cranioclast (krā'nĭ-ŏ-klăst). An instrument used in effecting cranioclasis.

craniotomy (krā"nĭ-ŏt'ŏ-mĭ). The opening of the fetal skull when necessary to effect delivery.

  c. scissors, strong S-shaped scissors for use in craniotomy.

Credé's method (krā-dā'). 1. Method of expelling placenta by kneading and pressing the uterus. 2. The installation of silver nitrate solution in the eyes of the newborn.

crib cap. See *seborrhea capitis.*

crowning (kroun'ĭng). That stage in the delivery of the baby's head when the wrinkled scalp becomes visible.

cul-de-sac (kool'dĕ-săk') **of Douglas.** A pouch between the anterior wall of the rectum and the uterus.

curd (kûrd). The coagulum which separates from milk upon the addition of acid, rennet or wine. It consists of casein with most of the fatty elements of the milk.

curettage (kū-rĕt'ĭj). The act of using a curette.

curette (kū-rĕt'). [French.] 1. A sort of scraper or spoon used in removing granulations, foreign bodies, incrustations, etc., from the walls of normal or other cavities in the body. Most commonly used for removing diseased tissue or foreign matter, such as retained placental tissue, from the walls of the uterus. 2. To use a curette.

cutaneous (kū-tā'nĕ-ŭs). Pertaining to the skin.

cutis (kū'tĭs). The skin, consisting of the cutis vera and the epidermis. Also, the cutis vera, or true skin.

cyanosis (sī"ă-nō'sĭs). A blue color of the skin resulting from congenital malformation of the heart or from some defect of the respiratory mechanism by which the venous blood is not wholly oxygenated.

cyclopropane (sī-klŏ-prō'pān). A colorless gas used as a general anesthetic; produces rapid and deep anesthesia; it is inflammable and should be guarded from contact with flame or electric spark.

cyesis (sī-ē'sĭs). Pregnancy.

cystitis (sĭs-tī'tĭs). Inflammation of the bladder.

cystocele (sĭs'tŏ-sēl). Hernial protrusion of the urinary bladder into the vagina.

cytoplasm (sī'tŏ-plăsm). The protoplasm of a cell exclusive of that of the nucleus.

decapitation (dĕ-kăp"ĭ-tā'shŭn). The removal of the head of the fetus in embryotomy.

decidua (dĕ-sĭd'ū-ā). The membranous structure produced during gestation and thrown off from the uterus after parturition. It consists of the greatly changed uterine mucous membrane.

  d. reflexa (rĕ-flĕk'să), that portion of the decidua which is reflected over and surrounds the ovum.

  d. serotina (sĕr-ŏ-tī'nă), "late decidua," that portion of the decidua vera which becomes maternal part of the placenta.

  d. vera (vē'ră), that portion of the decidua which lines the interior of the uterus.

decomposition (dē"kŏm-pŏ-zĭsh'ŭn). 1. The separation of compound bodies into their constituent parts or principles; analysis. 2. Putrefactive decay.

decrement (dĕk'rē-mĕnt). Decrease; also the stage of decline.

delirium (dĕ-lĭr'ĭ-ŭm). A derangement of the functions of the brain characterized by incoherent and wandering talk, illusions and unsteady gait.

delivery (dĕ-lĭv'ēr-ĭ). [French, *délivrer*, to free, to deliver.] 1. The expulsion of a child by the mother, or its extraction by the obstetric practitioner. 2. The removal of a part from the body; as *delivery* of the placenta.

denudation (dĕn"ū-dā'shŭn). The laying bare of any part of an animal or plant; the stripping off of the integument, whether by a surgical or by a pathologic process.

desquamation (dĕs-kwă-mā'shŭn). The shedding of epithelial elements, chiefly of the skin, in scales or sheets.

diagnosis (dī″ăg-nō'sĭs). The art or science of signs or symptoms by which one disease is distinguished from another.

diameter (dī-ăm'ĕ-tēr). A straight line through a center, joining opposite points of a periphery.

Baudelocque's d., the external conjugate diameter of the pelvis.

diaphoresis (dī″à-fō-rē'sĭs). A state of perspiration; profuse perspiration; sweat.

diaphoretic (dī'à-fō-rĕt'ĭk). 1. Stimulating the secretion of perspiration; sudorific. 2. A medicine that increases the perspiration.

diastasis (dī-ăs'tà-sĭs). The lateral separation of the abdominis recti muscle due to the overdistention of the abdominal wall.

diastolic pressure (dī″ăs-tŏl'ĭk). Pertaining to the pressure during diastole or relaxation of the heart. The point at which the pulse becomes inaudible as the pressure in the sphygmomanometer drops after the systolic pressure is noted.

diathesis (dī-ăth'ĕ-sĭs). A particular habit or disposition of the body which renders it peculiarly liable to certain diseases; constitutional predisposition.

diethylstilbestrol (dī-ĕth″ĭl-stĭl-bĕs'trŏl). A synthetic product which is not related to the natural estrogens but which has estrogenic activity similar to but greater than that of esterone. It is used in treating menopausal symptoms, vaginitis and suppressed lactation. Also called *stilbestrol.*

differential (dĭf″ēr-ĕn'shăl). Making a difference; showing a difference; distinguishing.

d. diagnosis, the determining of the distinguishing features of a malady when nearly the same symptoms belong to two different classes of disease, as in gout and rheumatism or epilepsy and eclampsia.

diffusion (dĭ-fū'zhŭn). The process of becoming widely spread; dialysis through a membrane.

disintegration (dĭs-ĭn″tĕ-grā'shŭn). The separation of the integrant parts or particles of a body.

disproportion (dĭs'-prō-pōr'shŭn). In obstetrics, refers to the condition in which the head of the fetus is larger than normal in relation to the pelvis of the mother.

diuresis (dī″û-rē'sĭs). Increased discharge of urine, from whatever cause.

dizygotic (dī″zī-gŏt'ĭk). Pertaining to or proceeding from two zygotes (ova).

Döderlein's bacillus (ded'er-līnz). The large gram-positive bacterium occurring in the normal vaginal secretion.

dormant (dor'mănt). Sleeping; inactive; quiescent.

Douglas' cul-de-sac (kōōl'dĕ-săk'). A sac or recess formed by a fold of the peritoneum dipping down between the rectum and the uterus. Also called *pouch of Douglas* and *recto-uterine pouch.*

dry labor (drī' lā'bēr). Labor during which the membranes rupture prematurely and the liquor amnii escapes.

ductus (dŭk'tŭs). A duct.

d. arteriosus (är-tē″rĭ-ō'sŭs), "arterial duct," a blood vessel peculiar to the fetus, communicating directly between the pulmonary artery and the aorta.

d. venosus (vĕ-nō'sŭs), "venous duct," a blood vessel peculiar to the fetus, establishing a direct communication between the umbilical vein and the descending vena cava.

Duncan (dŭng'kăn) **mechanism.** The position of the placenta, with the maternal surface outermost; to be born edgewise.

dysmenorrhea (dĭs″mĕn-ŏ-rē'à). Difficult and painful menstruation.

dyspnea (dĭsp-nē'à). Difficult or labored breathing.

dystocia (dĭs-tō'shĭ-à). Difficult, slow, or painful birth or delivery. It is distinguished as *maternal* or *fetal* according as the difficulty is due to some deformity on the part of the mother or on the part of the child.

d. placental, difficulty in delivering the placenta.

ecbolic (ĕk-bŏl'ĭk). An agent which accelerates labor, causing parturition.

ecchymosis (ĕk'-ĭ-mō'sĭs). An extravasation of blood; also a discoloration of the skin caused by the extravasation of blood.

eclampsia (ĕk-lămp'sĭ-à). A toxemic condition which may occur before, during or after labor and generally associated with convulsions and coma.

e. puerperal, a convulsive attack occurring in women during or after labor and due probably to toxemia.

ectoderm (ĕk'tŏ-dûrm). The outer layer of cells of the primitive embryo.

ectopic (ĕk-tŏp'ĭk). Out of place.

e. gestation, gestation in which the fetus is out of its normal place in the cavity of the uterus. See *extra-uterine pregnancy.*

e. pregnancy, same as *ectopic gestation.*

e. sac, the amniotic sac in ectopic gestation.

eczema (ĕk'zĕ-mà). A superficial affection of the skin characterized by a smarting eruption of small vesicles, generally crowded together. It is without fever and is not contagious.

edema (ĕ-dē'mà). A swelling from effusion of serous fluid into the cellular substance; a dropsical swelling.

effacement (ĕ-fās'mĕnt). Obliteration. In obstetrics, refers to dilatation of the cervix.

ejaculation (ĕ-jăk″ū-lā'shŭn). A sudden act of expulsion, as of semen.

emaciation (ĕ-mā″sĭ-ā'shŭn). The state of being or becoming lean or wasted.

emanation (ĕm″à-nā'shŭn). An effluvium, usually noxious, characteristic of lochia.

embolism (ĕm'bŏ-lĭz'm). The obstruction of an artery or a vein by a clot of coagulated blood, or by any body brought from some point away from the site of ob-

struction. See *embolus* and *thrombus.*

e., air, embolism in which the obstruction consists of air-bubbles.

embolus (ĕm'bŏ-lŭs). A piece of blood clot which has been formed in the larger vessels in certain morbid conditions and has afterward been forced into one of the smaller arteries so as to obstruct the circulation.

embryo (ĕm'brĭ-ō). The product of conception in utero before the end of the third month of pregnancy; after that length of time it is called the fetus.

embryology (ĕm-brĭ-ŏl'ŏ-jĭ). The science which treats of the development of the embryo.

embryotomy (ĕm″brĭ-ŏt'ŏ-mĭ). The destruction or separation of any part or parts of the fetus in utero when circumstances exist to prevent delivery in the natural way.

emetic (ĕ-mĕt'ĭk). 1. Having the power to excite vomiting. 2. A medicine which causes vomiting.

emmenagogue (ĕ-mĕn'à-gŏg). A medicine having the power to promote the menstrual discharge.

empirical (em-pĭr'ĭ-kàl). Depending upon experience or observation alone, without using science or theory, especially in medicine.

emulsion (ĕ-mŭl'shŭn). An oily or resinous substance suspended in water through the agency of mucilaginous or adhesive substances. Milk is a natural and perfect emulsion.

emunctory (ĕ-mŭngk'tŏ-rĭ). 1. Excretory. 2. Any excretory duct of the body.

endocervical (ĕn'dŏ-sûr'vĭ-kàl). Pertaining to the interior of the cervix of the uterus.

endocrine (ĕn'dŏ-krīn). Pertaining to internal secretions; applied to organs the function of which is to secrete into the blood or the lymph a substance which plays an important role in metabolism.

endometrium (ĕn″dŏ-mē'trĭ-ŭm). The mucous membrane which lines the uterus.

enervation (ĕn″ēr-vā′shŭn). Weakness; languor; lack of nerve stimulus.

engagement (ĕn-gāj′mĕnt). In obstetrics, applies to the entrance of the presenting part into the superior pelvic strait and the beginning of the descent through the pelvic canal.

engorgement (ĕn-gôrj′mĕnt). Hyperemia; local congestion; excessive fullness of any organ or passage. In obstetrics, often refers to the breasts when over-distended with milk.

ensiform (ĕn′sĭ-fôrm). Like a sword; sword-shaped.

> **e. appendix, cartilage,** or **process,** the extremity of the sternum or breast bone.

entoderm (ĕn′tŏ-dûrm). The innermost layer of cells of the primitive embryo.

enzygotic (ĕn-zĭ-gŏt′ĭk). Developed from the same fertilized ovum.

epidemic (ĕp″ĭ-dĕm′ĭk). 1. A term applied to any disease which seems to affect the entire population of a country at one time, as distinguished, on the one hand, from *sporadic* disease (or that which occurs in isolated cases) and, on the other, from *endemic* disease (or that which is limited to a particular district). 2. An epidemic disease; the season of prevalence of any epidemic disease.

epigastric pain (ĕp-ĭ-găs′trĭk). One of the symptoms of preeclampsia toxemia.

epigastrium (ĕp′ĭ-găs′trĭ-ŭm). The epigastric region; the upper middle portion of the abdomen, over or in front of the stomach.

epilepsy (ĕp′ĭ-lĕp″sĭ). The falling sickness; a chronic nonfebrile nervous affection, characterized by seizures and loss of consciousness, with tonic or clonic convulsions ("fits"). The ordinary duration of a seizure is from five to twenty minutes. The frequency of the attacks varies immensely; in some cases they occur daily and in others at intervals of ten years or more.

episiotomy (ĕp″ĭs-ĭ-ot′ŏ-mĭ). Surgical incision of the vulvar orifice for obstetric purposes.

epithelium (ĕp′ĭ-thē′lĭ-ŭm). The covering of the skin and the mucous membranes, consisting wholly of cells of varying form and arrangement; derived from all three of the primitive germinal layers.

epitrochlear (ĕp″ĭ-trŏk′lĕ-ēr). Pertaining to the inner condyle of the humerus.

Erb's paralysis. Partial paralysis of the brachial plexus, affecting various muscles of the arm and the chest wall.

ergot (ûr′gŏt). A drug having the remarkable property of exciting powerfully the contractile force of the uterus, and chiefly used for this purpose, but its long-continued use is highly dangerous. Usually given in the fluid extract.

ergonovine (ûr′gŏ-nō′vĭn). The ergot alkaloid, variously known as ergobasine, ergometrine, ergostetrine or ergotocin. It combines the oxytoxic properties of other ergot alkaloids with rapid action when taken orally or by injection, complete freedom from immediate toxic effects and absence of gangrene-producing qualities.

ergotamine (ûr-gŏt′a-mĭn). A crystalline alkaloid with the characteristic action of ergot.

erosion (ĕ-rō′zhŭn). An irritation or ulceration.

erythema (ĕr′ĕ-thē′ma). A morbid redness of the skin of many varieties, due to congestion of the capillaries; rose rash.

erythroblastosis (ĕ-rĭth″rŏ-blăs-tō′sĭs). A disease of the newborn due to the Rh factor.

estrin (ĕs′trĭn). A generic term for estrus-producing substances, no longer in good usage.

estrogen (ĕs′trŏ-jĕn). A generic term for estrus-producing compounds.

estrone (ĕs′trōn). An estrogenic steroid isolated from the urine of pregnant animals.

estrus (es′trŭs). A recurrent, restricted period of sexual receptivity in female mammals, marked by intense sexual urge. The term is frequently used for the specific genital changes that can be induced in laboratory animals by the injection of ovarian and hypophysial substances.

etiology (ē-tǐ-ŏl'ŏ-jǐ). The study or theory of the causation of any disease; the sum of knowledge regarding causes.

eutocia (û-tō'sǐ-à). Normal labor and delivery.

evisceration (ĕ-vǐs"ēr-ā'shŭn). Taking the bowels or viscera out of the body.

e., obstetric, removal of abdominal or thoracic viscera of the fetus in embryotomy.

exacerbation (ĕg-zăs"ēr-bā'shŭn). 1. An increased force or severity of the symptoms of a disease. 2. The stage or time of periodical aggravation in certain fevers.

excoriation (ĕks-kō"rǐ-ā'shŭn). Abrasion or removal, partial or complete, of the skin.

excrement (ĕks'krĕ-mĕnt). Originally, anything that is excreted: usually applied to the alvine feces.

exosmosis (ĕk'sŏs-mō'sǐs). Diffusion or osmosis from within outward; movement outward through a diaphragm or through vessel walls.

expulsive (ĕks-pŭl'sǐv). Tending toward, promoting or causing expulsion.

e. pains, labor pains occurring during the expulsive stage and accomplishing the expulsion of the fetus.

e. stage, that stage of labor which follows complete dilatation of the uterine cervix, during which the expulsion of the fetus takes place; the second stage of labor.

exsanguination (ĕks-săng"gwǐ-nā'shŭn). The state of being without blood.

extension (ĕks-tĕn'shŭn). The reverse of flexion.

extraction (ĕks-trăk'shŭn). The process or act of pulling or drawing out. In obstetrics the term is frequently used in regard to difficult delivery. (Breech or forceps extraction.)

extraperitoneal (ĕks"trà-pĕr-ǐ-tŏ-nē'ǎl). Situated or occurring outside the peritoneal cavity.

extra-uterine (ĕks"trà-ū'tĕr-ǐn). Outside of the uterus.

e. life, life after birth.

e. pregnancy, pregnancy in which the fetus is contained in some organ outside of the uterus.

extravasation (ĕks-trăv"à-sā'shŭn). The escape of any fluid of the body, normal or abnormal, from the vessel, cavity or canal that naturally contains it, and its diffusion into the surrounding tissues.

exudate (ĕks'û-dāt). A substance thrown out. Any adventitious substance deposited in or on a tissue by a vital process or a disease.

facies (fa'she-ēz). Expression or appearance of the face.

fallopian (fǎ-lō'pǐ-ǎn). [Relating to G. *Fallopius*, a celebrated Italian anatomist of the sixteenth century.]

f. pregnancy, pregnancy occurring in the fallopian tubes—same as *tubal pregnancy.*

f. tubes, the oviducts—two canals extending from the side of the fundus uteri to the ovaries.

fecundation (fē"kŭn-dā'shŭn). The act of impregnating or the state of being impregnated; the fertilization of the ovum by means of the male seminal element.

fenestrated (fĕ-nĕs'trāt-ĕd). Pierced with openings.

fertility (fēr-tǐl'ǐ-tǐ). The ability to produce offspring; power of reproduction.

fertilization (fûr-tǐ-lǐ-zā'shŭn). The fusion of the spermatozoon with the ovum; it marks the beginning of pregnancy.

fetus (fē'tŭs). The baby in utero from the end of the third month of development till birth.

filmated gauze (fǐl'māt-ĕd). A trade name for gauze dressings with an inner layer of cotton.

fimbria (fǐm'brǐ-à). A fringe; especially the fringelike end of the oviduct.

fissure (fǐsh'ēr). A crack or narrow opening.

fistula (fǐs'tû-là). A deep sinuous ulcer, often leading to an internal hollow organ.

flaccid (flǎk'sǐd). Soft, limp, flabby.

flagellate (flăj'ĕ-lāt). Furnished with slender whiplike processes.

flex (flĕks). To bend, as a joint or a jointed limb.

flexion (flĕk'shŭn). The act of bending; the state of being bent.

f. stage, that stage of labor in which the head of the fetus bends forward.

follicle (fŏl'ĭ-k'l). A small secretory sac or gland.

fontanel, fontanelle (fŏn"tá-nĕl'). The quadrangular space between the frontal and two parietal bones in very young infants. This is called the *anterior f.* and is the familiar "soft spot" just above a baby's forehead. A smaller, triangular one (*posterior f.*) sometimes exists between the occipital and parietal bones.

foramen (fŏ-rā'mĕn). A hole, opening, aperture or orifice—especially one through a bone.

f. ovale (ŏ-vā'lē), an opening situated in the partition which separates the right and left auricles of the heart in the fetus.

foreskin (fōr'skĭn). The prepuce—the fold of skin covering the glans penis.

fornix (fôr'nĭks). Pl. *fornices* (fôr'nĭ-sēz). An arch; any vaulted surface.

f. of the vagina, the angle of reflection of the vaginal mucous membrane onto the cervix uteri.

fossa (fŏs'á). A pit, depression, trench or hollow.

fourchette (fōōr-shĕt'). [French, "fork."] The posterior angle or commissure of the labia majora.

frenum (frē'nŭm). Lingual fold of integument or of mucous membrane that checks, curbs or limits the movements of the tongue (ankyloglossia). Congenital shortening.

friable (frī'á-b'l). Easily pulverized or crumbled.

Friedman's test (frēd'măn). A modification of the Aschheim-Zondek test for pregnancy; the urine of early pregnancy is injected in 4-cc. doses intravenously twice daily for two days into an unmated mature rabbit. If,

at the end of this time, the ovaries of the rabbit contain fresh corpora lutea or hemorrhagic corpora, the test is positive.

F.S.H., FSH. Abbreviation for follicle-stimulating hormone.

function (fŭngk'shŭn). A power or faculty by the exercise of which the vital phenomena are produced; the special office of an organ in the animal or vegetable economy.

fundus (fŭn'dŭs). The base or bottom of any organ which has an external opening considered as the top.

f. uteri (ū'tĕr-ī), the base of the uterus, which is to be considered as upside down with the top (os) pointing downward.

funic souffle (fū'nĭc sōō'f'l). A soft, blowing sound, synchronous with the fetal heart sounds and supposed to be produced in the umbilical cord.

funis (fū'nĭs). A cord—especially the umbilical cord.

furuncular (fū-rŭng'kŭ-lēr). Pertaining to or of the nature of a boil.

galactagogue (gá-lăk'tá-gŏg). 1. Causing the flow of milk. 2. Any drug which causes the flow of milk to increase.

galactin (gá-lăk'tĭn). See *prolactin.*

gamete (găm'ēt). A sexual cell; a mature germ cell, as an unfertilized egg or a mature sperm cell.

gastrula (găs'trōō-lá). The early embryonic stage which follows the blastula.

gavage feeding (gá-vàzh'). Feeding by stomach tube. This term is often used for the feeding of premature babies by a soft rubber catheter passed down the esophagus.

gene (jēn). An hereditary germinal factor in the chromosome which carries on an hereditary transmissible character.

genesis (jĕn'ĕ-sĭs). The process of originating; creation.

genitalia (jĕn-ĭtăl'ĭ-á). The reproductive organs.

genupectoral (jĕn"û-pĕk'tŏ-răl). [Latin, *ge'nu,* knee, + *pec'tus,* breast.] Relating to the knees and the chest.

g. position, that posture in which the patient rests on the knees with the thighs upright, the head and the upper part of the chest being on the table or bed. The knee-chest position.

germicide (jŭr'mĭ-sīd). An agent that kills germs.

gertrude. A baby's pettiskirt.

gestation (jĕs-tā'shŭn). The condition of pregnancy; pregnancy; gravidity.

g. sac, the sac enclosing the embryo in ectopic pregnancy.

gland (glănd). An organ consisting of blood vessels, absorbents and nerves, for secreting or separating some particular fluid from the blood; an organ that produces a specific product or secretion; a secreting organ.

Bartholin's g's, two small reddish-yellow bodies in the vestibular bulbs, one on either side of the vaginal orifice.

bulbocavernous (bŭlb'ō-kăv'ēr-nŭs) **g's,** Cowper's glands.

Cowper's g's, two bulbo-urethral glands near the bulb of the corpus spongiosum in the male; homologous with the Bartholin glands in the female.

endocrine g's, organs of internal secretion; ductless glands.

mammary (măm'ă-rĭ) **g's,** the milk secreting glands, the breasts.

miliary (mĭl'ĭ-ĕr-ĭ) g., the sweat gland.

Montgomery's g's, sebaceous glands of the mammary areola.

Naboth's g's, distended mucous glands within the cervix and about the os uteri.

sex g's, the ovaries and the testes.

Skene's g's, two glands just within the meatus of the female urethra; regarded as rudimentary homologues of the prostate gland in the male.

glans (glănz). An acorn-shaped organ.

g. clitoridis (klĭ-tŏr'ĭ-dĭs), the bulbous extremity of the clitoris.

g. penis (pē'nĭs), the nutlike head or end of the penis.

glycosuria (glĭ-kŏ-sū'rĭ-ä). The presence of an abnormal amount of glucose in the urine.

gonad (gŏn'ăd). A gamete-producing gland; an ovary or testis.

gonadotropin (gŏn″ăd-ŏ-trō'pĭn). A substance having an affinity for or a stimulating effect on the gonads.

gonocyte (gŏn'ŏ-sīt). The primitive reproductive cell of the embryo.

gonorrhea (gŏn″ŏ-rē'ä). A contagious, catarrhal inflammation of the genital mucosa caused by the gonococcus organism and usually transmitted by coitus.

Goodell's sign (gōōd'elz). If cervix is soft (as the lips), the woman is pregnant; if the cervix is hard (as the nose), she is not. Softening of the cervix.

graafian follicles or **vesicles** (gräf'ĭ-ăn). Small spherical bodies in the ovaries, each containing an ovum.

gradient (grā'dĭ-ĕnt). The rate of increase or decrease of a variable magnitude; also a curve which represents it.

granulation (grăn″û-lā'shŭn). 1. The process by which little grainlike, conical, fleshy bodies form on ulcers and suppurating wounds, filling up the cavities, and bringing nearer together and uniting their edges. 2. One of the bodies thus formed.

gravida (grăv'ĭd-ä). A pregnant woman.

gravidity (gr*a*-vĭd'ĭ-tĭ). The condition of a woman who is pregnant; gestation; pregnancy.

gynecic (jĭ-nē'sĭk). Relating to female sex or to women.

gynecoid (jĭn'ĕ-koid). The term adopted for the normal female type pelvis.

gynecologist (jĭn″ĕ-kŏl'ŏ-jĭst). One who is skilled in gynecology.

gynecology (jĭn″ĕ-kŏl'ŏ-jĭ). The science which treats of the female constitution and particularly of the disease and injuries of the female genital organs.

habitus (hăb'ĭt-ŭs). Attitude, disposition or tendency; to act in a certain way, position acquired by frequent repetition.

harelip (hâr'lĭp'). A congenital slit of one or both lips, but usually the upper only; sometimes double.

Hegar's sign (hā'gärz). Softening of the lower uterine segment; a sign of pregnancy.

helio- (hē'lĭ-ō). Combining form denoting relationship to the sun.

Hellin's Law (hĕl'inz). One in 80 pregnancies is twins; one in 80 × 80, or 6,400, is triplets; one in 80 × 80 × 80, or 512,000, is quadruplets.

hematoma (hē'mȧ-to"mȧ). A tumor containing effused blood; an accumulation of blood in the tissues.

hemorrhage (hĕm'ŏ-rĭj). Escape of the blood from its natural channels; bleeding.

hemorrhoid (hĕm'ŏ-roid). A pile; a vascular tumor immediately within (*internal h.*) or just outside of (*external h.*) the anus. Hemorrhoids are termed *blind* when they do not cause hemorrhage and *bleeding* when they do.

hemostasis (hĕm-ŏs'tȧs-ĭs). The arrest of an escape of blood. The checking of the flow of blood through any part or vessel.

hepatization (hĕp-ăt-iz-ā'shun). Change of tissue into a liverlike substance.

hernia (hûr'nĭ-ȧ). The displacement, through an abnormal opening, of an organ or tissue, most commonly of a portion of the intestine from the cavity in which it is naturally contained; a "rupture."

heterogeneous (hĕt'ēr-ō-jē'nē-ŭs). Consisting of or composed of dissimilar elements or ingredients.

heterogenic (hĕt'ēr-ō-jĕn'ĭk). Occurring in the wrong sex.

hiatus (hī-ā'tŭs). Any gap, fissure or opening, such as the vulva or the hiatus to the caudal canal.

homogenized (hō'mŏ-jĕ-nīzd). Of a uniform quality throughout.

homologous (hŏ-mŏl'ŏ-gŭs). Corresponding in structure or origin; derived from the same source.

hormone (hôr'mōn). A chemical substance produced in an organ, which, being carried to an associated organ by the blood stream, excites in the latter organ a functional activity.

hydatiform (hī-dăt'ĭ-fôrm) mole. Cystic proliferation of chorionic villi, resembling a bunch of grapes.

hydramnios, hydramnion (hī-drăm'nĭ-ŏs) (hī-drăm'nĭ-ŏn). An excessive amount of amniotic fluid.

hydremia (hī-drē'mĭ-ȧ). Excess of water in the blood.

hydrocephalus (hī"drŏ-sĕf'ȧ-lŭs). A condition characterized by abnormal increase in the amount of cerebral fluid accompanied by dilatation of the cerebral ventricles. The disease is marked by the enlargement of the head, with prominence of the forehead, atrophy of the brain and mental weakness.

hydrometer (hī-drŏm'ĕ-tēr). An instrument for ascertaining the specific gravity of fluids.

hydrorrhea (hī-drō-rĭ'ȧ). A copious watery discharge

    h. gravidarum, a discharge of thin mucus from the pregnant uterus, due to excessive secretion of the uterine glands.

hymen (hī'mĕn). A membranous fold which partially or wholly occludes the external orifice of the vagina, especially in the virgin.

hyperemesis (hī"pēr-ĕm'ĕ-sĭs). Excessive vomiting.

hypersecretion (hī"pēr-sĕ-krē'shŭn). Excessive secretion.

hypertension (hī"pēr-tĕn'shŭn). Abnormally high tension; especially high blood pressure.

hypertonic (hī"pēr-tŏn'ĭk). Excessive tone, tension or activity.

hypertrophy (hī-pûr'trŏ-fĭ). Enlargement of a part of an organ, especially when due to overnutrition or overstimulation.

hypochondrium (hī"pŏ-kŏn'drĭ-ŭm). The region of the abdomen below the ribs on each side of the epigastrium.

hypogastric arteries (hī"pŏ-găs'trĭk). Same as the umbilical arteries which accompany and form part of the umbilical cord.

hypogastrium (hī"pŏ-găs'trĭ-ŭm). The

lower abdomen in the middle line—below the navel; the suprapubic region.

hysterectomy (hĭs″tēr-ĕk′tŏ-mĭ). The operation for the removal of the uterus.

hysteria (hĭs-tēr′ĭ-ȧ). A functional disease often observed in young unmarried women, in which there may be a simulation of almost any disease and a great lack of self-control.

hysterotomy (hĭs″tēr-ŏt′ŏ-mĭ). The operation of cutting into the uterus, *e.g.*, cesarean section.

icterus (ĭk′tēr-ŭs). Jaundice.

idio- (ĭd′ĭ-ŏ). Combining form denoting relationship to self or to one's own, or to something separate and distinct.

idiosyncrasy (ĭd′ĭ-ŏ-sĭng′krȧ-sĭ). Individual and peculiar susceptibility to some drug, protein or other agent.

iliac (ĭl′ĭ-ăk). Belonging to the ilium or the flanks.

   i. artery, either of two arteries, right and left, given off from the abdominal aorta and dividing to form the external and internal iliac arteries on each side of the body.

   i. fossa (fŏs′ȧ), a broad and shallow cavity at the upper part of the inner surface of the ilium.

iliopectineal line (ĭl″ĭ-ŏ-pĕk-tĭn′ē-ăl). An oblique ridge on the inner surface of the ilium, continued on the pubis and forming the lower boundary of the iliac fossa; it separates the true from the false pelvis.

ilium (ĭl′ĭ-ŭm). Pl. *ilia* (ĭl′ĭ-ȧ). The hip bone; the broad, flat, upper portion of the innominate bone.

illegitimate (ĭl′lĕ-jĭt′ĭ-mĭt). Unlawful; born out of wedlock.

imbricated (ĭm′brĭ-kāt′ĕd). Overlapping.

immature (ĭm′ȧ-tūr′). Not fully developed.

immunity (ĭ-mū′nĭ-tĭ). Security against any particular disease or poison, specifically, the power which an individual sometimes acquires to resist and/or overcome an infection to which most or many of its species are susceptible.

imperforate anus (ĭm-pûr′fŏ-rāt ā′nŭs).

Closure of the natural opening of the anus.

impetigo (ĭm″pĕ-tī′gō). An inflammatory skin disease characterized by isolated pustules.

implantation (ĭm″plăn-tā′shŭn). In obstetrics usually refers to the embedding of the fertilized ovum in the wall of the uterus.

impregnation (ĭm″prĕg-nā′shŭn). The act of making, or state of being, pregnant; fecundation.

inanition (ĭn′ȧ-nĭsh′ŭn). The physical condition that results from complete lack of food.

inborn (ĭn′bôrn). Formed or implanted during intra-uterine life.

incise (ĭn-sīz′). To cut, as with a knife.

incontinence (ĭn-kŏn′tĭ-nĕns). Inability to restrain a natural discharge.

increment (ĭn′krĕ-mĕnt). That by which anything is increased.

incubator (ĭn-kū-bā′tēr). See *couveuse*.

indolent (ĭn′dō-lĕnt). Causing little pain.

induction (ĭn-dŭk′shŭn). The act or process of inducing or causing to occur.

indurated (ĭn′dū-rāt-ĕd). Hardened; rendered hard.

inertia (ĭn-ûr′shĭ-ȧ). Inactivity; inability to move spontaneously. Uterisluggishness of uterine contractions during labor.

infant (ĭn′fănt). A babe or young child; a child under two years of age.

infanticide (ĭn-făn′tĭ-sīd). The murder of an infant.

infantile (ĭn′făn-tīl). In obstetrics usually refers to the underdevelopment of the generative organs.

infarct (ĭn′färkt). A white or reddish, hard lump in the placenta due to degeneration following interruption of blood supply.

infection (ĭn-fĕk′shŭn). 1. It is the local or general condition due to the growth or multiplication of a parasitic organism. 2. The agent by which a communicable disease is conveyed; a contagium.

   i., septic, infection caused by septic germs. See *septic*.

infertility (ĭn-fûr-tĭl′ĭ-tĭ). The quality of being unfruitful or barren; sterility.

infiltration (ĭn″fĭl-trā′shŭn). The accumulation in a tissue of substances not normal to it.

inflammation (ĭn″flă-mä′shŭn). A state of disease characterized by redness, pain, heat and swelling, attended or not with fever.

infundibulin (ĭn′fŭn-dĭb′û-lĭn). An extract of the posterior lobe of the pituitary body.

infundibulum (ĭn′fŭn-dĭb′û-lŭm). Any funnel-shaped passage; the cavity of the fimbriated end of an oviduct.

infusion (ĭn-fū′zhŭn). To pour in or upon. In surgery the injection of normal salt solution beneath the skin.
   i., arterial, saline injection made into an artery.
   i., subcutaneous (sŭb″kû-tā′nē-ŭs), saline injection made into the subcutaneous connective tissue, usually under the breast, over the shoulder blade, or in the outer side of the thigh.
   i., venous, saline injection made into a vein.

ingest (ĭn-jĕst′). To throw in, or put in, as food into the stomach.

ingesta (ĭn-jĕs′tä). Food taken into the body by the mouth.

ingestion (ĭn-jĕs′chŭn). The act of putting or taking food into the stomach.

inguinal (ĭng′gwĭ-năl). Pertaining to the groin.

inlet (ĭn′lĕt). The upper limit of the pelvic cavity (brim).

innominatum (ĭ-nŏm″ĭ-nā′tŭm). The innominate bone.

insemination (ĭn-sĕm-ĭ-nā′shŭn). Impregnation; fertilization of the ovum.
   artificial i., introduction of semen into the vagina by artificial means.
   donor i., artificial insemination in which the semen used is that of a man other than the woman's husband. A.I.D.
   homologous i., artificial insemination in which the husband's semen is used. Also called A.I.H.

insinuating (ĭn-sĭn′û-āt-ing). 1. Suggesting or hinting. 2. Instilling or infusing subtly or artfully. 3. Bringing or introducing into a position or relation by indirect or artful measures.

insomnia (ĭn-sŏm′nĭ-ă). Want of sleep; wakefulness; chronic or habitual privation of sleep.

insufflation (ĭn-sŭ-flā′shŭn). The act of blowing a powder, vapor, gas or air into a cavity.

integument (ĭn-tĕg′û-mĕnt). The covering of the body—the skin.

interstitial (ĭn-tĕr-stĭsh′ăl). Pertaining to or situated in the spaces or gaps of a tissue.

intertrigo (ĭn″tĕr-trī′gō). An excoriation or galling of the skin about the anus, axilla or other part of the body, with inflammation and moisture.

introitis (ĭn-trō′ĭ-tŭs). A term applied to the opening of the vagina.

inunction (ĭn-ŭngk′shŭn). The act of rubbing in an ointment, or simply of anointing. This is a method of applying certain substances to the cutaneous surface, the object being to promote their absorption.

in utero. Inside the uterus.

inversion (ĭn-vûr′shŭn). A turning upside down, inside out, or end for end.
   i. of the uterus, the state of the womb being turned inside out, caused by violently drawing away the placenta before it is detached by the natural process of labor.

involution (ĭn″vŏ-lū′shŭn). 1. A rolling or pushing inward. 2. A retrograde process of change which is the reverse of evolution: particularly applied to the return of the uterus to its normal size and condition after parturition.

ischium (ĭs′kĭ-ŭm). The posterior and inferior bone of the pelvis, distinct and separate in the fetus or the infant, or the corresponding part of the innominate bone in the adult.

ischuria (ĭs-kū′rĭ-ă). Retention or suppression of urine.

iso- (ī′sŏ). A prefix or combining form meaning equal, alike, or the same.

jaundice (jôn'dĭs). Yellowness of skin, eyes and tissues, and secretions generally from impregnation with bilepigment; icterus.

jelly (jĕl'ĭ). A soft substance which is coherent, tremulous and more or less transparent.

    j. of Wharton, the soft, pulpy, connective tissue that constitutes the matrix of the umbilical cord.

juxtaposition (jŭks″tá-pŏ-zĭsh'ŭn). An adjacent situation; apposition.

Kahn's test. A precipitation test for syphilis.

keloid (kē'loid). A new growth or tumor of the skin, consisting of whitish ridges, nodules, and dense tissue.

Kiddie-Koop (kĭd'ē-koōp'). A type of bed for a baby which may be used instead of a crib.

knee-chest position. See *genupectoral position.*

labia (lā'bĭ-á). The nominative plural of *labium.* Lips or liplike structures.

    l. majora (má-jō'rá), the folds of skin containing fat and covered with hair which form each side of the vulva.

    l. minora (mĭ-nō'rá), the nymphae, or folds of delicate skin inside of the labia majora.

labor (lā'bēr). Parturition; the process by which a fetus is separated and expelled from its mother.

    artificial l., that which is facilitated or induced by mechanical or other extraneous means.

    dry l., when there is a lack of amniotic fluid.

    false l., one in which no progress toward delivery is made.

    induced l., labor brought on by artificial means.

    instrumental l., labor which is facilitated with the use of instruments.

    multiple l., labor with two or more fetuses present.

    obstructed l., that in which there is some mechanical hindrance, as from a tumor or contracted parturient canal.

    prolonged or **protracted l.,** one which is prolonged beyond the ordinary limit.

    spontaneous l., one which requires no artificial aid.

lac (lăk). Milk; any milklike medicinal preparation.

laceration (lăs″ēr-ā'shŭn). The act of tearing; a rent or torn place in any tissue; a wound made by tearing.

lactagogue (lăk'tá-gŏg). See *galactagogue.*

lactation (lăk-tā'shŭn). The act or period of giving milk; the secretion of milk; the time or period of secreting milk.

lacteal (lăk'tē-ăl). Resembling or relating to milk.

    l. calculus, a concretion of thickened milk occurring in the breast.

    l. swelling, swelling of the breast from accumulation of milk due to obstruction of the lacteal ducts.

lactiferous (lăk-tĭf'ēr-ŭs). Practically the same as *lacteal.*

lactoglobulin (lăk'tō-glŏb'ū-lĭn). The globulin of milk

lactometer (lăk-tŏm'ē-tēr). An hydrometer for determining the specific gravity of milk.

laity (lā'ĭ-tĭ). The nonprofessional portion of the people.

lambdoid, lambdoidal (lăm'doid, lăm-doi'dăl). Having the shape of the Greek letter Λ.

    l. suture, the suture between the occipital and two parietal bones.

lancinating (lăn'sĭ-nāt-ing). Tearing, darting or sharply cutting.

lanugo (lá-nū'gō). The fine hair on the body of the fetus. The fine, downy hair found on nearly all parts of the body except the palms of the hands and the soles of the feet.

laparotomy (lăp'á-rŏt'ō-mĭ). Surgical incision through the flank; less correctly but more generally, abdominal section at any point.

laparotrachelotomy (lăp'á-rō-trā-kĕl-ŏt-ō-mĭ). Cesarean section done by incising the cervix and the lower uterine segment; low or cervical cesarean section.

legitimacy (lĕ-jĭt′ĭ-mȧ-sĭ). The condition of having been born in wedlock.

lesion (lē′zhŭn). A hurt, wound or injury of a part; a pathologic alteration of a tissue.

lethargy (lĕth′ẽr-jĭ). A state of marked drowsiness, stupor or sleep which cannot easily be driven off.

leukorrhea (lū″kŏ-rē′ȧ). A whitish discharge from the female genital organs.

L.H. Abbreviation for luteinizing hormone.

lightening (līt″n-ĭng). The sensation of decreased abdominal distention produced by the descent of the uterus into the pelvic cavity, which occurs from two to three weeks before the onset of labor.

linea (lĭn′ĕ-ȧ). Pl. *lineae* (lĭn′ĕ-ē). A line or thread.

l. **alba** (ăl′bȧ), the central tendinous line extending from the pubic bone to the ensiform cartilage.

l. **albicantes** (ăl″bĭ-kănt-ēs′), shining whitish lines upon the abdomen caused by pregnancy or distention; old striae gravidarum.

l. **nigra** (nī′grä). A dark line appearing on the abdomen and extending from the pubis toward the umbilicus—considered one of the signs of pregnancy.

lingua (lĭng′gwȧ). Tongue.

l. **frenum,** tonguetie.

liquor (lĭk′ẽr). A liquid.

l. **amnii** (lĭ′kwôr ăm′nĭ-ī), the fluid contained within the amnion in which the fetus floats.

lithopedion (lĭth-ŏ-pē′dĭ-ŏn). A dead fetus that has become stony or petrified.

lithotomy position (lĭ-thŏt′ŏ-mĭ). The position of a patient flat on the back with legs and thighs flexed and thighs separated widely; also called the *dorsosacral* posture.

lochia (lō′kĭ-ȧ). The discharge from the genital canal during several days subsequent to delivery.

lochial (lō′kĭ-ăl). Relating to lochia.

lues (lū′ēz). The plague; more frequently syphilis.

lumen (lū′mĕn). A transverse section of the clear space within a tube.

lutein (lū′tĕ-ĭn). A yellow pigment from the corpus luteum; from fat cells; and from the yolk of eggs.

lying-in. The puerperal state.

l. **fever,** puerperal fever.

l. **hospital,** a hospital where pregnant women are cared for before, during, and after labor.

maceration (măs′ẽr-ā′shŭn). The softening of a solid by soaking.

malaise (măl-āz′). A vague feeling of bodily discomfort.

malformation (măl-fôr-mā′shŭn). Defective or abnormal formation; deformity.

malposition (măl″pŏ-zĭsh′ŭn). An abnormal position, as of the fetus; a displacement.

malpractice (măl″prăk′tĭs). Practice contrary to good judgment, whether from ignorance or carelessness.

malpresentation (măl-prez″ĕn-tā′shŭn). A faulty, abnormal, or untoward fetal presentation.

mamma (măm′ȧ). Pl. *mammae*. ["Mama," the instinctive cry of an infant.] The breast of the human female.

maneuver (mȧ-nōō′vẽr). A planned and regulated movement; any dextrous proceeding.

mania (mā′nĭ-ȧ). A form of insanity marked by an exalted but perverted mental activity.

manual (măn′ū-ăl). Relating to, or performed by, the hands.

marasmus (mȧ-răz′mŭs). Wasting or emaciation.

mask (mȧsk) of pregnancy. See *chloasma*.

massage (mȧ-säzh′). The systematic therapeutic use of rubbing, kneading, stroking, slapping, straining, pressure and other passive exercises applied to the muscles and accessible parts.

mastitis (măs-tī′tĭs). Inflammation of the breast.

maternal (mȧ-tûr′năl). Relating to, or originating with, the mother.

maternity (mȧ-tûr′nĭ-tĭ). 1. Motherhood;

the condition of being a mother.
2. A lying-in hospital.

m. nurse, an obstetric nurse.

matrix (mā'trĭks). Uterus or womb. That which gives origin or form to a thing or serves to enclose it; a formative part.

maturation (măt″ū-rā'shŭn). In biology, a process of cell division during which the number of chromosomes in the germ cells is reduced to one half the number characteristic of the species.

meatus (mĕ-ā'tŭs). A passage; an opening leading to a canal, duct or cavity.

m. urinarius (ū″rĭ-nā'rĭ-ŭs), the external orifice of the urethra.

mechanism (mĕk'ȧ-niz'm). The manner of combinations which subserve a common function. In obstetrics refers to labor and delivery.

meconium (mĕ-kō'nĭ-ŭm). The dark-green or black substance found in the large intestine of the fetus or newly born infant.

melancholia (mĕl″ăn-kō'lĭ-ȧ). A form of insanity (and a condition of mind bordering upon insanity) in which there is great depression of spirits, with gloomy forebodings.

melena (mĕ-lē'nȧ). The passage of dark, pitchy, grumous stools stained with blood pigment.

m. neonatorum. Due to the extravasation of blood into the alimentary canal.

membrane (mĕm'brān). A skinlike tissue used to cover some part of the body and sometimes forming a secreting surface. *Mucous membranes* line cavities and canals which communicate with the external air, as the nose, the mouth, etc. *Serous membranes* line cavities which have no external communication, such as the pleural and the peritoneal cavities. They have a smooth, glossy surface from which exudes a transparent serous fluid that gives to them their name. When this fluid is secreted in excess, edema of those parts is the result. The word "Membranes" is also used to indicate the amniotic sac which surrounds the fetus.

menarche (mĕ-när'kĕ). The establishment or the beginning of the menstrual function.

menopause (mĕn'ō-pôz). The period at which menstruation ceases; the "change of life."

menorrhagia (mĕn″ō-rā'jĭ-ȧ). An abnormally profuse menstrual flow.

menses (mĕn'sēz). [Pl. of Latin *mensis*, month.] The periodic monthly discharge of blood from the uterus; the catamenia.

menstruation (mĕn″strŏŏ-ā'shŭn). The monthly period of the discharge of a red fluid from the uterus; the function of menstruating. It occurs from puberty to the menopause.

mentum (mĕn'tŭm). The chin.

mesial (mē'zĭ-ăl). Situated in the middle; toward the middle line of the body.

mesoderm (mĕs'ō-dûrm). The middle layer of cells derived from the primitive embryo.

metabolism (mĕ-tăb'ō-lĭz'm). The sum of all the physical and chemical processes by which living organized substance is produced and maintained, and also the transformation by which energy is made available for the uses of the organism.

m., basal, the minimal heat produced by an individual measured from fourteen to eighteen hours after eating and when the individual is at rest but not asleep.

metamorphosis (mĕt″ȧ-môr'fō-sĭs). Change of shape or structure; particularly the transition from one developmental stage to another.

metritis (mĕ-trī'tĭs). Inflammation of the uterus; several varieties according to the part affected.

metrorrhagia (mē-trō-rā'jĭ-ȧ). Abnormal uterine bleeding.

microcephalus (mī-krō-sĕf'ȧ-lŭs). Fetus with a very small head.

microscopic (mī″krŏ-skŏp'ĭk). So minute that it can be seen only by means of a microscope.

micturition (mĭk″tû-rĭsh′ŭn). The act of voiding urine.

midwife (mĭd′wĭf″). A woman who delivers women with child; a female obstetrician.

migration (mĭ-grā′shŭn). In obstetrics refers to the passage of the ovum from the ovary to the uterus.

milk-leg. See *phlegmasia alba dolens.*

miscarriage (mĭs-kăr′ĭj). The expulsion of the fetus at any time between the third and sixth month of gestation. More generally used to indicate the expulsion of the fetus at any time up to the period of viability of the fetus.

mitosis (mĭ-tō′sĭs). Indirect cell division; typical mode of division of the active somatic cells and germ cells.

molding (mōld′ĭng). The shaping of the baby's head so as to adjust itself to the size and shape of the birth canal.

mole. A fleshy mass in the uterus. Hydatidiform myxoma formed by cystic degeneration of villi of the chorion.

monozygotic (mŏn″ō-zī-gŏt′ĭk). Pertaining to or derived from one zygote.

   m. twins (mŏn″ō-zī-gŏ′tĭk). Pertaining to or derived from one zygote.

mons veneris (mŏnz vĕn′ĕ-rĭs). The eminence in the upper and anterior part of the pubes of women.

monster (mŏn′stēr). A fetus born with a redundancy or a deficiency, a confusion or transposition, of parts. For example, a child born with two heads or with but one eye.

monstrosity (mŏn-strŏs′ĭ-tĭ). A monster.

Montgomery's tubercles (mŭnt-gŭm′ ĕr-ĭz). Small, nodular follicles or glands on the areolae around the nipples.

morbid (môr′bĭd). Diseased or pertaining to disease. Morbid is used as a technical or scientific term in contradistinction to the term healthy.

morbidity, morbility (môr-bĭd′ĭ-tĭ, môr-bĭl′ĭ-tĭ). 1. The condition of being diseased. 2. The amount of disease or illness existing in a given community; the sick-rate.

morula (môr′û-lȧ). A stage of the segmented ovum; it forms a solid mass of cells.

mother's mark. Nevus; birthmark.

mucosa (mû-kō′sȧ). A mucous membrane.

mucous (mū′kŭs). Belonging to or resembling mucus; covered with a slimy secretion or with a coat that is soluble in water and becomes slimy.

   m. membrane. See *membrane.*

mucus (mū′kŭs). The viscid liquid secretion of a mucous membrane.

multigravida (mŭl″tĭ-grăv′ĭ-dȧ). A woman who has been pregnant several times, or many times.

multipara (mŭl-tĭp′ȧ-rȧ). A woman who has borne several, or many, children.

mummification (mŭm″ĭ-fĭ-kā′shŭn). The shriveling up and compression of a dead fetus.

myoma (mī-ō′mȧ). Any tumor made up of muscular elements.

narcosis (när-kō′sĭs). Unconsciousness produced by a drug.

nates (nā′tēz). The buttocks.

navel (nāv′ĕl). The umbilicus.

   n. string, the umbilical cord.

neonatal (nē″ō-nā′tăl). Pertaining to the newborn, usually considered the first two weeks of life.

nephritis (nē-frī′tĭs). Inflammation of the kidney.

neurosis (nû-rō′sĭs). A nervous affection, without obvious disease, hysteria.

neurotic (nû-rŏt′ĭk). Of or belonging to the nerves; nervous.

neutral (nū′trăl). Neither one nor the other; indifferent.

   n. reaction, a reaction which is neither acid nor alkaline.

nevus (nē′vŭs). A natural mark or blemish; a mole, a circumscribed deposit of pigmentary matter in the skin present at birth (birthmark).

nidation (nĭ-dā′shŭn). The implantation of the fertilized ovum (embryo) in the endometrium of the pregnant uterus.

nodule (nŏd′ūl). A little node; a small rounded mass.

normal (nôr′măl). Regular; without any deviation from the ordinary structure or function; according to rule.

nucleus (nū'klē-ŭs). The essential part or core of a cell.

nullipara (nŭ-lĭp'a-ra). A woman who has not borne children.

obstetric (ŏb-stĕt'rĭk). Belonging to midwifery or obstetrics.

obstetrician (ŏb-stĕ-trĭsh'ăn). An accoucheur, or man-midwife; a practitioner of obstetrics; one who is skilled in obstetrics.

obstetrics (ŏb-stĕt'rĭks). [Latin, *obstetrix*, midwife.] Art of assisting women in childbirth and treating their diseases in pregnancy and after delivery; midwifery.

obturator (ŏb"tū-rā'tēr). A disk or plate, natural or artificial, which closes an opening.

　o., Holmes, an instrument used in packing the uterus.

occipitobregmatic (ŏk-sĭp"ĭt-ō-brĕg-măt'-ĭk). Pertaining to the occiput (the back part of the head) and the bregma (junction of the coronal and sagittal sutures).

occiput (ŏk'sĭ-pŭt). The back part of the head.

oligohydramnios (ŏl"ĭ-gŏ-hī-drăm'nĭ-ŏs). Deficiency of amniotic fluid.

oliguria (ŏl"ĭg-ū'rĭ-a). Deficient secretion of urine.

omphalic (ŏm-făl'ĭk). Pertaining to the umbilicus.

oocyesis (ō'ŏ-sī-ē'sĭs). Ovarian pregnancy.

opacity (ō-păs'ĭ-tĭ). 1. Incapability of transmitting light; the reverse of transparency. 2. Any defect in the transparency of the cornea, from a slight film to an intense whiteness.

operculum (ō-pûr'kŭ-lŭm). Any lid or covering. Mucous plug which shuts off the contents of a gravid uterus from the vagina.

ophthalmia (ŏf-thăl'mĭ-a). Severe inflammation of the eye.

　o. neonatorum, purulent blennorrhea of the newborn.

orexia (ō-rĕk'sĭ-a). Appetite.

organ (ôr'găn). A part of an animal or vegetable capable of performing some act or office appropriate to itself, as, for example, the heart, the lungs or the stomach.

orifice (ŏr'ĭ-fĭs). The entrance or outlet of any bodily cavity; any foramen, meatus or opening.

os (ŏs). Pl. *ora* (ō'ra). Mouth.

　o. externum (*external os*), the external opening of the canal of the cervix.

　o. internum (*internal os*), internal opening of canal of cervix.

　o. uteri, "mouth of the uterus."

os. (Pl. *ossa*, ŏs'a.) A bone.

　o. innominatum, the innominate bone.

osmosis (ŏs-mō'sĭs). The power or action by which liquids are impelled through a moist membrane and other porous partitions.

ossification (ŏs"ĭ-fĭ-kā'shŭn). The formation of bone or of a bony substance.

osteomalacia (ŏs"tē-ŏ-ma-lā'shĭ-a). A disease marked by progressive softening of the bones from loss of their mineral constituents, so that they become flexible and fragile and unable to support the body. The disease affects adults, especially pregnant women, and frequently causes extreme pelvic contraction.

ova. Plural of ovum.

ovarian (ŏ-vâr'ĭ-ăn). Belonging to the ovary.

ovary (ō'va-rĭ). The sexual gland of the female in which the ova are developed. There are two ovaries, one at each side of the pelvis.

oviduct (ō'vĭ-dŭkt). The fallopian tube which conveys the ovum from the ovary to the uterus.

ovisac (ō'vĭ-săc). Same as *graafian follicle.*

ovulation (ō-vū-lā'shŭn). The growth and discharge of an unimpregnated ovum, usually coincident with the menstrual period.

ovule (ō'vūl). A "little egg." The ovum before its discharge from the graafian follicle.

ovum (ō'vŭm). 1. An egg, particularly a hen's egg. 2. The female reproductive cell. The human ovum is a round cell about $\frac{1}{120}$ of an inch in diameter, developed in the ovary.

oxytocic (ŏk″sĭ-tō′sĭk). 1. Accelerating parturition. 2. A medicine which accelerates parturition.

oxytocin (ŏk-sĭ-tō-sĭn). One of the two hormones secreted by the posterior pituitary.

palpation (păl-pā′shŭn). [Latin, *pal-pa′re*, to handle gently, to feel.] Examination by the hand or by touch; manipulation of a part with the fingers for the purpose of determining the condition of the underlying organs.

    p., obstetric, palpation of the abdomen of the pregnant woman to determine the size, position and presentation of the fetus.

palpitation (păl″pĭ-tā′shŭn). Convulsive motion of a part: applied especially to the rapid action of the heart, whether caused by disease or by excitement.

palsy (pôl′zĭ). A synonym for paralysis, used in connection with certain special forms.

    Bell's p., peripheral facial paralysis due to lesion of the facial nerve, resulting in distortion of the face.

    birth p., palsy due to injury occurring at birth.

    Erb's p., the upper-arm type of brachial birth palsy.

papilla (pá-pĭl′á). Pl. *papillae* (pá-pĭl′ē). Originally, a "pimple." Any minute, nipplelike eminence.

papyraceous (păp-ĭ-rā′shŭs). Like paper.

para (pär′ä). The term used to designate the number of viable babies the woman has delivered.

parametrium (păr-á-mē′trĭ-ŭm). The fibrous subserous coat of the supravaginal portion of the uterus, extending laterally between the layers of the broad ligaments.

parenchyma (pá-rĕng′kĭ-má). The essential or functional elements of an organ as distinguished from its stoma or framework.

parenteral (păr-ĕn′tĕr-ăl). In a manner other than through the alimentary canal; i.e., either subcutaneous or intravenous.

parietal (pá-rī′ĕ-tăl). Belonging to the parietes or walls of any cavity, organ, etc.

    p. bones, the two quadrangular bones that form the transverse arch of the cranium.

parity (păr′ĭ-tĭ). The condition of a woman with respect to her having borne children.

parovarian (pär-ŏ-vâr′ĭ-ăn). Pertaining to the residual structure in the broad ligament between the ovary and the fallopian tube.

paroxysm (păr′ŏk-sĭz′m). An evident increase of symptoms which, after a certain time, decline; a periodic fit or attack; the periodic fits or attacks which characterize certain diseases.

parturient (pär-tū′rĭ-ĕnt). Bringing forth; child-bearing.

    p. canal, the canal through which the fetus passes in childbirth: it consists of the uterus and the vagina regarded as one canal.

    p. woman, a woman about to give birth to a child.

parturition (pär″tū-rĭsh′ŭn). Expulsion of the fetus from the uterus; also the state of being in childbed; labor.

pasteurization (păs″tĕr-ĭ-zā′shŭn). The process by which disease and spoilage organisms are destroyed or checked by maintaining a temperature of 145° F. for one-half hour.

pathology (pá-thŏl′ŏ-jĭ). The doctrine or consideration of diseases; that branch of medical science which treats of diseases, their nature and effects.

patulous (păt′ū-lŭs). Spreading somewhat widely apart; open.

p.c. Abbreviation for after meals, also complementary feedings.

pelvimeter (pĕl-vĭm′ĕ-tĕr). An instrument for measuring the diameters and capacity of the pelvis.

pelvimetry (pĕl-vĭm′ĕ-trĭ). The obstetric measurement of the pelvis. It may be performed with the hand (*digital p.*) or with a pelvimeter (*instrumental p.*). When the measurements are made on the outside of the body it is *external p.*; when within the vagina, *internal p.*; and when both within the vagina and outside of the body, *combined p.*

pemphigus (pĕm′fĭ-gŭs). A skin infection found in the newborn.

penicillin (pĕn′ĭ-sĭl′ĭn). An antibiotic compound, obtained from cultures of *Penicillium notatum*, which is bacteriostatic for numerous bacteria and other micro-organisms.

penis (pē′nĭs). The male organ of copulation.

perforator (pûr′fŏ-rā″tēr). An instrument for boring into the cranium.

perineorrhaphy (pĕr″ĭ-nē-ŏr′a-fĭ). Suture of the perineum; the operation for the repair of lacerations of the perineum.

perineotomy (pĕr′ĭ-nē-ŏt′ō-mĭ). A surgical incision through the perineum.

perineum (pĕr″ĭ-nē′ŭm). The space between the genital organs and the anus.

periphery (pĕ-rĭf′ēr-ĭ). The circumference of a circle; the parts most remote from the center.

peristalsis (pĕr″ĭ-stăl′sĭs). The peculiar movement of the intestines and other tubular organs, like that of a worm in its progress, by which they gradually propel their contents. Peristalsis is produced by the combined action of circular and longitudinal muscular fibers.

peritoneum (pĕr″ĭ-tŏ-nē′ŭm). A strong serous membrane investing the inner surface of the abdominal walls and the viscera of the abdomen.

peritonitis (pĕr″ĭ-tŏ-nī′tĭs). Inflammation of the peritoneum.

pernicious (pēr-nĭsh′ŭs). Baleful; deleterious; highly dangerous: as pernicious anemia, or pernicious vomiting.

pessary (pĕs′a-rĭ). An instrument, usually in the form of a ring or a ball, for introduction into the vagina, to prevent or remedy the prolapse of the uterus.

phantom (făn′tŭm). The small effigy of a child used to illustrate the progress of labor.

p. pregnancy, feigned, hysterical, spurious or false pregnancy, pseudocyesis.

p. tumor, a tumor of the abdomen due to flatus or contraction of the abdominal muscles.

phenomenon (fĕ-nŏm′ĕ-nŏn). Pl. *phenomena*. An appearance; anything remarkable. In pathology it is synonymous with symptom.

phimosis (fĭ-mō′sĭs). Tightness of the foreskin.

phlebitis (flĕ-bī′tĭs). Inflammation of a vein.

phlebothrombosis (flĕb″ŏ-thrŏm-bō′sĭs). Presence of a clot in the vein, unassociated with inflammation of the wall of the vein.

phlegmasia alba dolens (flĕg-mā′zhĭ-a ăl′ba dō′lĕnz). Phlebitis of the femoral vein following delivery.

phlegmatic (flĕg-măt′ĭk). Dull; sluggish; cold; morose; not easily excited. The opposite of *nervous* when applied to one's disposition.

physiologic (fĭz″ĭ-ŏ-lŏj′ĭk). Belonging to physiology.

physiology (fĭz″ĭ-ŏl′ŏ-jĭ). The doctrine of vital phenomena, or the science of the functions of living bodies.

physique (fĭ-zēk′). Natural constitution; corporeal form; personal endowments; the physical or exterior parts of a person.

pigment (pĭg′mĕnt). 1. Any dye or paint. 2. The normal coloring-matter of the organs and fluids of the body.

pigmentation (pĭg″mĕn-tā′shŭn). The formation or deposition of pigment.

Pitocin (pĭ-tŏ′sĭn). A proprietary solution, the oxytocic principle of the posterior lobe of the pituitary. It is used to stimulate uterine contractions and to arrest postpartum bleeding.

placenta (pla-sĕn′ta). The circular, flat, vascular structure forming in the impregnated uterus forming the principal medium of communication between the mother and the fetus.

ablatio p., premature detachment of a normal placenta.

abruptio p., premature separation of the placenta.

accessory p., a portion of placental tissue distinct from the placenta.

accreta p., a form of adherent placenta in which, owing to the absence of decidua at the placental site, the villi penetrate the uterine muscle and make separation impossible.

adherent p., one which adheres so closely to the uterine wall that it is impossible to find any line of cleavage for placental separation.

battledore p., one with a marginal attachment of the cord.

fetal p., the exposed part of the placenta from which the cord arises.

maternal p., that part of the placenta which comes next to the uterine wall.

previa p., a placenta which develops in the lower uterine segment, in the zone of dilatation, so that it adjoins or covers the internal os.

retained p., a placenta usually either adherent or incarcerated by irregular uterine contractions which, in consequence, fails to be expelled after the delivery of the baby.

platypeloid (plăt″ĭ-pĕl′oid). Flat type of female pelvis.

plethora (plĕth′ō-ra). A condition characterized by fullness of the blood vessels, strong heart action and pulse, florid complexion and general plumpness of the body.

plethoric (plĕ-thŏr′ĭk). Relating to plethora; full of blood.

pleura (plŏŏr′a). A serous membrane, divided into two portions and lining the right and left cavities of the chest or thorax.

plexus (plĕk′sŭs). A network or tangle, chiefly of veins or nerves.

podalic (pŏ-dăl′ĭk). By means of or relating to the feet.

p. version, version by which the feet of the fetus are made to present.

pole (pōl). The extremity of the axis of a sphere.

polydactylism (pŏl-ĭ-dăk′tĭl-ĭz′m). The occurrence of more than the usual number of fingers or toes. It is usually familial.

polyhydramnios (pŏl″ĭ-hĭ-drăm′nĭ-ŏs). Hydramnion; excess in the amount of the amniotic fluid.

position (pŏ-zĭsh′ŭn). The situation of the fetus in the pelvis; determined and described by the relation of a given arbitrary point (of direction) in the presenting part to the periphery of the pelvic planes.

postnatal (pōst-nā′tăl). Occurring after birth.

postpartum (pōst-pär′tŭm). After childbirth; subsequent to childbirth.

p. chill, a chill, lasting several minutes, often following expulsion of the child.

p. hemorrhage, hemorrhage following delivery.

p. shock, the exhaustion immediately following labor.

postpuerperal (pōst″pū-ûr′pĕr-ăl). Occurring after childbirth.

Poupart's ligament (pŏŏ-pärts′). A fibrous band running from the anterior superior spine of the ilium to the spine of the pubis.

preeclampsia (prē-ĕk-lămp′sĭ-a). Toxic condition due to pregnancy.

pregnancy (prĕg′năn-sĭ). [Latin, *praeg′-nans*, literally "previous to bringing forth."] The state of being with young or with child. The normal duration of pregnancy in the human female is two hundred and eighty days, or ten lunar months, or nine calendar months.

pregnant (prĕg′nănt). With young or with child.

premature (prē″ma-tūr′). Before it is ripe.

premonitory (prē-mŏn′ĭ-tō″rĭ). Advising beforehand; giving previous warning; precursory; applied to symptoms which give an indication or warning of the advent or onset of certain diseases—for instance, chills, during the invasion of fever.

p. **pains,** painless uterine contractions before the beginning of true labor.

prepuce (prē'pūs). The fold of skin which covers the glans penis in the male.

p. **of the clitoris,** the fold of mucous membrane which covers the glans clitoridis.

presentation (prĕ"zĕn-tā'shŭn). Term used to designate that part of the fetus nearest the internal os; or that part which is felt by the physician's examining finger when introduced into the cervix.

primigravida (prī"mĭ-grăv'ĭ-dà). Pl. *primigravidae* (prī"mĭ-grăv'ĭ-dē). A woman who is pregnant for the first time.

primipara (prī-mĭp'à-rà). Pl. *primiparae* (prī-mĭp'à-rē). A woman who is bearing or who has brought forth her first child.

primordial (prī-môr'dĭ-ăl). Original or primitive; of the simplest and most undeveloped character.

prodromal (prŏ-drō'măl). Premonitory; indicating the approach of a disease.

progesterone (prō-jĕs'tēr-ōn). The pure hormone contained in the corpora lutea whose function is to prepare the endometrium for the reception and development of the fertilized ovum.

prognosis (prŏg-nō'sĭs). The foreknowledge of the course of a disease drawn from a consideration of its signs and symptoms; the art of forecasting the progress and termination of any given case of disease.

prognosticate (prŏg-nŏs'tĭ-kāt). To make a prognosis.

prognostic symptom (prŏg-nŏs'tĭk). A symptom from a consideration of which a prognosis of any particular disease is formed.

prolactin (prŏ-lăk'tĭn). A proteohormone from the anterior pituitary which stimulates lactation in the mammary glands.

prolan (prō'lăn). Zondek's term for the gonadotropic principle of human-pregnancy urine, responsible for the biologic pregnancy tests.

prolapse (prŏ-lăps'). A falling down, partial or complete, of some viscus, in its latest stage accompanied by protrusion so as to be partly external or uncovered.

p. **of the cord,** descent of the umbilical cord on the bursting of the bag of waters.

p. **of the uterus,** descent of the uterus, "falling of the womb."

proliferate (prŏ-lĭf'ēr-āt). To grow by the reproduction of similar cells.

promontory (prŏm'ŭn-tō"rĭ). A small projection; a prominence.

p. **of the sacrum,** the superior or projecting portion of the sacrum when in situ in the pelvis, at the junction of the sacrum and the last lumbar vertebra.

protein (prō'tē-ĭn). Any one of a class of organic compounds forming the important part of animal and vegetable tissue. The protein in milk is the part responsible for forming the curd.

pruritis (proo-rī'tŭs). An intense degree of itching.

pseudocyesis (sū"dō-sī-ē'sĭs). An apparent condition of pregnancy; the woman really believes she is pregnant when as a matter of fact she is not.

psychic (sī'kĭk). Belonging to the mind or intellect.

psychosomatic (sī'kō-sō-măt-ĭc). Pertaining to mind and body relationship; having bodily symptoms of a psychic or mental origin.

ptyalism (tī'à-lĭz'm). Increased and involuntary flow of saliva.

puberty (pū'bēr-tĭ). The age at which the generative organs become functionally active.

pubic (pū'bĭk). Belonging to the pubis.

pubiotomy (pū'bī-ŏt'ŏ-mĭ). The operation of cutting through the pubic bone lateral to the median line.

pubis (pū'bĭs). The os pubis or pubic bone forming the front of the pelvis. Sometimes, but incorrectly, written *pubes.*

pudendal (pū-děn′dǎl). Relating to the pudendum.

pudendum (pū-děn′dŭm). [Latin, *pude′re*, to have shame or modesty.] The external genital organs or parts of generation of either sex, but especially of the female: also used, perhaps more correctly, in the plural (*pudenda*).

puerpera (pū-ûr′pēr-ȧ). A woman in childbed, or one who has lately been delivered.

puerperal (pū-ûr′pēr-ȧl). Belonging to, or consequent on, childbearing.

  p. convulsions, epileptiform convulsions occurring immediately before or after childbirth.

  p. eclampsia, same as puerperal convulsions. See *eclampsia*.

  p. fever, a severe febrile disease which sometimes occurs in the puerperal state, usually about the third day after childbirth, accompanied by an inflamed condition of the peritoneum, due to septic infection.

  p. insanity or **mania**, insanity occurring in females toward the end of pregnancy or soon after delivery.

  p. state, the condition of a woman in, and immediately after, childbirth.

puerperium (pū″ēr-pē′rĭ-ŭm). The state or period of a woman in confinement.

pungent (pŭn′jěnt). Sharp or biting; acri t.

purpura (pûr′pū-rȧ). A disease in which there are small distinct purple specks and patches on the surface of the body, with general debility but not always fever.

purpuric (pûr-pū′rĭk). Relating to purpura.

purulent (pū′rŏŏ-lěnt). Consisting of pus; of the nature of pus.

pus (pŭs). A bland, creamlike fluid composed of cells and a thin fluid called liquor puris, found in abscesses or on the surface of sores; matter; "corruption."

pyelitis (pī-ě-lī′tĭs). Inflammation of the pelvis of the kidney.

pyrosis (pī-rō′sĭs). Heartburn; a burning sensation in the esophagus and the stomach, with a sour eructation.

quickening (kwĭk′ěn-ĭng). The mother's first perception of the movements of the fetus.

rabbit test. See *Friedman test*.

racemose (răs′ē-mōs). Resembling a bunch of grapes on its stalk.

rachitic (rȧ-kĭt′ĭk). Pertaining to or affected with rickets.

rachitis (rȧ-kī′tĭs). Rickets.

rational (răsh′ŭn-ǎl). Comformable to reason or to a well-reasoned plan; reasonable. Also applied to the mental state of a person.

  r. symptoms, symptoms communicated by the patient to the physician; subjective symptoms.

reaction (rē-ăk′shŭn). 1. Increase of the vital functions succeeding their depression. 2. The phenomena resulting from the action of two or more substances upon each other.

rectocele (rěk′tō-sēl). Prolapse of the rectum and the posterior vaginal wall.

reflex (rē′flěks). Reflected; caused by the conveyance of an impression to the central nervous system and its transmission through a motor nerve to the periphery without consciousness of individual.

regimen (rěj′ĭ-měn). A systematic regulation for some special purpose.

regurgitation (rē-gûr″jĭ-tā′shŭn). A flowing back; a flowing the wrong way: applied, for example, to the passive vomiting of infants and to the rising of food in the mouth of adults.

relaxation (rē″lăk-sā′shŭn). The reverse of contraction or tension; looseness; want of muscular tone or vigor.

remission (rē-mĭsh′ŭn). An abatement or diminution of symptoms.

renal (rē′nǎl). Belonging to the kidney.

restitution (rěs″tĭ-tū′shŭn). The act of restoring or returning something— particularly, rotation of the fetal head after its expulsion from the vagina, so that it looks in the same direction as it did before it entered the pelvic brim; external rotation of the fetal head.

resuscitation (rĕ-sŭs″ĭ-tā′shŭn). The act of restoring to life those who are apparently dead.

retained placenta. A placenta not expelled by the uterus after labor.

retention (rĕ-tĕn′shŭn). The keeping back or stoppage of any of the secretions, particularly the urine.

   r. of urine, a condition in which the urine is retained in the bladder and cannot be discharged voluntarily.

retroflexion (rĕt″rō-flĕk′shŭn). Bending backward, *e.g.*, retroflexion of the uterus when it is flexed backward.

retroversion (rĕt′rō-vûr′shŭn). Of the uterus when it is turned back.

Rh. Abbreviation for *rhesus*, a type of monkey. This term is used for a property of human blood cells, because of its relationship to a similar property in the blood cells of *rhesus* monkeys.

Rh factor. A term applied to an inherited antigen in the human blood.

rhachitic (rà-kĭt′ĭk). Relating to or affected with rhachitis or rickets.

   r. pelvis, a pelvis deformed by rickets.

rhachitis (rà-kī′tĭs). Rickets.

rhomboid (rŏm′boid). Shaped like a rhomb or a kite; refers to the diamond-shaped area over the posterior aspect of the pelvis formed by the dimples of the posterior superior spines of the ilia, the lines formed by the gluteal muscles and the groove at the end of the spine.

rhythm (rĭth′m). Term applied to the so-called "safe period," at which time (theoretically) it is impossible to conceive.

rickets (rĭk′ĕts). A disease of childhood in which there is a lack of the salts in the bones, with resultant curvatures and deformities of them, affections of the liver and spleen, and a condition of general weakness. Vitamin D and sunshine furnish the best mode of treatment.

Ritgen maneuver (rĭt′gĕn). Delivery of the baby's head by lifting the head

upward and forward through the vulva, between pains; by pressing with the tips of the fingers upon the perineum behind the anus.

roentgenogram (rŭnt′gĕn′ō-grăm″). The photograph made by roentgen rays which shows the precise measurements of the pelvis with a clear picture of the inlet and general pelvic architecture.

roentgenology (rŭnt″gĕn-ŏl′ō-jĭ). The branch of radiology which deals with the diagnostic and therapeutic use of roentgen rays.

rotation (rō-tā′shŭn). The act of turning round; the motion of any solid body about an axis.

   r. stage of labor, that stage of labor at which the presenting portion of the fetus rotates or turns around.

rudimentary (rōō″dĭ-mĕn′tà-rĭ). Undeveloped, elementary.

rumination (rōō-mĭ-nā′shŭn). The regurgitation of food, part of it being vomited, and the rest swallowed: a condition seen in infants.

rupture (rŭp′tūr). 1. Bursting or breaking of a part. 2. Hernia.

sacrosciatic (sā″krō-sī-ăt′ĭk). Pertaining to the sacrum and the ischium.

sagittal (săj′ĭ-tăl). Relating to, or shaped like, an arrow.

   s. suture, the suture which unites the parietal bones.

salivation (săl″ĭ-bā′shŭn). An excessive flow of the saliva. The word is practically synonymous with ptyalism but, strictly speaking, describes the condition when produced by the action of medicines.

sanguineous (săng-gwĭn′ē-ŭs). Bloody, bloodstained.

sapremia (sà-prē′mĭ-à). Intoxication due to the presence in the blood of the products of saprophytic and nonpathogenic bacteria.

saturated solution (săt′ū-rāt″ĕd). A solution which, at a given temperature, cannot contain more of the substance than it already contains.

scalpel (skăl′pĕl). A small knife, usually

with a straight blade which is fixed firmly in the handle; used in dissection and in surgical operations.

scapula (skăp′ū-lȧ). The shoulder blade.

Schultze's mechanism (shōōlt′sĕz). The expulsion of the placenta with the fetal surfaces presenting.

scrotum (skrō′tŭm). [Latin, "bag."] A pouch at the base of the penis in the male, containing the testicles and other organs.

sebaceous (sĕ-bā′shŭs). Fatty; suety: applied to glands which secrete an oily matter resembling suet. Resembling or pertaining to sebum or fat.

seborrhea (sĕb″ŏr-ē′ȧ). An excessive discharge from the sebaceous glands, forming white or yellowish, greasy scales.

    s. capitis (kă′pĭ-tĭs), seborrhea of the scalp; often referred to as "cradle or crib cap."

sebum (sē′bŭm). A thick, semiliquid substance discharged upon the surface of the skin, composed of fat and broken-down epithelial cells.

secretion (sĕ-krē′shŭn). 1. A function of the body by which various fluids or substances are separated from the blood, differing in different organs according to their peculiar functions: thus, the liver secretes the bile, the salivary glands the saliva, etc. 2. The substance secreted.

secundines (sĕk′ŭn-dīn). The afterbirth; the placenta, etc., expelled after the birth of a child.

segmentation (sĕg″mĕn-tā′shŭn). The process of division by which the fertilized ovum multiplies before differentiation into layers occurs.

semen (sē′mĕn). 1. A seed. 2. The fluid secreted by the male reproductive organs.

seminal (sĕm′ĭ-năl). Pertaining to seed or to the semen.

sepsis (sĕp′sĭs). 1. Putrefaction. 2. Infection and poisoning by putrefactive matter.

septic (sĕp′tĭk). Tending to putrefy; causing or due to putrefaction.

septicemia (sĕp′tĭ-sē′mĭ-ȧ). A morbid condition due to the presence of pathogenic bacteria and their associated poisons in the blood.

septum (sĕp′tŭm). A dividing membrane.

sequela (sĕ-kwē′lȧ). Any lesion or affection following or caused by an attack or disease.

serous (sēr′ŭs). Of the nature of serum; secreting serum.

    s. membrane. See under *membrane.*

serum (sēr′ŭm). The clear, straw-colored liquid which separates, in the clotting of blood, from the clot and the corpuscles.

shock (shŏk). A condition of sudden depression of the whole of the functions of the body, due to powerful impressions upon the system by physical injury or mental emotion. The former is termed *surgical* and the latter *mental* shock.

show (shō). 1. Popularly, the red-colored mucus discharged from the vagina shortly before childbirth; called also "labor-show." 2. The vaginal discharge in menstruation.

sibling (sĭb′lĭng). One of two or more offspring of the same parents.

Sims' position. [J. Marion *Sims,* noted American gynecologist, deceased.] That position of the patient in which she lies upon the left side and the front of the left chest, with the right leg strongly flexed, or "drawn up": called also *semiprone position* and *side position.*

    S. speculum (spĕk′ū-lŭm), a vaginal speculum with duck-bill blades: by it the posterior wall of the vagina is held up, while the anterior is depressed, the patient being placed in Sims' position.

sinciput (sĭn′sĭ-pŭt). The anterior and upper part of the head.

Skene's duct (skēnz′). Opening of the Skene's glands on the surface of the vulva.

Skene's gland. Two glands just within the meatus of the female urethra; regarded as homologues of the seminal vesicles.

skim milk (skĭm). Milk from which the cream has been removed, leaving only one or two per cent of fatty matter.

smegma (smĕg′mȧ). [From a Greek word meaning *soap.*] Sebum, especially the offensive, soaplike substance produced from the sebaceous follicles around the glans penis and the prepuce and in the region of the clitoris and the labia minora.

   s. embryo′num. Same as *vernix caseosa.*

solution (sȯ-lū′shŭn). 1. The act of dissolving a solid body. 2. A clear, homogeneous liquid having particles of a solid, another liquid, or a gas uniformly diffused through it, so that the particles are invisible and do not separate upon standing.

somatic (sȯ-măt′ĭk). Pertaining to the body; especially to the framework of the body, as distinguished from the viscera.

sordes (sôr′dēz). Literally, "filth": applied to the foul matter which collects on the teeth, particularly in certain low fevers.

souffle (sōōf′f′l). A soft, blowing, auscultatory sound. A hissing souffle synchronous with the fetal heart sounds and supposed to be produced in the umbilical cord.

   fetal s., a blowing sound sometimes heard in pregnancy; supposed to be due to compression of the umbilical vessels.

   funic s., a hissing souffle synchronous with the fetal heart sounds and supposed to be produced in the umbilical cord.

   placental s., a souffle supposed to be produced by the blood current in the placenta.

   umbilical s., same as funic.

   uterine s., a sound made by the blood within the arteries of the gravid uterus.

sound. [French, *sonder*, to fathom, to try the depth of the sea; hence, to try or examine.] An instrument for introduction through the urethra into the bladder, or into any canal.

specific (spĕ-sĭf′ĭk). 1. Relating to a species; distinguishing one species from another. 2. Suited for a particular purpose: as, a *specific* remedy. 3. Produced by a special cause. 4. A specific remedy; a remedy supposed to have a peculiar efficiency in the cure of a particular disease, or one which has a special action on some particular organ.

   s. disease, any disease produced by a special cause; as syphilis and the eruptive fevers. (The term is frequently, but wrongly, restricted to syphilis.)

   s. gravity, the weight of a body compared with that of another of equal volume taken as a standard: hydrogen is the standard for gases, and distilled water for liquids and solids.

speculum (spĕk′ū-lŭm). An instrument for examining canals.

spermatozoon (spûr″mȧ-tȯ-zō′ŏn). Pl. *spermatozoa* (spûr″mȧ-tȯ-zō′ȧ). The motile, microscopic sexual element of the male, resembling in shape an elongated tadpole. The male element in fecundation.

sphincter (sfĭngk′tēr). A ringlike muscle which closes a natural orifice.

sprue (sprōō). Thrush; sore mouth of infants, with the formation of white patches and superficial ulcers.

spurious (spū′rĭ-ŭs). Simulated; not genuine; false.

stenosis (stĕ-nō′sĭs). Narrowing or stricture of a duct or canal.

   pyloric s., hypertrophic obstruction of the pyloric orifice of the stomach, usually congenital.

sterile (stĕr′ĭl). 1. Affected with sterility; barren. 2. Not containing micro-organisms; aseptic.

sterility (stĕ-rĭl′ĭ-tĭ). Inability, whether natural or as the result of disease, to procreate offspring.

stigma (stĭg′mȧ). A characteristic mark or sign of defect, degeneration or disease.

stillborn (stĭl′bôrn″). Born without life; born dead.

stimulant (stĭm′ū-lănt). 1. Stimulating. 2. A medicine having power to excite organic action or to increase the vital activity of an organ. A *stimulant* differs from a *tonic* in that its action is more speedy, more transitory, and usually followed by a reaction.

stimulate (stĭm′ū-lāt). To excite the organic action of a part of the animal economy.

stimulus (stĭm′ū-lŭs). Pl. *stimuli.* A Latin word signifying a "goad," "sting," or "whip." In physiology, that which rouses or excites the vital energies, whether of the whole system or only of a part.

stoma (stō′má). An opening on a free surface; usually refers to the mouth.

stomatitis (stō′má-tī′tĭs). Inflammation of the mouth, usually accompanied by pain and salivation.

stool (stool). The feces discharged from the bowels; a dejection; an evacuation.

streptococcus (strĕp″tō-kŏk′ŭs). A variety of micro-organism.

stria (strī′á). Pl. *striae* (strī′ē). A Latin word signifying a "groove," "furrow," or "crease."

   s. gravidarum (grăv-ĭ-där′ŭm), shining, reddish lines upon the abdomen caused by pregnancy or distention by abdominal tumors.

Stroganoff's treatment (strō-găn′ŏfs). The treatment of puerperal eclampsia by means of morphine and chloral hydrate according to a definite routine, the aim being to arrest the convulsions before they can develop.

stroma (strō′má). The tissue that forms the ground substance, framework or matrix of an organ.

stupor (stū′pēr). A suspension or diminished activity of the mental faculties; loss of sensibility.

styptic (stĭp′tĭk). Having the power of stopping bleeding through an astringent quality; hemostatic.

subcutaneous (sŭb″kū-tā′nĕ-ŭs). Situated just under the skin.

subinvolution (sŭb′ĭn-vō-lū′shŭn). Fail-

ure of a part to return to its normal size and condition after enlargement from functional activity, as subinvolution of the uterus.

succedaneum (sŭk′sĕ-dā′nĕ-ŭm). See *caput.*

sudorific (sū′dēr-ĭf′ĭk). Promoting the flow of sweat; diaphoretic; an agent that causes sweating.

sulfonamide (sŭl-fŏn′á-mīd). The term applied to the group of sulfonamide compounds, such as, sulfanilamide, sulfapyridine, sulfathiazole.

superfecundation (sū′pēr-fē-kŭn-dā′-shŭn). The fertilization at about the same time of two different ova by sperm from different males.

superfetation (sū′pēr-fĕ-tā′shŭn). The fecundation of a woman already pregnant.

superficial (sū″pēr-fĭsh′ăl). On or near the surface.

suppository (sŭ-pŏz′ĭ-tō″rĭ). A preparation of some substance (usually cacao butter) fusible at the temperature of the body, and combined with some medicinal substance, for introduction into the rectum, the vagina, the urethra or other cavity of the body.

suppuration (sŭp″ū-rā′shŭn). The formation of pus or the processes giving rise to it.

suppurative (sŭp′ū-rā″tĭv). Producing or discharging pus.

suture (sū′tûr). 1. The junction of the bones of the cranium by a serated line resembling the stitches of a seam. 2. A stitch used to draw together the lips of a wound. 3. The thread or material used in making a stitch.

symphysiotomy (sĭm″fĭ-zĕ-ŏt′ō-mĭ). The operation of severing the ligaments and the fibrocartilages of the pubic symphysis; done in difficult labor.

symphysis (sĭm′fĭ-sĭs). The union of bones by means of an intervening substance; a variety of synarthrosis.

   s. pubis (pū′bĭs), "symphysis of the pubis," the pubic articulation or union of the pubic bones which are connected with each other by interarticular cartilage.

synchondrosis (sĭng″kŏn-drō′sĭs). A union of bones by means of a fibrous or elastic cartilage.

synchronous (sĭng′krō-nŭs). Occurring at the same time.

synclitism (sĭng′klĭ-tĭz′m). Parallelism between the planes of the fetal head and those of the pelvis.

syncope (sĭng′kō-pē). Literally a "cutting short" of one's strength; swooning or fainting; a suspension of respiration and the heart's action, complete or partial.

syndrome (sĭn′drōm). A set of symptoms which occur together.

systolic pressure (sĭs-tŏl′ĭk). The pressure in millimeters of mercury when the arterial impulse is heard or felt at the wrist at the time that the pressure on the arm band is released, after the pulse has been obliterated by pressure.

tactile (tăk′tĭl). Pertaining to the touch.

T-bandage. A bandage shaped like the letter T—especially one in which the transverse limb passes around the body, and the longitudinal one under the perineum. Used to hold dressings against the vulva.

tampon (tăm′pŏn). 1. A portion of gauze, sponge, etc., used in plugging a cavity or canal. 2. To apply a tampon to.

tenaculum (tĕ-năk′ū-lŭm). A small hook-shaped instrument.

   t. forceps, a volsella.

tenesmus (tĕ-nĕz′mŭs). A constant desire to go to stool or to urinate, with painful straining without the expulsion of feces or urine.

testicle (tĕs′tĭ-k′l). One of the two glands contained in the male scrotum.

tetany (tĕt′a-nĭ). A syndrome manifested by sharp flexion of wrist and ankle joints, muscle twitching, cramps and convulsions.

theca (thē′ka). A case or sheath, as the outer covering of the graafian follicle.

Theelin (thē′lĭn). A proprietary brand of estrone.

thelitis (thē-lī′tĭs). Inflammation of the nipple.

thermo- (thûr′mō). Combining form denoting relationship to heat.

thrombin (thrŏm′bĭn). The fibrin ferment of the blood: the enzyme, present in shed blood but not in circulating blood, which converts fibrinogen into fibrin.

thrombophlebitis (thrŏm′bŏ-flĕ-bī′tĭs). A condition in which inflammation of the vein wall has preceded the formation of the thrombus.

thrombosis (thrŏm-bō′sĭs). The formation or progress of a thrombus.

thrombus (thrŏm′bŭs). A clot formed in any part of the circulatory apparatus. It differs from an embolus in that it is developed at the point where it is found, while an embolus is brought from a distance through the blood vessels.

thrush (thrŭsh). Sprue; sore mouth attended by whitish spots in the mouth; may be followed by shallow ulcers.

tissue (tĭsh′ū). A weblike structure; a collection of cells or elements, of a constant structure and function, which go to make up the body. Examples: muscular tissue; brain tissue; bone tissue, etc.

toco- (tō′kō). Combining form denoting relationship to labor or delivery.

tocography (tō-kŏg′ra-fĭ). The graphic recording of uterine contractions.

tonguetie. See *freneum lingua.*

torsion (tôr′shŭn). A twisting.

   t. of the umbilical cord, the normal spontaneous twisting of the umbilical cord.

torticollis (tôr-tĭ-kŏl′ĭs). The contraction of the cervical muscles producing a twisting of the neck.

   congenital t., due to injury to the sternocleidomastoid muscle at the time of birth.

toxemia (tŏks-ē′mĭ-a). A general intoxication due to the absorption of bacterial products (toxins).

   t. pregnancy, toxemia due to poisons in the blood, derived presumably from the products of conception.

toxemic (tŏks-ē'mĭk). Relating to, or caused by, toxemia.

traction (trăk'shŭn). The act of drawing or pulling.

trauma (trô'mȧ). A wound or injury.

Trendelenburg's position or **posture** (trĕn'dĕ-lĕn-bōōrk). That position in which the patient is placed flat on the back with body and thighs elevated to an angle of about forty-five degrees, the legs hanging over the edge of the table. It is used in abdominal surgery so that the abdominal viscera may be kept out of the way by gravitation.

trichomonas (trĭk-ŏm'ŏ-năs). A genus of parasitic flagellate protozoa.

    t. vaginalis, a species found in the vagina, especially those with an acid secretion.

trophectoderm (trŏf-ĕk'tŏ-dûrm). The outer layer of cells of the early blastodermic vesicle; it develops the trophoderm—the feeding layer.

trophoblast (trŏf'ŏ-blăst) (nourishment). The epiblastic layers which line the chorionic villi in the fetal villi.

trophoblastic (trŏf″ŏ-blăs'tĭk). Pertaining to the epiblastic layers which line the chorionic villi in the fetal villi.

trophoderm (trŏf'ŏ-dûrm). A layer on the outside of the blastodermic vesicle by which attachment is made to the uterine wall and nourishment obtained therefrom.

tubercle (tū'bĕr-k'l). A rounded eminence.

tumor (tū'mēr). 1. A swelling. 2. A morbid growth of new tissue in any part of the body, not due to inflammation, and differing in structure from the part in which it grows. Tumors may be solid or hollow (*cystic t.*). When a tumor tends to recur after removal, and infect the system, it is called *malignant*; when it does not, *benign, innocent* or *nonmalignant*.

tympanites (tĭm″pȧ-nī'tēz). Distention of the abdomen by gas in the intestines or in the peritoneal cavity.

    t., uterine, distention of the uterus with gas; physometra.

ulcer (ŭl'sēr). A loss of substance on some internal or external surface from gradual disintegration and destruction of the tissue.

ulcerate (ŭl'sēr-āt). 1. To form an ulcer in. 2. To become affected with ulcers.

umbilical (ŭm-bĭl'ĭ-kăl). Pertaining to the umbilicus.

    u. arteries, the arteries which accompany and form part of the umbilical cord.

    u. cord [Latin, *funis umbilicalis*], the cord connecting the placenta with the umbilicus of the fetus, and at the close of gestation principally made up of the two umbilical arteries and the umbilical vein, encased in a mass of gelatinous tissue called "Wharton's jelly."

    u. hernia, hernia at or near the umbilicus.

    u. vein, forms a part of the umbilical cord.

undulant fever (ŭn'dū-lănt). Infectious disease marked by recurrent attacks of fever.

urachus (ū'rȧ-kŭs). A canal in the fetus which connects the bladder with the allantois, which persists in the adult as the medium umbilical ligament.

urea (û-rē'ȧ). The principal solid constituent of the urine. It is produced by the decomposition of proteins and carries off most of the nitrogenous products of the body. Urea is also found in the blood and the lymph.

uremia (û-rē'mĭ-ȧ). The presence of urinary constituents in the blood, due to the suppression of the urine, and marked by headache, nausea, vertigo, coma and a peculiar odor of the skin.

uremic (û-rē'mĭk). Relating to uremia; affected with uremia.

urethra (û-rē'thrȧ). The membranous canal forming a communication between the neck of the bladder and the external surface of the body. The female urethra does not exceed two inches in length, and the passage is considerably larger and more dilatable than is that of the male.

urethral (û-rē'thr*a*l). Belonging to the urethra.

urinalysis (ū″rĭ-năl'ĭ-sĭs). Chemical analysis of the urine.

urine (ū'rĭn). The saline secretion of the kidneys which flows from them through the ureters into the urinary bladder.

> **u., incontinence of** (ĭn-kŏn'tĭ-nĕns), inability to retain the urine in the bladder, so that it escapes without the knowledge or control of the patient.

> **u., retention of,** inability to pass the urine which accumulates in the bladder.

> **u., suppression of,** arrested secretion of urine from the kidneys.

urinometer, urometer (ū″rĭ-nŏm'ĕ-tẽr, û-rŏm'ĕ-tẽr). An hydrometer for ascertaining the specific gravity of urine.

urticaria (ûr-tĭ-kā'rĭ-*a*). A condition characterized by the sudden appearance of smooth, slightly elevated patches which are usually whiter than the surrounding skin and attended by severe itching.

uterine (ū'tẽr-ĭn). Relating to the uterus.

> **u. appendages,** the ovaries and the fallopian tubes.

> **u. colic,** paroxysms of pain in the uterus due to menstruation or to other causes, such as "false pains" or "after-pains."

> **u. gestation,** normal pregnancy.

> **u. inertia** (ĭn-ûr'sh*a*), deficiency of contractile power of the uterus in labor.

> **u. involution** (ĭn″vō-lū'shŭn), the process by which, after childbirth, the uterus reassumes its normal size and shape.

> **u. mole** (mōl), a mass sometimes occurring in the uterus, consisting of a dead fetus which has undergone degeneration.

> **u. phlebitis,** a form of puerperal fever.

> **u. pregnancy,** normal pregnancy occurring in the uterus, as opposed to ectopic pregnancy.

> **u. probe** (prōb), a long, flexible probe for exploring the cavity of the uterus.

> **u. sinuses,** cavities formed by the uterine veins in the walls of the uterus; they are especially conspicuous in the pregnant uterus.

> **u. souffle** (sōōf'f'l), a sound made by the blood within the arteries of the gravid uterus.

> **u. sound,** an instrument somewhat resembling a urethral sound, used in making examinations of the uterus; a uterine probe.

> **u. tubes,** the fallopian tubes.

> **u. wound,** the area of the uterus from which the placenta has been detached.

uterus (ū'tẽr-ŭs). The womb, a hollow muscular organ designed for the lodgement and nourishment of the fetus during its development until birth.

vagina (v*a*-jī'n*a*). [Latin, a sheath.] The curved canal, five or six inches in length, extending from the vulva to the uterus.

vaginal (văj'ĭ-n*a*l). Belonging or relating to the vagina.

> **v. examination,** examination of the vagina by introducing a finger.

> **v. speculum,** an instrument for keeping open the vagina in order that its interior may be viewed.

vaginismus (văj-ĭ-nĭz'mŭs). Painful spasm of the vagina.

vaginitis (văj-ĭ-nī'tĭs). Inflammation of the vagina, marked by pain and by purulent leukorrheal discharge.

varicose (văr'ĭ-kōs). Unnaturally dilated; relating to a varix.

varicosity (văr″ĭ-kŏs'ĭ-tĭ). 1. A varicose condition of the veins; varicosis. 2. A varicose vein; a varix.

varix (vâr'ĭks). Pl. *varices* (vâr'ĭ-sēz). A dilatation of a vein.

vas (văs). A vessel; especially a blood vessel or a lymphatic duct.

> **v. deferens,** the excretory duct of the testicle, passing from the testicle to the ejaculatory duct.

vascular (văs'kū-lẽr). Having, or relating to, vessels; full of blood vessels.

vectis (vĕk′tĭs). The lever. In obstetrics, an instrument resembling one blade of an obstetric forceps, for making traction upon the head of the fetus in retarded labor. Seldom if ever used and never seen now, as a single forceps blade adequately answers the same purpose.

veil (vāl). A caul or a piece of the amniotic sac occasionally covering the face of a newborn baby.

vein (vān). A tube conveying blood from the various tissues of the body to the heart.

venesection (vĕn″ĕ-sĕk′shŭn). Bloodletting by the opening of a vein.

venous (vē′nŭs). Relating to the veins; contained in the veins.

>**v. blood,** a dark-colored liquid collected in the veins from every part of the system. It is subsequently exposed to the influence of the air in the lungs and is converted into bright-red arterial blood. It contains more carbonic-acid gas and less oxygen than arterial blood.

>**v. circulation,** the circulation of the blood through the veins.

>**v. congestion,** the engorgement of an organ with venous blood caused by interference with its return to the heart.

ventricle (vĕn′trĭk′l). Any small cavity.

ventro-, ventri-, (vĕn′trō, vĕn′trĭ). Combining form denoting relationship to the abdomen.

vernix caseosa (vûr′nĭks kā″sĕ-ō′sȧ). "Cheesy Varnish." The layer of fatty matter which covers the skin of the fetus (smegma).

version (vûr′shŭn). The act of turning; specifically, a turning of the fetus in the uterus so as to change the presenting part and bring it into more favorable position for delivery.

vertex (vûr′tĕks). The summit or top of anything. In anatomy, the top or crown of the head.

>**v. presentation,** presentation of the vertex of the fetus in labor.

vertigo (vûr′tĭ-gō). Dizziness; swimming of the head; giddiness.

vesical (vĕs′ĭ-kăl). Pertaining to the bladder; having the appearance of a bladder.

vesico- (vĕs′ĭ-kŏ). Combining form denoting relationship to the bladder, as vesicovaginal.

vestibule (vĕs′tĭ-būl). A triangular space between the labia minora; the urinary meatus and the vagina open into it.

viability (vī″ȧ-bĭl′ĭ-tĭ). Ability to live.

viable (vī′ȧ-b′l). A term in medical jurisprudence signifying "able or likely to live"; applied to the condition of the child at birth.

villus (vĭl′ŭs). A small vascular process or protrusion growing on a mucous surface; such as the chorionic villi seen in tufts on the chorion of the early embryo.

virgin (vûr′jĭn). A woman who has never had sexual intercourse.

virulent (vĭr′ū-lĕnt). Poisonous; malignant; caused by virus or having the nature of virus.

virus (vī′rŭs). Any poisonous matter produced by disease and capable of propagating that disease by inoculation; a deleterious agent supposed to be a parasitic organism or germ.

viscid (vĭs′ĭd). Clammy; glutinous or sticky.

viscus (vĭs′kŭs). Pl. *viscera* (vĭs′ēr-ȧ). Any organ contained in the cavities of the body, especially within the abdomen.

visual (vĭzh′ū-ăl). Pertaining to, or used in, vision or sight.

vital (vī′tăl). Belonging or essential to life.

vitality (vī-tăl′ĭ-tĭ. The principle of life.

volsella (vŏl-sĕl′ȧ). A forceps, each blade of which has hooked extremities; a volsellum.

Voorhees' bag (vōōr′ēz). A rubber bag which can be inflated with water; used for dilating the cervix of the uterus.

vulsella, vulsellum (vŭl-sĕl′ȧ, vŭl-sĕl′-ŭm). See *volsella.*

vulva (vŭl'vȧ). The external genitals of the female.

Walcher position or **posture** (väl'kēr). That position of the patient in which she lies on her back with her buttocks raised and well over the edge of the table and her limbs hanging down as much as possible. In this position the true conjugate diameter of the pelvis is lengthened by nearly half an inch.

wet nurse (wĕt nûrs). A woman who breast-feeds someone else's baby.

Wharton's gelatin or **jelly** (hwôr'tŭnz). [Thomas *Wharton*, English anatomist, died 1673.] The jellylike mucous tissue composing the bulk of the umbilical cord.

whiteleg. See *Phlegmasia alba dolens.*

W.H.O. Abbreviation for World Health Organization.

Winckel's disease (vĭn'kĕlz). A very rare and extremely fatal disease of newborn infants, marked by icterus, hemorrhage, bloody urine and cyanosis. Malignant jaundice.

witches' milk (wĭch'ĕz). A milky fluid secreted from the breast of the newly born.

womb (wōōm). The *uterus*, which see.

wryneck (rī'nĕk'). See *torticollis.*

xerophthalmia (zē-rŏf-thăl'mĭ-ȧ). Conjunctivitis with atrophy and no liquid discharge, due to lack of vitamin A.

xerosis (zē-rō'sĭs). Abnormal dryness.

zona pellucida (zō'nȧ pĕll-ū'sĭd-ä). A transparent belt; translucent or shining through.

zygote (zī'gōt). A cell resulting from the fusion of two gametes.

Index

(Numerals in italic type refer to the page upon which pertinent illustrations appear.)